Fourth Edition

VETERINARY CLINICAL PATHOLOGY

EMBERT H. COLES, D.V.M., M.S., Ph.D.

Professor of Clinical Pathology and Immunology,
Department of Laboratory Medicine, College of Veterinary Medicine,
Kansas State University, Manhattan, Kansas

1986

W. B. SAUNDERS COMPANY

Philadelphia, London, Toronto, Mexico City, Rio de Janeiro, Sydney, Tokyo, Hong Kong

W. B. Saunders Company: West Washington Square
                          Philadelphia, PA 19105

Library of Congress Cataloging in Publication Data

Coles, Embert H.
  Veterinary clinical pathology.

  Include bibliographies and index.
  1. Veterinary clinical pathology.   I. Title.
SF772.6.C65   1986   636.089'607   85-11957
ISBN 0-7216-1828-6

Acquisition Editor: Darlene Pedersen
Manuscript Editor: Edna Dick
Production Manager: Frank Polizzano

Veterinary Clinical Pathology   ISBN   0-7216-1828-6

Last digit is the print number: 9   8   7   6   5   4   3   2   1

PREFACE
TO THE FOURTH EDITION

When we began the first edition of *Veterinary Clinical Pathology* over 20 years ago laboratory medicine was just beginning to assume a role in the diagnosis and prognosis of animal diseases. Today, data from the clinical pathology laboratory is indispensable. Information gained from laboratory tests is used by veterinarians in all professional activities, from private practice to the research laboratory.

The dedication of private practitioners, clinical pathologists, pathologists, physiologists, internal medicine specialists and other scientists has been essential in the development of new tests and understanding the significance of others. Without their continued efforts and willingness to share their observations, revision of this text would be unnecessary—to all of them go my heartfelt gratitude for a job well done.

This edition, as with previous editions, is designed for use by students, practicing veterinarians and veterinary technicians and is not an exhaustive literature review.

The section on hematology has been reorganized, and most black and white photographs have been replaced by color plates. The chapters on organ functions have been extensively revised. New tests are discussed if their usefulness is well documented. Two new chapters, avian clinical pathology and immunology, have been added. Many outdated references have been removed and the method of citation changed from a name-date to a numerical system. For more complete references the reader is referred to the third edition.

I am especially indebted to Dr. S. A. Ewing, Department of Parasitology, Microbiology and Public Health, Oklahoma State University, for revising the chapter on parasitology and to Dr. T. W. Campbell, Instructor, Department of Laboratory Medicine, Kansas State University, for his contribution of the chapter on avian clinical pathology. My thanks go to Drs. W. E. Moore, K. S. Keeton, W. E. Bailie and L. J. Rich for their suggestions and counsel.

I am also indebted to Robert W. Reinhardt, Darlene D. Pedersen, Lorraine Kilmer, Edna Dick, Frank Polizzano and other staff members at W. B. Saunders Company for their efforts, cooperation and patience.

E. H. COLES

COLOR PLATES

CONTENTS

1

INTRODUCTION

In modern veterinary medicine the availability of laboratory tests is as important to the clinician as are the history and physical examination of the animal. In some instances test results are more important, as they may provide absolute evidence regarding physiologic alterations resulting from a disease. Advances in diagnosis in veterinary medicine may depend to a large extent on development of more accurate and new laboratory determinations as well as an understanding of the capabilities and limitations of the tests. The correct evaluation of the physiologic status of an animal is dependent upon a knowledgeable blending of the results of laboratory examinations, physical examinations, and history. Wells and Halsted (1967) made the following statement: "A physician who depends on the laboratory to make his diagnoses is probably inexperienced; one who says that he does not need a laboratory is uninformed. In either instance the patient is in danger." This statement is also applicable in veterinary medicine.

In recent years there has been an enormous increase in the number of laboratory procedures available. Many of these tests have found a place in the veterinary clinical laboratory, whereas others remain an unknown quantity in terms of their reliability as an aid to the diagnosis of animal disease. Consequently, the veterinarian has assumed that the principles governing use of laboratory determinations associated with disease in man are applicable to comparable diseases of animals. Such transposition of laboratory data may or may not be appropriate. Practicing veterinarians and researchers dealing with problems of animal diseases must continue to critically evaluate laboratory tests under controlled conditions. Until

this end is accomplished the interpretation of clinical laboratory results in veterinary medicine will not achieve the status that similar determinations now have in human medicine.

Although veterinary practitioners often complain that they do not have the time or inclination to complete laboratory tests manually, every veterinary practice should have at least a small laboratory in which common tests can be made. Some large veterinary practices have a completely equipped laboratory for all types of determinations and find it feasible to employ a qualified medical technologist. Commercial laboratories now provide a readily available resource for the practicing veterinarian in many areas of the world. Such institutions will continue to play a significant role in providing laboratory information to the veterinarian, particularly in performing assays that require techniques not usually available in the hospital laboratory. Care should be taken in selecting a reference laboratory. Some laboratories are excellent and have personnel who are knowledgeable concerning problems associated with the peculiarities and acceptability of procedures used for animals. Others do not have this capability, and results from such laboratories can be misleading.

Most reputable laboratories cooperate with veterinarians in establishing normal values to be used in a given practice area. Because of the interest in the establishment of clinical pathology laboratories, we are including in this chapter a list of equipment, glassware, and chemicals required for the establishment of, first, a minimal laboratory and, second, a completely equipped clinical pathology laboratory. We have not included a specific source for purchase of these items, believing

1

that equipment and supplies should be purchased from a local source from which service and technical assistance are available.

The decision as to what type of laboratory should be developed in a given situation will depend greatly on the volume of tests to be conducted. The volume should be adequate to ensure accuracy. Tests conducted at infrequent intervals do not provide laboratory personnel with adequate opportunities to develop skills in performing procedures, and results are likely to be unreliable. Tests that are not done several times a week should be sent to an outside laboratory that works with a larger volume.

The availability of adequately trained personnel must be considered in deciding how extensive the veterinary hospital laboratory should be. With modern technologies and simplification of test directions it has been assumed that anyone who can read can do laboratory determinations. This may be true, but the ability to read and follow directions does not guarantee accuracy. Acceptable results can be obtained only if personnel performing tests are sufficiently acquainted with laboratory complexities to detect discrepancies in results. The responsibility for conducting laboratory tests should not be delegated to an incompletely trained paraprofessional. Unless there is a sufficiently large volume to justify employing a trained medical technologist, the veterinarian should assume active supervision of the laboratory.

Every hospital should have a laboratory capable of conducting the determinations required for a minimal data base that can be used in the problem-oriented approach to diagnosis. These would include urinalysis, routine hematology and parasitology studies, blood urea nitrogen determination, and total protein, fibrinogen, and glucose determinations.

THE BASIC CLINICAL PATHOLOGY LABORATORY

Certain items of equipment, supplies, and chemicals are necessary in all clinical pathology laboratories in order to complete the determinations considered absolutely necessary. The minimal clinical pathology laboratory should contain the following:

Equipment

1. Microscope with mechanical stage, substage condenser, substage illuminator, and low dry, high dry, and oil immersion objectives.
2. Microhematocrit centrifuge capable of 12,000 rpm.
3. Standard clinical centrifuge capable of spinning tubes with up to 15 ml volume.
4. Refractometer for determining urine specific gravity and assessing total solids, plasma protein, and fibrinogen concentrations.
5. Differential cell counter.
6. Hand tally.
7. Interval timer.
8. Hemocytometer.

The items listed represent the greatest bulk of equipment needed for the basic laboratory, although additional small items such as test tube racks, a staining rack, and some glassware—including transfer pipettes, serologic pipettes of various sizes, and test tubes—are also needed.

Chemicals, Drugs, and Miscellaneous Supplies

1. Red and white cell diluting fluids are best purchased as part of a plastic disposable pipette (Unopette, Becton-Dickinson, Rutherford, New Jersey).
2. Blood stains can be purchased in a prepared liquid form, which is preferable. A number of excellent quick dip-type stains are commercially available. However, if the laboratory is using large quantities, blood stains can be prepared from
   A. Powdered Wright, Giemsa, or Leishman's stain
   B. Powdered new methylene blue stain
   C. Sodium phosphate (Na_2HPO_4), potassium phosphate (K_2HPO_4), ethyl alcohol (95 per cent)
   D. Absolute methyl alcohol (acetone-free)
   E. Pure white glycerine
3. Stains for bacteria should be purchased in a "ready to use" form.
4. Kits can be purchased for use in specific blood chemistry analyses.
5. Commercial preparations are available for detection of protein, glucose, blood, bilirubin, ketone bodies, urobilinogen, and pH of urine.
6. Zinc sulfate, sodium chloride (NaCl), or sugar should be purchased for preparation of flotation fluid.
7. Additional supplies include
   A. Formalin, 10 per cent (dilute one part concentrated formalin with nine parts water)
   B. Anticoagulants such as ethylenediaminetetraacetic acid (EDTA), oxalates, citrates, and so forth, depending upon need or preferably prepackaged blood-collecting tubes containing the appropriate anticoagulant
   C. A quantity of distilled water
   D. Immersion oil

THE COMPLETE PATHOLOGY LABORATORY

In the clinical pathology laboratory prepared to conduct most laboratory procedures of value in veterinary medicine, the following additional equipment and supplies should be made available:

Equipment

1. Spectrophotometer. The selection of a spectrophotometer depends on the type of chemical examinations to be conducted. A variety of specially designed spectrophotometers are now available that permit use of prepared kits.
2. Controlled temperature water bath or heating block.
3. Flame photometer if large numbers of electrolyte determinations are conducted. Analyzers using ion-specific electrodes are available and have replaced the flame photometer in many laboratories.
4. Automatic cell counter. This piece of equipment should be purchased and used only in those laboratories routinely doing large numbers of cell counts. The purchaser must be sure that the counter is adjustable to permit accurate counting of erythrocytes from all animal species.
5. Blood gas pH unit.
6. Balance capable of measuring to tolerance of ±1.0 mg.
7. Incubator.
8. Bunsen burner.
9. Bacteriology inoculating loop.
10. Sensitivity disc dispenser (optional).

Glassware and Disposable Plastic Supplies

1. Cuvettes for spectrophotometer.
2. Volumetric flasks in the following sizes: 50 ml, 100 ml, 500 ml, and 1000 ml.
3. Volumetric pipettes in the following sizes: 0.5 ml, 1.0 ml, 2.0 ml, 5.0 ml, and 10.0 ml.
4. Micropipettes as needed for the determinations to be conducted.
5. Glassware for automatic cell counter.
6. Special glassware as needed for the flame photometer.

Blood Chemistry Kits, Chemicals, and Other Consumable Supplies

1. Prepared kits and chemicals
   A. Prepared kits
      (1) Alkaline phosphatase
      (2) Transferases—alanine-amino transferase (formerly GPT) and aspartate-amino transferase (formerly GOT)
      (3) Serum lipase
      (4) Serum amylase
      (5) Serum creatinine
      (6) Blood urea nitrogen (BUN) (according to method preferred)
      (7) Calcium
      (8) Glucose (as glucose oxidase or other techniques)
      (9) Cholesterol
      (10) Prothrombin time
      (11) Bilirubin (total and direct)
      (12) Others as developed
   B. Prepared chemicals
      (1) Cyanmethemoglobin reagent
      (2) Cyanmethemoglobin standard
      (3) Stable tungstic acid
      (4) Biuret reagent—total protein and albumin/globulin ratio (A/G ratio)
      (5) Reagents for phosphorus determination
      (6) Bromsulphalein (sulfobromophthalein)
      (7) Phenolsulfonphthalein
   C. Control serum for following determinations:
      (1) Routine blood chemistries
      (2) Cholesterol
      (3) Enzymes
      (4) Bilirubin (unless included in prepared kit)
   D. Standards

A standard for most chemical analyses can be purchased commercially and is essential for any determination using the spectrophotometer. If not available commercially, standards may be prepared in the laboratory.

   E. Other reagents that may be needed include
      (1) Sodium hydroxide solution
      (2) Sodium chloride
      (3) Sodium sulfate
      (4) Ether
      (5) Aerosol-OT
      (6) Picric acid
      (7) Trichloroacetic acid
      (8) Mercuric chloride
      (9) Sodium carbonate
      (10) Phenolphthalein
      (11) Paradimethylaminobenzaldehyde
   F. Additional reagents
      (1) Propylene glycol (total eosinophil count)
      (2) Phloxine (total eosinophil count)
      (3) Hematoxylin
      (4) Eosin
      (5) Shorr's stain (purchased as a prepared liquid)
      (6) Opal blue (live/dead semen stain)

The reagents listed represent the majority of those required for most analyses. The list, however, may not be complete, and the reader is advised to check the detailed technique for the determination as it appears in the appendix.

Bacteriology Media

Listed herein are media that may, on occasion, be useful in a veterinary diagnostic laboratory.

The selection of these media must be dependent on the extent of service performed by the laboratory, and in all probability only selected media will be used in all laboratories.

Media for Isolation

In addition to blood agar, the veterinarian may have occasion to use one or more of the following selective media for the isolation of a specific microorganism.

1. Streptococcus: Phenylethyl alcohol agar or Streptosel agar.
2. Staphylococcus: Staphylococcus 110 medium with 7.5 per cent sodium chloride, glycine-tellurite medium, or mannitol-salt agar.
3. Listeria: Bile esculin agar.
4. Erysipelothrix: Blood agar containing sodium azide and crystal violet.
5. Salmonella: A variety of media for enrichment and isolation of salmonellae are available and include selenite broth, SS agar, MacConkey agar, brilliant green agar, deoxycholate agar, and bismuth sulfite agar.
6. Brucella: Base medium with a 1:200,000 concentration of gentian violet.
7. Campylobacter (Vibrio): Thiol medium.
8. Fungi: Sabouraud medium, mycobiotic medium.

Media for Bacterial Differentiation

Most, if not all, of the following are available commercially in a prepared form ready for use.

1. Carbohydrates. The number of carbohydrates utilized for bacterial identification will depend upon the genus and species. In general, four basic carbohydrates—dextrose, lactose, maltose, and sucrose—are used, but the laboratory may also find use for other carbohydrates such as salicin, mannite, inulin, trehalose, sorbitol, xylose, raffinose, glycerol, dulcitol, adonitol, rhamnose, and dextrin.
2. MR-VP medium.
3. Nitrate reduction medium.
4. Motility medium.
5. Litmus milk.
6. Urea broth.
7. Triple sugar agar or Kligler iron agar.
8. Indole production medium.
9. Plasma for the coagulase test.
10. Media for the study of gelatin liquefaction.
11. Media for the "string of pearls" test (see appendix).
12. O-R medium.
13. Decarboxylase base with lysine, ornithine, and arginine.

For Serologic Testing

1. Brucella antigen and antiserum or card-test equipment.
2. Leptospira antigen. In testing for the presence of leptospiral antibodies, it may be wise to purchase antigens containing several serovars of *Leptospira*.
3. Salmonella group antiserum.
4. Kit for detecting feline leukemia virus by the ELISA method.

Chemicals Required for Detecting Biochemical Activity

1. Nitrate reduction. Acetic acid, sulfanilic acid, and N,N-dimethyl-1-naphthylamine.
2. Indole test. Xylene, paradimethylaminobenzaldehyde, hydrochloric acid.
3. Methyl red (MR) test. Methyl red and ethyl alcohol 95 per cent.
4. Voges-Proskauer (VP) test. Potassium hydroxide, creatine.

For Antibiotic Sensitivity Testing

Details of antibiotic sensitivity testing are presented in Chapter 18. Selection of the medium, concentration of the antibiotic discs, and Petri dish size will depend on the technique selected. Materials required will include the following:

1. Disposable (or glass) Petri dishes containing medium selected for test.
2. Sterile broth tubes for growth of isolated organism (alternatively, tubes of sterile saline for suspension of organism).
3. Sterile swabs.
4. Antibiotic sensitivity discs of appropriate concentration and selected according to preferences of clinician.
5. Sensitivity disc dispenser.
6. Forceps (an old pair that can be flamed).

PREPARATION AND SHIPMENT OF LABORATORY SPECIMENS

A laboratory diagnostic service may be of assistance to the veterinarian, as it will permit a more accurate diagnosis and may provide information of value in instituting therapy or preventive measures. However, the value of a diagnostic laboratory service is dependent upon the submission of adequately collected specimens that are shipped to the laboratory in such a manner that the necessary tests may be conducted. Veterinarians often blame the laboratory for not obtaining expected results when the fault may actually be in methods of collection, packing, and shipment. The following information includes most methods for collection, preservation, packing, and shipping of specimens for submission to a central laboratory. For specific requirements the veterinarian should contact the diagnostic laboratory. When possible, specimens should be delivered by the owner or the veterinarian, or sent by a messenger delivery service. If there is a possibility that the sample could be infectious to man it should be so labeled and extra precautions taken in packing and shipping.

General Considerations

Collection of the Specimen

1. For obtaining specimens, select an animal that is in a good state of preservation. An animal in the advanced stages of the disease is most desirable. If the disease is a flock or herd problem, specimens should be obtained from more than one diseased animal. In such flocks or herds submit specimens from one or two animals that have died recently and samples from animals that are in various stages of illness.
2. Be sure that the specimens submitted are characteristic of the disease as seen in the field.
3. In collecting specimens make every attempt to avoid contamination with intestinal contents, hair, and dirt.

Identification of the Sample

A complete history including the following should be submitted with each sample:

1. Owner's name and address.
2. Description of the animal including species, age, and sex.
3. Duration of the condition or outbreak.
4. Mortality rate.
5. Number of animals affected.
6. Clinical signs observed.
7. Necropsy findings.
8. Treatment history and vaccination record.
9. Tentative clinical diagnosis.
10. Nature of feed including any change of feed that has occurred.
11. Possibility of contact with animals on neighboring farms.
12. Veterinarian's name, address, and phone number. (If a quick reply is essential, request that the results be reported by telephone.)
13. Type of preservative used on specimen prior to or during shipment.

Preservation of Specimens

REFRIGERATION

NATURAL ICE. This method of refrigeration is adequate only if the samples are properly packed and the distance to the laboratory is not great. Ice will preserve specimens for 18 to 24 hours during the winter months but for only a few (8 to 12) hours during the heat of the summer. Specimens packed in ice should either be placed in a watertight container and surrounded by ice in the form of frozen cans of water or packed in a small watertight container and placed into a larger one containing ice.

DRY ICE. This method of refrigeration is preferred if the specimen can be frozen without interfering with the laboratory procedures to be conducted. The specimen should be placed in a plastic bag or other watertight container and the dry ice wrapped in paper and placed in the box. Do not place the dry ice in direct contact with the specimen unless freezing is not a problem. DO NOT SEND DRY ICE IN AN AIRPROOF METAL OR GLASS CONTAINER AS THE ICE WILL VOLATILIZE, AND PRESSURE MAY RESULT IN AN EXPLOSION.

CHEMICAL PRESERVATIVES

FIXING SOLUTION. The fixing solution of choice for samples submitted for histologic examination is 10 per cent formalin. This preservative is prepared by diluting one part formalin to nine parts water. In fixing tissues a sufficiently large quantity of formalin should be used, approximately 10 times as much preservative as tissue.

BACTERICIDAL SOLUTIONS. DO NOT USE ON SPECIMENS FOR BACTERIAL EXAMINATION. These solutions are used when bacterial growth is to be kept to a minimum.

1. Formalin: 10 per cent for fecal material.
2. Phenol (0.5 per cent).
3. Merthiolate (1:10,000).

For viral isolations, frozen specimens are preferred. A good viral transport medium is normal saline (0.85 per cent sodium chloride) containing 1 per cent gelatin. This solution should be placed in screw-cap tubes and sterilized at 120° C for 15 minutes.

Specimens for Specific Diseases

Bacterial Diseases

SUBMIT ORGANS OR TISSUES IN INDIVIDUAL CONTAINERS.

ABORTION. Frozen tissues should include placenta, adrenal gland, kidney, liver, spleen, tied-off stomach, half of the brain, and serum. Sections of the placenta, lung, liver, kidney, brain, lymph nodes, and skin should be placed in 10 per cent formalin and submitted at the same time. If tissues are not available, submit paired serum samples (one taken at the time of abortion and a second sample 7 to 10 days later). Indicate which serologic tests you want to have run.

ABSCESSES. Collect material on a sterile swab or collect purulent exudate in a sterile tube. Make swab from the margin of the abscess. Submit specimen under refrigeration in a transport medium.

ACTINOMYCOSIS OR ACTINOBACILLOSIS. Submit portions of the affected tissue in 10 per cent formalin. Pus may be collected in a test tube. Avoid pus in the center of the lesion and collect material from the edge of the lesion if possible. Slides prepared from the exudate may also be submitted for examination for the presence of sulfur granules. The slide should be air dried before packing.

ANTHRAX. Saturate a piece of umbilical tape (approximately 4 inches) in venous blood and allow it to air dry. Carefully pack into a sterile test tube. May be forwarded with no refrigeration if the tape is dry. Label the specimen ANTHRAX SUSPECT. A cotton swab may be used but is more likely to contain complicating contaminants, as it is more difficult to dry. DO NOT SEND AN EAR.

ARTHRITIS. Collect a swab from the affected joint and forward in transport medium or send unopened affected joint under refrigeration.

BLACKLEG AND MALIGNANT EDEMA. Remove a 2-inch cube of affected muscle, freeze, pack in a sealed container, and forward under refrigeration. The specimen should be collected as soon as possible after death.

BRUCELLOSIS. If diagnosis is based on serologic evidence, submit a serum sample collected 10 to 20 days following abortion. If an aborted fetus is available, the stomach should be tied off, frozen, and shipped in a sealed container under refrigeration.

CASEOUS LYMPHADENITIS. Preserve a portion of the lymph node in 10 per cent formalin. Place remaining affected lymph nodes in a sealed container, freeze, and submit under refrigeration. A swab of the exudate may be substituted for the frozen lymph node.

COLIBACILLOSIS. If possible, the entire carcass should be delivered to the laboratory. If this is not practical, package sections of duodenum, mesenteric lymph nodes, spleen, liver, and kidney (each in a separate package) and forward frozen or under refrigeration.

CONTAGIOUS EQUINE METRITIS (CEM). Swabs from the clitoral fossa and cervix of mares or swabs from the sheath and urethra of stallions should be placed in Amies transport medium and shipped under refrigeration.

ENTEROTOXEMIA OF LAMBS. Tie off 12 to 14 inches of ileum from a recently destroyed lamb, or place duodenal contents in a clean container, freeze immediately, and forward to the laboratory packed in dry ice in sufficient quantity to prevent thawing.

ERYSIPELAS. Collect a section of the spleen, kidney, liver, lymph nodes, or affected joints; freeze, and ship under refrigeration with each organ in a separate container.

HAEMOPHILUS. A live sick animal is best if there is respiratory infection. Alternately, forward a large section of lung or pleural fluids under refrigeration. Sections of lung and adjacent normal tissue in 10 per cent formalin should be included. If the problem is in the reproductive tract, collect a saline flush from the dam and submit this plus fetal tissues under refrigeration.

JOHNE'S DISEASE. Submit frozen lesion from near ileocecal valve and the adjacent mesenteric lymph node. Duplicate specimens should be placed in 10 per cent formalin. Make a scraping of the rectal mucosa and prepare a thin smear on a clean glass slide, air dry, and submit slide requesting an acid-fast stain.

LEPTOSPIROSIS. Collect blood 10 to 20 days following acute disease and submit the serum from this collection plus serum collected at the time of the clinical signs of disease. In the case of a dead animal, forward $\frac{1}{4}$ inch thick sections (in 10 per cent formalin) from the kidney.

LISTERIOSIS. Submit half the brain following freezing and forward under refrigeration. The other half of the brain should be placed in 10 per cent formalin (a wide mouth quart jar filled with formalin should be used).

MASTITIS. Collect 5 to 10 ml of milk in a sterile container, using aseptic precautions. The sample should be refrigerated or frozen and shipped under refrigeration.

MYCOPLASMOSIS. Joint fluid, lung, fibrin, exudate, or milk should be frozen and shipped so that it will remain frozen.

NOCARDIOSIS. Collect a sample of the exudate on a sterile swab and ship to the laboratory under refrigeration. In addition, several $\frac{1}{4}$ inch thick sections of tissue should be preserved in 10 per cent formalin.

PASTEURELLOSIS. Collect a 3-inch square of affected lung tissue and mediastinal lymph nodes, freeze, and ship under refrigeration. Thin sections of affected tissues may also be preserved in 10 per cent formalin for histopathologic study.

PINK EYE (INFECTIOUS KERATITIS). Using a sterile swab, collect material from the conjunctiva of the eye, place it in a sterile tube in transport medium or freeze and ship under refrigeration.

PNEUMONIA. As for pasteurellosis. Tracheal washings and nasal swabs may be helpful.

SALMONELLOSIS. Collect sections of liver, spleen, kidney, and tied-off section of intestine and package each organ in a separate container; freeze and ship under refrigeration.

SWINE DYSENTERY. Tie off a section of large intestine and freeze. Portions of the liver, kidney, and spleen may also be forwarded.

TEME (THROMBOEMBOLIC MENINGOENCEPHALITIS). Collect brain and stem and submit half under refrigeration and the other half in 10 per cent formalin.

TOXOPLASMOSIS. For serology submit 1 ml of clear serum; for tissue analysis, liver, kidney, brain, eye, and lymph nodes in 10 per cent formalin. To check a cat, submit fecal sample refrigerated or in 10 per cent formalin.

TRICHOMONIASIS. Flush reproductive tract with saline, collect mucus from reproductive tract or swabs from cervix, refrigerate and deliver immediately to the laboratory.

TUBERCULOSIS. CONTACT FEDERAL REGULATORY OFFICIALS.

VIBRIOSIS (CAMPYLOBACTER). If an aborted fetus is

available, the stomach should be tied off, frozen, and shipped under refrigeration. In the cow, specimens of vaginal mucus may be obtained and submitted under refrigeration for bacterial examination. Liver sections from an aborted lamb may be preserved in 10 per cent formalin.

Viral Diseases

The specimens submitted will depend on the procedures used in the laboratory. Some viral diseases are identified by microscopic examination of tissues, others by the fluorescent antibody (FA) technique, virus isolation, electron microscopy, or serologic examination of paired serum samples. Because of the serologic methods applied to the diagnosis of viral diseases, extreme care must be used in blood collection. Sterile techniques should be utilized, but liquid disinfectants should not be used in the syringes or needles employed in collecting the blood. Tubes in which the serum is collected should be free of all detergents. Vacutainers (Becton-Dickinson, Rutherford, New Jersey) are the best receptacles for virus serology. Blood should be maintained at 4° C until clotted, then the serum should be removed, frozen or stored in the refrigerator, and shipped under refrigeration.

For virus isolation, tissue samples must be taken from animals dead less than two hours. Tissues should be immediately cooled to 4° C or below and maintained at that temperature until delivered to the laboratory. In respiratory diseases, nasal swabs and tracheal washings are often good specimens. They should be frozen and maintained frozen or at a temperature not above 4° C. Feces should be frozen and maintained under refrigeration. For additional details for specific viral diseases contact your local laboratory.

CANINE DISTEMPER. Collect ¼ inch sections of lung, liver, bladder, trachea, stomach wall, and half of brain and stem and preserve in 10 per cent formalin. No refrigeration is required for shipment. Frozen lung, urinary bladder, and cerebellum should be submitted for virus isolation.

INFECTIOUS BOVINE RHINOTRACHEITIS (IBR). Serum samples may be collected for use in the serum neutralization test. In animals submitted to necropsy, two or three rings of trachea and a portion of the turbinates are preserved in 10 per cent formalin. If FA study or virus isolation is possible, nasal, ocular, and vaginal swabs plus frozen trachea, lung, and kidney tissue can be used. Fetal material should include liver and kidney.

INFECTIOUS CANINE HEPATITIS (ICH). Several thin sections through the liver, gallbladder, and kidney are preserved in 10 per cent formalin and submitted in a sealed container with no refrigeration. Liver, lung, and kidney are required for FA study or virus isolation.

ENCEPHALOMYELITIS. Preserve half of brain and stem in 10 per cent formalin and forward the other half frozen.

HOG CHOLERA. If no total leukocyte count has been made, submit 5 ml of blood containing EDTA. If the laboratory is equipped to complete FA studies, submit tonsil, lymph nodes, spleen, and kidney that are refrigerated but not frozen. Half of the brain and stem should be preserved in 10 per cent formalin.

PANLEUKOPENIA (FELINE). If no total leukocyte count has been completed, send a sample of blood containing EDTA. Such a blood sample will be satisfactory if in transit not more than 24 hours. If the animal is dead, submit sections from several areas of the small intestine and mesenteric lymph nodes preserved in 10 per cent formalin. If isolation is desired, submit frozen intestine.

CANINE PARVOVIRUS. Feces, small intestine, lung heart, and blood should be submitted under refrigeration.

RABIES. Submit unopened head. The head should be frozen if it will be in transit more than 24 hours and must be labeled and shipped only by common carrier. A SUSPECTED RABIC HEAD MAY NOT BE SENT THROUGH THE UNITED STATES MAIL. If human exposure has occurred, the head should be delivered to the laboratory. The head should be placed in a metal container and sealed with tape.

RHINOPNEUMONITIS (EQUINE VIRAL ABORTION). Thin sections (¼ inch) of liver and lung from the aborted fetus should be preserved in 10 per cent formalin. Specimens for virus isolation should include nasal swabs and fetal lung and liver.

SCRAPIE. Submit half of brain and stem preserved in 10 per cent formalin.

BOVINE VIRUS DIARRHEA. If a mature animal is affected, nasal and fecal swabs, spleen, lymph node, and intestine should be submitted for virus isolation. If the fetus is thought to be involved, heart, heart blood, kidney, lung, and liver should be submitted.

PARAINFLUENZA VIRUS. Identification of parainfluenza-3 virus (PI_3) can be made from nasal swabs and lung of infected animals.

MALIGNANT CATARRHAL FEVER. The best tissue for isolation of this virus is the thyroid gland.

PSEUDORABIES. Brain, tonsil, lung, and lymph nodes should be forwarded to the laboratory.

PORCINE ENTEROVIRUS (SMEDI). Nasal swabs, feces, brain, and intestine are the preferred tissues.

ADENOVIRUSES. For bovine adenovirus isolation, nasal, ocular, and tonsillar swabs are indicated. For adenovirus of equine origin, lung and trachea are submitted, and for the canine form, lung is forwarded.

BOVINE REOVIRUS. Feces and small intestine should be submitted for identification of this agent.

BLUE TONGUE. Heparinized whole blood should be collected.

BOVINE CORONAVIRUS. This virus can be recovered from feces, small intestine, and colon.

TRANSMISSIBLE GASTROENTERITIS (TGE). The small intestine from infected swine should be forwarded for virus isolation.

EQUINE INFLUENZA. Specimens submitted should include nasal swab and lung tissue.

EQUINE ARTERITIS. Nasal swabs and blood are required for isolation.

FELINE RHINOTRACHEITIS. Nasal swabs, trachea, and lung tissue may be forwarded for virus isolation.

Other Diseases

ANAPLASMOSIS. For the complement fixation or other serologic test submit 5 ml of serum. Prepare a thin film of blood on a glass slide that has been cleaned by immersion in methyl alcohol and wiped dry with a piece of soft cheesecloth. Fix the slide in absolute alcohol for three minutes and pack in such a manner as to avoid scratching or damaging the film. Several slides should be prepared from fresh blood.

CLAY PIGEON OR PITCH POISONING OF PIGS. Several ¼ inch thick sections of liver should be preserved in 10 per cent formalin and shipped in a sealed container.

MYCOTIC INFECTIONS (ASPERGILLOSIS, BLASTOMYCOSIS, COCCIDIOIDOMYCOSIS, HISTOPLASMOSIS). Sections of grossly affected tissue, liver, spleen, lung, and lymph nodes should be preserved in 10 per cent formalin and submitted in a sealed container. If cultural examination is requested, the specimens should be frozen and submitted under refrigeration.

CUTANEOUS MYCOTIC INFECTIONS. Forward a skin biopsy in 10 per cent formalin or freeze biopsies and forward under refrigeration.

PARASITES (INTERNAL). Ship feces preserved with 10 per cent formalin.

PARASITES (EXTERNAL). Collect deep skin scrapings and place them in a clean, dry test tube or other screwcap container.

TOXOPLASMOSIS. Serum for serologic testing plus liver, kidney, brain, and eye in 10 per cent formalin is required.

TRICHOMONIASIS. Aseptically collect uterine or vaginal exudate or preputial washings. Dilute small quantities of collected material in Ringer's solution and ship to the laboratory under refrigeration.

TUMORS. Submit a portion of the tumor mass and adjacent area of normal tissue in 10 per cent formalin. The tissue should be sliced into sections not more than ⅜ inch thick and must be placed in 10 per cent formalin immediately after removal.

TOXICOLOGIC EXAMINATIONS. Detection of toxic chemicals is a difficult task, and adequate specimens are necessary if accurate reports are desired. The veterinarian should always submit information relative to the type of poisoning suspected and should include a complete history, clinical and necropsy findings, and treatment history.

HEAVY METALS (MERCURY, LEAD, BISMUTH, ARSENIC). Ample quantities (50 to 100 grams) of liver, kidney, and stomach contents should be collected and submitted under refrigeration. Care must be taken to avoid contamination of the organs with stomach contents. A separate sealed container should be used for forwarding stomach contents.

STRYCHNINE. Stomach contents, liver, kidney, and urine may be submitted under refrigeration. Ship all stomach contents and urine available.

INSECTICIDES. Fatty tissues, liver, brain, stomach contents, and heparinized blood provide the best material for assay. Tissues must not be contaminated with hay or stomach content. Use chemically clean glass jars. Avoid plastic containers.

ALKALOIDS. Liver, stomach contents, and sometimes the brain are the best sites for demonstration of alkaloids.

HYDROCYANIC ACID. Plant material from the suspected field, stomach (rumen) contents, blood, and liver may be submitted. This is a volatile chemical, and identification of the toxic material is difficult unless the specimens are quite fresh. The specimen should be frozen promptly in an airtight container.

NITRATE. Samples should be forwarded from the material suspected of containing nitrate. Stomach contents and blood may also be forwarded.

AFLATOXIN. Suspected feed samples (200 grams) should be selected and kept dry and cool.

AMMONIA. Whole blood, composite stomach contents, and urine should be frozen and submitted. For rumen contents one or two drops of saturated mercuric chloride may be used instead of freezing.

ETHYLENE GLYCOL. In animals suspected of being poisoned, 10 ml of serum, the whole kidney in 10 per cent formalin and a minimum of 10 ml of urine should be submitted.

FLUOROACETATE (1080). A kidney, a portion of the liver, urine, and frozen stomach contents are suggested for submission to diagnose 1080 poisoning. For blood, use only heparin or citrate as the anticoagulant.

PHENOLS. Stomach contents and other tissues should be packed in an airtight container and forwarded to the laboratory.

THALLIUM. Kidney, liver, and urine provide the best specimens for identification of this chemical.

OXALATES. Fresh plants (do not chop) should be promptly frozen and delivered while still frozen.

RECORDS

Record keeping is a vital part of the activities of the clinical pathology laboratory just as it is for the business aspects of veterinary practice. Without a system of records much of the knowledge available by correlation of the results of laboratory examinations with clinical signs and results of treatment will be lost.

The design of laboratory record forms will depend on the particular requirements in each laboratory but should contain the following information:

1. Patient identification number.
2. Owner's name.
3. Species of animal.
4. Breed of animal.
5. Sex.
6. Age.
7. Tests requested.
8. Clinician's name.
9. Space for reporting results.
10. Area for remarks.

ERYTHROCYTES

Erythron is a term for the mass of circulating erythrocytes plus the erythropoietic tissue of bone marrow. In order for erythrocytes to be produced, certain requirements must be met. There must be an adequate supply of globin; elements such as iron, copper and cobalt; and the hematopoietic factor that is responsible for normal, orderly maturation. In addition, there must be a sufficient amount of protoporphyrin and certain vitamins. If all of these factors are present in normal quantities, erythrocyte precursors will mature in an orderly process, and cells will begin to synthesize normal hemoglobin molecules at the proper stage of growth.

In the absence of these factors, abnormal erythropoiesis may occur, appearing as production of incompletely hemoglobinated erythrocytes or atypical cells that are deficient in number and have morphologic abnormalities. Abnormal erythropoiesis may not always result in a lack of either red cells or hemoglobin production; under some circumstances, excessive numbers of erythrocytes may be produced.

Erythrocyte maturation takes place in an orderly fashion within the bone marrow. With a prolonged stimulus, extramedullary erythropoiesis may occur. A multipotential stem cell in bone marrow gives rise to the erythroid precursor, which in turn differentiates to become a rubriblast. The identifiable stages of development following rubriblast formation are the prorubricyte, rubricyte (basophilic, polychromatic, and normochromatic), metarubricyte, reticulocyte, and erythrocyte. The characteristic morphology of these cells is discussed in Chapter 4.

The rubriblast responds to the body's need for erythrocytes, under normal or abnormal circumstances, by dividing and maturing. Each rubriblast will give rise to eight to 16 erythrocytes. Division may continue until the nucleus becomes pyknotic, usually at the late rubricyte to early metarubricyte stages. Estimates of turnover times for cells at different stages of the erythrocytic series have been calculated. In the normal cow, turnover time for the prorubricyte is 10 hours, for the basophilic rubricyte 17 hours, for the polychromatic rubricyte 31 hours, and for the metarubricyte and reticulocyte 42 to 52 hours.[1,2] Total transit time for erythroid cells in bovine bone marrow was estimated to be four to five days. Transit time for erythrocytes in the dog is estimated to be seven days.[3] The rate at which erythrocytes are produced is determined by the rate of cell division. Maturation time appears to remain constant, although normal marrow has the ability to increase production four- to fivefold when properly stimulated. Transit time in the marrow is prolonged if hemoglobin synthesis is reduced. When transit time is reduced erythrocytes released into the blood are larger than normal (macrocytes), while a delayed transit time may result in smaller erythrocytes (microcytes).

Under normal conditions, the erythron is maintained in a steady state of production that exactly matches the rate of destruction.

The erythron may be affected by certain pathologic and physiologic alterations that result in (1) hypertrophy or polycythemia, (2) atrophy or anemia, (3) hydremia or hemodilution, or (4) dehydration or hemoconcentration.

Anoxia stimulates production of an erythrocyte-stimulating factor (ESF) that is referred to as erythropoietin. This hormone stimulates normal bone marrow to increase production and release erythrocytes by accelerating differentiation of stem cells into prorubricytes. After this stimulation, maturation and multiplication of differentiated nucleated erythrocytes proceed at fixed rates independent of anoxic stimulation.

Erythropoietin is a heat-stable hormone normally present in small amounts in plasma. The kidney plays a dominant role in the production of erythropoietin. In response to anoxia the kidney is stimulated to produce erythrogenin (renal erythropoietic factor); this factor then activates inactive erythropoietin (erythropoietinogen) of hepatic origin. The activated erythropoietin stimulates erythropoiesis, causing an increase in the circulating erythrocyte mass. In the dog, the kidney is the sole source of erythropoietin; consequently the activity of this hormone is greatly reduced in severe kidney disease. In the cat, the carotid body has also been shown to control erythropoiesis.

Erythropoietin production may be induced in an animal by repeated bleedings, which create anemia, or stimulated by use of erythrocyte-destroying chemicals. Injection of plasma from erythrocyte-depleted animals stimulates production of erythrocytes, reticulocytes, and hemoglobin in normal animals.

Iron, which is an essential mineral in the hemoglobin molecule, is contained in a closed system in the animal body. The total body pool is replenished by iron absorption from the gut. Such absorption is regulated in part by the iron concentration in the diet and in part by the body's needs. Iron loss from the body, except in cases of blood loss anemia, is negligible and occurs primarily through the respiratory and intestinal tracts. The majority of body iron is contained in hemoglobin. The remainder is stored as ferritin or hemosiderin, a small quantity is incorporated into myoglobin, and a very small amount exists as tissue iron. When aged erythrocytes are destroyed, iron is liberated. Transported by a beta-globulin called transferrin, iron is incorporated into the hemoglobin of developing erythrocytes or is stored.

Proper diet is essential for erythrocyte production and must include adequate quantities of protein; minerals, including iron, copper, and cobalt; and vitamins, particularly those in the B series—riboflavin (B_2), pyridoxine (B_6), niacin or nicotinic acid, folic acid, thiamine, and B_{12}. Although not all of these vitamins are required by every species of animal, deficiencies may lead to anemia in one or more animal species.

The erythrocyte is composed of 60 to 70 per cent water, 28 to 35 per cent hemoglobin, and a matrix of inorganic and organic materials. The cell membrane is essentially nonelastic, but it is flexible. The erythrocyte of mammals is anuclear. Except in the dog, erythrocytes in domestic animals appear in a blood film as distinctly flat discs with little or no depression near the center of the cell. In contrast, the erythrocyte of the dog is distinctly biconcave and in stained smears has a distinct central pallor. In the deer family, some animals may have sickled red cells with an elongated shape. Members of the camel family have oval erythrocytes.

The primary function of the erythrocyte is to serve as a carrier of hemoglobin. Hemoglobin, in turn, functions as a carrier for oxygen and carbon dioxide and is, therefore, known as a respiratory pigment. In addition, the erythrocyte contributes to blood volume by means of its mass and consequently affects blood flow dynamics.

The life span of erythrocytes varies according to the species of animal. Several techniques for measurement of erythrocyte life span have been devised, but probably the most accurate of these involves labeling erythrocytes with isotopes. The isotopes most commonly used are ^{55}Fe, ^{59}Fe, ^{15}N, ^{14}C, and ^{51}Cr. The average erythrocyte life span in various species of animals as determined by the use of isotopes is presented in Table 2–1.

The destruction of erythrocytes is a continual process affecting cells that have completed their life span as well as a few cells that are inadvertently destroyed as part of normal physiology. The exact method by which overaged cells are destroyed in the normal animal has not yet been fully determined. Fragmentation without the loss of hemoglobin may be one method of erythrocyte destruction. Fragmented portions of cells continue to become smaller until they are only dust-like particles, referred to as hemoglobin dust, that are subsequently removed by reticuloendothelial cells. An abnormal shape may be suggestive of a cell that is soon to be destroyed. Abnormally shaped cells (poikilocytes) are not produced as such by bone marrow but are frequently found in the spleen and occasionally in other organs. The occurrence of poikilocytes in peripheral blood in association with anemia may be interpreted as a sign of early destruction of cells and may also be an indication of the existence of a cycle of pro-

TABLE 2–1. Average Life Span of Erythrocytes

Species	Isotope Method	Mean Life Span (Days)
Bovine	^{14}C	160
Ovine (adult)	^{59}Fe	70–153
Ovine (3 mo)	^{59}Fe	46
Caprine	^{14}C	125
Equine	^{14}C	140–150
Porcine	^{14}C	62
Porcine	^{59}Fe	63
Canine	^{59}Fe	107
Canine	^{14}C	115
Feline	^{59}Fe	68

duction and destruction of red cells. Excessive destruction accompanied by poikilocytosis occurs in haemonchosis in the sheep, in chronic lead poisoning in the dog, and in congenital porphyria of cattle.[4] Phagocytosis of intact erythrocytes may be another method of removal of senescent erythrocytes.

The function of the spleen in the removal of abnormal red cells that pass through its sinusoids is a well-known feature in some diseases. In certain hemolytic diseases the spleen becomes engorged with abnormal erythrocytes that have been removed from the blood by reticuloendothelial cells.

After erythrocytes are removed from the blood, the reticuloendothelial system breaks down hemoglobin to iron, globin, and protoporphyrin. Iron goes into the storage system of the body and may be reutilized. Globin is degraded, and the polypeptide chains are returned to the amino acid pool. Protoporphyrin is split, converted to bilirubin, and excreted.

When the protoporphyrin is cleaved at the alpha-methene bridge, the carbon atom is oxidized to carbon monoxide, which appears in the blood as carboxyhemoglobin. Estimation of the concentration of carboxyhemoglobin has been used as a determinant in estimating endogenous destruction of hemoglobin.

EVALUATION OF THE ERYTHRON

One method for determining the functional state of the erythron is the total erythrocyte count. However, this count reflects only the total number of red blood cells (RBC) in the circulating blood and does not indicate the oxygen-carrying capacity or amount of hemoglobin (Hb). The various techniques for determining hemoglobin content will be discussed later in this chapter. Another procedure for evaluating the total erythrocyte count is the hematocrit tube method, which is used to determine packed cell volume (PCV). These three determinations (total RBC, Hb, and PCV) can be utilized to calculate the mean corpuscular volume (MCV), the mean corpuscular hemoglobin (MCH), and the mean corpuscular hemoglobin concentration (MCHC). These corpuscular values, which are discussed in detail elsewhere in the chapter, are helpful in elucidating the type of anemia.

INDICATIONS FOR DETERMINATION

No hematologic examination is complete without one or more of the tests just mentioned for assaying the condition of the erythron. The most frequently used determination is estimation of PCV. If we wish to estimate erythrocyte size and

hemoglobin content, the total erythrocyte number, hemoglobin content, and PCV must be computed, and calculations must be made.

LIMITATIONS OF LABORATORY TECHNIQUE

Total Erythrocyte Count. The limitations of the laboratory technique for total erythrocyte count made using a hemocytometer are the same as those for a total white cell count calculated by this method (see Chapter 3). In hemocytometer determinations of total erythrocyte number, the inherent error is approximately ±20 per cent. Electronic methods for evaluating erythrocytic parameters are more accurate.

Hemoglobin Content. Precise determination of hemoglobin quantity is difficult, and some techniques are not sufficiently accurate. In the practice of veterinary medicine chemical methods for hemoglobin determination are of value in elucidating the condition of the erythron and are sufficiently accurate to permit correct interpretation.

Deficiencies in hemoglobin determination may be, in part, a consequence of the inadequacy of a chosen method, but limitations more commonly result from manipulative errors in measurement or processing of blood samples. The problems associated with technical deficiencies are entirely in the control of the individual making the analysis.

Spectrophotometric determinations of hemoglobin are affected by the presence of substances that are not lysed by the reagent. Such substances increase optical density and thus overestimate the concentration of hemoglobin. The presence of lipemia or large numbers of Heinz bodies increases optical density.

Although hemolysis does not increase the total hemoglobin value of a sample, the relationship between hemoglobin and packed cell volume as well as that between hemoglobin and total RBC count is affected. If hemolysis has resulted from RBC destruction by heating, freezing, or shear effects from mishandling of samples, total RBC and PCV are decreased while the MCH and MCHC are increased. In samples that have hemolyzed as a result of aging (samples 72 to 96 hours old or those exposed to a high environmental temperature) the remaining erythrocytes swell. If erythrocytes swell the MCV will be large even though total RBC counts are decreased because of cell death. The MCH and MCHC are also increased as outlined earlier.

Packed Cell Volume. The hematocrit method for determination of the percentage of blood composed of erythrocytes is one of the most valuable techniques in the clinical laboratory. The only limitation placed upon its use is the availability of a centrifuge with sufficient speed to completely pack the erythrocytes. In order for the determination to be accurate, erythrocytes must be packed so that additional centrifugation does not reduce packed cell volume. If centrifugation is insufficient to pack red blood cells completely, plasma will be trapped, and the hematocrit reading will be increased. The lower the relative centrifugal force, the larger the amount of trapped plasma. Therefore, the amount of plasma trapped in a hematocrit tube is greater in individuals having high packed cell volumes than in those with packed cell volumes that are lower than normal. Use of the microhematocrit will, for the most part, reduce the error caused by trapped plasma.

Other technical errors include failure to mix blood adequately prior to sampling, inclusion of the buffy coat as a part of erythrocyte packed cell volume, or improper reading of the level of packed cells. With good technique and adequate equipment, the precision of the hematocrit method in determining packed cell volume is ±1 per cent.

Calculations of the erythrocyte mass can be made by electronic particle counters. These are based on the measurement of the number of erythrocytes and their mean cell volume. Most of these calculations are accurate if the counter is properly adjusted to account for species differences in erythrocyte size. Some of the less sophisticated counters do not have this capacity and erroneous results may ensue. Clinical laboratories that routinely set their equipment for measurement of human cells and do not alter the equipment to account for the smaller size of some animal erythrocytes may report erroneous values.

Normal values for the red cell mass may be slightly different with particle counters from those established by centrifugation. These discrepancies are not great but may overestimate the MCHC in comparison to values obtained when the MCV is determined by centrifugation. These differences are related to variable amounts of trapped plasma and erythrocyte shape.

NORMAL VALUES

Normal values for the various determinations conducted on erythrocytes are summarized in Table 2-2. These values represent average determinations. In most geographic areas, normal values for total erythrocyte count, hemoglobin content, and packed cell volume must be determined, as altitude, temperature, and humidity may cause variation from the established ranges for these parameters. This is particularly true of high altitudes, as the values for total erythrocyte count, hemoglobin determination, and packed cell volume are higher in these areas.

Values in Table 2-2 are meant only as guidelines for the clinician. In order to interpret the various parameters for measuring the erythron, veterinarians should establish normal values for their own practice situation. As indicated earlier, estimations of the total erythrocyte count, hemoglobin determination, and packed cell volume all have limitations related to the proficiency of the laboratory technician and equipment and the technique being utilized. All variations must be considered in interpretation of laboratory results.

Physiologic alterations in the erythron must be considered in interpretation of laboratory results. Factors of significance include age, breed, environment, and method of handling an animal.

Age. Dog. The erythrocyte of the dog is large at birth, but the total count is less than that found in the older dog. These large cells are replaced by smaller erythrocytes during the first three weeks of life. The total erythrocyte count, packed cell volume, and hemoglobin content progressively increase with age, stabilizing when animals are six months old. MCHC, MCH, and MCV tend to increase with age. Nursing puppies have smaller erythrocytes with less hemoglobin, whereas in puppies that are weaned and placed on solid food, the total number of erythrocytes increases rapidly. Packed cell volumes reach adult values in dogs about eight months of age and remain constant thereafter.

Cat. At birth, kittens also have a large erythrocyte with a cubic volume almost twice that of the adult cell. The total number of red blood cells per microliter is lower in the kitten than in the adult. As with puppies, the MCHC and MCH of kittens may be lower than adult values during the

TABLE 2-2. Normal Values for Erythrocytes of Domestic Animals*

Species	Total RBC × 10^6/μl	Packed Cell Volume %	Hemoglobin (Gm/dl)	MCV† (fl)	MCH (pg)	MCHC‡ (Gm/dl)
Bovine	5–8(7.0)	26–42(34)	8–14(11)	40–60(52)	11–17(14)	26–34(31)
Ovine	8–15(12)	24–45(35)	8–16(12)	23–48(33)	8–12(10)	29–35(32)
Caprine	8–17(13)	20–38(28)	8–14(11)	16–25(19)	5–8(6.5)	28–34(32)
Porcine	5–8(6.5)	32–50(45)	10–16(13)	50–67(63)	17–21(19)	30–34(32)
Equine	7–13(9)	32–52(42)	11–18(15)	34–58(46)	14–18(16)	31–37(35)
Canine	6–9(6.8)	37–54(45)	12–18(15)	60–77(70)	20–25(23)	31–34(33)
Feline	5–10(7.5)	24–45(37)	8–15(12)	39–55(45)	13–17(16)	31–34(33)

* Values represent range (and average) for each species.
† Values may be higher if calculated on an automated counter not adjusted for the animal species.
‡ Normals may be 1.5–2.0 gm/dl higher if determined by an automated counter.

nursing period, only to increase as the animal is placed on solid food.[4] These reactions may reflect the lack of iron in the nursing diet and its influence on hemoglobin synthesis.

CATTLE. In cattle, erythrocyte counts are highest in calves and decrease gradually until the adult level is reached in animals that are between $1\frac{1}{2}$ and 3 years of age. Erythrocytes decrease in size for three to four months, then gradually increase as the total number decreases. The PCV and MCHC remain fairly stable throughout this time.

SHEEP. In sheep, erythrocyte counts change with age, following the same pattern as in cattle. The number of erythrocytes increases from approximately 7.5 million/μl at one week of age to over 14 million/μl at eight weeks of age. The erythrocyte in newborn animals is larger than that in adult animals.

GOAT. In the goat, the total erythrocyte count is relatively low at birth (7 to 8 million/μl), reaches its highest level at about eight months of age and gradually falls to stabilize at about 11 million/μl by three years of age. The MCV is higher at birth (45 fl) and declines as the animal ages.

HORSE. In the horse, packed cell volume, hemoglobin content, and erythrocyte count decline during the first three weeks of life, only to increase after that time. During the three-week interval the MCV decreases from about 40 to between 30 and 32 fl and remains at this level through the weanling age. In the adult animal, MCV approaches 45 to 46 fl. Similar findings have been reported in the burro,[5] as the total erythrocyte count, hemoglobin level, and PCV decrease during the first week, then stabilize with a slightly downward trend during the first year.

PIG. In the pig, the total erythrocyte number varies with age and husbandry during the suckling and growing period. Pigs at birth have a total erythrocyte count of between 5 and 6 million/μl. A marked reduction in the count occurs by the tenth day of life as a consequence of rapid growth and lack of a significant iron reserve. If piglets are in contact with a source of iron, the erythrocyte count increases, and by two months of age adult levels are reached. Immature forms of erythrocytes are commonly found in the peripheral blood of suckling pigs and disappear when the erythrocyte count approaches the adult level.

Breed Variations. Breed variations appear to be of little practical significance in interpretation of erythrocyte counts except in the horse. In the hot-blooded horse, erythrocytes are smaller and present in larger numbers per unit volume of blood. The total erythrocyte count of the hot-blooded horse will be from 2 to 3 million more per microliter of blood than in that of the cold-blooded animal. At the same time, hemoglobin concentration is 2 to 4 gm higher in the hot-blooded horse. The packed cell volume follows a similar pattern.

Erythrocyte values in Zebu and Scotch Highland cattle have been compared.[6] The Zebu is normally found in a warm climate and the Scotch Highland in a colder climate. Zebu cattle have more erythrocytes, smaller mean corpuscular and packed cell volumes, and a lower hemoglobin level than the Scotch Highland breed.

Environmental Influence. Animals at a high altitude have a greater number of erythrocytes, larger packed cell volume, and higher concentration of hemoglobin than comparable animals raised at a lower altitude.

Handling Influence. In most species, excitation, apprehension, and exercise dramatically increase values for total red cell count, packed cell volume, and hemoglobin determination. These alterations are probably consequences of splenic contraction and release of erythrocytes into the peripheral circulation. This is particularly true of the horse, which has a large splenic reservoir of erythrocytes that are released into the circulation within a few minutes following excitement or strenuous exercise. An increase in PCV ranging from 14 to 64 per cent as a consequence of excitement in the horse has been reported.[4] Strenuous exercise also produces a significant increase in PCV.

The influence of exercise and excitation in the horse is of such great significance that it has been suggested that a hemoglobin determination made on a horse at rest is a poor measure of the total amount of hemoglobin and does not reveal any abnormality other than an advanced pathologic change in the body's total hemoglobin content. It has been recommended that a horse be exercised until the pulse rate at 30 seconds following exercise exceeds 100 beats per minute and that the blood sample be taken within one minute after the end of the exercise. Such a standardization of sample collection might be helpful in obtaining a truer evaluation of the horse erythron.

Increases in PCV that occur with handling can be reduced when animals become conditioned to the environment and handling procedure.

TECHNIQUES OF ERYTHROCYTE EXAMINATION

COLLECTION

Blood for erythrocyte evaluation is obtained and preserved in the same manner as blood for a total leukocyte count. Extreme care must be taken to avoid hemolysis, as such an alteration will affect determinations. One must avoid using a syringe that contains water or chemicals that might destroy red blood cells. Determinations should be made on fresh blood, since hemolysis may occur in blood that is allowed to stand too long.

If the microhematocrit is being utilized, capillary blood may be obtained by puncturing the ear of a small animal or clipping a toenail into the vascular area. In such determinations a heparinized capillary tube is used, and the sample is collected directly from the free-flowing blood. In utilizing this technique extreme care must be taken to avoid contaminating the blood with dirt or other particles.

TOTAL ERYTHROCYTE COUNTS

Hemocytometer Method. The same basic method used for total leukocyte counts is employed in total erythrocyte determinations. However, the dilution factor and diluting fluid are different, and the red blood cell–diluting pipette is marked differently from the white cell pipette. The red cell pipette gives a dilution of 1:200 when blood is drawn to the 0.5 mark and diluted. Blood should be carefully drawn to the 0.5 mark of the pipette, and an isotonic solution, such as saline or Hayem's solution (see Appendix for formula), should be drawn to the 101 mark to dilute the blood. After being well mixed, the diluted blood is discharged onto the hemocytometer counting chamber and allowed to settle for several minutes. Erythrocytes require more settling time to assume a single level than do leukocytes. Before the areas in the chamber are counted, the slide should be examined under low power to check distribution of cells in the ruled area. If an obvious discrepancy in distribution occurs, the pipette should be shaken again, and a clean counting chamber used. The high dry objective of the microscope is employed in making a total erythrocyte count. The total number of cells in five squares in the center of the counting chamber is determined and multiplied by 10,000. This value represents the total number of erythrocytes per microliter. Precautions similar to those for counting leukocytes should be utilized to avoid duplicate counting of cells. Unopettes (Becton-Dickinson, Rutherford, New Jersey) are also available for preparing blood dilutions for total erythrocyte counts. If properly used these units provide an easy method for making accurate dilutions.

The inherent errors common to hemocytometer counts for white blood cells (see Chapter 3) also apply to erythrocyte counts. However, these errors may have a greater effect, since the quantity of blood counted in a total erythrocyte determination is less than that in a white cell count. Thus, minor errors in dilution or counting are multiplied many times in a total erythrocyte count. This undoubtedly is partially responsible for the fact that there is a large inherent error (±20 per cent) in such determinations. Such an inherent error means that if the true red cell count is 5 million/μl, one might expect a range of variations from 4 million to 6 million/μl to be reported. Since red cell counts are time-consuming and probably the least accurate procedure used to de-

tect anemia, they are rarely included in routine or screening procedures unless an automated electronic counter is used.

Electronic Counting Methods. Erythrocytes and leukocytes may be counted electronically, and a number of manufacturers construct such equipment. The high cost of some units may preclude their use in most veterinary hospital laboratories. However, the accuracy of erythrocyte counts completed by this technique is much greater than can be attained by the hemocytometer method. In some medical laboratories electronic counters are calibrated for human blood and can be used for animal bloods only if adjusted to account for the different sizes of animal erythrocytes.

HEMOGLOBIN DETERMINATIONS

As previously mentioned, hemoglobinometry is notable for its inaccuracies. In spite of this fact, hemoglobin determinations in veterinary practice are indicated, as they directly reflect the ability of the erythron to carry oxygen. Several practical techniques have been developed that provide the veterinarian with information relative to the amount of this respiratory pigment present in a blood sample. Many techniques are criticized because they require the veterinarian to compare a

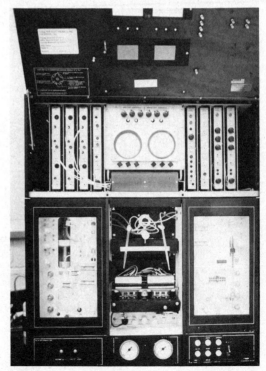

Figure 2–1. Automated cell counters such as this will count the total number of leukocytes and erythrocytes/μl, determine the hemoglobin (g/dl) and packed cell volume (per cent), as well as calculating MCV, MCH, and MCHC.

treated sample of blood with a standard color. Such matching of colors is inaccurate. Information obtained, however, may enable a practitioner to detect gross abnormalities in hemoglobin concentration.

Acid Hematin Methods. These methods depend upon the conversion of hemoglobin to acid hematin, which is usually accomplished by the use of dilute hydrochloric acid. The resulting brownish-yellow mixture is matched with a standard in a colorimeter or comparator. In these techniques 0.1 normal hydrochloric acid is added to whole blood, and the mixture allowed to stand until acid hematin has developed. In all of these methods, the color of the blood and acid mixture is compared with a standard, and the reading is made either in percentage of normal or in grams per deciliter of blood. Since each technique may have a different hemoglobin concentration as 100 per cent, hemoglobin should always be reported in grams per deciliter.

Sources of error in the acid hematin methods are numerous and include the following: (1) nonhemoglobin substances such as proteins and lipids normally present in plasma and cell stroma may influence the color of the diluted blood. (2) It is difficult to match the sample accurately with a brown glass standard, although this is probably the simplest glass standard available. (3) The variation in ability of individual operators in matching colors is a common source of error. (4) Each match must be made after the same interval for which the instrument was standardized; failure to observe this rule introduces another error. (5) Some hemoglobin present in blood is in an inactive form as methemoglobin, sulfhemoglobin, or carboxyhemoglobin; in acid solutions these are not converted into hematin and, consequently, are not included in values obtained by this technique. For these reasons the acid hematin methods for hemoglobin estimation are rarely used.

Direct Matching Methods. Two principal types of direct matching methods are used, the Tallqvist hemoglobin scale and the Dare hemoglobinometer. With the Tallqvist method, a drop of blood is placed on a piece of white absorbent paper, and the paper with its drop of blood is inserted in the central perforation of a serial red color chart. The intensity of red is matched with the most suitable color on the paper scale, and hemoglobin is read as the value that this scale represents. This rapid, simple, and inexpensive technique should be used only as a screening procedure under field conditions, when a more accurate method is not practical. Abnormalities should be confirmed by more accurate methods.

The Dare hemoglobinometer is somewhat different in that a drop of blood is placed in a capillary chamber between small glass plates and matched with a permanent red glass standard. This has some advantage over the Tallqvist technique, as the thickness of the drop of blood can be more carefully controlled, but comparison of red colors remains a difficult problem. The error for both the Tallqvist hemoglobin scale and Dare hemoglobinometer is estimated to be between ±10 and 40 per cent. Both techniques must be considered screening tests only.

Oxyhemoglobin Method. One of the simplest methods of determining oxyhemoglobin employs

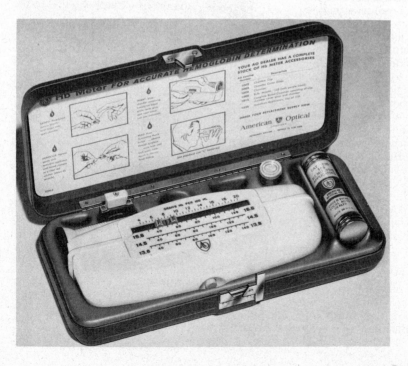

Figure 2–2. The Spencer hemoglobinometer is used to determine the quantity of hemoglobin in a blood sample. Photograph courtesy of American Optical Company, Buffalo, New York.

the Spencer hemoglobinometer (Fig. 2–2). This instrument uses a green filter to measure oxyhemoglobin by light absorption. A drop of blood is placed on a glass plate, and cells are laked by a hemolytic agent. The usual hemolytic agent is saponin, which is dried on the end of an applicator stick. The thickness of the drop of blood is controlled by placing a second glass plate over the one containing laked blood and pressing the two together. This glass chamber is inserted into the hemoglobinometer, and the green color is matched with that of a standard. Green colors are somewhat easier to match than other shades, consequently this technique is relatively more accurate than those involving other colors. Green also has the advantage that the maximum absorption of hemoglobin under visual light occurs in the green band of the spectrum.

Cyanmethemoglobin Method. This is probably the most accurate and widely used technique for determining hemoglobin concentration. It has its limitations in routine practice, as it must be done on a photoelectric colorimeter at a wave length of 540 mμ. The advantages of this technique are (1) solutions of cyanmethemoglobin are the most stable of the various hemoglobin pigments. (2) These solutions can be accurately standardized. (3) The absorption band of cyanmethemoglobin is broad in the region of 540 mμ, and its solutions can be used both in filter photometers and in narrow band spectrophotometers. (4) All forms of hemoglobin likely to be found in blood, except sulfmethemoglobin, are quantitatively converted to cyanmethemoglobin by addition of this single reagent.

To perform this technique, place exactly 5 ml of diluent (cyanmethemoglobin reagent) into a clean cuvette and add exactly 0.02 ml of blood to the diluent. Care should be taken to preserve the accuracy of this measurement by wiping off excess blood from the tip of the pipette. Since the quantity of blood used is small, even a slight excess of blood will influence results. After the blood is expelled into a cuvette, the pipette is rinsed several times with diluent. Cyanmethemoglobin diluent can be purchased commercially in a stable form, and it is recommended that this material be used. After blood is added, the tube is stoppered and inverted two or three times. Allow the mixture of blood and reagent to stand for approximately 10 minutes for maximum conversion of hemoglobin to cyanmethemoglobin. The cuvette is wiped clean and placed into a spectrophotometer for reading.

The per cent transmission or optical density at 540 mμ is recorded and compared either with the readings obtained using a standard solution of cyanmethemoglobin, or with the values on a previously prepared standard curve. This will, in effect, convert the reading to grams of hemoglobin per deciliter of blood. Commercially prepared standards and controls for hemoglobin estimation by this method are readily available.

For preparation of a standard curve, contents of a tube containing a known quantity of cyanmethemoglobin are placed in a cuvette that has been previously matched for light transmission. The cuvette containing the standard is placed into a previously warmed and zeroed spectrophotometer, and per cent transmission or optical density recorded. This reading represents the known quantity of cyanmethemoglobin in the standard solution. Similar readings can be made on other concentrations of a standard solution and a standard curve can be made.

Several manufacturers have special kits available for determining hemoglobin concentration. These usually include a precalibrated capillary tube for dispensing blood into a standard quantity of reagent. The accuracy of most of these kits is acceptable.

Sources of Error. As is true in any chemical determination, each step in the estimation of hemoglobin and preparation of a standard curve is a potential source of error. Each new batch of cuvettes should be matched, as there are variations in different groups of tubes, and there is even a variation within a single tube due to flaws in the glass. Pipettes used to measure fluids should be accurate, having a margin of error less than ± 0.5 per cent. Purchase of pipettes that meet specifications of the National Bureau of Standards is recommended. Pipettes of a cheap grade should not be utilized for this or any other chemical determination. Autopipettes with disposable tips are available and are sufficiently accurate. Cuvettes should be stored and handled individually, as a scratch on the glass may cause diffusion of light in the photoelectric cell system that could result in erroneous readings. Disposable cuvettes are also available. In addition, the photoelectric cell itself is subject to error and variation. Some precautions to be observed in utilizing any photometer are mentioned in Chapter 6.

Abnormally high hemoglobin values may be obtained with lipemic blood or if large numbers of Heinz bodies are present. Both will add optical density to the specimen and give erroneous readings. Heinz bodies can be removed by centrifugation and the sample re-evaluated. Lipemia is more difficult to eliminate. Occasionally lipemic samples can be clarified by centrifugation. The fat is removed from the top of the sample and the remainder used for obtaining a reading. Care must be used in interpretation as centrifugation may not remove all of the fat.

DETERMINATION OF PACKED CELL VOLUME

Hematocrit. Literally, the word hematocrit means to separate blood, and in the laboratory this is most readily accomplished by centrifugation. In a centrifuge, blood is separated into three distinct parts including (1) the mass of erythrocytes at the bottom, which is referred to as packed cell volume; (2) a white or gray layer of leukocytes and thrombocytes immediately above the red cell mass that is referred to as the buffy coat; and (3) the blood plasma. The macrohematocrit determination can be done by use of a Wintrobe tube. The microhematocrit method is preferred.

Blood utilized must be preserved with an anticoagulant that will not cause distortion in cell size. Recommended anticoagulants are EDTA and the formula of Heller and Paul (see Chapter 3).

Adequate centrifugation, with respect to both duration and speed, is an important consideration for accurate hematocrit readings. Red cells must be packed to the point at which further centrifugation does not reduce the packed cell volume. The time and speed for any centrifuge can be calculated by centrifuging a sample for a given period of time and recording the reading, then repeating the process. This procedure is continued until no further decrease in packed cell volume occurs. The time and speed necessary for maximum packing should be recorded and utilized as standards.

Wintrobe Method. At one time the Wintrobe tube was routinely used for determination of PCV. Today it has been almost completely replaced by the capillary tube.

Blood for testing should be thoroughly mixed by gently and slowly inverting the tube. After adequate mixing, the Wintrobe tube is filled, using a 5-ml syringe and a 16- or 18-gauge needle measuring 5 or 6 inches that has been blunted at the end. The needle is introduced into the bottom of the tube, and blood is expelled as the needle is slowly withdrawn. Care should be taken so that the opening in the needle always remains below the surface of the blood, since air bubbles in the blood will interfere with results. In this manner, the tube is filled to exactly the zero mark on the left hand scale. If prolonged centrifugation is necessary to achieve complete packing, the tube should be stoppered with a small rubber cap to combat evaporation. The filled tube is placed in the centrifuge and processed for the prescribed length of time.

In a reading of the Wintrobe hematocrit tube, the exact level of the erythrocytes immediately beneath the buffy coat should be recorded, as should the thickness of the layer of leukocytes.

Microhematocrit Method. This is the preferred method for measuring the PCV. For this determination, a capillary hematocrit tube approximately 7 cm in length and having a bore of about 1 mm is recommended. Capillary tubes containing anticoagulant can be purchased and used to collect blood directly from a venous or capillary puncture. Plaintubes are available for use on blood already containing an anticoagulant. The tubes are filled by capillary action, the outside is carefully dried with a piece of gauze, and the opposite end of the tube is sealed with a special clay. These sealed tubes are placed in a special high-

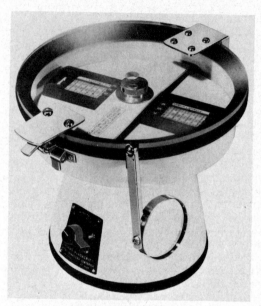

Figure 2–3. The Clay-Adams Readacrit, a microhematocrit centrifuge in which the packed cell volume can be read without removing the capillary tubes. Photograph courtesy of Clay-Adams, Inc., New York, New York.

speed centrifuge (Fig. 2–3) so that the sealed end is near the outside rim of the centrifuge. In order to avoid breakage, it is wise to spin the head by hand for a few revolutions to ensure that there will not be a sudden movement of the tube toward the outside rim when the centrifuge is turned on. The cover is tightened into place, and the centrifuge turned on for the length of time prescribed by the manufacturer for maximum packing.

After centrifugation, carefully place the tube on a special reader for determining the per cent of red cells (Fig. 2–4).

Automated Estimation of PCV. Most commercial clinical pathology laboratories and some veterinary hospitals utilize an automatic particle counter that calculates PCV using total erythrocyte count and mean cell volume. These results generally correlate well with those obtained by the microhematocrit method, although they may be slightly lower as there is no trapped plasma between erythrocytes. Erroneously high PCV values may occur in old samples, particularly those subjected to a higher than normal environmental temperature. As mentioned previously, these cell counters must be properly adjusted to account for variations in erythrocyte size according to animal species. Counters adjusted for determining the characteristics of the erythron in man are not suitable for making the same evaluations in all species of domestic animals. Therefore care should be taken in interpreting such values. If in doubt consult the laboratory manager.

Limitations of Techniques. The most signifi-

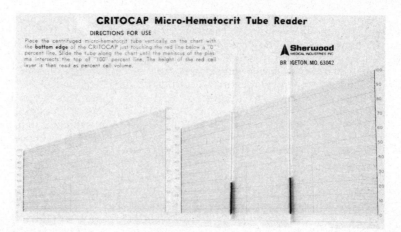

CRITOCAP Micro-Hematocrit Tube Reader

DIRECTIONS FOR USE

Place the centrifuged micro-hematocrit tube vertically on the chart with the **bottom edge** of the CRITOCAP just touching the red line below a "0" percent line. Slide the tube along the chart until the meniscus of the plasma intersects the top of "100" percent line. The height of the red cell layer is then read as percent cell volume.

▲ **Sherwood**
MEDICAL INDUSTRIES INC
BRIDGETON, MO. 63042

Figure 2–4. Spun microhematocrit capillary tubes are placed on a special reader to determine the packed cell volume.

cant source of error in packed cell volume determinations using the hematocrit tube is centrifugation. In the process of centrifugation, platelets, plasma, and leukocytes are trapped between the red cells. The proportion of packed cell volume that is due to trapped plasma is somewhat greater than that due to the presence of either platelets or leukocytes. This error is increased by a lack of proper centrifugal force and an insufficient length of time for centrifugation. Microhematocrit tubes that are properly centrifuged have an error of ±0.5 per cent. Errors with the Wintrobe tube macrohematocrit are from 2.0 to 8.0 per cent.

The microhematocrit has several advantages in comparison to the Wintrobe method in addition to the one just mentioned. These include: (1) The microhematocrit requires a considerably smaller amount of blood than does the macrohematocrit. (2) Less time is required for the entire procedure. (3) Results obtained for PCV are more accurate and reproducible. The disadvantages of the microhematocrit technique include: (1) A special reader is required for determining the packed cell volume values. (2) It is impossible to determine the erythrocyte sedimentation rate in such small tubes. (3) It is more difficult to evaluate the depth of the buffy coat.

Improper use of anticoagulant can also be a source of error. If EDTA is used as the anticoagulant, care must be taken not to use it in excess, as the PCV will be decreased if too much EDTA is present.

MEAN CORPUSCULAR VALUES

Utilizing the total erythrocyte count, hemoglobin content, and packed cell volume, it is possible to calculate the volume of an average erythrocyte and its hemoglobin concentration. These values are of particular importance in determining the morphologic type of anemia and may be of assistance in selecting therapy and monitoring an established therapeutic procedure. With some automated counters these calculations are made automatically.

Mean Corpuscular Volume (MCV). MCV is determined by dividing the volume of packed red cells per 1000 ml of blood by the total red cell count in millions per microliter. The result of this calculation is expressed in femtoliters (fl); for example, in a sample of blood having a PCV of 45 per cent and a total erythrocyte count of 5 million/µl, the formula is expressed as follows:

$$MCV = \frac{450}{5.0} = 90 \text{ fl}$$

Values for average mean corpuscular volume in the various species of domestic animals are summarized in Table 2–2.

TABLE 2–3. Normal Values for Erythrocyte Sedimentation Rate (ESR) in Various Species of Domestic Animals (Wintrobe Method)

| Species | Mm in Fall | | | | |
	10 MIN	20 MIN	30 MIN	1 HOUR	24 HOURS
Cattle			0	0	2.25–4.0
Sheep			0	0	3.0–8.5
Goat			0	0	2.0–2.5
Pig			0–6	1–14	
Horse	2–12	15–38			
Dog			1–6	5–25	
Cat				7–23	

Mean Corpuscular Hemoglobin (MCH). MCH is determined by dividing the hemoglobin present in grams per 1000 ml of blood by the total erythrocyte count in millions per microliter. With a blood sample that has a hemoglobin value of 15 gm and a total red cell count of 5 million/μl, the formula is completed as follows:

$$MCH = \frac{150}{5.0} = 30\ pg$$

Mean Corpuscular Hemoglobin Concentration (MCHC). MCHC is calculated by dividing the hemoglobin in grams per 10,000 ml of blood by the volume of PCV per 100 ml of blood. Results are expressed in grams of hemoglobin per deciliter. Using the same value for hemoglobin as previously indicated and a PCV of 50, the formula is expressed as follows:

$$MCHC = \frac{1500}{50} = 30.0\ gm/dl$$

The average values for the MCHC in the various species of domestic animals are presented in Table 2–3.

Interpretation of Mean Corpuscular Values. Mean corpuscular values are utilized to classify anemias morphologically. Morphologic classification has little reference to the cause of anemia; instead it represents an estimation of alterations in size and hemoglobin concentration of individual red blood cells. Erythrocytes are *normocytic* if the cells are of normal size, *macrocytic* if cells are larger than normal, or *microcytic* if cells are smaller than normal. Mean hemoglobin content is designated by the terms *normochromic* for normal hemoglobin content and *hypochromic* for cells having less than the normal amount of hemoglobin. True hyperchromic cells do not exist. However, cells larger than normal may contain quantitatively larger amounts of hemoglobin than are found in normal cells. In such cells the MCHC is within normal limits.

In anemic conditions, alterations in the average size of red cells (MCV) may be paralleled by similar changes in the MCH and often the MCHC. With microcytic cells hemoglobin may be decreased, and this is referred to as a microcytic hypochromic anemia. Such alterations are specific for iron deficiency or failure to properly utilize iron in the formation of hemoglobin. Microcytic hypochromic anemia may also appear in association with chronic blood loss; copper and pyridoxine deficiencies may also produce this type of anemia. When the MCHC of an anemic animal is calculated by an automated particle counter, the small size of the erythrocytes is easily detected; however, because the calculated PCV is somewhat less than might be obtained by a microhematocrit centrifuge, the MCHC may be within the normal range for the species. Therefore one should always consider the methodology used before interpreting laboratory results.

Normocytic anemias have normal MCV, MCHC, and MCH and are detected only by a decreased number of erythrocytes, a low packed cell volume, and a reduction in total hemoglobin. Such anemias occur when there is a depression of erythrogenesis. This is the most common anemia found in domestic animals and is often a sign that other disease conditions are present. Whenever a normocytic anemia is detected, every effort should be made to determine the primary disease condition.

Macrocytic anemias may be hypochromic or normochromic. Most macrocytic anemias are transitory and are observed in the recovery stages in animals that have had an acute blood loss or in which there is an acute hemolytic anemia. An increase in the number of reticulocytes in the peripheral circulation usually results in macrocytosis. This, however, soon disappears as cells mature and assume their normal size. Macrocytosis is indicative of a good bone marrow response. Persistent macrocytic anemias seldom occur. However, when they do, they are usually associated with an arrest of the maturation cycle and an increase in the size of erythrocytes released into peripheral circulation.

SEDIMENTATION RATE

When blood containing anticoagulant is allowed to stand in a perpendicular tube, the erythrocytes sink because they are heavier than the plasma in which they are suspended. The speed with which erythrocytes fall in the blood of normal animals is relatively slow, but in animals with inflammatory diseases in which there is tissue necrosis and degeneration, speed is increased. This alteration in suspension stability probably results from changes that occur in the physiochemical properties of the erythrocyte surfaces and the plasma. Alterations in these properties of the erythrocyte surfaces cause red cells to aggregate and form rouleaux. The larger the aggregation and the more aggregations that occur, the more rapid is the fall of erythrocytes. Increases in plasma fibrinogen are probably responsible for these changes.

The erythrocyte sedimentation test is most applicable to dog blood. Normal values for erythrocyte sedimentation rate (ESR) are summarized in Table 2–3.[4]

Technique for Conducting Erythrocyte Sedimentation Rate (ESR). The ESR is easily and accurately determined by filling a Wintrobe hematocrit tube as if for a packed cell volume determination or by using a disposable sedimentation tube and a special rack that holds the tube absolutely perpendicular to the surface of the table. This rack should be placed in an isolated area in the laboratory that is free from vibrations. Since temperature may influence ESR, every at-

TABLE 2–4. Relative Anticipated Erythrocyte Sedimentation Rates (One Hour) of Canine Blood for PCV Values from 9 to 50 per cent

PCV %	Sed. Rate mm	PCV %	Sed. Rate mm	PCV %	Sed. Rate mm
9	82	24	38	39	11
10	79	25	36	40	10
11	76	26	34	41	9
12	73	27	32	42	8
13	70	28	30	43	7
14	67	29	28	44	6
15	64	30	26	45	5
16	61	31	24	46	4
17	58	32	22	47	3
18	55	33	20	48	2
19	52	34	18	49	1
20	49	35	16	50	0
21	46	36	14		
22	43	37	13		
23	40	38	12		

Record results as follows: Compare observed ESR to anticipated ESR and record difference as + or −.

tempt should be made to standardize the room temperature. The filled tube is allowed to stand for one hour, and the level of the top of the erythrocyte column is recorded. If a Wintrobe tube is used, the scale on the left hand side is read, and measurement is recorded as the number of millimeters of fall. If a disposable tube is used, the ESR is recorded by reading the millimeters of fall inscribed on the special rack.

The total number of erythrocytes in a given blood specimen will influence the rate of fall of erythrocytes in an ESR determination. In anemic animals, the ESR is considerably increased. Tables of expected ESR determinations for various PCV values in the dog and in horse have been developed. These data are presented in Tables 2–4 and 2–5.[4] Thus, interpretation of ESR is dependent upon the number of erythrocytes as determined by the PCV.

In evaluation of the effect that disease may have on ESR, the value obtained must be corrected by subtracting it from the rate of fall anticipated for the packed cell volume. For example, a dog with a packed cell volume of 40 per cent had a sedimentation rate of 18 mm. The anticipated ESR for this packed cell volume is 10 mm. Subtraction of observed ESR from anticipated ESR gave a difference of plus 8 mm. Negative ESR values may also occur and are expected in young growing dogs that have low levels of plasma fibrinogen. Negative ESR values are also recorded in animals with macrocytic erythrocytes.

Diphasic Sedimentation. Occasionally in an ESR determination there is no definite line between the settling erythrocytes and the plasma. The plasma is clear except for a stream of red cells that seems to be following along behind the red cell mass much as a tail follows a dog. This phenomenon is the result of the presence of reticulocytes or other young forms of erythrocytes. It may also occur if there are large numbers of abnormally shaped erythrocytes. This trailing out of erythrocytes occurs because these cells are larger and do not actively participate in rouleau formation. Whenever diphasic sedimentation occurs, it suggests the presence of an erythrogenic alteration.

Sources of Error. Sources of error that may occur in ESR determinations include the following: (1) If the concentration of anticoagulant is not

TABLE 2–5. Anticipated Erythrocyte Sedimentation Rates (ESR) in Equine Blood for PCV Values from 10 to 50 per cent

PCV %	Anticipated ESR/20 Minutes mm	PCV %	ESR/20	PCV %	ESR/20
10	86	26	58	41	8
11	85	27	55	42	5 ± 4
12	84	28	53 ± 4	43	4
13	83 ± 1	29	50	44	3.0
14	82	30	47	45	2.5
15	80	31	44	46	2.0 ± 1
16	78	32	40 ± 5	47	1.5
17	76	33	36	48	1.0
18	74	34	32	49	0.5
19	72 ± 2	35	28	50	0.0
20	70	36	24 ± 15		
21	68	37	20		
22	66	38	17		
23	64 ± 3	39	14 ± 8		
24	62	40	11		
25	60				

exact, results may be affected. (2) If the tube is not clean, the presence of substances such as dirt, alcohol, or ether will influence rate of fall. (3) If the tube is not placed absolutely vertically, ESR will be increased, and an abnormal value will be obtained. (4) If bubbles of air are present, the settling of cells will be affected. (5) If the blood sample undergoes hemolysis, sedimentation may be modified. (6) If the blood is collected too long before the determination is made, age of the blood sample may affect results. (7) If the sample has been refrigerated, it should be allowed to reach room temperature before the test is set up, as temperature will influence settling. (8) If the blood sample is from an anemic animal, this condition is of considerable significance in interpretation of ESR, as discussed previously. (9) If tubes other than the Wintrobe hematocrit tube are utilized, different normal values must be established, as the dimensions of the tube utilized will also affect the ESR.

Interpretation. Many of the various factors influencing ESR have not yet been established. However, it has been ascertained that ESR is increased in association with tissue damage and inflammation. This increase, however, is a nonspecific response and as a tool for making a definite diagnosis is of limited value. The greatest importance of ESR is probably in following the course of a disease, particularly in evaluating the response of the individual to inflammatory or necrotic processes.

As most increases in ESR are associated with an increase in plasma fibrinogen, quantitative estimation of this protein has almost completely replaced the ESR as a laboratory test.

FIBRINOGEN

Fibrinogen is a plasma protein produced by the liver. It functions in the clotting mechanism and plays a significant role in the body's defense by moving into extravascular spaces to assist in localization of disease processes. Because of fibrinogen's association with inflammatory conditions, estimations of fibrinogen level have been found useful in evaluation of the inflammatory response.

Technique for Estimating Amount of Fibrinogen. Fibrinogen will precipitate at a temperature of 56 to 58° C. At this temperature other plasma proteins remain in solution. We can take advantage of this physical characteristic to measure fibrinogen concentrations.

A simple method for quantitating fibrinogen begins by filling two 75-mm capillary tubes with blood to at least three-fourths of their capacity. Both are centrifuged as for a microhematocrit determination. One tube is broken, just above the erythrocyte line, and a refractometer is utilized to estimate total proteins in the plasma. The Goldberg refractometer was designed specifically for use in providing an accurate measurement of total solids in body fluids such as urine, plasma, or serum. The TS meter (American Optical Company, Buffalo, New York) has a direct reading scale for total protein in grams per deciliter (a second scale is used in estimating urine specific gravity). This instrument is especially useful in veterinary laboratories, as it has a built-in temperature compensation between 60 and 100° C. The refractometer is reliable in estimating concentration of total solids in plasma and serum if the fluids are clear. Lipemic plasma or serum will give false high readings.

In using the refractometer a single drop of plasma, such as that obtained by breaking a microhematocrit capillary tube just above the red cell line, is placed on the prism of the TS meter and viewed through the eye piece. The total protein level is read from the right hand column at the point where the dividing line between dark and bright crosses that scale.

After the total protein concentration of one sample is determined, the second centrifuged capillary tube is placed in a water bath at 56 to 58° C for three minutes to precipitate the fibrinogen. The tube is then recentrifuged and broken just above the fibrinogen layer. A drop of this fibrinogen-free plasma is placed on the prism of the TS meter, and the plasma protein is again estimated. The amount of fibrinogen is the difference between the protein content of the heated and unheated tubes.

If plasma is available from other centrifuged specimens, it can be treated in a similar fashion. Other chemical methods are available for estimating fibrinogen levels and are probably more accurate for an absolute determination. However, the simplicity of the heat precipitation method, its relative accuracy, and its reproducibility make it the method of choice in most veterinary laboratories.

Normal Values. Plasma fibrinogen levels in the dog and horse are normally between 100 and 500 mg/dl. Normal levels in the cat range from 100 to 300 mg/dl, whereas for the cow the normal range is from 300 to 700 mg/dl.

In order to compensate for dehydration, the ratio of plasma proteins to fibrinogen (PP:F) is calculated. The fibrinogen value is subtracted from the total plasma protein and the quantity of fibrinogen divided into the remainder. Ratios of 15:1 or greater are normal, whereas ratios of 10:1 or less reflect an absolute increase in plasma fibrinogen. Only in cases of very severe hypoproteinemia would the normal plasma protein:fibrinogen ratio be less than 10:1.

Interpretation. Estimations of plasma fibrinogen have been compared to total leukocyte and neutrophil counts in dogs. It was concluded that fibrinogen increases indicated the presence of an inflammation that was not detected by increases in total leukocytes or neutrophils. Many of these animals had a PP:F ratio of less than 10:1 while leukocyte counts were normal.[7] The increase in fibrinogen associated with inflammatory and suppurative diseases is not always in direct relationship to disease severity. For example, a massive liver disease may reduce fibrinogen levels in dogs.

Similar studies have been performed in horses. Fibrinogen levels of 500 to 600 mg/dl occur during developmental stages of a severe inflammation and with mild inflammation may not rise above these values. Levels of 1000 mg/dl or more reflect a serious and more advanced stage of disease.[4]

In the cow normal plasma fibrinogen levels range from 300 to 700 mg/dl. Increases above 800 mg indicate the presence of inflammation or tissue destruction. A total fibrinogen concentration of 1000 mg/dl or greater that persists is an unfavorable sign. PP:F ratios less than 10:1 indicate an absolute increase in fibrinogen and support the presence of inflammation or necrosis.

In sheep the normal fibrinogen level is 100–500 mg/dl of plasma. Increases of fibrinogen in disease range from 600–900 mg/dl.

Because of its value in identifying the presence of diseased tissues a fibrinogen estimation should be considered as an integral part of any hematologic evaluation.

ERYTHROCYTE MORPHOLOGY

The morphology of erythrocytes is most readily observed by examination of smears, such as those utilized in making differential leukocyte counts, or wet mounts. Use of wet mounts has the advantage of detecting alterations in size and shape since artefacts, which may appear when a blood film is prepared, do not occur. Scanning electron microscopy reveals that erythrocytes of the cow, sheep, and dog are typically biconcave, whereas those of the horse and cat have a shallow concavity and those of the goat are rather flat. The existence of concavities is not obvious in a routinely prepared blood film except in the dog. The erythrocyte of the dog is a distinct biconcave disc, as is the erythrocyte found in humans. Consequently, these cells have a distinct central pallor in stained smears. Noticeable alterations in the shape of erythrocytes may occur. In general, these abnormalities of morphology fall into three categories: (1) abnormalities in size, (2) abnormalities in shape, and (3) the appearance of erythrocyte inclusions.

Judgments of erythrocyte morphology are subjective and thus rating the severity of change is subject to the experience and bias of the technologist. An attempt to semiquantitate these morphologic changes has been developed and is presented in Table 2–7. Use of this information will

TABLE 2–6. Diameter of Erythrocytes in Various Species of Domestic Animals

Species	Range of Erythrocyte Diameter (Microns)
Catttle	4.0–9.6
Sheep	3.5–6.0
Goat	3.2–4.2
Pig	4.0–8.0
Horse	5.6–8.0
Dog	6.9–7.3
Cat	5.4–6.5

aid in standardization of reports and is recommended. The clinician judging a report must be careful in interpreting these assessments. If the laboratory has accepted these standards the evaluation can be made with more confidence. Check with the laboratory to see if they have adopted these recommendations. If they have not, encourage them to do so.

ABNORMALITIES IN SIZE

Erythrocytes of domestic animals vary in size depending upon the species. The average size of an erythrocyte in various species of animals is presented in Table 2–6. As will be noted from the data, the erythrocyte of the dog is the largest, and that of the goat and sheep is the smallest. Variation in the diameter of erythrocytes may be readily observed in some species upon examination of direct smears; however, the minute variations that occur between some species of animals are not readily observable in a smear of peripheral blood. A slight variation in size among erythrocytes is considered normal. Anisocytosis (variation in size) occurs commonly in blood smears of cattle and is seen with less frequency in blood from the cat, sheep, and goat. Anisocytosis is relatively common in bovine blood as erythrocytes in normal cattle vary from 3.6 microns to 9.6 microns. The greatest differences usually occur in young animals. Cells that are 8 microns in size or larger are not frequent and are not seen in increased numbers in diseased cattle. These cells are normal, and are macrocytes that have no relationship to large corpuscles of embryonal blood formation. Anisocytosis occurring in sheep blood is usually slight, with only an occasional very large cell being observed in smears from normal animals. It must be emphasized that there is no direct relationship between MCV and anisocytosis, since anisocytosis may be present with high, normal, or low values for MCV.

Anisocytosis occurs in the animal with a regenerative anemia when macrocytes are being released into the peripheral circulation. Some poikilocytes, as we will see later, are of smaller size

TABLE 2–7. Semiquantitative Evaluation of Erythrocyte Morphology Based on Average Number of Abnormal Cells/1000 × Microscope Field

	1+	2+	3+	4+
Anisocytosis				
Dog	7–15	16–20	21–29	>29
Cat	5–8	9–15	16–20	>20
Cow	10–20	21–30	31–40	>40
Horse	1–3	4–6	7–10	>10
Polychromasia				
Dog	2–7	8–14	15–29	>29
Cat	1–2	3–8	9–15	>15
Cow	2–5	6–10	11–20	>20
Horse	- - - - - - - - - - Rarely observed - - - - - - - - - - -			
Hypochromasia				
All species	1–10	11–50	51–200	>200
Poikilocytosis				
All species	3–10	11–50	51–200	>200
Codocytes				
Dogs only	3–5	6–15	16–30	>30
Spherocytes				
All species	5–10	11–50	51–150	>150
Echinocytes				
All species	5–10	11–100	101–250	>250
Acanthocytes, schizocytes, keratocytes, elliptocytes, dacryocytes, depranocytes, and stomatocytes				
All species	1–2	3–8	9–20	>20

From Weiss, D. J.: Uniform evaluation and semiquantitative reporting of hematologic data in veterinary laboratories. Vet. Clin. Pathol. XIII(No. II):27, 1984. Reprinted with permission.

than the usual erythrocyte and may tend to give an overall impression of anisocytosis.

ABNORMALITIES IN SHAPE

Poikilocytosis is defined as a major deviation from the normal shape of the erythrocyte. Some minor alterations in the shape of an erythrocyte may be normal. However, marked deviations in shape may be a sign of abnormal erythrogenesis. Care must be taken in evaluating poikilocytosis because improperly prepared blood films may contain abnormally shaped erythrocytes. Erythrocytes in the thinnest or thickest portions of a blood smear may not exhibit abnormalities of shape. If there is any question regarding the presence or absence of poikilocytosis a wet blood film should be examined. A phase microscope is preferred but most alterations in erythrocyte shape can be detected with an ordinary light microscope. The degree of illumination should be reduced by adjusting the position of the substage condenser and the amount of light emitted. The slide should be viewed as these adjustments are made in order to establish the amount of light that permits best visualization of erythrocytes.

With the advent of scanning electron microscopy, several new terms have been coined to identify the various abnormally shaped erythrocytes present in human blood. Some of these terms may have applicability in identification of abnormally

shaped erythrocytes of other mammals.[8] Terms considered acceptable in the identification of canine erythrocytes include *leptocyte*, *codocyte*, *spherocyte*, *keratocyte*, *schizocyte*, *knizocyte*, *stomatocyte*, and *torocyte*.

Leptocytes are thin erythrocytes in which surface area is increased but cell volume is not changed. Consequently, it is possible for the cell membrane to fold and become distorted. These cells are usually more resistant to hemolysis in a hypotonic saline solution. Since such cells have a larger diameter, they usually do not participate in rouleau formation and do not clump readily with other cells. Consequently, in ESR determinations they do not always fall readily and may lead to a minus value in a corrected sedimentation rate. Such cells may become entrapped in the buffy coat and give a pinkish tinge to this normally white layer.

The folded leptocyte has a raised fold that crosses the cell transversely. In a stained blood smear there appears to be a bar of hemoglobin extending across the center of a cell in which little hemoglobin is demonstrated.

A target cell (codocyte) is a form of leptocyte. The target cell is characterized by a dark-staining center section surrounded by a clear, unstained area that is surrounded by a peripheral ring of stained cytoplasm. Occasionally, a bridge of hemoglobin may be observed between the central mass and the peripherally stained hemoglobin. Target cells are most commonly seen in canine blood. In wet films these cells do not have a central condensation of hemoglobin. It is possible that target cell formation may be an artefact resulting from fixation and staining. Although the appearance of such cells in a stained smear may be artefactual, these cells are nevertheless abnormal erythrocytes, as the ratio of surface area to volume is greater than in a normal red blood cell. Leptocytes are more commonly found in an animal having a chronic disease process, and this should be considered when evaluating the morphology of erythrocytes in individuals having a characteristic nonresponding anemia.

Spherocytes are recognized by their morphology and staining characteristics. They are most frequently found in the dog, appear smaller than normal erythrocytes, stain more intensely, and have no central pallor. They can be readily identified in a wet mount and when present in large numbers can be recognized in a stained blood film. These cells may also occur in feline blood but because of the smaller size of feline erythrocytes are less easily recognized.

Spherocytes have a more rigid membrane and therefore resist deformation. Because of this rigidity the intravascular life span is shortened, as these cells are rapidly removed from the peripheral circulation.

Spherocytosis is not common in domestic animals. In humans, spherocytosis is a congenital disease. Spherocytosis occurs in dogs with autoimmune hemolytic anemia. Stored erythrocytes tend to become spherical. Dogs transfused with large quantities of stored blood may have a detectable spherocytosis. The veterinarian must be careful in assigning significance to the presence of spherocytes in such patients.

Erythrocyte fragmentation may occur in hemolytic anemias or diseases in which there is an alteration in the microcirculation. Some fragmentation occurs naturally and is thought to be one of the methods of normal erythrocyte destruction. This may be an important mechanism for the removal of abnormal erythrocytes. Erythrocyte frag-

mentation may occur because of a loss of cell membrane plasticity as a consequence of antibody coating, as in immune-mediated anemia. It is also seen in association with iron deficiency, Heinz body formation, and sickle cell disorders. It has been suggested that hypercholesterolemia and lipemia may also cause erythrocytes to become more rigid and thus be subject to possible fragmentation. Fragmented erythrocytes also occur with disseminated intravascular coagulation. In a blood smear, fragmented erythrocytes appear as partial red cells and are known by the terms *keratocyte* if there are one or more incomplete cuts, *schizocyte* if there is a complete cut, and *knizocyte* if the shape is triconcave. Knizocytes are frequently seen in hemolytic anemias.

Acanthocytes are erythrocytes with rounded projections. Such cells have been demonstrated in blood from healthy cows[4] and in blood from dogs with liver disease. Evidence in humans suggests that acanthocytes result from plasma abnormalities such as decreased phospholipid and cholesterol levels, depressed triglycerides, free fatty acids, and abetalipoproteinemia.[8]

Crenation (the appearance of projections on the erythrocyte surface), which is usually not clinically significant, results from delayed drying, exposure to a lytic agent, or the presence of hypertonic solutions. It also occurs when blood is allowed to stand. Crenation does not take place readily in dog blood; however, in the cat it may happen with some frequency, and the cells appear to have a few blunt processes. In smears from pig blood, crenation is characterized by sharp points appearing on processes emanating from the cell. Although not clinically important, crenation must be distinguished from the significant alterations in erythrocyte morphology.

ERYTHROCYTE INCLUSIONS

Reticulocytes. Reticulocytes (Fig. 2–5) are not recognized as such in a smear of peripheral blood

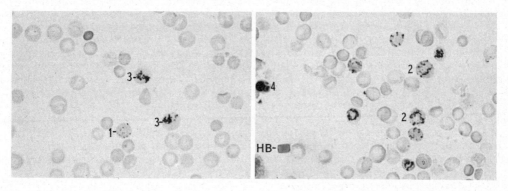

Figure 2–5. Reticulocytes in feline blood. A punctate form of reticulocyte (1) is shown as well as are classic reticulocytes (2 and 3). A metarubricyte is also illustrated (4). A hemoglobin crystal is present (HB).

stained by routine methods. They may, however, be identified by size and staining characteristics, as they are macrocytic and polychromatophilic. If present in large numbers, they may increase the MCV. A reticulocyte differs from a mature red cell in that it is more resistant to crenation, does not participate in the formation of rouleaux, has a lower specific gravity, is a larger cell, and is more resistant to hypotonic saline solutions.

Reticulocytes are not found in the blood of healthy horses, sheep, goats, or cows. Reticulocytes mature in the bone marrow of these animals. In the dog and cat as many as 0.5 to 1.0 per cent reticulated cells may appear in peripheral blood. In the pig there may be up to 2 per cent reticulocytes in peripheral blood. Many laboratory animals, including the guinea pig, rat, rabbit, and mouse, have a reticulocyte level between 2 and 4 per cent.

Reticulocytes are best demonstrated by use of a supravital stain. The most commonly used stains are a 1.0 per cent solution of brilliant cresyl blue in physiologic saline and a 0.5 per cent solution of new methylene blue in a 1.6 per cent solution of potassium oxalate. Reticulocytes stained in this manner have a bluish stippling in the center of the cell. The quantity of bluish-staining material in any reticulocyte may vary depending upon the stage of maturation.

Three distinct types of reticulocytes have been demonstrated in cat blood (Fig. 2–5). Those classed as type I are lightly reticulated and have a faint blue stippling with new methylene blue stain. Type II reticulocytes have isolated dark granules and one or two threads of reticulum. Type III are characterized by the appearance of a heavy dark blue granular network. In evaluating the reticulocyte response in the cat it is important to differentiate among these various types of reticulocytes.

Under the influence of increased levels of erythropoietin there may be a premature release of reticulocytes from the bone marrow. These are termed *shift* or *stimulated* reticulocytes, which are larger and contain more reticulum than do the more mature reticulocytes. These cells require more time to mature in the peripheral blood. Estimation of the total number of reticulocytes includes those recently released in response to marrow stimulation as well as those previously liberated as shift reticulocytes. Taking these facts into consideration, it is obvious that an approximation of the percentage of reticulocytes in peripheral blood might overestimate true marrow response. It has been suggested that the observed per cent reticulocyte count should be corrected for variations in the number of circulating erythrocytes and for changes in maturation time. Correction for variations in the number of circulating red cells can be made by determining the absolute number of circulating reticulocytes per microliter of blood. This is done by multiplying the per-

centage of reticulocytes by the total erythrocyte count. If the total red blood cell count is not known, the absolute per cent reticulocyte count is obtained by the following formula:

$$\text{Absolute \% reticulocyte count}$$

$$= \frac{\text{Observed \%}}{\text{reticulocyte count}} \times \frac{\text{Observed PCV}}{\text{Normal PCV}}$$

For example: in a dog with a packed cell volume of 20 per cent and a reticulocyte count of 32 per cent the formula would be:

$$\text{Absolute count} = 32 \times \frac{20}{45} = 14.2\%$$

In humans, an additional correction is made based upon the estimated reticulocyte maturation time. This has been utilized somewhat in animals, although there is not definite evidence that the same figures are true

Reticulocytosis. The degree of reticulocytosis is proportional to erythropoietic activity, as an increased reticulocyte count indicates increased erythrogenesis. An acute hemorrhage is usually followed by a reticulocyte shower, which indicates accelerated erythropoiesis. Chronic hemorrhage is usually followed by a reticulocytosis, but it is not as high as that occurring in association with acute hemorrhage. In hemolytic anemias, persistent reticulocytosis results from a constant demand for new erythrocytes. Except in the horse, reticulocyte counts may be used to evaluate the response of an individual to an existent anemia. Reticulocyte counts may also be used as a method of evaluating therapy for anemia. Under optimal conditions, the reticulocyte count increases by the fourth or fifth day after therapy has begun and reaches a maximum on the ninth or tenth day. Reticulocytes usually return to normal by the end of the second or third week of therapy. Failure to obtain a satisfactory response to hemopoietic preparations in the treatment of anemia should lead the clinician to search for localized or systemic infections or other factors that are known to interfere with the efficacy of such therapy. One must also consider the possibility that the therapy being utilized is not adequate.

Discovery of a reticulocytosis in an animal may lead to detection of an otherwise occult disease such as hidden hemorrhage or unrecognized hemolysis of erythrocytes. A persistent lack of reticulocytes in the peripheral blood of an anemic animal subsequent to therapy generally indicates a poor prognosis. At the same time, if a persistently elevated reticulocyte count is the rule in chronic anemias, a sudden drop to very low values may indicate impending or existing marrow failure.

Reticulocyte Response. In the early stages of active reticulocyte response in the cat increased numbers of cells containing large amounts of reticulum can be expected. In the later stages, cells with a punctate form of reticulum are commonly found. Reticulocytes have a rather lengthy maturation time in cats, and an increased reticulocyte count does not necessarily indicate active erythrocyte production at that time. Large numbers of reticulocytes of the punctate type may be present without any bone marrow activity. Such cells probably represent erythrocytes produced at an earlier time in response to anemia but that have not yet completed their development to maturity.

The effect of epinephrine on reticulocyte count, red blood cell count, and packed cell volume has been evaluated. There is a marked increase in reticulocytes following epinephrine treatment, which suggests that sequestration is a factor to be considered in assessing the cat reticulocyte response. If a cat struggles and becomes excited during sampling, this could elevate the apparent reticulocyte response by as much as 60 to 80 per cent.

A slight reticulocyte response for the dog would be 1 to 4 per cent and for the cat, 0.5 to 2 per cent; a moderate response is 5 to 20 per cent in the dog and 3 to 4 per cent in the cat; a marked reticulocyte response would be 21 to 50 per cent in the dog and greater than 5 per cent in the cat. Values for the cat were based on type II and III reticulocytes (sometimes referred to as classical reticulocytes), as these cells characteristically stained polychromatophilically in a Wright-stained smear. In the dog and cat counts of the polychromatophilic erythrocytes are comparable to reticulocyte counts.

Reticulocytosis is also seen in cattle and sheep following massive blood loss or erythrocyte destruction and the subsequent erythrogenic stimulation. Basophilic stippling can also be seen in cattle and sheep in responding anemias.

Reticulocytes are not seen in the peripheral blood of horses, even in very severe anemias. In the horse erythrocytes mature in the bone marrow and are not released until the reticulum has disappeared.

Punctate Basophilia. Punctate basophilia (basophilic stippling) (Fig. 2–6) is characterized by the appearance of punctate aggregations of basophilic-staining material in the form of large numbers of fine or coarse granules in the erythrocyte. The number of granules in an erythrocyte usually varies in inverse ratio to the size of the granules. They stain a deep blue with Wright's stain. Erythrocytes containing these granules may stain normally in other respects, or they may exhibit polychromatophilia. Basophilic stippling may also be seen in some nucleated red cells. Stippling is generally attributed to degenerative changes in the cytoplasm involving ribonucleic acid (RNA) in the young cells.

Punctate basophilia occurs in anemias of the bovine and ovine species and is characterized by an accumulation of small, basophilic-staining particles in the erythrocytes. It also may occur in certain anemic conditions in the cat. Care must be taken to differentiate these granules in an erythrocyte from possible blood parasites.

Basophilic stippling of erythrocytes also occurs in dogs with lead poisoning. In a study of dogs with lead poisoning, 94 per cent had basophilic stippling with a mean count of stippled erythrocytes of 80 per 10,000 red blood cells. Fixation of the blood film with alcohol or staining with acidic stain buffers resulted in fewer detectable basophilic-stippled red blood cells. Exposure to excessive quantities of ethylene-diaminetetraacetic acid (EDTA) reduces the percentage of detectable basophilic-stippled erythrocytes. Potassium oxalate has a similar effect, but sodium citrate does not.

Basophilic stippling is sometimes seen in healthy dogs, but the numbers are low.

Polychromasia. Diffuse basophilia is characterized by an overall bluish-red color to the normally red-staining erythrocyte. After the metarubricyte loses its nucleus, a small amount of basophilic substance remains in the cytoplasm. This remnant of cellular maturation is composed of RNA and protoporphyrin, the latter being responsible for the fluorescence of erythrocytes under ultraviolet light. In addition to the overall distribution of this basophilic substance, in fixed preparations the cell may have bluish basophilic areas that give it a patchy appearance. This condition is known as polychromatophilia. Such cells occur in association with anemia and are usually reticulocytes.

Howell-Jolly Bodies. Howell-Jolly bodies are remnants of nuclear material after the nucleus has been extruded. In Wright-stained smears Howell-Jolly bodies appear as refractile single, and at times double, bluish spherical bodies within red blood cells. In the bovine these must be distinguished from *Anaplasma marginale*. Howell-Jolly bodies may appear anywhere within a cell and are not confined to the periphery as are anaplasma organisms. In addition, anaplasmata are usually uniform in size, whereas Howell-Jolly bodies may vary considerably in size.

Howell-Jolly bodies are common in any severe anemia, and their occurrence may vary within the erythrocytes of a given species of animals. About 1 per cent of the erythrocytes of cats regularly have an eccentric body closely resembling a Howell-Jolly body. These bodies may be seen occasionally in canine blood and are common in young pigs up to three months of age. Howell-Jolly bodies are seen occasionally in the horse erythrocyte. In the horse, this body varies considerably in size and is generally black and located eccentrically.

Heinz Bodies. Heinz bodies are small, round to irregularly shaped refractile inclusions that may occur singly or multiply within a single cell. These bodies occur in horses having an anemia

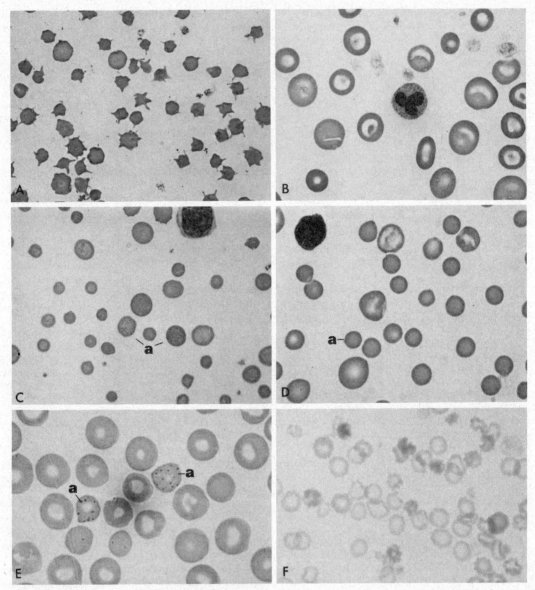

Figure 2–6. Changes in erythrocyte morphology associated with anemias. A, Many poikilocytes in the blood of an anemic cow. B, Very large erythrocytes in the blood of a basenji dog with a pyruvate kinase deficiency. Note the size of the erythrocytes in comparison with the size of the segmented neutrophil. C, Blood of a sheep with a regenerative anemia. There is marked anisocytosis and basophilic stippling can be seen at (a). D, A blood film from a dog with autoimmune hemolytic anemia. Note the anisocytosis with a spherocyte (a). E, Basophilic stippling (a) in erythrocytes of a dog with lead poisoning. F, Hypochromic erythrocytes in the blood of a dog with chronic external hemorrhage. The presence of these pale-staining cells is typical in an iron-deficiency anemia.

resulting from phenothiazine therapy or wild onion poisoning. These bodies are thought to consist of a denatured protein and are most commonly associated with hemolytic anemias produced by agents toxic to erythrocytes. Their presence is indicative of erythrocyte injury and may occasionally indicate an unsuspected hemolytic anemia. Heinz bodies are not readily visible in Wright-stained preparations but may easily be seen in reticulocyte smears and in unfixed and unstained smears. They disappear after fixation with either ethyl or methyl alcohol. In a stained blood film, Heinz bodies may appear as blunt projections of the erythrocyte membrane. In humans, appearance of these bodies may follow exposure to chemicals such as naphthalene, sodium nitrate, sodium chlorate, sulfanilamide, paraaminosalicylic acid, isoniazid, nitrofurantoin, certain antimalarial drugs, and phenacetin.

Heinz bodies are found in the blood of healthy

cats as well as in cats in which there is active red cell destruction. It has been suggested that formation of these bodies may represent a disease-associated intensification of the normal aging process of the feline erythrocyte.[4] In healthy cats the spleen may remove these structures, but in diseased animals the action of the spleen may be retarded, resulting in an increase in the size and number of these bodies.

In some animals the concentration of Heinz bodies may be so great that it will interfere with the normal hemoglobin determination. Heinz bodies are not destroyed by the reagent used in hemoglobin assays and consequently must be removed by centrifugation in order to get a true hemoglobin value.

Hemolytic anemia characterized by the formation of Heinz body inclusions in mature erythrocytes has been reported to occur in the cat treated with a urinary antiseptic containing methylene blue. The anemia was believed to be caused by methylene blue contained in urinary antiseptics used for treatment of cystitis and urolithiasis.

Heinz bodies, hyperbilirubinemia, and hemoglobinuria have been observed in cows fed kale, and in those fed wild and domestic onions. Similar erythrocyte inclusions were observed in cattle with postparturient hemoglobinuria.[9]

Small numbers of Heinz bodies have been seen in some dogs receiving daily doses of prednisolone.[4]

Hemoglobin Crystals. Hemoglobin crystals have been reported in the dog and cat. They occur within and between erythrocytes. The crystals vary in shape; some are square and others rectangular or polygonal. On a smear prepared with Wright's stain, crystals have the same staining characteristics as hemoglobin but are usually darker. Long crystals in cells stretch the membrane and in such cells there is frequently no noncrystalline hemoglobin present.

The significance of these crystals is unknown. They have been demonstrated in collie dogs with cyclic neutropenia and in cats, particularly those that have had splenectomy.

NUCLEATED ERYTHROCYTES

Nucleated red blood cells (NRBC) do not occur normally in any species of domestic animal, with the exception of the suckling pig up to three months of age and, occasionally, the normal dog. In healthy adult animals of other species, nucleated erythrocytes are confined to the bone marrow and appear in circulating blood only in disease. In these instances their presence usually denotes an excessive demand on blood-forming organs to regenerate erythrocytes. As a response to this demand, imperfectly formed and immature cells are released into circulation. Reticulocytes (polychromatophilic erythrocytes) usually accompany the nucleated erythrocytes as part of a normal regenerative response.

Any time that nucleated erythrocytes and reticulocytes are reported, one should consider that the animal currently has or has had an anemia and that the presence of these cells represents a bone marrow response.

Unless nucleated erythrocytes are present in extremely large numbers, they should be considered a favorable sign, as they indicate activity of bone marrow. If, however, they are present in excessively large numbers, persist for long periods of time without a compensatory increase in mature erythrocytes, or appear without a concomitant increase in reticulocytes, they should be considered an unfavorable sign. Persistence of NRBC without a corresponding elevation in total erythrocytes suggests abnormal erythrogenesis and should be thoroughly investigated. Nucleated erythrocytes are present in blood if there is extramedullary erythropoiesis and are frequently seen in the blood of animals that have been anoxic for any reason. Neoplasia of the erythron is characterized by the presence of nucleated erythrocytes in the blood. Many of these are very large and are referred to as megaloblastoid rubriblasts.

Nucleated erythrocytes and reticulocytes are seldom, if ever, observed in peripheral blood of the horse, even in severe anemia.

ERYTHROCYTE FRAGILITY

Although veterinarians do not routinely utilize erythrocyte fragility as a hematologic evaluation test, it is a well-known fact that the resistance of erythrocytes to hemolysis may be increased or decreased in disease. The use of such an evaluation should be considered in prolonged deficiency and dietary studies when the hematopoietic system might be adversely affected.

Erythrocyte fragility is tested by exposing freshly drawn erythrocytes to hypotonic saline solutions of various strengths. The resultant swelling and hemolysis in lower dilutions are an index of cell stability in relation to hypotonic solution. The hypotonic saline solutions are prepared from a 1.0 per cent sodium chloride solution in increments of 0.02 per cent extending beyond both the maximum and minimum values for the species in question. Details of the technique are presented in the Appendix.

The normal values of average osmotic fragility in hypotonic solutions are presented in Table 2–8. In general, dogs and chickens have the greatest resistance among domestic animals, whereas goats have the least.

Although little is known about osmotic fragility of erythrocytes in animal diseases, there are literature reports to indicate that it is increased in anaplasmosis of cattle, isoimmune hemolytic ane-

TABLE 2–8. Average Osmotic Fragility of Normal Erythrocytes in Hypotonic Saline Solutions

Species	% Saline Minimum Resistance*	Maximum Resistance†
Cattle	0.59–0.66	0.40–0.50
Sheep	0.60–0.76	0.40–0.55
Goat	0.62–0.74	0.48–0.60
Pig	0.70–0.74	0.45
Horse	0.42–0.59	0.31–0.45
Dog	0.45–0.50	0.32–0.36
Cat	0.69–0.72	0.46–0.50
Chicken	0.41–0.42	0.28–0.32

* The point of initial hemolysis
† The point of complete hemolysis.

TABLE 2–9. Comparison of the Morphologic and Etiologic Classifications of Anemia

Morphologic Classification	Etiologic Classification
Normocytic normochromic	1. Depression of erythrogenesis A. Chronic inflammation B. Nephritis with uremia C. Endocrine deficiencies (thyroid, adrenal medulla) D. Neoplasia E. Marrow hypoplasia as with Bracken fern poisoning, radiation, ehrlichiosis, chloramphenicol toxicity F. Acute hemorrhage after fluid volume has been restored and before regeneration occurs G. Feline leukemia virus infection
Macrocytic normochromic	1. Dietary deficiencies A. Vitamin B_{12} deficiency B. Folate deficiency C. Cobalt deficiency in ruminants 2. Erythremic myelosis in cats 3. Poodle macrocytosis
Macrocytic hypochromic	1. During recovery from large loss of RBC A. Hemorrhage following injury or in animals with coagulation defects B. Massive destruction of RBC as with immune-mediated anemia, hemoprotozoan infections, drug toxicity, congenital anemia of the basenji dog
Microcytic hypochromic	1. Iron deficiencies A. Lack of dietary iron B. Chronic blood loss to the exterior 2. Defect in utilization of iron stores A. Copper deficiency B. Molybdenum poisoning 3. Vitamin B_6 deficiency

mias of newborn pups and autoimmune hemolytic anemia in dogs. Osmotic fragility also increases in dogs given an intravenous injection of anti–canine red cell immune serum. In contrast, there is an increased resistance to osmotic lysis of erythrocytes from porphyric cows that could be attributed to the presence of young erythrocytes.

ANEMIA

Anemia is a reduction in the number of erythrocytes, hemoglobin, or both in the circulating blood. In domestic animals, anemia is seldom primary; it is most often a secondary response following or associated with disease. Since this condition is often an enigma to practicing veterinarians, it behooves them to search for the underlying cause rather than to attempt to treat it as a distinct entity. Treatment of anemia per se without an understanding of the cause of the condition is often unsuccessful. It is important that the practitioner understand the various methods of classifying anemias and their relationship to other disease conditions.

CLASSIFICATION

Many classifications for anemia have been proposed. The two most common and widely accepted are: (1) morphologic classification and (2) etiologic classification.

Anemias are classified morphologically by utilizing the MCV, MCH, and MCHC.

These morphologic alterations may be found in association with certain etiologic factors as indicated in Table 2–9.

Etiologically, anemias may be placed in four general categories: (1) blood loss, (2) excessive destruction of erythrocytes or shortened erythrocyte life span, (3) depression of bone marrow, and (4) nutritional deficiencies.

Additionally, anemias can be classified as responding or nonresponding. In general, macrocytic anemias are responding, normocytic anemias are usually nonresponding, and microcytic anemias can be either responding or nonresponding.

Blood Loss Anemias. Blood loss anemias are associated with acute, subacute, or chronic hemorrhage. Acute hemorrhage usually follows trauma or surgical procedures unless blood loss is adequately controlled. Anemia is not manifested immediately following peracute hemorrhage but appears when blood volume returns to normal. Severe coagulation defects may also produce acute hemorrhage such as that occurring in poisoning associated with sweet clover, warfarin or bracken fern, and in animals with coagulopathies.

Anemias associated with chronic hemorrhage to the exterior are usually microcytic and hypochromic. Chronic blood loss anemias are almost always microcytic and usually are hypochromic because of a lack of iron for formation of new hemoglobin. In most instances of chronic hemorrhage, the iron reserve is depleted, and there is insufficient quantity of this important element to permit adequate hemoglobin synthesis. In addition to microcytes, nucleated erythrocytes and reticulocytes may be observed in the peripheral circulation if there is adequate erythrogenesis.

A common cause of chronic hemorrhagic anemia is parasitism. Internal parasites such as hookworms, stomach worms, coccidia, nodular worms, and liver flukes produce anemia by a combination of blood loss and poor nutrition. External parasites such as ticks, blood-sucking lice, and certain types of fleas may also produce anemia. Chronic blood loss resulting in anemia may occur in association with gastrointestinal lesions such as hemorrhagic gastritis and enteritis. Ulceration of the digestive tract may also result in gradual blood loss. Bleeding into the genitourinary tract may occasionally produce anemia, as will hemorrhage into a body cavity from a neoplasm. Occasionally, coagulation defects that are not extremely severe will result in sufficient blood loss to cause persistent anemia.

Laboratory findings associated with acute and subacute hemorrhages are rather typical. Nucleated erythrocytes appear in the peripheral circulation usually within 72 to 96 hours following hemorrhage. An increase in reticulocytes customarily occurs on the fourth to seventh day subsequent to blood loss. Hemorrhagic anemias are not typically accompanied by a marked alteration in morphology of the erythrocytes, although regenerative reticulocytosis is associated with anisocytosis and polychromasia. One of the characteristics of such a hemorrhage, particularly if it occurs into a body cavity, is the almost immediate bone marrow response with a leukocytosis and left shift. If acute hemorrhage is followed by a continuing but lesser blood loss, reticulocytosis may persist. If the blood loss ceases, reticulocytosis will disappear in a few days, but may persist for a few days after the erythrocyte count returns to normal.

Laboratory findings associated with peracute hemorrhage into the abdominal or thoracic cavity are influenced by autotransfusion. Much of the red cell mass deposited in either of these cavities is recirculated, and the blood volume is returned to near normal. Peracute loss to the exterior is soon reflected in laboratory evaluations. Immediately following hemorrhage to the exterior, all erythrocyte parameters may be normal, but as hypovolemia is corrected by the movement of fluids from extravascular to intravascular spaces, the anemia becomes evident. Hemorrhage into tissues is not followed by restoration of the erythrocyte mass, as most extravasated erythrocytes are destroyed before they can be reabsorbed.

Hemolytic Anemias. Hemolytic anemias associated with the excessive destruction or shortened erythrocyte life span may be caused by a variety of diseases. Blood parasites, bacterial infections, viral infections, chemical agents, poisonous plants, and metabolic diseases may all result in destruction of erythrocytes. In addition, hemolytic anemia may be associated with isoimmunization phenomena or autoimmune reactions.

Blood parasites causing anemia include organisms from the genera *Anaplasma*, *Piroplasma*, *Haemobartonella*, and *Eperythrozoon*. The conditions caused by these organisms are characteristically diagnosed by demonstration of typical inclusions or parasites on or in red blood cells. Parasitized erythrocytes are most easily detected during acute stages of disease when the erythrocyte count is falling rapidly. Methods for diagnosing these diseases are discussed in detail in Chapter 20.

Bacterial Infections. The two most common bacterial diseases in which anemia occurs are leptospirosis and *Clostridium haemolyticum* infection.

LEPTOSPIROSIS. Hemolytic anemia due to infection with *Leptospira* occurs iin cattle, sheep, and dogs. In the canine, infection with *L. icterohaemorrhagiae* frequently results in a hemolytic process. However, infection with *L. canicola* is not commonly associated with a hemolytic condition. The characteristic hematologic findings in dogs infected with *L. icterohaemorrhagiae* include moderate to marked anemia and the appearance of aberrant forms of erythrocytes. Clinically, the animal is icteric and hemoglobinuria is present. Care must be taken to properly evaluate erythrocyte changes, as dehydration may be present and mask the anemia. In addition to alterations in the number of erythrocytes, the ESR is increased. The increased ESR is due to the inflammatory processes and the anemia. Certain blood, chemical, and urine alterations that are also associated with this disease will be discussed in later chapters.

Infection in the canine with either species of

Leptospira is accompanied by a marked increase in mature and immature neutrophils. The total leukocyte count may reach as high as 50,000/μl with as many as 50 per cent immature neutrophils.

Leptospira infection in the bovine is often accompanied by anemia and hemoglobinuria. In experimentally induced infections with L. pomona, variation in number of erythrocytes was the most significant hematologic finding.[10] Between the fourth and eighth days post inoculation there was a trend toward a decrease in erythrocyte count, hemoglobin concentration, and PCV. This decrease varied in rapidity and was most marked and abrupt in animals in which it was associated with hemoglobinuria.

BACILLARY HEMOGLOBINURIA. Infection caused by *Clostridium haemolyticum* in sheep and cattle is a specific infectious disease characterized by high fever, rapid hemolysis of erythrocytes, and hemoglobinuria. This disease is found endemically in certain of the western United States and occurs most frequently in pastures where drainage is not adequate. Since there is a rapid hemolysis of erythrocytes, anemia is characteristic. The total erythrocyte count may fall below 2 million/μl, and the hemoglobin may be as low as 3.5 gm/dl. Death sometimes occurs rapidly, and the clinician has no opportunity to acquire laboratory specimens for examination. Some cases are prolonged and a typical remission state of anemia is observed. This remission state is characterized by polychromasia (reticulocytosis), macrocytosis, basophilic stippling, and the appearance of nucleated erythrocytes.

Viral Infections. Equine infectious anemia (EIA) is characterized by a long chronic illness following an acute initial attack. Animals infected with this virus become carriers and serve as a source by which the disease can be introduced into previously uninfected areas.

Clinically, the disease is characterized by an intermittent fever, jaundice, edema, and petechial hemorrhages in the mucosa. Many animals temporarily recover from the acute stage, whereas others become progressively weaker and may die after 10 to 14 days of illness. Animals that temporarily recover may appear normal for two to three weeks before a relapse occurs. Such relapses may continue to occur, often coinciding with periods of stress.

During the initial acute attack, there is a marked fall in the total erythrocyte count, the degree of fall being proportional to the severity of the attack. Immature and nucleated red cells are usually absent in such acute episodes. A single hematologic examination is not diagnostic; a series of examinations should be run and compared with a temperature curve in order to correlate erythrocyte alterations with temperature fluctuations in animals that have continual stages of relapse.

Today the diagnosis of equine infectious anemia is almost exclusively dependent upon use of an immunodiffusion test.

The life span of erythrocytes in infected horses ranges from 28 to 113 days, whereas normal equine erythrocytes have a mean life span of 136 days. This decreased life span correlates with increased indirect bilirubin levels, increased plasma hemoglobin content, and decreased serum haptoglobin values. Such results indicate that both intra- and extravascular hemolysis are significant factors in the production of the anemia in EIA.

The anemia associated with EIA may occur as a consequence of the initiation of a series of immunologic events culminating in hemolysis and premature removal of sensitized cells from the circulation.[11] It appears probable that viral activation of an immunologic mediation system may result in erythrocyte destruction.

Chemical Agents. A wide variety of chemical agents are capable of causing hemolytic anemia in domestic animals. Among the most common are: copper, lead, phenothiazine, saponins, naphthalene, and certain drugs such as acetanilid, nitrofurantoin, neoarsphenamine, phenacetin, and some sulfonamides. Fortunately, the majority of the drugs capable of producing an anemia do not do so if utilized at the recommended dose and over the recommended period of time.

Methylene blue has also been implicated in hemolytic anemia.

COPPER. Sheep are the animals most susceptible to excessive intakes of copper, either from the consumption of plants containing a high level of copper or from excessive worming using copper sulfate drench. This element accumulates in the liver and under certain conditions of stress may be released into the bloodstream, resulting in rapid hemolysis of the erythrocytes. Hemoglobinuria is a consistent clinical sign and is accompanied by a typical hemolytic crisis. Bone marrow is characteristically hyperplastic as a result of response to acute blood destruction. Hemolytic anemia from excess copper has also been reported in swine and calves.

LEAD. Consumption of lead results in an often fatal disease characterized hematologically by the appearance of a variable type of anemia in which the erythrocytes may be normochromic or hypochromic, macrocytic or normocytic. Nucleated red blood cells, basophilic stippling, and Howell-Jolly bodies are frequently observed.

Lead poisoning in the dog should be suspected when a routine hematologic examination reveals the presence of a significant number of immature erythrocytes, particularly nucleated erythrocytes, out of proportion to the apparent need as indicated by the PCV. When lead is present, hemoglobin synthesis is deficient, leading to an accumulation of metarubricytes in the bone marrow. These are released and account for the sometimes extremely high nucleated erythrocyte count in blood. Frequently there are no other signs of erythrogenesis such as polychromasia and anisocytosis.

Acute lead poisoning in the dog is not usually accompanied by the erythrocyte changes just described. Lead poisoning in the dog produces a typical basophilic stippling. Finding 15 basophilic-stippled erythrocytes per 10,000 RBC in a dog is suggestive of lead poisoning and 40 or more basophilic stippled erythrocytes per 10,000 RBC nearly pathognomonic. Basophilic stippling is most readily demonstrated if the blood film is prepared under optimal conditions, especially regarding use of the anticoagulant, fixation of the film, and pH of the buffer. Sodium citrate is the anticoagulant of choice—a staining technique that does not involve alcoholic fixation of the film, and a stain buffer that is not acidic should be used.

Lead poisoning in the horse produces a modest anemia with PCV values between 21 and 28 per cent.[4] Basophilic stippling of the erythrocytes or the presence of large numbers of nucleated erythrocytes in the peripheral circulation is not characteristic of lead poisoning in the horse. Occasional stippled erythrocytes are observed, but these are rare.

Lead poisoning in cattle is usually an acute disease. Cattle appear to have more resistance to poisoning by lead than do horses, as it requires a much greater intake of lead to poison a cow than it does to poison a horse. Hematologic values have not been extensively studied, but anemia occurs if lead intake is extended for several weeks.

PHENOTHIAZINE. Anemia associated with the use of this anthelmintic may occur in the horse. Although such anemia is not common, certain individuals appear to be susceptible to this drug and a characteristic hemolytic anemia results. It has been suggested that this anthelmintic accelerates the lytic action of a naturally occurring lysolecithin present in horse blood. Heinz bodies occur in association with this condition.

METHYLENE BLUE. A severe hemolytic anemia may develop in cats receiving a urinary antiseptic containing methylene blue. This anemia is characterized by the presence of Heinz bodies that appear within 24 hours of drug administration and rapidly increase until they are present in all erythrocytes. A severe Heinz body hemolytic anemia has been experimentally produced. Within 24 hours after animals received methylene blue, Heinz bodies appeared, and by 48 hours following the initial dose all erythrocytes were involved. The packed cell volume dropped from 40 to 13 per cent within six days, and the color of the plasma suggested the presence of free hemoglobin and bilirubin. Seven days following the initial dose, the percentage of erythrocytes containing Heinz bodies declined as they were removed and replaced by newly formed erythrocytes. A similar hemolytic anemia was observed in a cat receiving acetaminophen.

Poisonous Plants. A wide variety of poisonous plants are capable of producing hemolytic anemia in domestic animals. Included are: castor beans, oak shoots, frosted turnips, broom, ranunculus, convolvulus, colchicum, ash, privet, hornbeam, hazel, hellebore, and wild onion. Fortunately, the majority of these plants are not appetizing to most animals. Consequently, poisonings due to toxic plants are seldom observed as clinical entities except when animals are forced to consume such plants because of lack of other foods.

Onions, both wild and domestic, produce Heinz body anemia in cattle, sheep, horses, cats, and dogs. The anemia is typically regenerative and accompanied by macrocytosis and reticulocytosis.

Kale produces a Heinz body hemolytic anemia accompanied by hemoglobinuria in both cattle and sheep.

Metabolic Diseases. Postparturient hemoglobinuria is a disease usually found in high-producing dairy cows and occurs two to three weeks following parturition. It is characterized by anemia in addition to the hemoglobinuria. The total erythrocyte count may drop below 2 million/μl and hemoglobin may decrease accordingly. Heinz bodies are often present.[9] The etiology of this disease is unknown. However, the fact that inorganic phosphorus values in blood plasma are low suggests a possible relationship between this disease and phosphorus deficiencies. The condition may occur in cattle grazing on lush pastures and those consuming cruciferous plants. The bone marrow responds in a typical fashion, and the blood picture is characteristic of that observed in any hemolytic disease.

Consumption of cold water has the capacity to produce a hemoglobinuria in calves and occasionally in older cattle. It is characterized by an intravascular hemolysis as well as hemoglobinuria.

IMMUNOHEMOLYTIC DISEASE OF THE NEWBORN. Hemolytic disease of the newborn occurs in the horse, the pig, the dog, the cat, and the calf. It resembles erythroblastosis fetalis in the human. However, there is a difference between these two entities. The human mother and her fetus are separated by a single placental barrier that allows antibodies possessed by the mother to pass into the developing fetus. Consequently, antibodies formed by the mother against an Rh factor that the fetus may have inherited from the father are able to cross the placental barrier, and fetal blood destruction may result. The domestic animal and its fetus are separated by many placental membranes. Antibodies do not traverse these membranes to any great extent; consequently the fetus is in little danger of receiving harmful antibodies in situations in which blood incompatibilities are present. The newborn animal must receive these antibodies from the colostrum during the first few hours of life. Blood destruction of the newborn occurs only after colostral antibodies are received.

Hemolytic disease in foals appears within 12 to

96 hours after birth. Hemolytic icterus occurs in newborn foals when mares sensitized to certain types of erythrocytes are bred to stallions that transfer that type of blood cell to their offspring. The disease appears in seemingly normal newborn foals after they absorb erythrocyte-destroying antibodies from the colostrum of the dam. Once a mare becomes sensitized to a certain type of erythrocyte, from that time on her foals will become icteric if sired by a stallion transmitting that type of erythrocyte. The process of sensitization of the mare is not understood, but it is possible that it occurs as a result of breakdown and absorption of parts of the fetal placenta. Exposure to the foal's blood cells at parturition or the use of incompatible blood transfusions might also sensitize the mare. Mares bred to a stallion whose erythrocytes are compatible with theirs do not produce icteric foals.

The colostral antibody titer drops to a level too low to be detected by ordinary agglutination tests 12 hours following birth. In addition, a newborn foal loses its ability to absorb antibodies approximately 24 to 36 hours after birth. A foal susceptible to hemolytic disease may be removed from its mother and allowed to nurse a mare having no erythrocyte-destroying antibodies. Such foals may be returned to their own mothers 48 to 72 hours following birth. Some horse breeders maintain a supply of frozen colostrum to feed to newborn foals if they suspect the possibility of hemolytic disease.

Laboratory procedures may be utilized in identifying such incompatible conditions. A mate for a sensitized mare may be selected by a test of the mare's serum with the red blood cells of the stallion. A simple cross match is utilized in which the red blood cells of the stallion are suspended in various dilutions of the mare's serum. If the stallion's erythrocytes do not clump in a 1:2 dilution of the mare's serum, such a mating will not produce a foal subject to hemolytic disease. Cross matching is a rather simple procedure, as equal quantities of a 50 per cent cell suspension and the proper dilution of the serum or plasma in saline are mixed, and an agglutination test is made on a cross-lined glass plate. If antibodies to the erythrocytes are present, clumping of the erythrocytes is readily visible.

If premating cross agglutination tests are not possible, the probability of the development of hemolytic icterus can be tested in the newborn foal prior to the time that it first nurses. This is accomplished by cross agglutination of the foal erythrocytes and serum from the dam as already described. Another procedure that may be utilized is a test of the colostrum and the foal's erythrocytes. A procedure similar to that utilized with serum and blood is conducted. If specific antibodies to the foal's erythrocytes are present in the colostrum, the erythrocytes will agglutinate rapidly.

A hemolysin test may be utilized. In this assay the mare's serum or plasma is diluted 1:10, 1:100, and 1:1000, and 1 ml of each dilution is placed in a small test tube. To each tube is added 0.2 ml of a 1:20 dilution of active guinea pig complement and 0.01 ml of a 50 per cent suspension of the foal's red blood cells. The tubes are incubated in a water bath at 37°C for 15 minutes, then read. The appearance of hemolysis in any tube indicates a potentially hemolytic condition.

Hemolytic anemia was produced in baby pigs by immunizing a sow with erythrocytes from the boar to which she was bred and permitting the newborn piglets to suckle her. As with the foals, the disease appeared in seemingly normal newborn piglets after they received the specific erythrocyte-destroying antibodies from the colostrum.

A naturally occurring hemolytic disease in pigs was apparently associated with a blood group incompatibility. The results of tests conducted on the blood samples indicated that there was an incompatibility in the F system. Sows giving birth to affected piglets had been immunized with a modified live virus vaccine and simultaneous administration of antiserum. It is possible the antiserum contained antigens that resulted in the development of antibodies responsible for producing the hemolytic crisis.

Hemolytic icterus in pups has been produced experimentally by immunization of bitches whose erythrocytes lacked the canine A factor with intravenous injections of A-positive canine red blood cells. These bitches were mated with A-positive sires. All A-positive pups born to such dams developed hemolytic icterus if they suckled the immunized dam during the first day of life. There was no evidence of transplacental isoimmunization or of transfer of antibody across the placenta from mother to pup.

The degree of anemia in the A-positive pups varied widely. The minimum PCV for the group was 10 per cent 48 hours after birth. Nucleated erythrocytes, reticulocytes, and spherocytes were present in most of the severely affected pups. The osmotic fragility of the erythrocytes was substantially increased in all A-positive pups exposed to the anti-A factor.

Isoimmunization may also occur following multiple transfusions between animals having incompatible blood types. Such reactions seldom, if ever, occur following the first transfusion. However, if transfusions are separated by a period of several days, antibodies to certain erythrocytes develop and can be detected by cross matching serum from the recipient and erythrocytes from the donor.

AUTOIMMUNE HEMOLYTIC ANEMIA (AIHA). Naturally occurring autoimmune hemolytic anemia in the dog, cat, and horse have been reported.

In autoimmune hemolytic anemia antibodies or complement (C3) are present on erythrocytes and can be detected by means of an antiglobulin test

(Coombs' test). Such coated erythrocytes can be destroyed by direct cytolysis mediated by complement or as opsonized erythrocytes that are removed by phagocytosis.

The method of erythrocyte removal is dependent upon the type of antibody involved and its action on the erythrocytes. With the *saline-acting autoagglutinins*, clumping of erythrocytes is observed upon withdrawal of the blood. Agglutination is obvious when a drop of blood is deposited on a glass slide. In order to differentiate autoagglutination from excessive rouleau formation, the blood can be diluted with a drop of saline. If clumping is associated with rouleau formation the erythrocyte aggregation will disperse, whereas, in the presence of agglutinating antibodies, clumping persists. In such animals it is unnecessary to conduct additional tests for the presence of erythrocyte antibodies. Antibodies of immunoglobulin classes IgG and IgM have been identified in patients with this type of AIHA.

Other animals affected with AIHA will have *hemolytic antibodies*. Some erythrocyte antiglobulins, particularly of class IgM, have the ability to fix complement after attaching to erythrocytes and produce intravascular hemolysis. Although these are usually of immunoglobulin class IgM, IgG molecules have the capacity to initiate the same type of reaction. It requires two IgG molecules to activate complement whereas one IgM molecule will accomplish the same effect.

Incomplete antibodies also coat erythrocytes but are unable to cause direct cytolysis or agglutination. In this form of AIHA, antibody-coated erythrocytes are removed by the phagocytic system. Antiglobulin tests are needed to detect the presence of incomplete erythrocyte antibodies. These are usually of class IgG.

Cold-agglutinating hemagglutinins of class IgM act at a temperature below that of the body. These hemagglutinins can be detected by cooling the blood to 4°C. When cooling is completed the erythrocytes autoagglutinate; agglutination is reversed by warming the blood to body temperature.

Cold-acting nonagglutinating antibodies have also been detected. These antibodies do not cause agglutination but can opsonize erythrocytes and cause them to be removed by phagocytosis. These antibodies are detected by conducting an antiglobulin test at 4°C.

Autoimmune hemolytic anemia can be primary as antibodies to erythrocytes develop in the absence of any other underlying disease process. AIHA may occur secondarily to other disease entities. With the primary form of AIHA, specific antierythrocyte antibodies develop. With the secondary type of AIHA, cross-reacting antibodies that share specificity for erythrocytes and foreign antigens can develop. Some drugs or infectious agents may induce chemical modification of the erythrocyte membrane. The immune system recognizes this new antigen determinant as foreign and antibodies arise that have the capacity of attaching to erythrocytes.

If immune complexes become attached to erythrocytes the effects are identical to those seen when a specific antibody is attached. Coombs'-positive anemias in the dog and cat have been found in association with a variety of diseases. Included among them are lymphoid and myeloid neoplasia, hemangiosarcoma, feline leukemia virus infection, haemobartonellosis, ehrlichiosis, dirofilariasis, leishmaniasis, piroplasmosis, and other autoimmune diseases including systemic lupus erythematosus and immune-mediated thrombocytopenia. Because of the great diversity of conditions in which a patient may have a positive Coombs' test, the clinician must evaluate each patient carefully in an attempt to determine and treat the underlying cause of the positive Coombs' reaction.

The anemia that develops is characterized by spherocytosis in most but not all patients. These are small dense erythrocytes that, in the dog, have no central pallor. Erythrocytes assume a spherical shape because of immunologic damage to the cell membrane. Because of the smaller size of the erythrocytes, spherocytes are difficult to identify in the cat. The anemia is usually regenerative, and polychromatophilia, marked anisocytosis, poikilocytosis, and reticulocytosis are present. The MCV and MCHC in dogs with AIHA are usually normal. Spherocytes appear to be small but their cell volume is usually within the normal range. Remember that these cells are spherical rather than disc-shaped. If there is regeneration the MCV is increased and the MCHC may be slightly decreased because newly formed cells may not be completely hemoglobinated.

Occasionally a nonregenerative anemia is encountered. Although not proved in domestic animals, in humans it is thought that such nonregenerative immune-mediated anemias occur as a consequence of antibody-mediated damage to erythrocyte precursors in the bone marrow.

If the Coombs'-positive patient has a nonregenerative anemia a bone marrow examination should be completed in order to rule out other bone marrow disorders or myeloproliferative diseases.

In addition to the anemia, affected animals generally have leukocytosis. The principal increase is in neutrophils and there is a characteristic increase in immature cells. As similar leukocyte alterations are seen with infection these changes in the leukogram can be misinterpreted.

The clinical manifestations of AIHA are, in part, dependent on the type of autoantibody produced. Almost all patients exhibit clinical signs that result from the anemia. These include pale mucous membranes, weakness, anorexia, lethargy, tachycardia, and tachypnea. If there has been a massive intravascular hemolysis such as seen in patients in which erythrocytes have been destroyed by the activation of complement, icterus, hemoglobinuria, and fever are often present. If the antibody is a cold hemagglutinin, cutaneous lesions of the extremities can be observed. These lesions frequently appear following cold weather. The lesions occur at the tip of the ears and tail, the feet, and nose. They occur as a consequence of ischemia resulting from erythrocyte agglutination in small vessels.

Hemoglobinuria is not confined to patients with intravascular hemolysis but is occasionally seen in other forms of AIHA. Its appearance depends on the amount and rapidity of red cell destruction. If destruction occurs over a fairly short time span and the quantity of free hemoglobin exceeds the binding capacity of haptoglobin, hemoglobin may appear in the urine.

In some cases of AIHA in the dog, erythrophagocytosis may be seen in the blood (Fig. 2–7). Although this is not a constant finding, when phagocytosed erythrocytes are observed in neutrophils or monocytes, one should suspect the presence of an autoimmune reaction.

Systemic lupus erythematosus (SLE) occurs in the dog and occasionally in the cat. Systemic lupus erythematosus is characterized clinically by the presence of hematologic, dermatologic, renal, and joint lesions. Hematologic changes are those of a typical AIHA and an idiopathic thrombocytopenic purpura. The kidney lesion is principally glomerulonephritis, whereas the joint lesions are presented as symmetric (rheumatoid) polyarthritis.

Laboratory abnormalities include anemia, with hemoglobin levels as low as 2 gm/dl; reticulocytosis; spherocytosis; positive Coombs' test; a leukocytosis with a left shift; thrombocytopenia; and bilirubinemia with an accompanying urobilinuria. An increase in serum globulins is common, and antibodies to deoxyribonucleic acid (DNA), ribonucleic acid (RNA), thyroglobulin, erythrocytes, and 7S gamma globulins are found in various combinations in infected dogs. The LE test is frequently positive. This phenomenon occurs as a result of the action of an antinuclear serum factor upon the nuclei of dead or injured leukocytes.

TESTING FOR AIHA AND SLE. Two techniques can be utilized for detection of antiglobulins in confirming a diagnosis of autoimmune hemolytic anemia. The direct Coombs' test is conducted in such a fashion as to detect the in vivo coating of erythrocytes. The indirect Coombs' test is used to detect the presence of antiglobulins present in plasma or serum. Details for conducting these tests are presented in the Appendix.

Diagnosis of systemic lupus erythematosus can be made by demonstrating LE cells in the peripheral blood.

The LE cell test is based upon the principle that antibodies present in plasma or serum of affected patients react with the nucleoprotein of leukocyte nuclei. A nucleoprotein transformed by the presence of this LE factor acquires chemotactic properties and attracts phagocytes, which are usually segmented neutrophils but occasionally monocytes. These phagocytes with ingested nuclear material are referred to as LE cells. Morphologically, the LE cell contains two nuclei. The nucleus of the cell that has been actively phagocytic is found at the periphery of the cell and is often flattened. The chromatin structure of this nucleus is usually well preserved. The cytoplasmic portion of the cell is occupied by the ingested nuclear mass of nucleoprotein. The chromatin structure of the ingested material is indistinct and appears as a purplish, homogeneous, amorphous, round mass that varies in size but is usually larger than an erythrocyte in the same preparation. In some cases, multiple nuclei can be observed, indicating that the phagocytic cell has engulfed more than one nucleus.

Details for completing an LE cell test are presented in the Appendix.

The antinuclear antibody (ANA) test is conducted using an immunofluorescent technique. A kit is available that contains the needed reagents. As this test requires a microscope equipped for fluorescence microscopy, it is best completed in a diagnostic or commercial laboratory. The latex particle test does not compare favorably with the detection of ANA by immunofluorescence or LE cell demonstration and is not recommended.

Bone Marrow Depression. Nonregenerative anemias associated with depression of the bone marrow are caused by several factors including physical, chemical, and infectious agents. Such anemias also occur as secondary reactions associated with a primary disease condition. These anemias are spoken of as hypoplastic or aplastic and are not uncommon. They are characterized by the lack of adequate reticulocyte response.

Physical Agents. Irradiation resulting from exposure to roentgen rays, radium, or radioactive isotopes may result in selective depression of

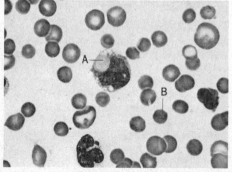

Figure 2–7. Erythrophagocytosis, particularly by monocytes (*A*), is sometimes associated with anemias. One erythrocyte shown here (*B*) is a spherocyte.

bone marrow. Such bone marrow depression is characterized by anemia, marked granulocytopenia, lymphopenia, and thrombocytopenia. In dogs exposed to 300 roentgens, a white blood cell count as low as 900 cells/μl has been reported. The erythrocyte count was depressed at the same time. Bone marrow examination of animals several days following irradiation revealed an almost complete lack of hematopoiesis.

If the amount of irradiation is not lethal, the development of new cells will begin 15 to 20 days following exposure to irradiation.

Chemical Agents. Chemical agents responsible for development of a hypoplastic anemia include trichloroethylene-extracted feeds, bracken fern, certain antibiotics, estrogens, and phenylbutazone.

Trichloroethylene-extracted soybean oil meal may produce a clinical picture characterized by high temperature, anorexia, depression, and bleeding from the body openings. The primary alteration is a marked reduction of thrombocytes. This diminution in thrombocytes is followed by a rapid reduction in the numbers of leukocytes and erythrocytes. Bone marrow examination reveals an inactive marrow with few immature forms.

Bracken fern poisoning occurs in cattle following prolonged consumption of bracken ferns when other dietary substances are in short supply. Experimental bracken fern poisoning has also been produced in sheep. In horses, this condition may take the form of staggers. The clinical picture observed is almost identical with that associated with trichloroethylene-extracted soybean oil meal poisoning. The unknown toxic substance associated with this plant is accumulative, and clinical signs do not develop until after one to three months of continuous feeding on the plant. Initially, thrombocytopenia and leukopenia occur and are later followed by a reduction in total erythrocyte count.

Chloramphenicol may produce a mild nonregenerative anemia when administered orally or parenterally at therapeutic doses. High doses administered to a cat may result in a severe disease leading to death. Experimental exposure of cats for 21 days to a dose of 50 mg of chloramphenicol/kg of body weight produced vacuolation of precursor cells of both the erythrocytic and granulocytic series.[12] Chloramphenicol can also produce bone marrow depression in the dog if administered at a high dosage (225–275 mg/kg/day).

Estrogens cause a hypoplastic marrow in dogs when administered in excess. Some animals given an excessive dose of estrogen, including synthetics such as diethylstilbestrol, develop marrow depression characterized by anemia, thrombocytopenia, and leukopenia. Anemia results from a reduction in erythrocyte production and hemorrhage associated with the thrombocytopenia.

There is some individual variation in the susceptibility of dogs to the effects of estrogen. Development of marrow aplasia is also dependent upon the dose of estrogens. Recommended estrogen doses should never be exceeded and should never be given to animals that are anemic.

Phenylbutazone may induce marrow dyscrasias in dogs. Early laboratory findings include thrombocytopenia and leukopenia followed by a nonregenerative anemia. The mechanism for this effect is unknown.

Secondary Anemias. Anemias occurring secondary to a variety of disease conditions are probably the result of metabolic inhibition of the bone marrow itself. Some disease conditions in which a secondary anemia is obvious include: chronic infections, chronic nephritis, chronic liver disease, endocrine deficiencies, parasitic diseases, myeloproliferative disease, and other hematopoietic malignancies.

CHRONIC INFECTIONS. Many chronic infections have an associated normocytic normochromic anemia, although microcytic normochromic and microcytic hypochromic cells do occur. (The erythrocyte and hemoglobin values are not extremely low, but a borderline anemia occurs, with the total erythrocyte count and hemoglobin values being slightly below normal.) The mechanism or mechanisms of this anemia are not firmly established. However, one hypothesis suggests that as a result of an inflammatory reaction, iron is diverted to tissues and is not available for hemoglobin synthesis.

More recently the term "anemia of inflammatory disease" has been used to describe this low-grade anemia.[13] Experimental evidence suggests that there is a disturbance of iron metabolism as evidenced by depressed serum iron concentration, total iron-binding capacity, percentage saturation of transferrin, and decreased numbers of bone sideroblasts, while there is an increase in bone marrow reticuloendothelial cell iron.

There may be a moderate decrease in erythrocyte life span, although red cell production may be normal or slightly increased. However, erythropoiesis is insufficient to compensate for the decreased red cell survival.

CHRONIC NEPHRITIS. This disease in the dog is usually accompanied by a normocytic normochromic anemia, which is more typically found in dogs with uremia. The degree of anemia is somewhat dependent upon the severity of the condition and may range from a borderline anemia in animals not having severe uremia to a total erythrocyte count as low as 3 million/μl in animals suffering an acute attack of uremic poisoning. The anemia in severe renal disease may include a shortened life span of erythrocytes and failure of production to keep pace with demand. Erythropoietin synthesis may be diminished as a consequence of kidney disease. There appears to be some correlation between the severity of anemia and the degree of elevation of blood urea nitrogen levels, but this does not always hold true.

CHRONIC LIVER DISEASE. Detailed information on blood alterations associated with chronic liver disease indicates that the anemia is most commonly macrocytic. This is probably the result of a partial deficiency of hematopoietic factor. Anemia associated with liver diseases is not often observed in domestic animals. Erythrocyte aplasia in a dog with hepatic cirrhosis has been reported. This animal had a severe anemia without evidence of reticulocyte release, and erythrocyte precursors were not observed in the bone marrow. If liver damage is severe, coagulation factor production may be reduced enough to interfere with blood clotting and permit development of anemia.

ENDOCRINE DEFICIENCIES. Hypothyroidism and hypopituitarism in the canine may have an associated anemia. The anemias are usually borderline with the packed cell volume being from 30 to 37 per cent, although in some instances the PCV may be considerably below normal. With hyperthyroidism, the anemia is usually normocytic and normochromic, and large numbers of leptocytes are observed. A macrocytic anemia due to hypopituitarism has been reported to occur in the dog.

PARASITISM. A severe normocytic normochromic anemia that has all the appearances of a selective depression of erythrogenesis may occur in association with trichostrongyloid parasites of sheep and cattle. The packed cell volume has been reported as low as 12 per cent with no evidence of reticulocyte increase occurring to compensate for the anemia.

Canine ehrlichiosis is accompanied by a severe nonregenerative anemia. Infected animals also have a thrombocytopenia and leukopenia. Diagnosis of ehrlichiosis is made by demonstration of the parasite (see Chapter 20).

MYELOPROLIFERATIVE DISEASE AND OTHER HEMATOPOIETIC MALIGNANCIES. Myeloproliferative diseases of the cat are uniformly accompanied by abnormal erythrogenesis. The severe anemia is usually explained on the basis of ineffective erythropoiesis. The anemia of myeloproliferative disease in the cat is characterized by a sharp decrease in packed cell volume to 8 to 12 per cent. This anemia is unresponsive to treatment, and varying numbers of normal and abnormal nucleated erythrocytes are frequently identified in peripheral blood.

Lymphocytic leukemia in the cat is also characterized by an anemia. The packed cell volume ranges from 10 to 20 per cent, is accompanied by the appearance of varying numbers of nucleated erythrocytes that are rarely less mature than metarubricytes. Although the definitive cause of this anemia is not known, it is regularly seen in cats, even those with no increase in lymphocytes in either blood or marrow. The feline leukemia virus will induce a nonregenerative normocytic normochromic anemia. The anemia may be present when there is no other evidence of neoplasia including a negative blood test for the feline leukemia virus. If the clinician suspects feline leukemia an FA test for the virus should be conducted on bone marrow smears prepared from fresh marrow. Although some cats have a bone marrow infection, the virus does not escape into the blood. Anemia is also a consistent finding in granulocytic leukemia.

Erythremic myelosis and erythroleukemia are also characterized by severe anemia and neoplastic proliferation of immature erythrocytes. In these cases, rubriblasts and more mature nucleated erythrocytes dominate the blood picture. Abnormally large cells, some with severe disparity in maturation of nuclei and cytoplasm, as well as cells with double nuclei may be found in blood and marrow.

Lymphocytic neoplasia in the dog is characterized by a moderate anemia usually of the chronic type. Occasionally, if the bone marrow is infiltrated with neoplastic cells, a typical aplastic anemia may occur. Myelogenous leukemia is invariably accompanied by a marked anemia. Lymphocytic leukemia in the cow may have an associated anemia, but it is not characteristic of the disease.

A severe macrocytic anemia was reported in a horse with plasma cell myelomatosis. Anemia has also been reported in cases of myeloma in other animal species.

IDIOPATHIC APLASTIC ANEMIA. Erythrocyte aplasia is occasionally observed in which no underlying cause can be identified. These nonregenerative anemias may be associated with immune-mediated depression of erythrogenesis but this has not been confirmed in animals. It has been associated with SLE in man and animals but may also occur when there is no other evidence of an immune-mediated disease.

Hereditary Anemias. Hereditary anemias are not uncommon in humans, but there are few reports in the veterinary literature concerning similar conditions. Hereditary conditions resulting in anemia include porphyria in cattle and swine, familial anemia in the basenji dog, and hemolytic anemia of the chondrodysplastic malamute.

In porphyria of cattle, the hematologic picture of the majority of cases includes increased erythrogenesis in response to an anemic process similar to that observed in hemolytic anemias. The anemia is normochromic and, if the degree of response is adequate, may be macrocytic. Microscopically typical findings of a responding anemia include polychromasia, anisocytosis, basophilic stippling, reticulocytosis, and the presence of nucleated erythrocytes. In newborn porphyric calves there is also an erythrogenic response that persists for the first three weeks of life. Nucleated erythrocyte counts during the first day of life have ranged from 5000 to 63,500/μl.[1]

The research findings associated with porphyria suggest that a high porphyrin content induces a defect in the synthesis of heme. It is thought that this biochemical abnormality is expressed as a maturation defect, and the morphologically defective and altered cell is more susceptible to hemolysis.[1]

Porphyria has also been reported in swine and cats.

A familial anemia occurs in the basenji dog. This condition is characterized by a severe anemia of the responding type with the presence of nucleated erythrocytes in the peripheral circulation accompanied by a remarkable reticulocytosis, polychromasia, anisocytosis, and poikilocytosis. These findings support a conclusion that the mechanism of the anemia in these dogs is hemolysis or hemorrhage. The possibility of hemorrhage can be ruled out by repeated studies of the urine and feces and by careful physical examination. This is a hemolytic anemia resulting from a shortened erythrocyte life span.

Hemolytic anemia in basenji dogs is caused by a deficiency of erythrocytic pyruvate kinase (PK).[14] This deficiency results in an impairment of erythrocytic energy metabolism leading to a progressive unremitting anemia within the first year of life. In the late stages of disease many dogs develop myelofibrosis and osteosclerosis.[15] A similar PK deficiency has been reported in a beagle.[16] Peculiar spiculated erythrocytes have been reported to occur in PK-deficient dogs.[17]

A hereditary anemia has also been reported in the Alaskan malamute. This condition occurs in association with chondrodysplasia. The anemia is characterized by stomatocytosis in which the erythrocytes have a pale slit-like center. There is an increase in MCV and a decrease in MCHC with a normal MCH. The PCV is usually normal.

Nutritional Anemias. Anemias due to nutritional deficiencies seldom occur as single entities in domestic animals. They are more commonly associated with disease conditions that result in anorexia, debilitation, or a metabolic alteration affecting either digestion or absorption of nutrients.

Mineral Deficiencies. The principal mineral deficiencies that may lead to an anemia include insufficiencies of iron, cobalt, and copper. With the exception of anemia in piglets, iron deficiency anemias rarely occur as a result of dietary deficiency. Occasionally, however, a dietary iron deficiency may be observed in animals grazing on pastures deficient in iron and in nursing calves that are not provided with additional supplements.

Severe chronic hemorrhage to the exterior may deplete the store of iron in the body. The resultant anemia has many of the characteristics observed in iron deficiency. The lack of iron absorption due to intestinal disturbances may also be a factor. One cause of iron deficiency is inadequate utilization of readily available iron. Molybdenum poisoning interferes with copper metabolism, which, in turn, may interfere with iron utilization.

Although the fundamental defect in these deficiencies is reduced hemoglobin synthesis, there is an accompanying erythrocyte deficit. In general, hemoglobin synthesis is more deficient than erythrocyte production, and the red cell count is not as markedly lowered as hemoglobin concentration. The erythrocytes are usually hypochromic and microcytic.

The anemia in copper deficiencies is similar to that observed in iron deficiency. Deaths from a microcytic hypochromic anemia due to copper deficiency have been reported in four- to seven-week-old pigs in England.[18] Anemia stemming from experimental copper deficiency in dogs was normocytic and normochromic.[19]

Copper deficiencies may occur in grazing ruminants in areas in which the land is deficient in this element. Copper-deficient areas have been identified in the United States (Florida), Sweden, New Zealand, Norway, Australia, England, Scotland, and Ireland.[20] An excessive quantity of molybdenum interferes with copper utilization, affecting the availability of iron and its utilization in hemoglobin synthesis. Cattle pastured on soil with a high molybdenum content suffer from profuse scours, a decrease in the pigmentation of the hair, and are debilitated. Areas of high molybdenum content in soil are present in certain counties in California. The signs and effects of the disease may be controlled by administration of copper.

Cobalt deficiency is accompanied by a decrease in synthesis of vitamin B_{12}. A profound anemia may develop in cattle or sheep feeding on soils deficient in cobalt, since synthesis of vitamin B_{12} is dramatically decreased.[21] Cobalt-deficient areas have been reported to occur in the United States (Michigan, Wisconsin, Florida), Kenya, the British Isles, New Zealand, and Australia. In sheep, the morphology of the blood cells suggests an aplastic condition of the bone marrow; as the disease progresses, a marked macrocytic anemia with an accompanying poikilocytosis and polychromasia develops.

Vitamin Deficiencies. With modern feeding programs vitamin deficiencies rarely occur as clinical problems. The extent to which vitamin B_{12} and folic acid are necessary for erythropoiesis in domestic animals is not entirely known. Although macrocytic anemias occur in domestic animals, their relation to vitamin B_{12} and folic acid has not been established.

A case of spontaneous folic acid deficiency in the dog has been reported. However, the dog is normally capable of obtaining folic acid as a result of intestinal bacterial action.

Restriction of niacin (nicotinic acid) in the diet may decrease folic acid synthesis. Niacin is important to the dog, as it is essential for normal metabolism. In the presence of low protein and nicotinic acid intake, black tongue may develop. The signs of this disease include infection of the oral mucosa accompanied by necrosis, ropy salivation, anorexia, and marked dehydration. There may be a concomitant loss of body weight and bloody diarrhea. In dogs fed an experimental diet deficient in nicotinic acid, severe macrocytic anemia and leukopenia developed. It has been found that nicotinic acid is essential for normal erythropoiesis in pigs fed a low-protein diet. Lack of niacin may be associated with the development of a normocytic anemia with no leukopenia. If tryptophan intake is adequate, niacin deficiencies do not develop.

Riboflavin deficiencies rarely occur in animals. Experimental riboflavin deficiencies resulting in microcytic hypochromic anemia have been produced in dogs.[22] Experimental riboflavin deficiency in pigs did not lead to an anemia but did result in a marked increase in neutrophils.[23]

Pyridoxine (B_6) deficiency is rare and probably does not occur as a clinical deficiency in domestic animals under normal circumstances. It has been demonstrated, however, that pyridoxine is required by the dog for utilization of iron in hemoglobin synthesis.[24] The anemia resulting from an experimental pyridoxine deficiency is similar to that resulting from iron deficiency. In swine, experimental anemia has been produced by a pyridoxine-deficient regimen.[23] Significant anemia appeared and in a few weeks became severe with the total erythrocyte count falling as low as 3.2 million/μl. The anemia was primarily microcytic. Following treatment with pyridoxine, an immediate reticulocyte response occurred, accompanied by an increase in erythrocytes. Red blood cells soon returned to normal size. During the course of these anemias in swine, an extensive deposition of iron pigment was found in the liver, spleen, and bone marrow.

Protein Deficiencies. A deficiency of protein in the diet may interfere with hemoglobin production and result in development of an anemia. Such conditions might be seen clinically in animals in which there has been a marked serum protein loss or in which there is inadequate intake or digestion of protein. Lysine deficiency in swine reportedly produces a normocytic normochromic anemia.

LABORATORY FINDINGS RELATED TO CAUSES OF ANEMIA

The diagnostic and prognostic value of laboratory examinations associated with anemia depends upon the ability of the clinician to interpret results in relation to the cause of anemia. Although there are many findings attributed to all anemias regardless of the underlying cause, there are some differences that should be considered.

Hemolysis. Laboratory findings associated with hemolytic anemia differ, depending upon the amount of blood destroyed and the rate of destruction. If destruction is rapid and the number of destroyed erythrocytes is great, free hemoglobin may be present in the plasma, and hemoglobinuria may or may not appear. The most consistent finding in association with hemolytic anemias is the presence of icterus. Icterus is not always present and varies from slight to marked, depending on the rate of erythrocyte destruction.

The existence of hemoglobinuria depends upon the action of haptoglobin, a hemoglobin-binding globulin. The complex of hemoglobin-haptoglobin is normally removed from the circulation and catabolized by the reticuloendothelial system. Activation of this normal process prevents hemoglobin from appearing in the urine. However, in some circumstances, this reaction does not operate normally if the plasma hemoglobin level exceeds 100 to 130 mg/dl or if the plasma haptoglobin has been depleted. Under such circumstances, the plasma hemoglobin exceeds the resorptive capacity of the proximal tubules and passes the renal barrier into the urine, resulting in a hemoglobinuria.

Hemolytic anemias are almost always accompanied by signs of increased bone marrow activity. Observations made using a blood smear reflect the activity and capacity of the marrow to compensate for blood that has been destroyed. This activity is manifested morphologically by anisocytosis, poikilocytosis, reticulocytosis, polychromatophilia, basophilic stippling (in some species), and by the appearance of nucleated erythrocytes in the peripheral circulation. Reticulocytosis (polychromasia) is frequently greater in hemolytic than in blood loss anemias. As a rule, this anemia is normocytic. If large numbers of reticulocytes are present in the peripheral blood, there is a tendency toward macrocytosis.

Reticulocytes and other forms of immature erythrocytes are rarely observed in equine blood regardless of the severity or cause of anemia.

In response to excessive blood destruction, the call for increased production reaches the bone marrow, which reacts as an organ and releases not only erythrocytes but also younger forms of leukocytes and blood platelets. This, of course, results in a leukocytosis with a left shift and thrombocytosis. The compensatory increase in the rate of blood flow also tends to increase the total leukocyte count as cells move from the marginal granulocyte pool (MGP) to the circulating granulocyte pool (CPG).

Hemorrhage. Anemia due to blood loss typically occurs following acute and subacute hemorrhages and is characteristically normocytic. As with hemolytic anemias, signs of increased bone marrow activity are present. Nucleated erythrocytes appear in the peripheral circulation 72 to 96 hours following blood loss. An increase in the number of reticulocytes occurs on the fourth to seventh day following hemorrhage. The morphologic characteristics include minimal anisocytosis and poikilocytosis. Achromia is not marked, although the total hemoglobin content may be diminished. The degree of drop in total hemoglobin level is dependent upon the quantity of blood cells lost.

Acute and subacute hemorrhages are usually followed by a rising total erythrocyte count. If hemorrhage has occurred into a body cavity, a dramatic and marked leukocytosis and shift to the left appear. Regeneration following an acute blood loss is usually progressive, with the red cells returning to a normal level in three to five weeks. The morphologic changes disappear in approximately 10 days, and the elevated leukocyte count usually returns to normal in two to four days. The persistence of reticulocytosis and leukocytosis may be indicative of continued bleeding. One must, however, rule out the possibility of a concurrent infection before assuming that the persistent leukocytosis is due to continuing hemorrhage.

Blood loss should be suspected as the cause of anemia in any animal having a large number of immature erythrocytes in the peripheral circulation if no clinical or laboratory evidence of icterus is present. In such cases, an immediate attempt should be made to determine the cause of the blood loss. In cases of chronic blood loss, iron storage in the body may be reduced, and signs of iron deficiency may then be present. Such a state is recognized by the presence of microcytic hypochromic cells.

Bone Marrow Depression. A decrease of erythropoiesis in the bone marrow is usually accompanied by a progressive fall in the total erythrocyte count and hemoglobin content. Occasionally, a simultaneous decrease in total leukocytes is observed. This is particularly true if the bone marrow is severely aplastic. Close examination of a hematocrit tube will often reveal clear, colorless, and watery plasma. Since there is a general bone marrow depression, a decrease in thrombocytes also occurs. Leptocytes occasionally appear in smears from peripheral blood and probably are due to malfunctioning of the marrow and improper maturation of the erythrocytes. Anemias due to bone marrow depression are characterized by decreases in all erythrocyte parameters with no evidence of regeneration. Reticulocytes and nucleated erythrocytes are not observed in the peripheral circulation. Such anemias are often refractory to treatment until the underlying cause of the bone marrow depression can be determined.

POLYCYTHEMIA

Although the most common abnormality associated with erythrocytes is a decrease in cell number or hemoglobin content, or both, polycythemia, although rare, has been reported in domestic animals. This increase in red cell mass may be absolute, as in polycythemia vera and hypoxia-stimulated erythropoiesis, or relative, as a consequence of hemoconcentration.

Polycythemia vera is a disease characterized by an absolute increase in the number of erythrocytes accompanied by an increase in total blood volume. Laboratory findings are characterized by a marked increase in total circulating erythrocytes, packed cell volume, and hemoglobin content.

Polycythemia vera has been reported in the dog, cat, and cow.

An apparently primary familial polycythemia of calves in an inbred Jersey herd has been reported. The condition was characterized hematologically by marked elevations in erythrocyte count, hemoglobin content, and packed cell volume. There was no increase in thrombocytes, reticulocytes, nucleated erythrocytes, or immature neutrophils.[25] These calves had a consistently increased rate of transfer of iron from the plasma compartment, which supported the abnormally accelerated erythropoiesis.

Recently a case of polycythemia was reported in a dog with renal carcinoma.[26] The dog was dehydrated and had a PCV of 72 per cent upon admission. Following rehydration the PCV dropped to 68 per cent. Following removal of the diseased kidney the PCV returned to normal (43 per cent three weeks after surgery). The blood level of erythropoietin was high before surgery and decreased following unilateral nephrectomy, suggesting that the renal carcinoma was in some fashion producing an excess of erythropoietin.

A true increase in circulating erythrocytes (polycythemia) may also occur following hypoxic stimulation of the marrow. The underlying mechanism for this erythrocyte increase is erythropoietin stimulation of the marrow. In animals, such an increase in erythrocytes can be seen in relationship to (1) exposure to high altitudes, which results in a mild polycythemia; (2) any disease that interferes with oxygenation of the erythrocytes, as might occur in obstructive lesions in the air passageways; (3) congenital heart disease in which there is a right-to-left shunting of blood; or (4) a circulatory insufficiency that permits stagnation of blood and accompanying hypoxia. In the polycythemic animal, the clinician must carefully analyze laboratory data to determine whether polycythemia is true or a consequence of hypoxia.

True polycythemia is rare; however, it is not uncommon to find a relative increase in erythrocytes in disease in which there is fluid loss or in animals that are excited or have been exercised. In the latter case, the increase in erythrocytes is a consequence of splenic contraction. Hemoconcentration is apparent in animals in a state of shock due to the reduction in plasma volume. A comparable alteration occurs in plasma volume in animals that have had a low water intake either because of lack of supply or as the result of a disease condition in which water intake is limited. Hemoconcentration resulting from these various alterations may mask the existence of anemia and interfere with proper interpretation of both total erythrocyte and total leukocyte counts.

REFERENCES

1. Kaneko, J. J.: Porphyria, heme and erythrocyte metabolism: The porphyrias. In: *Clinical Biochemistry of Domestic Animals*, edited by Kaneko, J. J. and Cornelius, C. E., Vol I, 2nd ed., Academic Press, New York, 1970.
2. Rudolph, W. G., and Kaneko, J. J.: Kinetics of erythroid bone marrow cells of normal and porphyric calves in vitro. Acta Haematol., 45:330, 1971.
3. Morley, A., and Stohlman, F., Jr.: Erythropoiesis in the dog: The periodic nature of the steady state. Science, 165:1025, 1969.
4. Schalm, O. W., Jain, N. C., and Carroll, E. J.: Veterinary Hematology, 3rd ed., Lea & Febiger, Philadelphia, 1975.
5. Brown, D. G. and Cross, F. H.: Hematologic values of burros from birth to maturity: Cellular elements of peripheral blood. Am. J. Vet. Res., 30:1921, 1969.
6. Olbrich, S. E., Martz, F. A., Tumbleson, M. E., Johnson, H. D., and Hilderbrand, E. S.: Serum biochemical and hematological measurements of heat tolerant (Zebu) and cold tolerant (Scotch Highland) heifers. J. Anim. Sci., 33:655, 1971.
7. Sutton, R. H., and Johnstone, M.: The value of plasma fibrinogen estimation in dogs: A comparison with total leukocyte and neutrophil counts. J. Small Anim. Pract., 18:277, 1977.
8. Schall, W. D., and Perman, V.: Diseases of the red blood cells. In *Textbook of Veterinary Internal Medicine, Diseases of the Dog and Cat*, edited by Ettinger, S. J., W. B. Saunders Company, Philadelphia, 1983.
9. Martinovich, D., and Woodhouse, D. A.: Post-parturient hemoglobinuria in cattle: A Heinz body haemolytic anemia. N. Z. Vet. J., 19:259, 1971.
10. Reinhard, K. R.: A clinical pathological study of experimental leptospirosis of calves. Am. J. Vet. Res., 12:282, 1951.
11. Henson, J. B., and McGuire, T. C.: Immunopathology of equine infectious anemia. Am. J. Vet. Res., 56:306, 1971.
12. Penny, R. H. C., Carlisle, C. H., Prescott, C. W., and Davidson, H. A.: Further observations on the effect of chloramphenicol on the haemopoietic system of the cat. Br. Vet. J., 126:453, 1970.
13. Feldman, B. F., Kaneko, J. J., and Farver, T. B.: Anemia of inflammatory disease in the dog: Clinical characterization. Am. J. Vet. Res., 42:1109, 1981.
14. Searcy, G. P., Miller, D. R., and Tasker, J. B.: Congenital hemolytic anemia in the Basenji dog due to erythrocyte pyruvate kinase deficiency. Can. J. Comp. Med., 35:67, 1971.
15. Searcy, G. P.: Myelofibrosis and osteosclerosis as sequelae to congenital hemolytic anemia in the Basenji dog. Bull. Am. Soc. Vet. Clin. Pathol., 2:9, 1973.
16. Prasse, K. S., Crouser, D., Beutler, E., Walker, M., and Schall, W. D.: Pyruvate kinase deficiency anemia with terminal myelofibrosis and osteosclerosis in a beagle. J.A.V.M.A., 166:1170, 1975.
17. Chandler, F. W., Jr., Prasse, K. W., and Callaway, C. S.: Surface ultrastructure of pyruvate kinase-deficient erythrocytes in the Basenji dog. Am. J. Vet. Res., 36:1477, 1975.
18. Brooksbank, N. H.: Anemia in piglets associated with a copper deficiency. Vet. Rec., 66:322, 1954.
19. Van Wyk, J. J., Baxter, J. H., and Motulsky, A. G.: The anemia of copper deficiency in dogs compared with that produced by iron deficiency. Johns Hopkins Hosp. Bull., 93:41, 1943.
20. Marston, H. R.: Cobalt and molybdenum in the nutrition of plants and animals. Physiol. Rev., 32:66: 1952.
21. Maynard, L. A.: Animal species that feed mankind: The role of nutrition. Science, 120:164, 1954.
22. Spector, H., et al.: The role of riboflavin in blood regeneration. J. Biol. Chem., 150:75, 1943.
23. Mitchell, H. H., Johnson, B. C., Hamilton, T. S., and Haines, W. T.: The riboflavin requirement of the growing pig at two environmental temperatures. J. Nutr., 41:317, 1942.
24. McKibben, J. M., Schaeffer, A. E., Frost, D. V., and Elvehjem, C. A.: Studies on anemia in dogs due to pyrodoxine deficiency. J. Biol. Chem., 142:77, 1942.
25. Tennant, B., Asbury, A. C., Laben, R. C., Richards, W. P. C., Kaneko, J. J., and Cupps, P. T.: Familial polycythemia in cattle. J.A.V.M.A., 150:1493, 1967.
26. Peterson, M. E.: Inappropriate erythropoietin production from a renal carcinoma in a dog with polycythemia. J.A.V.M.A., 179:996, 1981.

LEUKOCYTES

Leukocytes utilize the bloodstream much as one uses a highway to travel from home (bone marrow) to work (tissues). Thus, examination of peripheral blood to determine the number and types of leukocytes is similar to watching traffic flow on a busy highway, analyzing it with respect to the types of vehicles present at a given time, and attempting to judge from this information the state of business in the community toward which the traffic is directed. If this analysis is made during the busy rush hours of the day, one conclusion might be reached, whereas if the analysis is made during the middle of the afternoon, a modified conclusion could be drawn. Accurate interpretation of such an analysis is possible only if the entire situation is reviewed and results are considered in light of all the facts. Interpretation of a total and differential leukocyte count without completing a physical examination of the animal would be an analogous situation. It is difficult, if not impossible, to accurately interpret results in the absence of all available information.

Total and differential leukocyte counts, if properly interpreted, are of value in confirming or eliminating a tentative diagnosis and aid in making a more accurate prognosis. The results may also serve to guide therapy. Such findings reflect (1) susceptibility of the host, (2) virulence of the infecting organism, (3) nature and severity of the disease process, (4) systemic response of the individual, and (5) duration of the disease process. Although a single blood count incorporating total and differential leukocyte counts may be of value when considered in association with a complete physical examination, more valuable information is obtained when a series of counts is completed.

INDICATIONS FOR LEUKOCYTE EXAMINATION

Total and differential leukocyte counts are often part of a routine physical examination of a sick animal. Such studies may be used as part of the initial examination of an animal presented for routine immunization or surgical procedure.

Total and differential leukocyte counts should be completed whenever the history and physical examination reveal an abnormality that could result in changes in the leukocyte picture that might be of value in confirming a diagnosis, in making a prognosis, or in selecting a proper therapy. Such determinations are helpful in animals with generalized, systemic, or localized disease. An absolute diagnosis is seldom, if ever, made as a consequence of leukocyte examinations. The only exceptions might be disorders such as leukemias, localized pyogenic processes, or viral diseases during the incubating stages.

LIMITATIONS OF LEUKOCYTE EXAMINATION

As with any laboratory determination, certain factors must be considered that produce deviations as a consequence of technical error rather than of physiologic or pathologic change occurring with disease. The most common errors encountered in the examination of leukocytes include those associated with (1) collection, (2) dilution, and (3) counting.

Collection Errors. If liquid anticoagulants are used, care must be taken to avoid excessive specimen dilution. Significant dilution is most likely to occur when less blood is obtained from small dogs and cats than was anticipated when anticoagulant was placed in the syringe. Dilution errors can be avoided if dry anticoagulants are used, but this may present an additional problem as it is often difficult to obtain adequate mixing of anticoagulant with blood, and small clots may form that interfere with leukocyte determinations. This latter error can be solved by complete and adequate mixing of blood with anticoagulant.

Hemolysis will interfere with determinations and is most commonly the result of (1) a wet syringe, (2) too much syringe vacuum in relation to needle size, (3) forcibly expelling blood through the needle, (4) contamination by a chemical substance in the syringe or collection tube, or (5) violent agitation of the specimen following collection. Most collection errors can be solved by use of special vacuum collecting units containing a premeasured quantity of anticoagulant. These units, along with a special holder and disposable needle, can be used to obtain blood. Alternatively, blood can be collected in a clean dry syringe and added to these tubes.

If blood specimens are collected by puncture of a capillary bed rather than by venipuncture, contamination of the sample with animal dander, dirt, and hair presents an additional problem to the technician. This can be avoided by careful cleansing of the area prior to puncture.

Dilution Errors. Although the majority of the white blood cell (WBC) diluting pipettes are accurately manufactured, selection of pipettes should not be based entirely on the cost of the equipment but on the error inherent in the pipettes. It is preferable to employ pipettes and hemocytometers that have been certified by the National Bureau of Standards or are guaranteed by the manufacturer to meet specifications designated by that agency. The most common error associated with dilution of blood for a total leukocyte count, however, is not due to equipment but to human error. Extreme care must be taken in making blood dilutions in order to ensure accurate results. Use of a disposable unit with a calibrated capillary tube and the proper amount of diluting fluid will reduce dilution errors.

Counting Errors. Counting errors in a determination of total leukocytes are most commonly due to improper lighting of the microscope field or careless examination and enumeration of cells. As it is difficult to differentiate leukocytes from particles of debris, use of dirty equipment or diluting fluid will result in erroneously high counts. Care must be taken to avoid contaminating dilution fluids, as fluids containing even a small quantity of a previous specimen will alter results.

A factor limiting the accuracy of a differential leukocyte count is correct cell identification. Cell identification is dependent upon the ability of the individual making the count and the quality of the stained film. It is difficult, if not impossible, to properly identify cells if the staining technique is poor. If the stain is too light, nuclear characteristics are indistinct, and neutrophils are so pale that identification is almost impossible. If the stain is too dark, the nuclei stain intensely, and minor alterations in the chromatin-parachromatin patterns of significance in cell identification are obliterated.

In addition to poorly stained slides, improperly prepared blood films that are too thick or too thin, in which excessive pressure has been used in making the slides, or in which the spreader slide has been moved too quickly or too slowly, are also difficult to evaluate. Only properly prepared films should be examined in making a differential leukocyte count. Erroneous results may be obtained if the technician examines only limited sections of a blood film. If the end or edges are examined and the center section of the film is ignored, different results are obtained from those reported when the entire film is examined in a systematic manner. If insufficient numbers of cells are identified, the accuracy is affected. A minimum of 100 cells should be located, and their identity should be recorded. Accuracy can be greatly improved by counting 200 cells.

NORMAL LEUKOCYTE VALUES

Values for total leukocyte counts are incorporated in Table 3–1. These represent the compilation of data from several sources and, in general, represent the range and average of total leukocyte counts as reported by various authors. Values for differential leukocyte counts are presented in Table 3–2.

Bovine. The normal total leukocyte count for the cow is influenced by age of the animal. Many investigators report a higher leukocyte count in calves than in adult animals. Others report little variation in total leukocyte counts in animals

TABLE 3–1. Total Leukocyte Values for Various Species of Domestic Animals

Species Counts × 10^3	Range of Total Leukocyte Counts × 10^3	Average Total Leukocytes
Bovine	4–12	7.6
Ovine	4–12	7.6
Caprine	4–13	12.0
Porcine	10–22	16.0
Equine (thoroughbred)	5.5–14	10.0
Equine (draft)	6–12	8.8
Canine	6–15	11.0
Feline	5.5–19	12.5

* These values are adapted from the literature and the data accumulated in our laboratory. Age, sex, and other physiologic factors may influence total leukocyte counts.

TABLE 3–2. Differential Leukocyte Values for Various Species of
Domestic Animals

Species	Per Cent of Cells (Range)					
	BAND	SEG.	LY.	MONO.	EOS.	BASO.
Canine	0–4	60–75	12–30	3–9	2–10	Rare
Feline	0–2	35–75	20–55	1–4	2–10	Rare
Bovine	0–1	15–45	48–75	2–7	2–15	0–2
Equine						
(thoroughbred)	0–2	30–65	25–70	1–8	1–10	0–3
(draft)	0–2	35–75	15–50	2–10	1–10	0–3
Ovine	0–2	10–50	40–75	1–5	1–8	0–3
Porcine	0–5	28–47	39–60	2–10	1–11	0–2
Caprine	0–2	30–48	50–70	1–4	3–8	0–2

Seg. = segmented neutrophil, Ly. = lymphocyte, Mono. = monocyte, Eos. = eosinophil, Baso. = basophil.

under one year of age and mature cattle. There is good evidence, however, that aged cattle have a normal total leukocyte count considerably lower than that of younger animals. Apparently healthy aged cows may have leukocyte counts as low as 5000/µl. Breed variations have been reported, but most alterations can be attributed to the physiologic leukocytosis that occurs in beef cattle, which resist the sampling procedure more vigorously than more docile dairy breeds.

The number of circulating lymphocytes is low in the newborn calf and increases as the animal begins to grow, only to decrease slightly with age. At birth lymphocytes represent only about 33 per cent of the total leukocytes and rise to 72 per cent in four months, then gradually decrease until the normal adult level of 50 to 60 per cent is reached at about two years of age. There is a decrease in neutrophils and an increase in eosinophils as animals age. There is an accompanying decrease in absolute numbers of lymphocytes with age.

Band neutrophils are uncommon in the peripheral blood of the healthy bovine. Estrus may result in a slight increase in total leukocyte count accompanied by an increase in neutrophils and a decrease in eosinophils on the day of heat and the day after. The blood picture associated with parturition closely resembles that observed under conditions of stress in the bovine: namely, a leukocytosis due to an increased number of neutrophils and a decrease in lymphocytes and eosinophils. The differential count of peripheral blood returns to normal within five days following parturition. Pregnancy has a more limited effect on the number of leukocytes, but an increase in total leukocyte count has been reported for the first four months of pregnancy. Neutrophils have a tendency to increase during this period, only to decrease until the time of parturition.

Sampling in an unnatural environment may cause sufficient stress to reduce the lymphocyte count without affecting neutrophil and eosino-

phil counts. This fact must be taken into consideration in interpreting differential and total leukocyte counts on cattle that become excited during the sampling procedure.

Equine. A variation in the total leukocyte count occurs in different breeds of horses. The thoroughbred or so-called "hot-blooded" horse has a total leukocyte count somewhat higher than that of the "cold-blooded" animal.[1] Leukocyte values in Arabian horses are consistent with both "hot blooded" (thoroughbred, standardbred, and saddlebred) and "cold-blooded" (draft) horses. Younger thoroughbreds have leukocyte counts lower than mature animals, and the mature stallion has a lower total count than the mare.

In thoroughbred horses there is an approximate 1:1 ratio between neutrophils and lymphocytes, whereas in the "cold-blooded" horse this ratio is more nearly 5:3. A neutrophil:lymphocyte ratio of 6:4 exists in the thoroughbred horse up to two months of age and is followed by a decrease in neutrophils until the 1:1 ratio in the mature animal is reached. The 1:1 ratio persists for one to two years, and as the horse ages, the ratio increases as lymphocyte numbers decrease and the neutrophil count stabilizes.

In burros the total leukocyte count increases from birth to 10 months and then decreases to reach a plateau at about 18 months of age. The agranulocyte count follows the total leukocyte count. Eosinophils increase at a relatively constant rate through two years of age, whereas mature neutrophils and basophils increase during the first week and then remain stable. The ratio of neutrophils to lymphocytes changes inversely with age as segmented neutrophils decrease from birth through 10 months of age and then increase to normal values by 18 months of age.

Canine. Normal counts for leukocytes in the dog have been determined for the most part by investigations using groups of dogs maintained for medical research. The total leukocyte count in the healthy dog has not been found in our laboratory to be as high as 19,000/μL (Table 3–1). The lower range given by several authors would, in general, agree with the results in this laboratory. Although sex and age of the dog have been reported not to affect the total leukocyte count, more recent results suggest that there are age and sex influences. A statistical difference between males and females has been reported but is of little practical significance in interpretation of sample variations except in well-defined populations of experimental animals.

Total leukocyte counts are highest in young dogs and decrease with age. Most of the decrease is in lymphocytes while neutrophils remain fairly constant; eosinophils may increase slightly and monocytes tend to decrease. These changes must be taken into consideration in interpreting total leukocyte counts. In a young dog a total count of 15,000 to 16,000/μl may be normal while in an older animal it may represent leukocytosis. Conversely, a total count of 7,000/μl may be normal in an older dog but may represent leukopenia in a dog 15 to 18 months of age.[2]

The percentage of lymphocytes in the normal adult dog seldom is over 20 to 25, but in dogs under six months of age a lymphocyte percentage of 30 is not uncommon. In these younger animals there is a simultaneous decrease in the percentage of neutrophils. As the animal becomes older, there is also an increase in circulating eosinophils.

Feline. The normal total leukocyte count in the cat is difficult to establish, as this animal is excitable, and excitation markedly influences total leukocyte counts. Physiologic leukocytosis occurs most commonly in cats under one year of age.

These facts may explain why the normal total leukocyte count in the cat has been reported to be as high as 40,000/μl. As physiologic leukocytosis is important in the cat, interpretation of results is dependent upon knowing how much resistance and excitement were manifested as a blood sample was drawn.

The differential leukocyte count in the cat is dependent upon the degree of excitation and apprehension exhibited by the animal as the blood sample is drawn. Physiologic leukocytosis due to fear or emotional stress should be suspected when neutrophils are in the high normal absolute range and lymphocytes are in excess of the maximum normal value and may exceed neutrophils in number. Emotional disturbance is indicated when all leukocyte types are at the high normal or above the maximum normal levels.[3]

The mean marginal neutrophil pool of clinically normal cats has been estimated to be three times greater than the circulating pool. The movement of cells from this large marginal pool into the circulating pool in animals stimulated by excitement and muscular activity may explain the great increase in total leukocytes seen in apparently healthy cats.

Porcine. The normal total leukocyte count in the pig is considerably higher than in any other species of domestic animal. The normal range of total leukocyte counts in piglets (six to 12 weeks of age) is between 10,000 and 40,000/μl with a mean of approximately 20,000. In adults the normal total leukocyte count is from 12,000 to 23,000 with a mean of about 16,000. A total leukocyte count of less than 10,000 in a pig over six weeks of age should be considered a leukopenia.[1]

The differential leukocyte count in the young pig is characterized by a high percentage of neutrophils (70 per cent) at birth followed by a decrease to approximately 45 per cent by the end of the first week of life. This percentage of neutrophils increases to approximately 55 per cent in the mature animal.[1] Total and differential leukocyte counts in the sow at parturition are characteristic of the stress pattern observed in the bovine and may include a left shift 24 to 36 hours postpartum.

Caprine. The influence of age on leukocyte counts in goats has been studied by a number of workers. For the first two weeks of life the total count averaged 8371/μl, then increased to slightly over 19,000/μl by four months of age and fell to approximately 11,000/μl at 2½ years of age. Lymphocyte numbers gradually increased from 3590/μl at birth to 11,570/μl at three months of age. Neutrophils remained fairly constant at less than 4000/μl for the first three months of life but by six months of age had increased to 4200/μl and remained nearly at this level until maturity. The number of lymphocytes observed was greatest at six months of age (13,840/μl) but declined to 4700/μl at 36 months of age. Band neutrophils were uncommon after the fourteenth month, and no metamyelocytes were seen after the fourth month.

Ovine. The normal total leukocyte count for sheep is similar to that of cattle. The normal range is 4000 to 12,000/μl with a mean of around 8000. There is a slight downward trend in total leukocytes as sheep mature. Most of this decrease is due to a fall in the number of lymphocytes. In newborn lambs the lymphocyte:neutrophil ratio is 1.61, and as lymphocytes increase the ratio is altered and at maturity is between 2.0 and 3.0.

COLLECTION OF BLOOD SAMPLES

The usual procedure in large animals is to collect blood directly from the jugular vein into a test tube or vial containing an adequate amount of anticoagulant for the amount of blood desired. Five ml of blood is sufficient for most hematologic examinations. An alternate technique in the cow is to utilize the caudal vein or artery as a source of peripheral blood, and in this instance a clean, dry syringe or Vacutainer (Becton-Dickinson, Rutherford, New Jersey) is utilized (Fig. 3–1). Blood

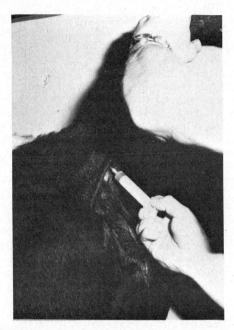

Figure 3–1. Blood can be drawn from the caudal vein in the cow. A ¾- to 1-inch 14- to 16-gauge needle is attached to a syringe and directed toward the vein on the midline of the tail. Care must be taken to avoid entering the vertebra.

sampling from the dog is best accomplished by use of a Vacutainer or, alternatively, a dry syringe into which has been placed one drop of anticoagulant; this is allowed to coat the inside of the syringe and the excess is discharged. Care must be taken in obtaining blood, as improper collection procedures may cause cellular distortion. Obtaining venous blood from a cat using a Vacutainer or dry syringe may prove difficult because of the size of the vein and the necessity for restraint. Adequate samples can be collected from the jugular vein. Some veterinarians prefer this method for the collection of blood from dogs and cats. There are certain advantages in using the jugular; it is relatively easy to locate, there is no excessive resistance to restraint, the vein is large and easy to penetrate, and adequate quantitites of blood are readily obtained, even from small animals. Blood may be obtained from the ear vein of dogs and cats by first cleaning the surface of the ear followed by placing a thin layer of petrolatum over the vein to be punctured. The vein should be punctured by quickly thrusting a sharp, pointed scalpel blade or sterile disposable needle through the petrolatum and into the vein. The blood forms a drop on the petrolatum and is not contaminated with hair or dander from the ear. An adequate flow of blood usually results, and the sample can be either collected in diluting pipettes or utilized for other techniques. Most animals do not object too violently to this procedure. An alternate technique is to clip a toenail into the vascular area.

The quantity of blood collected from the ear or toenail is usually inadequate for use in automated cell counters but may be adequate for hemacytometer counts and for samples diluted in a Unopette. Blood samples from swine are removed from either an ear vein or the anterior vena cava (Fig. 3–2).

In collecting blood, care should be taken to ensure that the needle is of sufficient diameter. A needle of too small gauge may cause disruption of erythrocytes and damage leukocytes. Blood should flow smoothly with a minimum of vacuum, and if a syringe is used, one should avoid pumping the syringe barrel. If it is necessary to transfer the blood from a syringe into a test tube, the needle should be removed, as forcing blood through the needle may damage cells.

ANTICOAGULANTS

A great variety of anticoagulants may be used in preserving a sample of blood for hematologic examinations.

EDTA. Dipotassium and disodium salts of ethylenediaminetetraacetic acid (EDTA) act as chelating agents and prevent the coagulation of blood by combining with calcium. Ether salt is the anticoagulant of choice when the preservation of cells and cellular characteristics are important criteria. EDTA may be used in either a liquid or dry form. If used as a liquid, one drop of a 10 per cent solution is sufficient to prevent the coagulation of 5 ml of blood. In the dry powder form, a concentration equivalent to 1 mg of powder/ml of blood should be used. It is convenient to prepare test tubes containing 5 mg of the powder by designing a small metal scoop that will hold approximately this amount and dispensing the powder into test

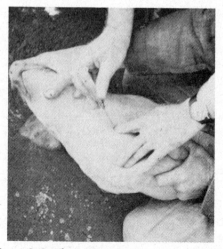

Figure 3–2. The anterior vena cava is the desired site for collecting blood from a pig. A small pig is placed on its back with the head extended.

tubes. If the disodium salt is used, it is advisable to measure the powder into the tubes and dissolve it in a small amount of water, then to dry it in an oven prior to use. Disodium salt is not readily soluble, and this procedure will give better results. Soluble tablets containing sufficient EDTA to prevent coagulation of 5 ml of blood are available.

EDTA has the advantage of preserving the stainability and morphologic characteristics of leukocytes. These qualities are altered less with EDTA than with most other anticoagulants. Samples of blood have been preserved in the refrigerator overnight in our laboratory with minor effects on cellular characteristics or stainability. However, bovine lymphocytes may become monocytoid if held in EDTA for several hours. Leukemic neutrophils may develop cytoplasmic vacuoles in blood containing EDTA. EDTA is suggested as being the anticoagulant most compatible with saponification of erythrocytes for use in the Coulter Electronic Cell Counter.

Care must be taken not to exceed the recommended level of EDTA, as it has been shown that excess EDTA adversely affects the determination of packed cell volume (PCV). The packed cell volume is decreased if EDTA is present in excess. This occurs as a consequence of cell shrinkage.

Oxalates. Oxalates also prevent coagulation of blood by combining with calcium. The oxalate preparation of Heller and Paul[4] has been used for the prevention of blood coagulation. A stock solution is prepared by dissolving 1.2 gm of ammonium oxalate and 0.8 gm of potassium oxalate in 100 ml of water. One ml of this mixture is placed in a suitable container and allowed to dry in a hot air oven at 60° C. This is sufficient to prevent coagulation of 10 ml of blood. Oxalate is an inexpensive anticoagulant that is easy to prepare and use. Little cellular distortion occurs if the sample is examined within the first hour after collection. If more time elapses, leukocytic degeneration may render accurate readings difficult. This double salt cannot utilized in drawing samples for nitrogen determinations, as the presence of the ammonium ion will interfere with the results. Either of these salts may be used alone to prevent coagulation of blood, but this method is not recommended as ammonium oxalate produces an increase in cell size, and potassium oxalate a decrease. These alterations influence cell morphology, making identification difficult. Oxalate artefacts in leukocytes are manifested by karyorrhexis. Lithium oxalate may be used as an anticoagulant in a concentration of 10 mg/dl of blood. This anticoagulant is particularly adapted for use in blood collected for a nonprotein nitrogen determination.

Heparin. Heparin prevents coagulation of blood by interfering with the conversion of prothrombin to thrombin. It is most commonly used in the liquid or dry form in a test tube. A syringe may be rinsed with a stock solution (1 per cent) of heparin and will contain sufficient anticoagulating activity to preserve 5 ml of blood. Although an excellent and convenient anticoagulant for use in small animal practice, it has the disadvantage of adversely affecting leukocyte stainability. If heparin is present in excess, as will occur if one intends to draw 5 ml of blood but obtains only 2 ml, staining of the leukocytes is difficult and occasionally the cells are unstainable. Heparin is the most expensive of the anticoagulants commonly used and is effective for only 10 to 12 hours. Plasma collected from heparinized blood is not acceptable for use in automated chemical analyses.

Sodium Fluoride. Sodium fluoride at a concentration of 10 mg/dl is used as an anticoagulant and preservative of glucose. Both sodium citrate and potassium citrate may be used as anticoagulants but are not commonly adopted for the preservation of blood for hematologic determinations.

ENUMERATION OF TOTAL LEUKOCYTES

HEMOCYTOMETER METHOD

Equipment necessary for performing a total leukocyte count (Fig. 3–3) includes:

1. Counting chamber.
2. Special coverglass for the counting chamber.
3. Diluting pipette.
4. Diluting fluid.
5. Microscope and lamp.
6. A hand tally for enumeration of cells.

The counting chamber most commonly used is made of a single piece of glass with two elevated platforms, each having etched on it the improved Neubauer ruling (Fig. 3–4). Each platform on which the rulings are engraved is surrounded by a moat, and on each side of the platform there is an elevated glass support at a height that will allow for a distance of 0.1 mm between the bottom of the coverglass and the ruled area. The improved Neubauer ruling of the platform consists of a system of squares in which there is a square measuring 3 by 3 mm that is divided into nine equal squares, each containing 1 sq mm. The four corner squares are divided into 16 intermediate squares measuring 0.25 by 0.25 mm. These four corner squares are used for the total leukocyte count. The center square millimeter is subdivided into 25 squares, and each of these is subdivided into 16 small squares that measure 0.05 by 0.05 mm. As a rule, five of the middle-sized squares are used in making the total erythrocyte count (see Fig. 3–4).

Diluting pipettes for a total leukocyte count have two markings that are used in making a dilution of blood for counting. These are the 0.5

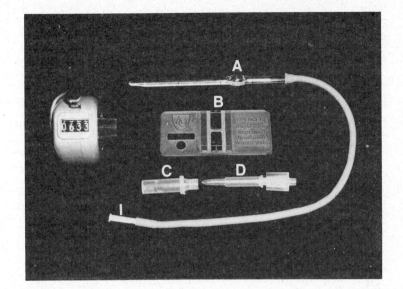

Figure 3–3. Equipment used in completing a total leukocyte count. *A*, White blood cell–diluting pipette. *B*, Hemocytometer. *C*, Unopette reservoir containing a premeasured quantity of leukocyte-diluting fluid. *D*, Unopette capillary pipette (25/μl).

mark on the capillary tube portion of the pipette and an 11 mark just over the bulb of the pipette. These marks do not represent any given or standardized quantity of fluid but represent a ratio of 1:20 or a dilution of 0.5 part to 10 parts.

The pipette is filled by using a rubber tube fitted with a glass or plastic mouthpiece that can be attached to the stem end of the pipette above the bulb. With gentle suction blood is drawn to the 0.5 mark, and excess blood clinging to the exterior of the pipette is removed by wiping it with a piece of cheesecloth. Care must be taken to stop the level exactly on the 0.5 mark or slightly above it.

This is most easily accomplished by slightly parting the lips as the blood reaches this mark on the pipette. If blood is drawn into the diluting pipette slightly above the 0.5 mark, it can be lowered to the proper level by carefully touching the end of the capillary tubing containing the blood to the finger. The proper diluting fluid is then drawn to the 11 mark, and the blood and diluting fluid are mixed by shaking the pipette vigorously for two to three minutes.

Diluting fluids most commonly used include:

1. Glacial acetic acid, 2 ml in 100 ml of dis-

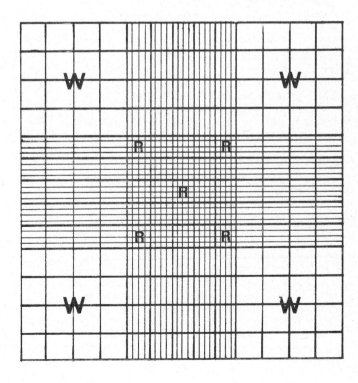

Figure 3–4. Ruled area on improved Neubauer hemocytometer. For total leukocyte count, the WBC in the area (W) are counted. The total erythrocyte count is completed by counting all cells in the squares labeled R.

tilled water to which has been added 1 ml of a 1 per cent aqueous solution of gentian violet.

2. N/10 hydrochloric acid (HCl), which is prepared by adding 1 ml of concentrated HCl to 100 ml of water. This is approximately 0.1 normal HCl and is sufficiently accurate for this test.

These diluting fluids should be carefully filtered prior to use to remove particles that might be confused with leukocytes.

Care must be taken in cleaning diluting pipettes following use, as they may serve as a source of contaminating particles that interfere with accurate leukocyte counts. After use, pipettes should be washed in clear water or a weak solution of a mild detergent and then dried by drawing acetone through them. This is most easily accomplished by use of a water pump. After cleaning, air is drawn through the pipette until it is completely dry. Dryness is indicated if the glass bead in the pipette rolls freely in the bulb. Occasionally, it is impossible or impractical to clean equipment immediately after use, and if this is the case, the pipettes should be stored in a beaker of water to prevent drying. Dried material is difficult to remove from these pipettes but sometimes can be dislodged by use of a horse hair or very fine long stylet. If pipettes become stained, they can be cleaned by drawing a solution of sodium hypochlorite into them and allowing them to stand for several minutes prior to washing in water and drying with acetone.

A rapid method for making dilutions for white blood cell counts by means of a plastic disposable pipette has been developed. This disposable plastic equipment is manufactured by Becton-Dickinson, Rutherford, New Jersey, and is identified by the trade name "Unopette." This unique equipment includes a capillary pipette into which a measured quantity of blood is automatically drawn when touched to a drop of blood. The measured quantity of blood is then discharged into a premeasured quantity of white cell–diluting fluid, and the erythrocytes are lysed. The dilution factor is 1:100, and the total leukocyte number is determined by counting all cells in the entire ruled area of a hemocytometer. The total count is calculated using the formula:

Total cells in 9 squares + 10% of total cells
× 100 = WBC/μl

This Unopette can also be used to enumerate thrombocytes. In addition, Unopettes calibrated for the 1:20 dilution are also available.

Charging the counting chamber may influence the results of a total leukocyte count if improperly done. Before diluted blood is placed into the chamber for counting, the chamber should be carefully cleaned to remove any grease, lint, or dust particles. After the diluted blood is thoroughly mixed, several drops of fluid are discarded, and the end of the pipette is dried with a piece of clean cheesecloth or other lint-free absorbent material. The tip of the pipette is touched to the side of the counting chamber, and a drop of fluid will run under the coverglass. This is best accomplished by removing the rubber tubing from the pipette and handling it much as one would handle a pipette in any standard chemical procedure. The flow of diluting fluid is more easily controlled if the finger is not completely removed from the end of the pipette but only partially lifted from it. Retaining a finger on the pipette enables the operator to halt the flow of fluid when the chamber is completely filled. If fluid escapes into the moats surrounding the chamber, it should be cleaned and recharged, as an accurate count is impossible if the fluid flows into these trenches. The chamber should be filled without any hesitation. If the flow of liquid is halted before the chamber is completely charged, there is a tendency for the leukocytes to settle out, and an uneven distribution of cells may result.

Counting of the leukocytes should be started after the cells have settled for one to two minutes in order to allow them to assume a position in the same plane. Using the low power objective of the microscope, locate the corner ruled square and adjust the light intensity, diaphragm, and substage distance so that the cells and marking lines are readily observed. While focusing up and down slightly with the fine adjustment of the microscope, use a meandering system to count all the cells in the 16 squares within the larger ruled area in the corner (Fig. 3–4). Some difficulty may be encountered in counting the same cell twice. This is particularly true of cells resting on one of the lines. One method of avoiding duplicate counting of a single cell is to count only those cells that touch the lower and right boundaries. After all the cells are counted in one corner square, the results should be recorded, and each of the other three corner squares counted in the same manner and the number of cells in each square recorded. Thus, a count of the total cells in 4 sq mm will be completed. These four counts are totaled; the calculation is completed by applying the formula:

$$\frac{\text{Total leukocytes in 4 sq mm}}{4} \times 20 \times 10$$

$$= \text{Leukocytes/μl}$$

A simpler method of calculation is to multiply the total of the four corner squares by 50, or divide by two and add two zeros.

The most common sources of error in making a total leukocyte count by this method include the following:

1. Errors in dilution.
2. Errors in counting.
3. Errors in calculation.

4. Inaccurate calibration of pipettes and counting chambers.

5. Inadequate or improper shaking of the pipette after dilution.

6. Contamination of diluting fluid with yeasts, molds, or other cells.

7. Failure to wipe excess blood from the end of the pipette.

8. Drying of the sample during or prior to counting.

9. Overflow of fluid into the moat.

10. Improper adjustment of light source, which may make leukocytes difficult to observe.

11. Failure to allow the cells to settle into a single plane prior to counting.

12. Inadequate cleaning of glassware.

13. Failure to discharge diluting fluid from the capillary prior to charging the chamber.

14. Chipped pipettes.

15. Failure to focus microscope up and down during counting. Even if the cells are allowed to settle, a single focus adjustment will not make all cells visible.

The inherent error in making total leukocyte counts is ± 10 per cent.

Occasionally it becomes necessary to correct the total white cell count if the differential count shows the presence of nucleated erythrocytes. These cells are not lysed by the usual white cell diluting fluid and therefore cannot be distinguished from a leukocyte. The formula for correcting the total leukocyte count in the presence of nucleated red blood cells (RBC) is:

$$\frac{100 \text{ Leukocytes}}{100 + \text{Number of nucleated RBC/100 WBC}}$$

$$\times \text{ Uncorrected WBC count}$$

$$= \text{ Corrected leukocyte count}$$

For example: a sample of blood is examined, and a total uncorrected leukocyte count of 15,000/μl is obtained. On the differential count, 25 nucleated erythrocytes are found as 100 leukocytes are observed. This information is then placed in the formula as follows:

$$\frac{100}{100 + 25} \times 15,000 = 12,000$$

$$= \text{ Corrected leukocyte count/μl}$$

ELECTRONIC METHODS

Development of semiautomated electronic methods for determining total blood cell counts has greatly improved the accuracy of such estimations. These techniques are rapidly replacing the hemocytometer method in larger laboratories in which the daily load is sufficient to justify the expense of purchasing such equipment. Several such instruments are now available. Some of the more sophisticated models are computerized to provide calculations of hemoglobin concentration, packed cell volume, mean corpuscular volume, and mean corpuscular hemoglobin concentration in addition to counting blood cells.

TECHNIQUES FOR RAPID ESTIMATION OF LEUKOCYTES

If absolute values for total leukocyte counts are not required, several methods can be utilized for estimating such counts. These methods are not meant to replace the more accurate hemocytometer technique but do have their place in veterinary clinical pathology either in the field or in laboratories not equipped to complete the more sensitive total leukocyte count. Methods found acceptable include (1) deoxyribonucleic acid (DNA) viscosity technique, (2) examination of wet blood film stained with new methylene blue, and (3) estimation of total leukocyte count from a stained blood film.

DNA Viscosity Technique. A rapid indirect method for estimation of leukocyte numbers has been described. This method involves the use of a 30 per cent solution of alkyl aryl sulfonate containing bromcresol purple in a 1:1000 concentration. This same reagent at a lower concentration has been used as a screening test to detect leukocytes in milk.

This method utilizes a special funnel having a capacity of 4.5 ml and a stem 2.0 cm long with a 1.3 mm bore. The reagent, blood, and alkaline tap water are mixed, and the length of time required for the mixture to flow through the funnel is recorded. Flow time is influenced by the viscosity, which, in turn, is dependent upon the quantity of DNA of leukocyte nuclei present in one drop of blood. Conversion tables for the estimation of total leukocyte counts are consulted to convert the flow time to total leukocyte count/μl.

The technique for this test is as follows:

1. Dispense 3.0 ml of alkaline tap water into a graduated centrifuge tube.

2. Add three drops of the concentrated reagent (California Mastitis Test Reagent) and mix well with the water. A blue color indicates that the water pH is satisfactory.

3. Add one drop of well-mixed blood and start a stop watch. Mix the blood and reagent by slowly and gently inverting the tube *exactly five times.*

4. Press the stem of the special funnel (Dairy Research Products Inc., Brunswick, Maine) onto a rubber stopper, and at 20 seconds from addition of the drop of blood pour the reagent-blood mixture into the funnel without the loss of any fluid.

5. At exactly 30 seconds from addition of the blood, raise the funnel, and return the stop watch to zero and start it again. When the fluid level has

fallen to the top of the funnel stem, stop the watch and record the elapsed time in seconds.

6. Compare the flow time with the conversion table and record the approximate leukocyte count.

Results obtained by the DNA viscosity test have been reported to be comparable to standard hemocytometer counts.[5] This method may have limitations in animals with anemia when large numbers of nucleated erythrocytes are present in peripheral blood. Limited numbers of observations on leukemic blood suggest that the test may overestimate the number of leukocytes if there is a significant number of immature cells. Lipemic blood and an excessive amount of anticoagulant (EDTA) appear to affect the accuracy of the method.

Extreme care must be taken to perform the test exactly as described, as any variation in this technique will affect the results.

Examination of Wet Blood Film Stained with New Methylene Blue. Equipment required includes the following:

1. Scrupulously clean coverglasses 22 × 22 mm and glass slides. These slides should be carefully cleaned, dipped in alcohol, and dried with a lintless cloth prior to use.

2. A 0.5 per cent new methylene blue solution in 0.85 per cent sodium chloride (NaCl) to which has been added 1 ml of formalin per 100 ml.

3. A 26 gauge Nichrome wire loop having an inside diameter of about 2 mm.

The film to be examined is prepared as follows: (1) using a clean, dry loop, transfer one loopful of stain to the coverglass. (2) Dry the loop completely, add one loop of blood, and mix blood and stain by a gentle circular movement of the loop. Do not attempt to spread the mixture over the coverslip. (3) Free the surface of the slide of dust and lint by blowing on it gently. Bring the coverslip with the mixture of blood and stain as close to the surface of the slide as possible; invert it and gently drop it onto the slide, permitting the blood film to spread between the glass surfaces. If large numbers of air bubbles occur or the film fails to spread under the entire area of the coverslip, the preparation should be discarded and a new one made. (4) Place the film under the high dry objective of the microscope, and examine it carefully.

Leukocyte nuclei stain intensely, and a rough estimate of the number of leukocytes can be obtained by computing the average number of cells seen in ten high power fields. More than 13 cells per field indicate a leukocytosis with a total leukocyte count above 20,000/μl. If the average number of leukocytes per field is less than two, a leukopenia is indicated.

Erythrocytes can also be observed in this manner.

Estimation of Total Leukocyte Count from a Stained Blood Film. This method of estimating leukocytes is based on three premises: (1) an animal with a normal PCV has an approximate erythrocyte count of 7 million RBC/μl. (2) In a normal animal there is approximately one leukocyte for every 1000 erythrocytes. Thus if there is one leukocyte for every 1000 erythrocytes the animal would have a total leukocyte count of 7000. (3) In the monolayer area of a blood film examined at 1000 (oil immersion) there are approximately 1000 erythrocytes in three oil immersion fields while at 400 (high dry) there are approximately 2000 erythrocytes per field.

A blood film should be prepared and stained as discussed later in the chapter. Total leukocytes can be estimated by a careful examination of a properly prepared blood film. This method of estimation is valid only for blood films in which leukocytes are evenly distributed.

Counting is done in the monolayer area of the blood film. The density of erythrocytes in this area should be such that individual cells are easily detectable and there are 20 to 22 red cells in the diameter of an oil immersion field or 50 to 55 red cells in the diameter of a high dry field. If the blood is from an anemic animal there may be fewer erythrocytes and with blood from an animal with very small erythrocytes there may be many more cells per diameter. In order to accommodate these discrepancies count the erythrocytes in several field diameters and calculate the average per field. If it is significantly different from 20 at oil immersion or 50 at high dry, the number of erythrocytes in a field can be calculated as follows: Using the average number of cells in a field diameter, divide by half to obtain the number of cells in the radius. Use the formula for the area of a circle substituting the number of cells in the radius for the length of the radius. This will give you the number of erythrocytes per field. For example, the monolayer area of a blood film from an anemic dog has an average of 16 red cells in one diameter. Thus the radius is 8 RBC. To determine the number of cells in a oil immersion field the following calculations are made:

$$3.14 \text{ (pi)} \times 8 \times 8 = 200$$
$$= \text{Number of RBC/oil immersion field}$$

Estimation of the total leukocyte count is completed as follows:

1. Count all of the leukocytes in 30 adjacent fields using the oil immersion objective or 10 fields if you are using the high dry objective.

2. Find the average number of leukocytes per 1000 erythrocytes. If you have used the oil immersion objective, divide the total leukocytes counted in 30 fields by 10. If you used the high dry objective, divide the total number of leukocytes counted by five.

3. Multiply the number of leukocytes per 1000 erythrocytes by 7000.

For example, using the oil immersion lens 30 leukocytes were counted in 30 adjacent fields of a monolayer of a blood film from a dog. Make your calculation as follows:

$$\frac{30}{10} = 3 \times 7000 = 21000$$

$$= \text{Estimated leukocyte count}$$

If the packed cell was normal this calculation is all that is needed. If the animal was anemic the count can be corrected by substituting the number of erythrocytes per field into the formula:

$$\frac{\text{Leukocytes counted}}{10}$$

$$\times \frac{\text{Calculated No. RBC/3 fields}}{\text{Normal No. RBC/3 fields}} \times 7000$$

$$= \text{Corrected WBC count}$$

In the example used we found that three fields contained 600 erythrocytes instead of the 1000 we would normally expect to find. Therefore we must adjust our count to account for this fact. Our calculations would be:

$$\frac{30}{10} = 3 \times \frac{600}{1000} = 1.8 \times 7000 = 12600$$

$$= \text{Corrected WBC count}$$

The estimated leukocyte count can also be corrected for anemia by using the observed packed cell volume and the normal packed cell volume for the species. The formula for this adjustment is:

$$\frac{\text{Observed PCV}}{\text{Normal PCV}} \times \text{Calculated count}$$

$$= \text{Corrected WBC count}$$

Thus, as in the example above, if the calculated leukocyte count is 21000, the observed PCV in the dog is 27 and the normal PCV is 45 our formula would be:

$$\frac{27}{45} = 0.6 \times 21000 = 12600$$

$$= \text{Corrected WBC count}$$

It must be remembered that this technique and the examination of a wet blood film stained with new methylene blue are only estimates intended to provide information relevant to marked changes in the total leukocyte count and cannot be substituted for more accurate laboratory counting methods. Borderline results should be treated as such and not read too closely. It would be wise to have these methods checked by a laboratory as a control.

THE BLOOD FILM

Examination of a smear of peripheral blood is one of the most informative laboratory procedures. It is of particular value to the practicing veterinarian in aiding diagnosis and prognosis of acute, generalized, and localized infections. Blood diseases such as leukemia can be diagnosed by examination of a blood smear, and information relative to the status of the erythrocytes and an associated anemia may also be obtained. Blood parasites such as eperythrozoa, trypanosomes, microfilaria, and *Anaplasma, Haemobartonella,* and *Babesia* organisms are demonstrated by use of a blood smear. Since the examination of blood is often made by practitioners, or in their laboratories, it is essential that satisfactory smears be made, as no degree of skill or diagnostic ability in the analysis of the results will compensate for a poorly made blood film.

The blood film should be made as soon as possible after collection of the specimen, as leukocytes and other cells have a tendency to degenerate rapidly. More time can elapse without interfering with results if EDTA is used as the anticoagulant, although bovine lymphocytes may be adversely affected by EDTA. Blood films prepared from bovine samples that are a few hours old often contain abnormal-appearing lymphocytes. When possible, films should be made from fresh blood containing no anticoagulants. Films of blood may be prepared either on a microscope slide or coverslip. For routine laboratory work, the microscope slide is preferable to the coverslip, which is not as practical owing to the difficulty of preparing the film. Coverslips are difficult to clean and store and have the disadvantage of being awkward to identify and file.

Cleanliness of slides is a "must" if adequate films are to be prepared. Precleaned slides are available commercially and are preferred but should be dipped in alcohol and dried with a lintless cloth prior to use. Care must be taken not to touch the surface of the slide, as deposition of grease left by fingers interferes with making the smear. Used slides should be left in water or a solution of mild detergent until they can be cleaned. Cleaning is best accomplished by boiling the dirty slides in a solution of Hemosol, Alconox, or sodium bicarbonate followed by scrubbing with a scouring powder or concentrated detergent. Slides should be rinsed thoroughly and allowed to stand in 95 per cent ethyl alcohol until used and dried carefully with a lintless cloth before use. Unless exceptionally large numbers of slides are used, it is better to use new slides for all blood smears.

In preparing the blood film, a precleaned slide should be placed on a flat surface or held by the edges between the forefinger and thumb with the little finger supporting the other end of the slide (Fig. 3–5). A small drop of blood is placed on one

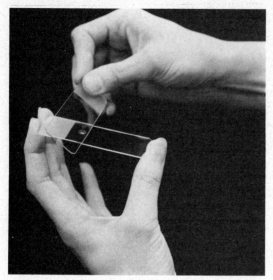

Figure 3–5. Preparation of a blood film using the long edge of a glass slide. The slide is pushed into the drop of blood and immediately after it contacts the blood is quickly pulled toward the operator.

end of the slide. This may be accomplished by use of an applicator stick, or if a microhematocrit determination is made, the capillary tube may be utilized to place a drop of blood on the slide. The tendency for the inexperienced operator is to use too large a drop of blood.

Immediately after placing blood on the slide the spreader should be grasped by its edges at one end. The spreader *must* be a slide with a perfectly smooth edge. The spreader slide is placed in front of the drop of blood at an angle of approximately 30 degrees and pushed back until it just touches the drop (Fig. 3–5). Care should be taken not to push the spreader back into the drop too far. As soon as the spreader touches the drop of blood, the blood spreads by capillary action along the edge of the spreader, which should immediately be pulled forward smoothly and quickly at an angle of about 30 degrees. If the spreader slide is pulled too rapidly, leukocytes will be concentrated on the edges or near the end of the film. Proper speed is gained only by experience. No pressure should be applied to the spreader, as its weight is sufficient. The angle at which the spreader is pulled influences the thickness of the blood smear: the greater the angle the thicker and shorter the film, and the smaller the angle the thinner and longer the smear.

The slide should be waved in the air to dry and identified by writing either the identifying number or the owner's name on the thick end of the blood film with a pencil or with the edge of the spreader slide. This method has the advantage that the marking is neither destroyed by chemicals, nor easily rubbed off the slide as is the case with some other marking methods. If the slide is

not stained immediately, it should be fixed in alcohol and placed in a slide box and covered or wrapped in paper for protection.

Some laboratory workers prefer to make the smear while the slide is resting on the smooth surface of a table top; however, this is often impossible in the field, and veterinarians should learn to make the blood film in their hands for the sake of convenience.

A good blood film should be thick at one end and thin and feathered at the other. The edge of the film should be at least 2 mm from the slide edge. The film should have a smooth, even appearance and should be free from holes. Holes indicate the presence of grease on the slide, and long streamers at the end of the smear are usually caused by dirty or chipped spreaders. A wavy film is due to jerky movements as the blood is pushed along in front of the spreader.

One should avoid blowing on the slide or placing it near a radiator or sink or in an area where steam might reach the slide. Hemolysis of the erythrocytes is likely to occur if the slide is exposed to water vapor.

Coverslip preparations are desired if a careful examination of the cellular characteristics is required. Coverslip preparations are superior because leukocytes are better distributed, there are usually more suitable fields for examination, there are more leukocytes per field than with the slide method, and there is generally better cell definition.

Coverslips to be used for blood films should be carefully cleaned and stored in 95 per cent ethyl alcohol and dried with a lintless soft cloth immediately before use. Square coverglasses 22 by 22 mm of No. 1 thinness are used. Holding the clean, dry coverslip by its edges in one hand, place a small drop of blood on the center of the slide. The drop should be small enough so that on spreading, it will not reach the edges of the coverglass. Place a second clean, dry coverglass diagonally on the first, forming an eight-pointed star; the blood will immediately spread by capillary action (Fig. 3–6). Grasp the top coverglass by its corners and using a smooth motion slide the two apart. Wave the coverglasses in the air to enhance drying. The coverslips should be identified by placement in a small box with the name of the owner or number of the case on it.

Staining the Blood Smear. Several stains and staining techniques can be used. Most are of the Romanowsky type, incorporating basic and acid aniline dyes that bring out the contrasting colors red and blue. The best known and most widely used stains of this type are Wright and Giemsa stains. Both these stains are available in a powder form and can be purchased in a liquid form from most laboratory supply companies. Stock stains purchased in a liquid form must be stored in tightly stoppered bottles and dispensed into smaller dropper bottles for routine laboratory use.

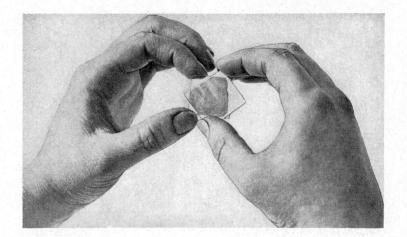

Figure 3–6. Coverslip preparation of blood film. (From Davidsohn, I., and Henry, J. B.: *Todd-Sanford Clinical Diagnosis by Laboratory Methods*, 15th Ed., Philadelphia, W. B. Saunders, 1974.)

Exposure to air will cause evaporation of the methyl alcohol, resulting in precipitation of stain particles.

Wright's stain may be utilized in the conventional manner or in a dip technique. Methods for preparation and use of Wright's stain are presented in the Appendix.

A Wright-Leishman stain[1] has proved to be an excellent stain for routine use in the laboratory (see Appendix for formula and staining method).

Commercial dip technique stains that are generally acceptable for routine use are available. In these stains, the blue and red stains are separated, and the film is dipped alternately into each solution. Such stains have been used by students in our laboratory for several years, and the results have been generally good. These techniques might be criticized for lack of clarity in staining cytoplasmic granules and giving a slightly muddy look to the nucleus. However, the ease of use and speed with which a slide can be stained tend to overbalance these minor defects.

Unfixed dry blood films can be stained with new methylene blue. This provides a method ideally suited for rapid estimations of a leukocyte differential count. A blood film is prepared as described earlier and new methylene blue stain consisting of 0.5 per cent new methylene blue in 0.85 per cent saline to which 1 ml of formalin has been added as a preservative is utilized. A large drop of stain is applied to a clean, dry coverglass that is inverted and carefully dropped on the feathered end of the dry blood film. Both slide and coverglass should be dust- and lint-free in order to permit stain to spread evenly over the blood. This is not a permanent preparation and should be examined as soon as possible. The specimen can be preserved for a longer time if the coverglass is ringed with petrolatum (Vaseline) or immersion oil to prevent evaporation of the staining solution. Such a preparation can be retained for several hours. This staining technique is not limited to blood films but can be used for cytologic examinations and examinations of other types of direct smears, as will be discussed later.

Only material containing nucleic acids will take on the dark color. Mature erythrocytes do not stain but appear in outline form. The nuclei of leukocytes are readily seen, as are nuclei of immature erythrocytes, Howell-Jolly bodies in erythrocytes, and the reticulum of reticulocytes. Erythrocyte parasites such as *Babesia*, *Anaplasma*, *Trypanosoma*, and *Haemobartonella* are readily demonstrated. Heinz bodies are visible when present in erythrocytes.

Leukocyte nuclei stain intensely, and characteristic shapes can easily be observed. Although cytoplasmic granules do not stain, eosinophils can be identified by the granules, which appear as refractile structures. Basophils from the horse and the cow stain intensely, but the basophil of the dog is seldom detected with the new methylene blue stain.[1] There may be some difficulty in distinguishing metamyelocyte neutrophils from monocytes, especially when the cytoplasm of the metamyelocyte is basophilic as a consequence of toxic effects resulting from disease. The various cytoplasmic manifestations of toxicity are readily demonstrable in new methylene blue–stained preparations from cat blood.

Thrombocytes can also be demonstrated, appearing as small, rounded structures of varying sizes and staining pale lavender.

Reticulocytes stain readily and are identified by the presence of dark-staining reticulum within erythrocytes.

Special Blood Stains. Staining and counting reticulocytes may be an adjunct to diagnosis and prognosis. Since this cell represents a more immature form of erythrocyte, its presence in peripheral blood is of importance in assessing bone marrow response.

Several techniques for the demonstration of reticulocytes have been described and are of value. The method most commonly used in this laboratory is presented in the Appendix, pp. 434–436.

If reticulocytes are present in peripheral blood, they appear as erythrocytes containing a granulo-reticular-filamentous network that stains baso-philically with the supravital techniques usually used. Reticulocytes are usually larger than mature erythrocytes.

Reticulocytes may also be enumerated by use of a properly stained wet blood film. This technique, which was described earlier in the chapter, is also useful in determination of other alterations in blood, including anemia, leukopenia, leuko-cytosis, thrombocytopenia, erythrocyte aggluti-nation, and abnormal morphology of the erythro-cytes and in the demonstration of certain blood parasites. The wet blood film staining method is of limited value in determining minor variations, but the more obvious pathologic alterations are apparent.

Two other special stains occasionally employed are oxidase and alkaline phosphatase stains, which are used principally in detecting or iden-tifying certain types of leukemic cells.

Examination of Stained Smear. Although some individuals examine a stained blood smear under high dry magnification of the microscope, it is advisable to use the oil immersion objective if accurate cell identification and careful study of abnormal blood cells are indicated. Irrespective of the magnification, the examination should start at the thin end of the smear, and a systematic meander of the slide should be made. If such a system of examination is used, a recount of the same field is avoided. Fields selected for exami-nation should be those in which erythrocytes are well separated and the leukocytes thinly spread. Avoid fields in which the erythrocytes are stacked up or in rouleaux. Accurate identification of leu-kocytes in the thick portion of the smear is dif-ficult, as cells are smaller and less readily iden-tified. Care should be taken when using the meander system to examine the edges of the smear as well as other areas. One meander system that has been found to be excellent is presented in Fig-ure 3–7.

As cells are identified a record should be made and the presence of abnormal cells noted. If a sin-gle unit tally counter is used as an aid in recording the number of cells, the following technique has proved adequate. Record each individual cell type on a piece of scratch paper, ignoring the seg-mented neutrophils. When a total of 100 cells has been counted, as indicated on the tally counter,

the number of segmented neutrophils may be de-termined by subtracting the sum of all other cells from 100. A multiple unit tally counter is helpful in recording results, as it eliminates the need for a tally mark to identify each cell.

In almost all blood smears there are a few dis-torted, degenerated, and atypical cells that cannot be classified accurately. If few such cells are pres-ent, they should be classified simply as atypical. However, if these cells appear to be immature or abnormal forms of leukocytes, a note should be made of them. At the end of the differential count the operator can state that these abnormalities exist and should be able to estimate the approx-imate percentage of cells having these abnormal features.

The minimum number of leukocytes counted in arriving at the differential count is 100. For greater accuracy 200 or more cells should be enumerated. It has been suggested that 100 cells should be clas-sified on the differential count for every 10,000 total leukocytes.

One common error encountered in differential examinations is failure by the operator to observe the characteristics of the erythrocytes and the number and nature of the thrombocytes. A search should be made for the presence of stippled eryth-rocytes, diffuse basophilia, and other erythrocytic abnormalities. In case of an anemia, the smear should be carefully examined for the presence of blood parasites. If nucleated erythrocytes are pres-ent, they should be classified according to the stage of development and enumerated in relation to the number of leukocytes examined. In the ex-amination of peripheral blood smears, nucleated erythrocytes are reported as the number observed in relation to 100 leukocytes.

DESCRIPTION OF CELLS IN PERIPHERAL BLOOD

The description of cells present in bone marrow (Chapter 4) applies to cells of the peripheral blood. There are certain characteristics of the leu-kocytes of various species of domestic animals that warrant discussion here.

Canine. Various types of canine leukocytes are shown in Plate 3–1.

Canine segmented neutrophils have an irregu-larly lobed nucleus without the true formation of

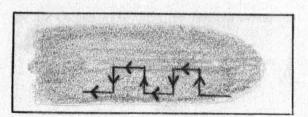

Figure 3–7. Meander system for examining stained blood film. This will ensure that all areas of the slide are examined.

filaments connecting the lobes. The majority of the segmented cells are lobated by a narrowing of the nucleus between lobes, although occasionally a true filament may be seen. In the female dog a small nuclear sex bud may be observed. The nuclear membrane is often irregular, the cytoplasm stains a faint pinkish-gray, and the granules appear as fine, dust-like particles. Toxic granules, such as these occurring in humans and cattle, rarely appear, but the toxic neutrophil has an irregular, foamy, vacuolated gray-blue cytoplasm and is enlarged. Holding blood in EDTA may alter the morphology of some neutrophils.[6] In healthy dogs a few discrete, clear cytoplasmic vacuoles may appear within three hours and vacuolation reaches a maximum at 24 hours. The cytoplasm of these cells is not basophilic and the foamy vacuolation typical of a toxic neutrophil does not appear. A few hypersegmented neutrophils may appear if circulation time is increased. Such cells are observed in dogs with excess glucocorticoids (endogenous or exogenous) and occasionally in association with chronic suppurative infections.

The severity of degenerative changes in neutrophils is usually qualitative; evaluations on the same blood smear by different technologists will often vary. A protocol that permits a more uniform evaluation has been developed.[7] The severity of degenerative changes is graded as follows: 1+ = cytoplasmic basophilia or presence of Döhle bodies; 2+ = muddy cytoplasm; 3+ = toxic neutrophils with foamy basophilic cytoplasm; and 4+ = indistinct nuclear membrane, karyolysis, or giant degenerated nonsegmented neutrophils. The number of cells with degenerative changes is reported as: few = 5 to 10 per cent; moderate = 11 to 30 per cent; and many = more than 30 per cent.[7] The clinician must be careful in judging reports of cell toxicity as not all laboratories use this method for assessment of toxic neutrophils. The laboratory should be contacted to determine if it has adopted this method for rating toxicity. If not, it should be encouraged to do so as this method will make report evaluation more constant.

The band neutrophil is seen in the peripheral blood only in small numbers in health but may appear in response to infectious or inflammatory conditions. The nucleus of this cell is a curved band with a smooth nuclear membrane. The nucleus may occasionally appear in the shape of an S. The sides of the nucleus are parallel, and the chromatin is less dense than in the mature segmented neutrophil and consequently is less intense in color. The pale gray cytoplasm contains pale-staining neutrophilic granules. If the nuclear membrane is irregular or nuclear indentation occurs the cell should be classified as a segmenter.

The canine eosinophil may be overlooked in making a differential leukocyte count, as it contains varying numbers of eosinophilic-staining granules that are irregular in size, shape, and staining characteristics. All granules in a single cell may be small and regular in shape, or there may be only one to three large, irregularly shaped granules. In general, eosinophilic granules stain lightly, and all granulocytes should be carefully inspected, as it is easy to miss these cells if a rapid examination is conducted. Occasionally, eosinophilic granules may appear to be vacuolated. This is particularly true in the adult greyhound, in which vacuoles predominate.

Basophils contain granules that vary in number, size, and color. Most basophils have numerous granules that are definitely basophilic although in some cells the granules are gray. If slides are overwashed, granules may be removed and the cell confused with a vacuolated monocyte.

Canine lymphocytes are commonly of the small type with a narrow rim of slightly basophilic cytoplasm, and have an eccentrically located nucleus containing clumped chromatin that stains intensely. Antigenic stimulation may alter the appearance of a lymphocyte. The cytoplasm becomes more intensely basophilic, whereas the nucleus is unchanged and retains its characteristic staining qualities. Azurophilic granules occur occasionally but when present are small and few in number.

The monocyte in the dog is characterized by its size, frequently being the largest cell in peripheral blood. The cytoplasm is basophilic and has a light blue, ground-glass appearance. In some cells, very small dust-like, pinkish granules may be observed in the cytoplasm. Cytoplasmic vacuoles are frequently seen, and occasionally one will be observed in the nucleus. The nucleus is extremely variable and can assume a number of different shapes. At times the nucleus will have an appearance similar to that of a band neutrophil or a metamyelocyte. Most immature neutrophils have a relatively colorless cytoplasm in comparison to the slightly basophilic cytoplasm of the monocyte. If there is systemic toxemia, mature and immature neutrophils have a basophilic cytoplasm and may be difficult to differentiate from monocytes. The nuclear chromatin pattern of the monocyte is characteristically diffuse and lacy. Heavy chromatin condensation occurs infrequently, which assists in differentiating the monocyte from the neutrophil. Nuclear folds can sometimes be detected and are characteristic of this cell.

Feline. Various types of feline leukocytes are shown in Plate 3–1.

Feline segmented neutrophils are similar to those of the canine, having an irregular nuclear membrane with only occasional cells having distinct filament formation. Small sex buds are sometimes present in the nucleus of neutrophil from the female. Granulation in the cytoplasm is indistinct, but occasionally small, dark-staining granules may be seen singly or in larger numbers.

The eosinophil has rod-shaped granules that may partially cover the nucleus.

The basophil of the cat, unlike that of other an-

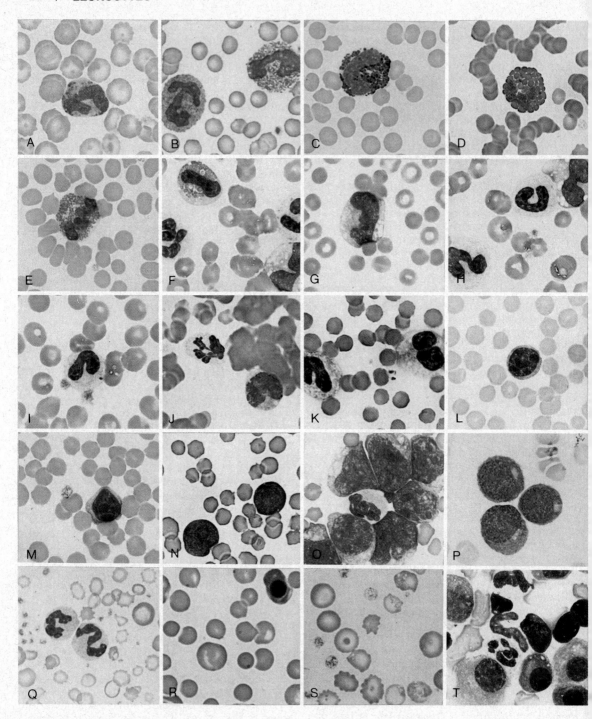

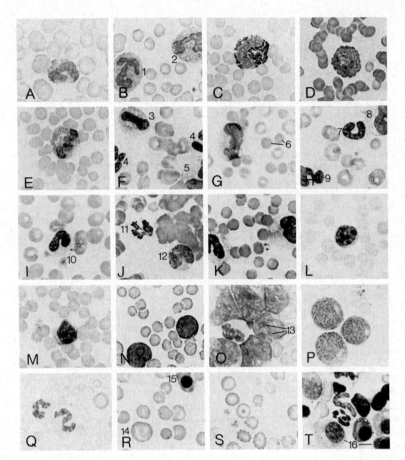

Plate 3–1   Key

A. Basophil—dog. Some dog basophils contain characteristic dark-staining granules while others, like this one, contain only a few granules that stain less intensely.

B. Cat blood. (1) Basophil with its characteristic pale-staining granules. (2) Eosinophil with rod-shaped granules.

C. Basophil—horse. The granules stain intensely, and are small and variably shaped.

D. Eosinophil—horse. Note the rouleaux formation of the erythrocytes. This is characteristic of horse blood.

E. Eosinophil—cow. The granules are very small and stain intensely.

F. Dog blood. (3) Eosinophil with pale-staining granules and a vacuolated cytoplasm. (4) Neutrophils. Note the larger granules (Dohle bodies) in the cytoplasm of these cells. (5) Monocyte with cytoplasmic vacuoles.

G. Dog blood. A monocyte with its pale blue vacuolated cytoplasm. Note the spherocytic erythrocytes (6). Spherocytes are commonly observed in immune-mediated anemias. They are small and stain more intensely than normal erythrocytes.

H. Dog blood. (7) Band neutrophil. (8) Monocyte. (9) Segmented neutrophil.

I. Band neutrophil. Notice the one dark-staining body in the cytoplasm and the thrombocytes (10).

J. Horse blood. (11) Segmented neutrophil. The nuclear membranes of horse neutrophils often have a jagged appearance. (12) Monocyte.

K. Dog blood. Two very toxic neutrophils. The cytoplasm appears foamy and the granules are darker than normal.

L. Cow blood—typical small lymphocyte.

M. Cow blood—lymphocyte with more cytoplasm.

N. Two reactive (antigen-stimulated) lymphocytes.

O. Lymphosarcoma—cow. The lymphocytes are abnormal and contain many distinct nucleoli (13).

P. Cat with myeloproliferative diseases. These are very immature cells.

Q. Pig blood. Note the hypochromia of most of the erythrocytes. There is some anisocytosis (size variation) and some poikilocytes are present. Note the clump of thrombocytes to the left of the neutrophils.

R. Regenerative anemia. Note the anisocytosis and the polychromatic erythrocyte at 14. The cell at 15 is a metarubricyte.

S. Poikilocytosis with many abnormally shaped erythrocytes including a typical target cell.

T. Bone marrow from a dog with an IgA myeloma. There are several plasma cells (16).

imal species, does not have intensely staining granules. Mature basophils are characterized by the presence of large numbers of oval, lavender to pale pinkish granules with an occasional larger dark granule. Unless care is taken in completing a differential count, these cells can be easily mistaken for eosinophils or vacuolated neutrophils.

Lymphocytes are usually of the small type with a round to bean-shaped nucleus containing uniformly dispersed chromatin. There is very little blue-staining cytoplasm, which has a tendency to form a perinuclear halo. Azurophilic granules are sometimes present in the cytoplasm.

Unlike in the dog, granulation of the cytoplasm of the monocyte is seldom observed, but vacuolation is fairly common and the cytoplasm is grayish. The nucleus of the monocyte is typically lacy in appearance, and folding of the nucleus is observed only occasionally. Monocytes can be differentiated from toxic neutrophils by their irregular nuclear membranes as compared to the smooth membranes usually seen in immature neutrophils.

Bovine. Bovine neutrophils of the mature type frequently have filaments connecting the lobes, although many segmented neutrophils are identified only by an indentation of the nucleus. The nuclear membrane has a tendency to be smooth, although irregular nuclear membranes may be observed. The cytoplasm is indistinctly granular and more often appears as a homogeneous pale pink color. Toxic neutrophils, particularly the bands and metamyelocytes, have a basophilic cytoplasm and frequently have reddish granules. Occasionally, dark-staining, irregular granules may be present.

The nucleus of the band neutrophil is fat and curved with widely dispersed chromatin clumps and a pale-staining cytoplasm.

Eosinophils of the bovine are filled with small, intensely staining, round, regular granules that completely fill the cytoplasm to the extent that the gray-staining cytoplasm is seldom observed. Eosinophils usually have a two-lobed or band-shaped nucleus. (See Plate 3–1.)

Bovine basophils contain numerous dark-staining granules that completely fill the cytoplasm and cover the nucleus. Thus, the basophil may occur as a dark-staining mass, and the nucleus may not be visible. This cell is infrequently seen in the peripheral blood of the cow.

Lymphocytes of the cow vary in size, and one smear may have all sizes from small to large. Small lymphocytes have an intensely staining, almost pyknotic nucleus with very little blue-staining cytoplasm. A large lymphocyte may be confused with the monocyte, as its nucleus is rather pale-staining. Some large lymphocytes may have a deeply indented nucleus or one that appears folded. Aging of bovine blood after collection seems to enhance the development of such cells.

Occasionally the nucleus will have such a deep cleft that the cell appears binucleate. These are referred to as Reider type cells and are most frequently seen in lymphocytic leukemia. Azurophilic granules are often present in the cytoplasm and vary in size and shape, some being rod-shaped, others oval, and some round.

Monocytes are variable in size, have an irregular nucleus sometimes in the shape of a cloverleaf but more commonly folded and lacy in appearance. The cytoplasm is blue and granular. Occasionally the cytoplasm may be foamy and filled with vacuoles of varying size.

Ovine. Ovine neutrophils frequently have a distinctly multi-lobed nucleus with typical chromatin clumping and distinct filaments connecting the lobes. The cytoplasm is faintly staining and contains a few very small granules throughout. Characteristically, a few darker and larger cytoplasmic granules may be present.

The nucleus of the band neutrophil is usually U-shaped and relatively thick. Chromatin clumping is less intense than in the mature neutrophil, and the cytoplasm may be slightly basophilic. Basophilia of the cytoplasm of a band cell may be an indication of a maturation defect and is consequently associated with toxemia.

Eosinophils of the ovine stain orange-red and are ovoid, uniform in size, and refractile. The granules are numerous in the cytoplasm, frequently filling it so that the usual pale-blue–staining cytoplasm is not visible.

The basophil typically contains a varying number of dark granules with halos. Ovine lymphocytes vary in size, but the range of variation is less than that seen in the bovine. The nuclear chromatin has a relatively smooth appearance and on occasion may have a reddish cast. The cytoplasm stains blue, and a perinuclear halo is sometimes seen. Azurophilic granules may or may not be present. The ovine monocyte is characteristic for this cell type, having a lacy nucleus and an ameboid shape.

Caprine. Mature neutrophils in the goat are less lobated than in the sheep, and the nuclear membrane is irregular. The cytoplasm is similar to that found in other ruminants, and distinct granules are seen only rarely.

The eosinophil of the goat usually has a band-shaped nucleus, although occasionally there may be sufficient indentation to give a true lobed appearance. The granules are small, round, and distinctly eosinophilic, completely filling the cytoplasm.

Basophils from goat blood have dark-staining granules that completely fill the cytoplasm and push the nucleus to one side. Lymphocytes resemble those of other ruminant animals. Monocytes are also characteristic, frequently containing cytoplasmic vacuoles and small azurophilic cytoplasmic granules.

Equine. Equine segmented neutrophils have a nuclear chromatin arrangement characterized by the presence of dark-staining plaques that may make the nucleus appear almost granular. This results in an irregular nuclear membrane. Small pinkish granules are present in the cytoplasm, which in animals with toxemia is frequently basophilic and may contain darker-staining toxic granules.

Because of the same plaquing of the nuclear chromatin, the band neutrophil has a jagged edge and can be mistaken for a mature cell unless care is taken in examination of the blood film. The band neutrophil can be distinguished from the mature cell by its lack of definite indentation and the thickness of the nucleus.

The distinguishing feature of the eosinophil of the horse is the presence of large, round, irregular-sized granules that stain orange-red. The eosinophil is usually tightly packed with these granules to the extent that it causes an irregular bulging of the cytoplasm, as if the cell were filled with oranges (Plate 3–1).

The horse basophil contains dark-staining granules that are irregular in shape with some being round to oval and others rod-shaped. The number of granules varies; in some cells there are a few widely scattered granules, and in others the granules fill the cytoplasm and almost cover the nucleus.

The majority of lymphocytes are of the small type with a small amount of cytoplasm and a dark-staining nucleus. Occasionally larger lymphocytes may be observed. Azurophilic granules sometimes occur and are few in number in a single cell.

The nucleus of the monocyte is most commonly bean-shaped and not often folded. As with monocytes of the blood of other animal species, the nucleus has a lacy appearance and stains poorly. The cytoplasm has fine pinpoint granulation throughout. The granules stain pink.

Porcine. Porcine neutrophils are characterized by an irregularly but intensely staining nucleus that seldom has filaments. The nuclear outline is irregular, and the nucleus is often coiled, making positive identification difficult. The cytoplasm is filled with small granules that take a pink stain.

Eosinophils have round to ovoid granules that stain orange and completely fill the cytoplasm of the cell. The nucleus is commonly of the band type. Basophil granules stain darkly and are coccoid- to dumbbell-shaped.

Lymphocytes of the pig are similar to those found in other species of domestic animals. Azurophilic granules are occasionally present. They are of small size and usually located on the periphery of the cell.

The nucleus of the monocyte is folded and convoluted with a lacy chromatin arrangement. Granulation of the cytoplasm is not obvious.

KINETICS AND FUNCTIONS OF LEUKOCYTES

Accurate interpretation of leukocyte counts is dependent upon an understanding of the functions of and the kinetics associated with the various types of leukocytes.

Granulocytes. Under normal conditions, granulocytopoiesis is a cell renewal system in which cell production equals cell death. Granulocytopoiesis normally progresses in an orderly fashion from the blast cell to the mature granulocyte, which makes morphologic identification of cellular compartments relatively easy. Granulocytes are produced in the bone marrow and subsequently released into the peripheral blood, from which they migrate into the tissues in which they have their principal functions. Specific cellular compartments can be identified in the bone marrow and peripheral blood.

Bone marrow compartments include: (1) stem cell pool; (2) differential proliferating pool of myeloblasts, progranulocytes, and myelocytes; and (3) a nonproliferating (maturation) pool that consists of metamyelocytes, band cells, and mature segmented granulocytes.

Each compartment has several characteristics that are related to the ability of the body to respond to a stimulation requiring production and mobilization of granulocytes. The stem cell pool must be able to (1) maintain itself against continual removal of cells into the differential proliferating pool, (2) reconstitute itself if depletion occurs, and (3) increase cell production upon demand. The differential proliferating pool, however, is not self-sustaining. This pool consists of many large and small myelocytes, the larger cells forming a dividing pool that supplies cells to the small cell or maturation pool. It is not known whether small myelocytes continue to divide, or whether they mature and enter the next compartment. Myelocytes play a key role in granulocyte production, as it is generally believed that such production is expanded by an increase in the number of myelocytic divisions and possibly by shortening of generation time.

The nonproliferating or maturation pool, like the differential proliferating pool, is not self-sustaining. However, it differs from the differential proliferating pool in that there is no DNA synthesis in this compartment. Although there is no cell division, biochemical and morphologic changes occur in both the nucleus and cytoplasm of granulocytes. Morphologic changes are characterized by a progressive nuclear condensation and concomitant gross changes in the cytoplasm, particularly in the appearance of granules. Upon completion of maturation, granulocytes enter the granulocyte reserve of the bone marrow. Release of cells from this compartment is a function of the utilization rate of granulocytes.

When granulocytes enter the peripheral circulation, they immediately equilibrate between the circulating granulocyte pool (CGP) and the marginal granulocyte pool (MGP). Combined, these two pools are referred to as the total blood granulocyte pool (TBGP). The marginal pool consists of those granulocytes that marginate along and adhere to walls of small vessels throughout the body. These cells constitute an additional reserve that can be readily and quickly released into the circulating granulocyte pool when stimulated to do so by physiologic or pathologic alterations. The marginal granulocyte pool is not a static accumulation of cells; rather, there is rapid and continual exchange between the cirulating granulocyte pool and the marginal granulocyte pool. Cells are removed from the marginal granulocyte pool to the circulating granulocyte pool as a consequence of physiologic activities, such as exercise, or by a sudden release of epinephrine producing a physiologic leukocytosis or a pseudoleukocytosis. The same phenomenon may occur whenever the rate of blood flow increases.

Granulocytes are removed from the TBGP in a random fashion and at a single exponential rate. Most neutrophil loss in the healthy animal occurs in the digestive and respiratory tracts. In the normal animal there is no appreciable tissue pool of granulocytes, and there is no return of granulocytes from tissues to the bloodstream. In event of an increased demand, the large pool of cells in bone marrow serves as a reserve from which cells can be rapidly obtained.

The proliferation of granulocytes is controlled by a family of glycoprotein hormones that stimulate granulopoiesis. These hormones are designated colony-stimulating activity (CSA). Production of CSA is by the monocyte-macrophage and activated T lymphocytes. Blood monocytes as well as tissue macrophages in the lungs, liver, and peritoneum produce CSA. Intense antigenic stimulation may stimulate granulopoiesis and monocytopoiesis through the interaction of T lymphocytes and the production of CSA. The proliferation of granulocytes and mononuclear phagocytes is closely related.

It has also been postulated that there is a specific feedback inhibitor produced by mature granulocytes that affects leukopoiesis. Mobilizing factors responsible for release of granulocytes into the peripheral circulation have also been postulated. Leukotaxine, a polypeptide from inflammatory exudate, has been found to increase capillary permeability and will induce local migration of granulocytes. The existence of a leukocytosis-inducing factor has also been postulated.

The amount of time required for granulocytes to appear in the peripheral circulation seems to vary according to animal species. In all animals, activation and removal of cells from the marginal granulocytic pool are instantaneous. Release from the bone marrow pool may occur in as little as 15 minutes, and two or three times the number of cells in the circulating pool may be mobilized in one hour. It has been estimated that eight to 10 times the number of cells in the circulating pool can be released in six to seven hours. If the bone marrow reserve pool cannot supply the demand of the tissues, it may require two to three days, or perhaps longer in some animals, to make up the depletion of that reserve. It has been estimated that a maturation time of approximately six days is required for the bovine neutrophil.

Only relatively mature granulocytes (segmented and band cells) are normally released from the bone marrow. Occasionally, metamyelocytes are found in the peripheral circulation. However, they are usually present in small numbers and may indicate depletion of the storage pool if present in large numbers.

In tissues, the principal function of the neutrophilic granulocyte is phagocytosis of small particles. This function is primarily that of the mature segmented neutrophil, although metamyelocyte and band neutrophils have some phagocytic ability. Neutrophils are associated with inflammatory conditions and are found in large numbers in tissues infected with pyogenic microorganisms such as staphylococci, streptococci, and corynebacteria. In addition to their phagocytic capabilities, neutrophils elaborate powerful proteolytic enzymes that react within the cell to destroy phagocytosed particles or may be liberated and function outside the cell body.

Eosinophils primarily function as detoxifiers. Eosinophilic granules have an affinity for histamines and are therefore capable of removing these chemicals from tissues. They are mostly commonly encountered in the epithelial lining of the intestinal and respiratory tracts where they are also thought to function as detoxifiers. Eosinophils are mobilized at the site of antigen-antibody reactions in response to mediators released from mast cells and basophils. This mobilization is accompanied by an increase in the number of eosinophils in the blood.

The precise function of the basophil has not been delineated, although it is known that the granules contain heparin, histamine, a chemotactic factor for eosinophils, and a platelet-activating factor. It has also been suggested that the basophil may function in promoting the clearing of fat from the plasma. Basophils are important in initiating inflammation as they degranulate in response to activated complement factors, allergens, and particularly if IgE molecules are attached to their cell membrane. Mediators released activate platelets, attract eosinophils, cause smooth muscle contraction, initiate edema formation, and may affect coagulation. Mast cells function in a similar manner.

Lymphocytes. The sequence of development of lymphocytes is classically the same as that of other leukocytes. It begins as a stem cell, progresses from a lymphoblast through the prolymphocyte stage to the final development of the mature cell. The mature cell may be designated as either a large or small lymphocyte. Although all small lymphocytes appear to be identical morphologically, they are, in fact, different cells with different origins and physiologic functions. The original stem cell for the lymphocyte remains unknown, but it has long been thought to be the reticulum cell. It has been demonstrated that in mature animals lymphocytes can differentiate from reticuloendothelial cells, whereas in the embryo the lymphocyte comes from a bone marrow precursor.

In most species of animals, after birth the thymus is the most active lymphopoietic tissue in the body, having a mitotic rate five to 10 times that of other lymphoid tissue. Formation of lymphocytes in the thymus is independent of immunologic stimuli. In fetal and early postnatal life the thymus seeds lymphocytes to the lymph nodes and spleen. Two distinct populations of lymphocytes have been demonstrated in the thymus: those that are short-lived and stationary and those that are long-lived and appear to migrate. In the adult animal, peripheral lymphoid organs, such as the spleen, lymph nodes, and lymphoid structures related to the intestinal tract, appear to be responsible for a majority of lymphocytes. However, lymphopoiesis continues to occur in the bone marrow independently of antigen stimulation. The majority of the cells produced in the bone marrow are distributed by the blood to peripheral lymphoid organs.

The life span of lymphocytes varies from three to four days to some that have an extended life span. In man, it has been estimated that some lymphocytes may survive for up to 20 years. Distribution of long- and short-lived lymphocytes in the animal body varies. Those in the thoracic duct are mostly of the long-lived variety, whereas those in the bone marrow are short-lived. In the peripheral lymphoid tissues, many in the thymus-dependent areas are long-lived, whereas those appearing in follicles and in the medulla of lymphoid organs are of the short-lived variety. In the bloodstream both types can be demonstrated.

Lymphocytes in the animal body are constantly in a state of circulation and recirculation. Thoracic duct lymphocytes recirculate from the blood via postcapillary venules into lymph nodes and efferent lymphatics back into the thoracic duct. Recirculation occurs at a relatively constant rate so that the numbers of lymphocytes entering and leaving the blood are approximately equal, and the number in the blood remains fairly constant in the healthy animal. Because of this constant recirculation and the fact that there are populations of lymphocytes with different life spans, it is not possible to determine precisely the total number of lymphocytes in an animal body at any

given time. Little definitive information is known concerning the factors controlling growth and distribution of lymphoid masses. The most important single determinant of overall size of lymphoid organs is the degree of immunologic stimulation to which they are subjected. The factors regulating blood lymphocyte levels are also largely unknown, although antigen stimulation may result in an outpouring of reactive lymphocytes from lymphoid tissues. This is a transient phenomenon and not frequently observed as a clinical entity. It is also known that stress reduces the number of lymphocytes in blood, suggesting that there may be an adrenocortical regulating mechanism that appears primarily to affect the short-lived cells.

The principal function of the lymphocyte is its immunologic activity. Following exposure to an antigen the cellular events can be divided into stages of proliferation and differentiation. In terms of their response to the antigen, the thymus-dependent cells (T cells), which rely on the thymus gland for their maintenance and reactivity, are primarily responsible for the cell-mediated response of the animal. The bursa-dependent (chicken) or the equivalent of bursa-dependent (mammal) cells (B cells) are precursors for antibody-producing cells.

In addition to their function in the immunologic response of the body, it has been postulated that lymphocytes may perform a role in contributing essential metabolites to other proliferating cells. It has also been suggested that the lymphocyte may serve as a hematopoietic stem cell. At one time it was thought that lymphocytes might be precursors for monocytes and macrophages, but this hypothesis has been disproved.

Monocytes. Monocytes arise predominantly, if not exclusively, in the bone marrow from a system of progenerators that are comparable in behavior with those of other blood cells. The monocyte migrates into tissues and becomes a macrophage. Monocytes play an important role in inflammation as they contain or secrete numerous biologically active substances including proteolytic enzymes, interferon, interleukin 1, complement components, prostaglandins, and carrier proteins, to name a few. In such areas the primary function of the monocyte is phagocytosis. These cells play an important role in antigen processing. They also have the capacity to ingest and remove large particles of cellular debris that accumulate in tissues.

INTERPRETATION OF LEUKOCYTE COUNTS

Accurate interpretation of leukocyte alterations is dependent upon an understanding of the various factors that influence total and differential leukocyte counts in both healthy and diseased animals. Physiologic factors to be considered in the interpretation of leukocyte counts include:

1. Age of animal.
2. Breed or species of animal.
3. Degree of excitement and muscular activity exhibited by the patient at the time the blood was drawn.
4. Stage of pregnancy.
5. Stage of estrus.
6. Stage of digestion.

The age of an animal may influence both total and differential leukocyte counts. In general, the total leukocyte count in the dog and calf is high at birth. In young pigs the leukocyte count is low. In addition, young animals may have a differential count that varies from that normally found in the adult. The total lymphocyte count is greater in the young dog that in the adult. The blood of the young pig and calf has fewer lymphocytes than that of the adult.

Species variation is marked, ranging from a predominance of lymphocytes in bovine blood to a preponderance of segmented neutrophils in canine blood. An understanding of these variations is essential if an accurate interpretation is to be rendered. It is impossible to apply a single set of standards to fit blood alterations in all animal species.

Muscular exercise and apprehension influence total and differential leukocyte counts. A blood sample from an animal that has been subjected to excessive exercise or one that has become emotionally disturbed by restraint is not representative of the true state of the leukocytes in that individual. If in the process of blood sample collection the animal is mishandled or caused to exercise violently, as often occurs when restraint of an animal is attempted, the total leukocyte count may be increased, and the number of neutrophils will be greater than normal as cells move from the MGP into the CGP.

In some animals (cow, dog), pregnancy may influence the leukocyte picture. Approximately 75 per cent of cows have an increased leukocyte count in the later stages of pregnancy, and in dogs a similar increase occurs near term.

Limited changes have been reported to occur in the bovine in connection with estrus. Cows have a slight increase in both total leukocyte and neutrophil counts on the day of heat and the first day thereafter.

The stage of digestion apparently influences the total leukocyte and neutrophil counts in the dog, has a minimal effect in the horse, and exerts no influence in ruminants. Total leukocytes and neutrophils increase about an hour after eating. In the pig this change may be dramatic, with an increase in total count up to 5000/μl within $1\frac{3}{4}$ hours after a meal.

Absolute vs. Relative Leukocyte Counts. Although the differential leukocyte count is usually reported in percentages, interpretation should be based on the absolute numbers of the various cell types. Absolute numbers are obtained by multiplying the percentage by the total leukocyte count. If interpretation is based solely on the differential count with no consideration for the total count, erroneous conclusions may be reached. For example, assume that there are two cows with the following differential count:

Segmented neutrophils	56%
Lymphocytes	39%
Eosinophils	2%
Monocytes	3%

Such a differential leukocyte count indicates a percentage increase in neutrophils with an accompanying decrease in lymphocytes. Let us now assume that cow No. 1 had a total leukocyte count of 10,000/μl and cow No. 2, a total leukocyte count of 15,000/μl. If these figures are converted to absolute numbers, the results then indicate the following to be the case:

	Cow No. 1	Cow No. 2
Segmented neutrophils/μl	5600	8400
Lymphocytes/μl	3900	5850
Eosinophils/μl	200	300
Monocytes/μl	300	450

In the case illustrated, animal No. 1 does have an absolute increase in total segmented neutrophils (normal = 2240) and a decrease in total number of lymphocytes (normal = 4640). In cow No. 2 with the same differential count there is an increase in mature segmented cells, but in spite of the percentage decrease in lymphocytes the total number of these cells is almost normal. Therefore, an interpretation based solely on a differential count does not reflect the true alteration in cell distribution.

A guide for interpretation of the absolute differential counts for the various species of domestic animals is presented in Table 3–3.

Leukocytosis. Leukocytosis is an increase in total leukocyte count above the normal upper limit for the animal species. This increase is usually a consequence of an increase in the total number of circulating neutrophils, although in some circumstances other cell types may also be increased.

This alteration in the leukocyte picture can be the consequence of a normal physiologic response (Table 3–4) or a disease condition.

Pathologic leukocytosis as a rule is an increase in segmented neutrophilic granulocytes. This increase in neutrophils may be relative—an increase in the percentage of neutrophils—or absolute—an increase in the total number of cells—or both. Alterations observed are, for the most part, a reflection of the response of the animal spe-

TABLE 3–3. Interpretation of Absolute Differential Counts for Various Species of Domesticated Animals*

Condition	Absolute Differential Count (Cells/μl)						
	DOG	CAT	COW	HORSE	PIG	SHEEP	GOAT
Leukocytosis	>15,000	>19,000	>12,000	>12,500	>22,000	>12,000	>13,000
Leukopenia	<6,000	<5,500	<4,000	<6,000	<10,000	<4,000	<4,000
Neutrophilia	>11,800	>12,500	>4,000	>6,700	>10,000	>5,600	>7,200
Neutropenia	<3,000	<2,500	<1,500	<2,700	<3,200	<700	<1,200
Left shift†	>300	>300	>200	>100	>800	>100	>100
Lymphocytosis	>5,000	>7,000	>7,500	>5,500	>13,000	>9,000	>9,000
Lymphopenia	<1,500	<2,000	<3,000	<2,000	<4,500	<2,000	<2,000
Monocytosis	>800	>600	>850	>1,000	>2,000	>750	>550
Eosinophilia	>750	>750	>1,500	>1,000	>2,000	>1,000	>650

* These data (adapted from Schalm et al., 1975) are meant as guidelines only. Age, sex, and other physiologic factors may influence interpretation.
† Increase in the number of band or younger neutrophils.

cies to disease. In addition to an evaluation of the presence of increased numbers of neutrophils, the stage of maturation of these cells must also be taken into consideration, as must any alteration in numbers of monocytes, eosinophils, or lymphocytes. Demonstration of an increase in the number of leukocytes on its own is of little value as an aid to diagnosis unless it can be correlated to the clinical condition observed in the patient. Only when the two are considered together is a useful interpretation possible.

The general causes of leukocytosis, other than physiologic, are as follows:

1. Generalized infections.
2. Localized infections.
3. Intoxications, including those produced by metabolic disturbances, chemicals, drugs, and venoms.
4. Rapidly growing neoplasms.
5. Acute hemorrhage, particularly into one of the body cavities (thoracic, peritoneal, joint).
6. Sudden hemolysis of erythrocytes.
7. Leukemias.
8. Trauma.

Neutrophilia. Changes in the number of circulating neutrophils can occur by three mechanisms: (1) movement between the circulating and marginal blood pools, (2) change in the movement of cells from the storage pool into the blood pool, and (3) alteration in the rate of movement of cells out of the blood pool. In systemic infections neutrophilia is frequently preceded by a decrease in the total number of circulating leukocytes (leukopenia). Leukopenia is most likely to occur if there is an overwhelming microbial infection, viral-induced disease, or endotoxemia. This decrease occurs as neutrophils move into tissues. If tissue demand is great the storage pool is depleted and the total neutrophil count decreases. Neutrophilia occurring in systemic infections such as salmonellosis, pasteurellosis, leptospirosis, or other septicemias is usually not marked, but neutrophils do increase, and there may also be an increase in immature neutrophils.

In localized infections produced by pyogenic microorganisms such as staphylococci, streptococci, and corynebacteria, neutrophilia is usually much greater than with systemic diseases. However, the degree of neutrophilia is not always re-

TABLE 3–4. Physiologic Leukocytosis

Cause	Cell Type	Mechanism
Increased epinephrine with fear and excitement	Neutrophils. If marked (leukocytosis) also lymphocytes	Removal of cells from MGP to CGP.
Exercise	Neutrophils. If prolonged also lymphocytes	Accelerated blood flow. Also increased epinephrine
Anemia	Neutrophils	Increased blood flow cells from MGP to CGP.
Estrus (cow)	Neutrophils and lymphocytes	
Digestion (dog and pig)	Neutrophils	About one hour after eating
Stage of pregnancy (dog and cow)	Neutrophils	Occurs near term in dog. High in cow at parturition.

lated to the extent of the localized process; the pressure exerted within it is more important. For example, a small abscess under pressure but not yet organized by a limiting membrane will produce a greater neutrophilia than will a larger organized abscess with a limiting membrane.

Noninfectious diseases resulting in a neutrophilia are usually those that stimulate a stress reaction. Included in this category are metabolic disturbances, drugs, and toxic chemicals. Tissue destruction, irrespective of its cause, will produce an increase in the number of circulating neutrophils. Typical of this response is the neutrophilia seen following prolonged surgical procedures in which there has been considerable tissue damage. Hemorrhage is often followed by an increase in neutrophils, particularly if there has been bleeding into one of the serous cavities of the body (peritoneum, pleura, joint, subdural space).

Leukocyte Response to Corticosteroids. Endogenous or exogenous increases in glucocorticoids produce leukocyte alterations that are typical for each animal species.

Dog. In the dog increased glucocorticoids produce a three- to fourfold increase in neutrophils and a simultaneous 50 to 60 per cent reduction in lymphocytes along with the disappearance of eosinophils from the peripheral circulation. There is a concomitant two- to threefold increase in monocytes. The neutrophil increase is almost exclusively in mature cells, suggesting that the effect of excess glucocorticoids is primarily one of redistribution of cells already available in the vascular system. Band neutrophils are rarely increased.

Horse. A similar increase in neutrophils and decrease in lymphocytes has been observed in the horse. Lymphocytes of the horse appear to be less responsive to glucocorticoids than lymphocytes of the dog and monocytosis does not usually occur.

Cow. In the cow the leukocyte response to glucocorticoids is characterized by neutrophilia, lymphopenia, eosinopenia, and monocytosis. As with other species the neutrophil increase is in mature cells.

Cat. The cat responds in a similar manner with the appearance of neutrophilia, a fall in lymphocytes, and some elevation of monocytes.

Evaluating a hemogram from an animal being treated with ACTH or glucocorticoids may be difficult unless one understands the type of response that may occur as a consequence of therapy.

Factors Influencing Neutrophilic Leukocytosis. The neutrophilic response varies in different species of domestic animals. It is essential that the clinician understand these variations in order to accurately interpret leukocyte response to disease.

Dog. The total leukocyte response in the dog in infections and diseases of stress is often great. Total leukocyte counts of 30,000 to 50,000/μl

occur frequently, and total leukocyte counts of over 80,000/μl are not uncommon.[1]

Cat. Although the cat responds well to stress and infectious diseases by an increase in the number of circulating leukocytes, this animal is not as responsive as the dog in developing extremely high leukocyte counts in disease.

Neutrophilia exists in the cat when the total neutrophil count exceeds 12,500/μl of blood. A total leukocyte count in excess of 19,000/μl should be considered representative of a leukocytosis. Total leukocyte counts in excess of 75,000/μl are uncommon in the cat except in association with leukemia. Physiologic leukocytosis occurring as a consequence of fear or emotional stress should be suspected when neutrophils are in the high normal range and lymphocytes are in excess of maximum normal value and exceed the number of neutrophils.[3]

Cow. The cow is less responsive in terms of total leukocyte count than are other domestic animal species. The total leukocyte count in the cow may remain within normal range but with an increase in the absolute number of neutrophils. In the cow, a marked leukocytosis would be reported in animals having total counts of 15,000 to 25,000/μl, and an extreme leukocytosis would be noted with counts in excess of 25,000/μl. This may be explained in part by consideration of the normal leukocyte distribution in the cow. Normally, this species has a neutrophil:lymphocyte ratio of approximately 0.35:0.50. In response to stress and increased adrenal activity lymphocytes are destroyed in greater numbers than other cell types. As the cow normally has a high lymphocyte count, many cells are destroyed, and even if there is an increase in neutrophils, it is seldom sufficient to produce a marked leukocytosis. The usual bovine response to infection and stress is an initial fall in lymphocytes that may exceed the increase in neutrophils. It is possible for a cow to have fewer total leukocytes than normal but still have evidence of an infection or stress as manifested by the increased number of neutrophils.

Cattle do not have a large bone marrow reserve of mature neutrophils. If tissue demands are great the reserve is quickly mobilized, neutrophils leave the blood to enter tissues, and a neutropenia develops. Such marrow depletion is frequently followed by the appearance of relatively large numbers of immature neutrophils in the blood (marked left shift).

Horse. Leukocyte response in the horse is less than that in the cat or dog, but total leukocyte counts of 17,000 to 20,000/μl may be seen in infections. The general level of leukocyte response to infection is in the range of 15,000 to 25,000/μl. A marked leukocytosis in the horse would be 25,000 to 30,000/μl, but counts higher than this have been reported.

Pig. The pig with its higher normal total leukocyte count also responds to infections with a marked increase in neutrophils. Total leukocyte counts of 30,000 to 40,000/µl occur with some degree of frequency.

SHEEP. In the sheep, a total leukocyte count of 13,000/µl may represent a slight leukocytosis, whereas 20,000/µl would be indicative of a marked leukocytosis. An absolute neutrophil count of 5600/µl or greater is considered to be an absolute neutrophilia, whereas an absolute neutropenia occurs when the count falls below 700/µl.

GOAT. In the goat, band neutrophils occur commonly in association with neutrophilia and total leukocyte counts in diseased animals reach levels of 22,000 to 27,000/µl. These increases occur primarily as results of neutrophilia.

SUSCEPTIBILITY OF HOST

The total leukocyte response in an individual animal is directly related to its susceptibility to an infectious agent. Susceptibility is frequently highly specific for a certain microorganism and is dependent upon the immune status of the individual. Animals that have developed immunologic resistance as a result of previous experience with an organism are less likely to respond to a specific agent with a high degree of leukocytosis than are animals that have not had previous exposure to the infectious agent. The individual's general state of health may also be a factor influencing the severity of the condition as well as the extent of leukocyte response. Animals that are cachectic or otherwise debilitated may fail to show a leukocytic response to the infectious agent, as the marrow may be affected by the poor state of nutrition and the usual leukocyte response diminished.

Susceptibility of a host to an infectious process is closely related to the virulence of the infecting organism. If the organism has a low virulence and the individual a degree of resistance leukocytosis is usually minimal. The opposite may be true if a patient is highly susceptible and the organism exceptionally virulent. This may result in either a marked leukocytosis or a decrease in circulating neutrophils if marrow reserves are exhausted. The latter is most likely to occur as a consequence of an overwhelming infection or endotoxemia.

Another factor that must be taken into consideration is the ability of the individual animal to localize the infectious process, as a consequence of resistance to the organism or the characteristics of the infectious agent. Localization is likely to result in a pronounced neutrophilia, whereas general infections produce a less marked increase in circulating neutrophils. Pyogenic organisms belonging to the genera *Streptococcus*, *Staphylococcus*, *Corynebacterium*, *Actinobacillus*, and *Spherophorus* are most likely to produce a localized process and, as a consequence, a marked neutrophilia with a leukocytosis.

Leukopenia. Leukopenia is a reduction in the leukocyte count below normal values. Leukopenia either may be balanced (i.e., a decrease in all cellular elements) or may be confined to a single cellular element. The latter is referred to by the more specific name—neutropenia, lymphopenia, or eosinopenia. The general causes of neutropenia are related to alteration in the bone marrow and are known as the three D's:

1. Degeneration (ineffective granulopoiesis)
2. Depression (reduced granulopoiesis)
3. Depletion (reduced survival in blood)

If any of these alterations occur in the bone marrow, the number of neutrophils in the peripheral circulation is decreased.

Degeneration of the marrow is usually the result of a condition that causes deficiency in bone marrow activity that results in an inability to mature neutrophils (ineffective granulopoiesis). Such a condition is reflected by a large number of immature neutrophils in the peripheral circulation.

At the bone marrow level there is a maturation arrest, although the total number of granulocyte precursors may be increased. Myelocytes, promyelocytes, and myeloblasts predominate with a paucity of mature neutrophils in the marrow. It is almost impossible to differentiate ineffective granulopoiesis from reduced neutrophil survival neutropenia. Differentiation can be made only by following the clinical course of disease with periodic hematologic examinations.

Depression results when the marrow loses its ability to produce neutrophils in response to peripheral demands. This alteration is characterized by a diminished number of neutrophils with zero or very few immature neutrophils in peripheral blood. If the marrow recovers from this depressed state, immature neutrophils reappear as the total count increases.

Depletion (reduced survival neutropenia) occurs when the demand of leukocytes is such that the marrow's storage pool is exhausted and the compensatory functional reaction has not yet become manifest.

Marrow depletion is characterized by a low neutrophil count in peripheral blood and, depending on the marrow response, the appearance of immature neutrophils. Sequential blood examinations following depletion neutropenia will usually reveal a marked increase in immature neutrophils, followed by a comparable change in mature neutrophils, as a consequence of bone marrow activity. This response usually occurs within 48 to 72 hours following initial depletion. Neutropenia may persist if tissue demands exceed production.

Destruction of the marrow is usually the result of chemical or physical agents that destroy blood-forming elements in bone marrow. Bone marrow destruction is manifest by a decrease in all cell types formed in the marrow, and the animal often becomes anemic in addition to have a leukopenia. Immature forms of neutrophils are not usually seen in the peripheral blood.

Conditions that may produce leukopenia are as follows:

1. Viral infections such as canine distemper, infectious canine hepatitis, feline panleukopenia, hog cholera, swine influenza, mucosal disease, and others are often accompanied by a decreased total leukocyte count. The decrease is usually observed during the early stages of disease. Secondary infections following viral diseases are usually accompanied by a leukocytosis. Strictly neurotropic viruses seldom produce a leukopenia, but most pantropic viral diseases are accompanied by a distinct leukopenia.

2. Overwhelming bacterial infections also result in a leukopenia that is commonly accompanied by a diminution of mature neutrophils in the peripheral blood.

3. Endotoxins from gram-negative bacteria produce a significant leukopenia. Large doses of endotoxin have severe effects on formed elements of the blood, particularly thrombocytes and leukocytes, both of which decrease.[1]

4. Leukopenia is also associated with cachectic and debilitated states that may be caused by lack of certain nutritional factors or by exhaustion of the marrow.

5. Physical agents such as x-rays and radioactive substances produce a leukopenia by destroying the cellular elements of the bone marrow.

6. Chemical agents may also produce a leukopenia. Included are some of the antibiotics (chloramphenicol, penicillin, streptomycin, and oxytetracycline); analgesics such as phenacetin, antipyrine, and aminopyrine; inorganic chemicals including lead, benzene, bismuth, and mercury; cortisone products; antihistamines; and sulfonamides.

7. Anaphylactic shock and the early stages of a reaction to foreign protein may produce a leukopenia.

Lymphocytosis. Increases in the absolute number of circulating lymphocytes occur occasionally in domestic animals and may be caused by one or more of the following conditions:

1. All conditions that have an associated neutropenia may have a relative lymphocytosis, but this is rarely an absolute increase.

2. Physiologic leukocytosis in the cat may be accompanied by an absolute increase in lymphocytes. This is the most frequent cause of an absolute increase in lymphocytes in the dog and cat.

3. Lymphocytic leukemias are accompanied by a marked increase in lymphocytes.

4. During the recovery stages of certain infections, an increase in the total number of lymphocytes may be observed.

5. Adrenocortical insufficiency may be manifested by an increase in the absolute number of lymphocytes.

6. Lymphocytosis sometimes occurs following vaccination and in chronic infections when constant antigenic stimulation results in an increase in T lymphocytes. Some lymphocytes may be large with an increased cytoplasmic basophilia. These are often referred to as immunocytes or as reactive or stimulated lymphocytes.

7. Hyperthyroidism has been reported to have an accompanying lymphocytosis.

Lymphopenia. Interpretation of the results of a differential cell count may depend to a certain extent on the degree of decrease of the lymphocytes and the persistence of this decrease. A lymphopenia may be caused by:

1. Certain viral diseases such as canine distemper, infectious canine hepatitis, parvovirus gastroenteritis, panleukopenia, coronavirus enteritis, and leukemia virus infection of cats.

2. Stress, which produces a moderate to marked absolute decrease in lymphocytes. This results from the action of glucocorticoids.

3. The injection of adrenocortical hormones or ACTH.

4. Ionizing radiation or immunosuppresive drugs.

5. Loss of efferent lymph as with rupture of the thoracic duct and loss of lymph into the lumen of the intestine in some chronic enteric diseases.

Monocytosis. A monocytosis occurs in several conditions:

1. Chronic diseases, particularly those in which large amounts of particulate matter must be removed. Examples are fungal infections and most conditions accompanied by a granulomatous reaction. If there is considerable tissue debris to be removed, an increase in monocytes often occurs.

2. Certain infectious diseases such as erysipelas and listeriosis in swine and brucellosis in other animals.

3. A relative monocytosis is seen in conditions that also produce a leukopenia and neutropenia.

4. Monocytic leukemias.

5. ACTH and corticoid treatment in the dog, cow, and cat.

6. In association with acute stress reactions in the dog and cat.

7. Hyperadrenocorticism.

Eosinophilia. Eosinophilia is an increase in the number of circulating eosinophils in the peripheral blood. It is seen in the following conditions:

1. As a reflection of hypersensitivity in conditions such as parasitism and allergic reactions. Parasites that produce an increase in eosinophils

are those that penetrate the tissues of the animal body such as migrating ascarid larvae, trichinae, and occasionally hookworms. Parasites that produce only localized lesions do not usually induce an eosinophilia. Allergic reactions such as asthma, urticaria, allergic bronchitis, allergic dermatitis, and food allergies also produce an eosinophilia.

2. Anaphylactic reactions that are also a reflection of hypersensitivity are accompanied by an increase in eosinophils.

3. In adrenocortical insufficiency eosinophilia may occur but is not a usual finding.

4. In the recovery stages of some acute infections, a relative increase in eosinophils may be observed. This is usually a reappearance of eosinophils following the eosinopenia that accompanies stress associated with the more acute stages of disease.

5. Granulocytic eosinophilic leukemias have been reported.

6. Neoplasms of the ovary, serous membranes, and bone may have an associated absolute increase in eosinophils.

7. Eosinophilic myositis may also be accompanied by eosinophilia.

8. Splenectomy in the dog may be followed in about 30 days by an eosinophil increase.

9. Eosinophilic gastroenteritis in the dog.

10. Eosinophilic granuloma in the cat.

11. In association with estrus in some dogs.

Eosinopenia. A decrease in the number of circulating eosinophils is difficult to detect. Differential leukocyte accounts on normal animals may reveal no eosinophils. An absolute eosinopenia is best detected with a total eosinophil count (see Appendix, p. 436). Decreases may occur in:

1. Any stress condition (decrease only or complete disappearance).

2. After administration of ACTH or corticoids as a therapeutic measure.

3. Hyperactivity of the adrenal gland occurring as a consequence of hyperplasia or neoplasia.

Basophilia. An increase in the absolute number of basophils is rare. If it does occur, it is most probably associated with an eosinophilia or is the result of a basophilic granulocytic leukemia. Basophilia often is found in dogs with heartworms. It may occur in hyperlipoproteinemias.[8]

CLASSIFICATION OF THE LEUKOCYTIC RESPONSE

Certain terms are commonly used to describe alterations that occur in the total and differential leukocyte counts in domestic animals. These alterations are often referred to in interpreting counts, thus an understanding of these changes and their mechanisms is important in interpretation.

Shift to the left is a term used to denote an increase in the number of immature neutrophils in the peripheral circulation. Two types of shift to the left have been described.

A *regenerative left shift* is characterized by an absolute increase in neutrophils accompanied by the appearance of immature neutrophils in the peripheral circulation.

A slight left shift is manifested by a slight to moderate increase in the number of band neutrophils. A moderate left shift may include a few metamyelocytes and many band cells, whereas a marked shift is characterized by an increasing number of metamyelocytes with the occasional appearance of myelocytes and possibly some promyelocytes.[1]

A *degenerative left shift* is one in which there is a normal, low, or falling total leukocyte count accompanied by a moderate to marked shift to the left, with the absolute number of immature neutrophils frequently exceeding the number of mature neutrophils. This alteration is a result of the inability of bone marrow to produce mature cells in response to infection, and as a result there is a proportional increase in immature neutrophils in the blood.

Toxic neutrophils are abnormal, and their presence in the blood reflects a toxic condition. There are several criteria used to identify such cells:

1. The appearance of very few to many blue-black granules in the cytoplasm of the neutrophils (cattle, sheep, and horses).

2. In the dog and cat, a common indication of toxicity is the presence of vacuoles located in the cytoplasm along the periphery of the cell, usually accompanied by diffuse cytoplasmic basophilia. In toxic granulopoiesis in the cat, neutrophils are frequently larger than normal and have a bizarre nuclear pattern in addition to the cytoplasmic characteristics already described.

3. Under conditions of extreme toxicity in all animals, toxic neutrophils may be evidenced by the presence of diffuse cytoplasmic basophilia.

4. The neutrophil of the healthy cat may have a few dark bodies appearing in the cytoplasm. The number of such granules in neutrophils may be increased in disease conditions. These irregularly shaped, blue-staining structures are referred to as Döhle bodies.

Grading of the degree of toxicity is based on the extent of change occurring in the cells rather than on the number of cells affected. Grading should be on a 1 to 4 + basis and should be recorded along with the differential count, as these alterations are important in interpretation of leukocyte counts. Grading of toxicity is strictly qualitative and may vary depending on the individual making the evaluation. The presence or absence of toxic neutrophils is probably more important than a qualitative rating of the degree of toxicity.

A *leukemoid reaction* is similar to the left shift

of the regenerative type and is characterized by an extreme leukocytosis simulating that observed in leukemic leukemias. Such a reaction can be differentiated from a true leukemia by means of bone marrow examination.

INTERPRETATION OF LEUKOCYTE ALTERATIONS

In general, it may be said that the extent of leukocytosis indicates the degree of an individual's resistance and that the degree of left shift indicates the severity of the infection. In keeping with this concept, a simultaneous fall in total leukocyte count and an increase in immature neutrophils are unfavorable prognostic signs.

Essentially, three factors in relation to a disease condition can be elicited by interpretation of the leukocyte picture: (1) severity of the condition, (2) duration of the process, and (3) prognosis.

The severity of a disease is judged by the following:

1. A neutrophilia with a slight left shift and persistence of the eosinophils is suggestive of a mild infection that is being well handled by the body's defense mechanisms.
2. A high total leukocyte count consisting mainly of neutrophils is indicative of a more severe condition with good bone marrow response.
3. A neutrophilia with a coexistent lymphopenia and eosinopenia is indicative of a moderately severe to severe condition and reflects stress.
4. If toxic neutrophils are present, the condition is severe.
5. If immature neutrophils are present in excess of the number of mature neutrophils, the condition is severe.
6. If the animal has clinical evidence of illness of marked to moderate severity and there is no neutrophil response, the condition must be considered more severe than if a leukocytic alteration occurs.
7. A falling total leukocyte count with a diminishing proportion of neutrophils and a return of the lymphocytes and eosinophils indicates diminishing severity and probable recovery.

The duration of the disease process may be estimated by an examination of the leukocyte alterations. This, however, is probably the most difficult factor to evaluate accurately in interpreting a leukocyte count.

1. Acute disease conditions may be accompanied either by a regenerative shift to the left with the characteristic appearance of immature neutrophils or by a leukopenia. Acute, overwhelming bacterial infections and endotoxemias are accompanied by a leukopenia followed or accompanied by a regenerative left shift. Neutrophilia appears if the animal survives. If stress accompanies the disease, lymphopenia and eosinopenia accompany the neutrophilis and left shift. In some species there may be a monocytosis.
2. As the disease regresses, the number of immature neutrophils decreases; although the total neutrophil count may continue to be high, the majority of the cells are mature. As stress is alleviated lymphocyte and eosinophil absolute counts return to normal.
3. In chronic diseases, one of the most characteristic alterations is an absolute increase in monocytes. Some chronic conditions may also be typified by the appearance of a degenerative left shift or bone marrow depression.

The prognosis of disease is facilitated by proper interpretation of leukocyte counts. The prognostic significance of these determinations is of more value if several leukocyte counts of the patient's blood are available for evaluation. Unfavorable prognostic signs are:

1. Degenerative shift to the left that is indicative of ineffective granulopoiesis.
2. Persistent lymphopenia.
3. Severe intoxication as indicated by marked increase in the toxicity of neutrophils.
4. The absence of eosinophils over a long period of time.
5. An extremely high total leukocyte count with a high percentage of neutrophils.
6. A persistent leukopenia with decreased numbers of all types of cells.

Favorable prognostic signs are:

1. Falling total leukocyte count with reappearance of lymphocytes and eosinophils.
2. Disappearance of toxic neutrophils.
3. A decrease of immature neutrophils.
4. Reappearance of eosinophils.
5. Temporary increase of monocytes.
6. Occurrence of a regenerative left shift in an animal that has had a leukopenia.

DISEASES OF LEUKOCYTES (NON-NEOPLASTIC)

Pelger-Huet Anomaly. The Pelger-Huet anomaly is characterized by hyposegmentation of the granulocytes. Neutrophils and eosinophils have a nonlobed nucleus that is frequently round or oval. Although nuclear shape suggests immaturity, nuclear maturation appears to be complete because the chromatin is condensed, cell size is normal, and the cytoplasm does not contain immature granules.[8] This condition must be differentiated from the typical left shift as seen in response to active granulopoiesis. If the presence of immature cells is the consequence of active granulopoiesis, the signs of cell maturation are missing, the nuclear chromatin is less condensed, the cytoplasm may retain some of its basophilia, and primary granules may be present in the cytoplasm. Absolute confirmation of the existence of this anomaly is dependent upon sequential blood examinations in which granulocyte immaturity persists. Acquired hyposegmentation has also been reported and must be differentiated from the Pelger-Huet anomaly.[8] Acquired hyposegmentation is usually transitory and sequential counts will reveal reappearance of mature granulocytes.

This is not a common condition in animals but has been reported in the dog and cat. In the dog it has been reported in the foxhound,[9] cocker spaniel,[10] black-and-tan coonhound,[11] basenji, Boston terrier, and in a mixed-breed dog.[8] The anomaly has also been reported in cats with the classic nuclear changes in eosinophils and neutrophils.[12]

Cyclic Hematopoiesis of the Canine (Gray Collie Syndrome). This condition occurs only in the collie. This cyclic disease is inherited as a simple autosomal recessive trait. The condition is characterized by the appearance of neutropenic episodes that occur at 11- to 12-day intervals.[8] The neutropenia that accompanies the condition is of short duration, lasting approximately three days. This is followed by a slightly increased neutrophil count that may persist for a week. During the neutropenic stages of the condition many of the circulating neutrophils are immature. Reticulocyte, platelet, and monocyte numbers are also cyclic and decrease as neutrophils decrease.[13] The defect appears to be at the stem-cell level.

Affected animals are frequently subject to secondary infections during the intervals when they are neutropenic. Collies with this disease typically have a silver-gray hair coat but the color may vary, ranging from a pale tricolor to a dark charcoal gray.[14,15]

Granulocytopathy Syndrome. This condition has been reported in the dog and is characterized by a reduced functional capacity of the neutrophils.[16–18] Neutrophils from such animals have reduced bactericidal activity. This is a rare condition but affected animals frequently are unable to ward off infections because of the deficiency in normal leukocyte function. Such animals do have a responding neutrophilic leukocytosis, and the condition can be confirmed only by demonstration of a lack of normal bactericidal activity by neutrophils.

Chédiak-Higashi Syndrome. This syndrome was first described in mink but since then has been detected in cattle, cats, and the white tiger.[19] Affected animals exhibit varying amounts of albinism and have an increased susceptibility to infection. Enlarged granules are seen in neutrophils, eosinophils, basophils, and melanocytes.

The disease was reported in Persian cats bred to develop a blue-smoke coat.[19,20] These cats had bleeding tendencies following surgery, and hematomas at venipuncture sites were common. Platelet function has been reported to be abnormal.

Poodle Bone Marrow Dyscrasia. Miniature and toy breeds of poodles are sometimes affected by a marrow dyscrasia that results in abnormalities of neutrophils and erythrocytes.[1] The neutrophils are hypersegmented and sometimes quite large. The affected dog does not usually have any well-defined clinical problem that can be associated with the bone marrow problem, and the condition is discovered only when the animal is presented for some other disease condition and a hematologic examination is completed. Erythrocytes are characteristically larger than normal but have adequate concentrations of hemoglobin.

Leukocyte Inclusions. MUCOPOLYSACCHARIDOSIS. Cytoplasmic granules containing mucopolysaccharides have been reported in leukocytes of dogs and cats.[21–23] These are associated with heritable conditions characterized by deficits in central nervous function and skeletal deformities. In addition such animals have deficiencies in enzymes associated with mucopolysaccharide catabolism. The granules that accumulate in neutrophils stain purple on Romanowsky-stained blood smears and can be differentiated from toxic granules because the cytoplasm of toxic neutrophils is basophilic, whereas the neutrophil cytoplasm in animals with these enzyme deficiencies is normal. A final diagnosis of such a storage disease problem cannot be confirmed simply by demonstration of the cytoplasmic inclusions in leukocytes but depends on the demonstration of skeletal defects plus the presence of glycosaminoglycans in the urine.[23] Demonstration of typical granules should suggest these additional evaluations.

ABNORMAL NEUTROPHIL GRANULATION IN BIRMAN CATS. Affected cats have fine, eosinophilic neutrophil granules that are similar to azurophilic granules of the promyelocyte or to the granules of mature neutrophils in cats with mucopolysaccharidosis.[23a] The granules do not stain for acid-mucopolysaccharide, and have normal bactericidial, phagocytic, and oxidative activity. This anomaly is inherited as an autosomal recessive trait. As it does not influence neutrophil activity, affected cats do not present any unusual clinical problems.

INCLUSIONS ASSOCIATED WITH INFECTION. Distemper inclusion bodies can be found in any of the leukocytes, although they are not consistently found in infected dogs. These inclusions stain a light red and are relatively easily identified in leukocyte cytoplasm but may be difficult to see in erythrocytes. In erythrocytes they usually stain a shade of red different from hemoglobin. If blood is permitted to stand in anticoagulants too long these inclusions disappear. If one wishes to have an evaluation for distemper inclusions a freshly prepared blood smear should be examined using a routine Romanowsky-type stain.

Other infectious agents can sometimes be identified in the cytoplasm of blood and bone marrow leukocytes. Examination for the presence of such inclusions is simplified if a buffy coat smear is prepared, stained, and examined.

Included among the infectious agents that can be found in the cytoplasm of leukocytes are *Histoplasma capsulatum, Ehrlichia canis, Hepatozoon canis* gametocytes, and *Leishmania* sp. The morphology of these agents is described in later chapters.

Erythrophagocytosis occurs occasionally in which either intact or fragmented erythrocytes can be observed in monocytes and occasionally in neutrophils. These cells are described in the chapter on erythrocytes and the chapter on cytology.

NEOPLASIA OF HEMATOPOIETIC TISSUES

Neoplasia of hematopoietic tissue is either lymphoproliferative or myeloproliferative. Included in the lymphoproliferative neoplasias are lymphosarcoma, plasma cell myeloma, and reticulum cell sarcoma. The latter may represent a form of lymphosarcoma.

Myeloproliferative neoplasias are associated with cells produced in the bone marrow. Such neoplasias include the granulocytic leukemias (neutrophilic, eosinophilic, and basophilic), erythremic myelosis, erythroleukemia, reticuloendotheliosis, monocytic leukemia, myelomonocytic leukemia, and megakaryocytic leukemia. Mast cell neoplasia usually has its origin in tissues other than bone marrow, but metastasis to this tissue produces a typical leukemia.

Neoplasia of hematopoietic tissue is usually fatal, therefore care should be taken not to make a positive diagnosis unless it is well confirmed. In some cases, confirmation is made by blood examination and demonstration of typical alterations in peripheral blood. Bone marrow examination is often utilized to confirm peripheral blood findings. Absolute confirmation is often difficult because, although the term leukemia suggests the existence of an observable alteration in the blood and an increase in leukocytes, these findings do not always prevail. In identifying the type of leukemia, the cell type characterizing the condition should be stated. Leukemia may also be identified as aleukemic, subleukemic, or leukemic. An aleukemic leukemia is difficult to characterize by means of a peripheral blood examination, as it occurs without an accompanying increase in total white blood cells, and no, or only a very few, abnormal immature cells (less than one per 1000 cells) can be demonstrated. Aleukemic leukemia may be confirmed by bone marrow examination. A subleukemic leukemia is characterized by the presence of a few abnormal cell types with a normal or only slightly increased total leukocyte count. Leukemic leukemia is identified by the presence of a marked increase in total leukocytes with the presence of many abnormal and immature cells. Absolute confirmation of neoplasia of hematopoietic tissue usually depends on cytologic or histologic examination of affected tissues.

Canine. Leukemia in the canine is usually limited to the lymphocytic type, although cases of granulocytic and monocytic leukemia have been recorded. The term *lymphosarcoma* is commonly used to designate a neoplastic disease of the lymphoid organs of the dog, as peripheral blood alterations are often not typical of leukemia. Although leukemic, subleukemic, and aleukemic blood pictures have been reported, the most common alteration in the peripheral blood is a neutrophilic leukocytosis. Anemia may or may not be present.

It is not unusual to observe a dog with clinical signs of lymphosarcoma, including generalized lymphadenopathy and splenic enlargement, in which the hemogram is normal. Any animal that has clinical signs indicating the possibility of lymphosarcoma should have a careful blood examination, and careful analytical examination of the differential smear should be made in an effort to determine the presence of abnormal lymphocytes. Repeated careful scrutiny of several blood films over time may be helpful in confirming a diagnosis. Most abnormal cells observed in lymphosarcoma with an accompanying leukemia are of the immature type (Fig. 3–8). Immaturity is manifested by a dark-staining cytoplasm that is characteristic of the prolymphocyte or lymphoblast. The nucleus may contain nucleoli. Leukemic cells have a tendency to be more fragile than the mature cells of this series. Atypical, smeared, or smudged cells may appear on the blood film as cells that are not readily identifiable.

Caution must be utilized in reporting the presence of abnormal lymphocytic elements in dogs suspected of having lymphosarcoma. A technician having knowledge of the clinical signs is tempted to attribute abnormal characteristics to cells that may in reality be normal. Lymphocytes observed in a blood smear from such an animal should be judged with as little prejudice as possible. In the absence of a typical blood picture with the presence of increased numbers of lymphocytes or the observation of atypical lymphocytes, a lymph node biopsy or bone marrow examination may aid in establishing a diagnosis.

An example of typical leukemic lymphosarcoma was observed in our clinic in a three-year-old boxer dog. This animal had been presented to two practicing veterinarians because of a history of difficult breathing. Various treatments had been unsuccessful, and the dog continued to show evidence of strenuous breathing and a gradual weight loss accompanied by progressive weakness. When presented to the clinic as a referral

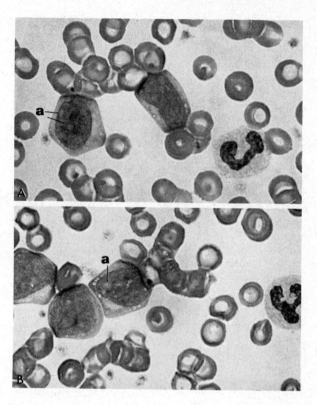

Figure 3–8. Peripheral leukocytes in the blood of a dog with lymphosarcoma. Note the size of the lymphocytes in comparison with the neutrophils. Nucleoli are shown (a).

case, the animal was emaciated and weak; dyspnea was evident, and there were clinical signs of anemia. Examination of the mouth and throat revealed a greatly enlarged soft palate that was thought to be responsible for the difficulty in respiration. There was no enlargement of the superficial lymph nodes, but palpation of the abdominal cavity revealed a greatly enlarged spleen. A complete blood count was requested with the following results:

RBC	3,320,000/μl
PCV	19%
Hemoglobin (Hb)	6.8 gm/dl
WBC	65,000/μl
Bands	1% (650/μl)
Segmented neutrophils	5% (3250/μl)
Lymphocytes	93% (60,450/μl)
	(many were immature as evidenced by an intensely basophilic cytoplasm and a nucleus containing nucleoli)
Monocytes	1% (650/μl)

In addition, atypical lymphocytes with bizarre nuclei were observed.

On the basis of the physical examination and the peripheral blood alterations a diagnosis of lymphosarcoma was made. The diagnosis was confirmed at necropsy and histologic examination.

The more common finding associated with lymphosarcoma in the dog is a hemogram not unlike that occurring with infectious disease. This type of blood count occurred in an eight-year-old boxer dog. This animal was presented with typical clinical signs of lymphosarcoma, including enlarged external lymph nodes and emaciation. Palpation revealed an enlarged spleen, and other large masses were present in the abdominal cavity. An examination of the blood was made on two occasions with the following results:

	I	II
RBC	7,500,000/μl	7,150,000/μl
PCV	48%	45%
Hb	15.6 gm/dl	15.0 gm/dl
WBC	21,500/μl	20,750/μl
Bands	215/μl	208/μl
Segmented neutrophils	19,135/μl	17,637/μl
Lymphocytes	1,720/μl	2,697/gml
Monocytes	215/μl	208/μl
	Hypersegmentation of the neutrophils	

In spite of the fact that the blood picture was not leukemic, a diagnosis of lymphosarcoma was made based on clinical observations. Euthanasia was recommended, and the diagnosis was confirmed at necropsy. Splenic hyperplasia was present; the mesenteric lymph nodes and most of the external lymph nodes were enlarged. This type of hemogram is more commonly observed in cases of lymphosarcoma than is the leukemic alteration reported in the previous case.

Granulocytic leukemia has been reported in the dog and is sometimes referred to in the literature as myelogenous leukemia.

One characteristic of a differential count from a dog with granulocytic (neutrophilic) leukemia is the disparity in the stages of developing granulocytes. In a normal responsive animal one would expect to find fewer myelocytes than metamyelocytes, fewer metamyelocytes than bands, and fewer bands than mature segmented neutrophils. With granulocytic leukemia this is not always true, and one frequently finds larger numbers of myelocytes than metamyelocytes or of metamyelocytes than bands, and immature neutrophils usually outnumber mature segmented neutrophils. Anemia, usually nonregenerative, is a constant finding in the myeloproliferative leukemias. Thrombocytopenia may also occur. There is usually an asynchrony of nuclear and cytoplasmic maturation. Leukemic cells frequently are extremely large and have a highly basophilic cytoplasm; nucleoli are present, sometimes even in the more mature forms of the granulocytes; and there is vacuolation of the cytoplasm. Unidentifiable immature cell types are not uncommon. Neoplastic neutrophils are susceptible to degenerative changes that take place after collection. Degenerating neoplastic neutrophils frequently assume the characteristics of monocytes and may be difficult to differentiate from them. Cytoplasmic vacuolation and cell shrinkage may also occur in the specimen that has been held for some time prior to preparation of the blood film. If leukemia is suspected, it is best to prepare a blood film immediately following collection.

Chronic myelogenous leukemia in the dog has been reported.[23b] Affected animals had a marked neutrophilia in the absence of any demonstrable infection. The total leukocyte counts ranged from 41,600/μl to 169,000/μl with a high percentage of immature cells of the myeloid series. The bone marrow M:E ratios ranged from 3.5:1 to 23.7:1 and an orderly progression of myeloid maturation was noted. All of the animals had a nonregenerative anemia. Five of the seven dogs were treated with hydroxyurea and three were still alive at the time of the report. Two untreated dogs later developed leukemic blast crises at 80 and 703 days, respectively, postdiagnosis. Necropsy confirmation was made on one animal that failed to respond to treatment and myeloid neoplasia was confirmed. Care must be taken in assuming that an animal has a chronic myeloid leukemia because localized, often undetected, pyogenic processes will produce similar leukocyte changes.

Monocytic leukemia is exceedingly rare in the canine. Blood studies reveal a marked increase in the total leukocyte count, and a high percentage of cells in the peripheral circulation are identified as monocytes. Similar cells are present in bone marrow. Histologic examination of tissue from affected dogs usually reveals accumulations of neoplastic cells in the lymph nodes and spleen. Similar cells have been reported as occurring extravascularly in the liver and kidney and perivascularly in the duodenum.

Acute myelomonocytic leukemia has been reported in the dog.[24-26] These cases were characterized hematologically by a mild to moderate nonregenerative anemia and a marked monocytoid leukocytosis. In the terminal stages, myelophthisic anemia and thrombocytopenia were present. There is frequently great difficulty in classifying the leukemic cells, in which case cytochemistry is of value. Peroxidase, alpha naphthol butyrate, Sudan black, alpha-naphthyl acetate esterase, and naphthol-AS-D chloroacetate esterase stains have been reported to be effective in assisting in differentiation.[25,26]

Mast cell leukemia is not infrequent in dogs. The criteria for the diagnosis are: (1) demonstration of mast cells in the blood and (2) active proliferation of these cells in the marrow. The percentage of mast cells in the circulation is variable. In some animals the typical mast cell with its intensely basophilic granules is present in sufficient numbers to be easily identified on a blood film. In other cases the number of mast cells in the blood is relatively low. If a diagnosis of mastocytoma has been made, examination of a smear made from the buffy coat of a hematocrit tube may reveal the presence of neoplastic cells. Bone marrow examination is also indicated. Dogs with confirmed mastocytoma should be periodically examined for the development of leukemia.

Multiple myeloma has been reported[27-29] in the dog. The disease is characterized by proliferation of plasma cells in the bone marrow. These cells are rarely found in the peripheral circulation. In some patients, lytic lesions of the bone are observed, whereas in others no bone changes can be demonstrated, probably because the condition is diagnosed prior to development of these bone changes. Paraproteins are routinely demonstrated in the blood plasma and are of significance in determining a final diagnosis. Hyperproteinemia often accompanies the disease. Bence Jones proteins may or may not be present in the urine.

Erythroblastic leukemia has been reported.[30] This disease was characterized by a severe nonregenerative anemia and the presence of large numbers of nucleated erythrocytes in the peripheral blood with no reticulocytosis. There was extensive erythroblastic proliferation in the bone marrow.

Bovine. Neoplasms of the hematopoietic tissues of the bovine are almost exclusively of lymphocytic origin. This condition has been reported in a stillborn fetus[31] and in animals of all ages. However, the majority of the neoplasms of lymphocytic origin occur in older animals. This condition has been reported frequently in the literature by various authors as lymphosarcoma, lymphoblastoma, lymphocytoma, malignant lymphoma, and simply as leukemia. The term *leukemia* is probably a misnomer, as many cases involving neoplastic lymphoid proliferation are not characterized by a leukemic alteration in the peripheral circulation. Since lymphoid neoplastic involvement occurs in many tissues of the body, the terms *malignant lymphoma, lymphocytoma,* and *lymphosarcoma* are probably more descriptive. Three clinicopathologic forms of lymphosarcoma have been identified: (1) mature, (2) thymic-adolescent, and (3) juvenile or calf.

The blood picture in the mature form of lymphosarcoma may vary from normal to leukopenia to obvious leukemia. Even though the total leukocyte count may not reveal a typical leukemia, the presence of abnormal lymphocytes may be of significance in making a final diagnosis. This alteration in lymphocyte morphology occurs as an increase in immature lymphocytes characterized by a dark-blue–staining cytoplasm and a nucleus containing nucleoli. Prolymphocytes, which are large cells with a considerable amount of cytoplasm and a nucleus with a nucleolar remnant, may be observed. Abnormally shaped lymphocytes, including those that are binucleate and those with mitotic figures, may be present; occasionally cells are seen that have a lobed nucleus, and the cytoplasm of these neoplastic cells may contain vacuoles. Such abnormal cells are not present in all cases of lymphosarcoma but do occur in a sufficient number of cases to be useful in diagnosis. Many neoplastic cells are fragile and have a tendency to become smudged and smeared in a routine film of peripheral blood (see Plate 3–1).

The hemograms observed in 10 cases of malignant lymphoma diagnosed at Kansas State University are presented in Table 3–5. It will be noted that in several instances no abnormal cells of the lymphocytic series and no immature lymphocytes were observed. In these cases, it was impossible to identify positively the existence of neoplasia from the blood count alone. In other animals, leukemia was obvious, and the diagnosis was confirmed by the hemogram.

Lymphosarcoma may become a herd problem. Observations made in Denmark and Germany pointed to this disease as a herd problem and suggested its contagious nature. In such instances it was suggested that a herd study utilizing both total and differential leukocyte counts could assist in identifying animals that may be affected or predisposed to lymphosarcoma. Keys were developed for identification of animals susceptible to or positive for lymphosarcoma. They were based on a combination of total leukocyte count percentage of lymphocytes and animal age.[32,33]

Surveys of the blood picture in herds in which lymphosarcoma is a problem might assist the owner in culling the animals that might be affected. However, this technique has not been widely accepted as a routine method for the positive diagnosis of such conditions. The availability of an immunologic test for the detection of lymphosarcoma in the bovine has replaced hematologic surveys of affected herds.

A thymic form of bovine lymphosarcoma has been described.[34] The outstanding clinical sign was a tumor involving the cervical thymus as evidenced by the presence of a large swelling in the lower neck, cephalic to the thoracic inlet. Hemograms were studied for eight of 14 affected animals. Only one animal had a frank leukemia, although four others had some increase in atypical lymphocytes and unclassified cells. Bone marrow examination revealed the presence of neoplastic cells in five of seven animals. Generalized lymphadenopathy is not common. This form usually occurs in cattle six to 30 months of age.

In the calf form of bovine lymphosarcoma, two of eight calves had frank lymphocytic leukemia. A third calf that did not have an elevated lymphocyte count did have atypical lymphocytes in its peripheral blood. Five calves had macrocytic anemia. All calves whose bone marrow was examined had massive neoplastic infiltration,

TABLE 3–5. Blood Findings in 10 Cases of Bovine Lymphosarcoma

Case No.	Age	Total WBC 10³/μl	Total RBC 10⁶/μl	HB Gm/dl	PCV %	Differential Leukocyte Count (Per Cent)						
						META.	BAND	SEG.	AL	LY.	MONO.	EOS.
1	7	71.3	3.75	7.1	23	0	1	2	+	93	3	1
2	7	37.7	4.80	8.5	27	0	0	11	+	89	0	0
3	3	71.8	3.94	7.0	25	0	1	5	+	94	0	0
4	6	21.5	5.25	9.8	32	0	0	16	+	83	1	0
5	8	29.6	2.30	4.3	13	0	20	49	−	31	0	0
6	9	5.4	5.88	12.6	40	0	6	34	−	58	2	0
7	2	12.4	2.00	3.9	12	0	4	61	−	35	0	0
8	6	8.25	2.90	5.1	17	1	1	19	+	69	9	0
9	7	9.60	5.20	9.6	32	0	1	39	−	27	1	31
10	5	3.90	5.16	9.5	31	1	16	7	+	76	0	0

Meta. = neutrophilic metamyelocyte, Seg. = segmented neutrophil, AL = atypical and/or immature lymphocytes, Ly. = lymphocyte, Mono. = monocyte, Eos. = eosinophil.

which rendered differential bone marrow counts unnecessary. There is usually a generalized lymphadenopathy in calves one to six months of age.

There is good evidence that bovine lymphosarcoma is associated with an oncogenic virus. Detailed studies of a "C-type" virus have revealed a relationship between the presence of this agent and lymphosarcoma. A serologic test for the identification of animals having had experience with or exposure to this agent has been developed and is now commercially available. Injection of a purified culture of this virus has resulted in the development of lymphosarcoma.

Myelogenous leukemia in the bovine is rare. A single case in a four-month-old calf has been described.[35] The leukocyte count was typical for the condition with a preponderance of immature forms of neutrophils. Examination of bone marrow impression smears showed that approximately 70 per cent of the cells were infiltrative blasts. The remainder of the cells observed were of the erythroid series and were markedly reduced in number.

Feline. Malignant conditions of the hematopoietic tissues of the cat occur with some frequency and usually are of one of the following types: lymphocytic, granulocytic (neutrophilic, eosinophilic, basophilic), or monocytic. Reticulum cell myeloma[36] and megakaryocytic myelosis have been recorded.[37] The most common neoplasia occurs in the lymphocytes.

Association of the feline leukemia virus with neoplasia of the hematopoietic system is a well-established fact. The virus is spread horizontally upon contact with infected cats. In addition to the production of frank neoplasia of the hematopoietic system, there is evidence to suggest that the virus is associated with immunosuppression aplastic anemia, and erythrocyte aplasia. This virus has also been demonstrated in a variety of other diseases of the cat. The association of the feline leukemia virus with a variety of infectious diseases may occur because of virus-induced immunosuppression of the cell-mediated immune response.

Fluorescent antibody (FA) and enzyme-linked immunosorbent assay (ELISA) tests for the detection of the feline leukemia virus are commercially available. The FA test is simple and easy for the practitioner, as all that is required is an unstained, unfixed blood film that is then submitted to a commercial laboratory. The ELISA test is made on serum from the patient. This test can be conducted in the hospital laboratory. A positive test indicates only that the virus is present and is not considered to be a diagnostic test for leukemia. Normal cats, particularly those in contact with other infected cats, may harbor the virus without having any evidence of leukemia. Some cats have the ability to develop neutralizing antibodies to the virus, thus eliminating it from their bodies.

Examination of blood or bone marrow is the most reliable, and sometimes the only, way of making an accurate diagnosis of leukemia.[38] As anemia is a progressive feature of practically all leukemias, evaluation of the erythron becomes an important part of the laboratory examination. The most valuable diagnostic tool available to clinicians in the confirmation of a diagnosis of feline leukemia is a well-made, properly stained blood film. The number of leukemic cells in feline blood can fluctuate greatly from day to day, and it is sometimes only after careful searching of the blood film that a few suspect cells are found. Nevertheless, examination of the blood smear remains the best confirmatory method for diagnosing leukemia in the cat. Leukemic cells, which may be larger than normal leukocytes, are often pushed to the sides or trailing edge of the blood film where they may be missed unless a careful examination is completed.

If leukemic cells are scant or absent in the blood, they can sometimes be found in a film from aspirated marrow. Unless these cells are relatively numerous, however, they may be difficult to identify in the marrow.

Anemia is the only consistent hematologic feature in cats with lymphocytic leukemia. Varying numbers of nucleated erythrocytes usually accompany the anemia. Less than one-fourth of the cats with lymphosarcoma have malignant cells in their circulating blood and therefore are classed as leukemic under the strict definition of the term. However, leukemic cells can often be demonstrated if the observer is willing to persevere in examining a blood film. As day to day fluctuations in the number of leukemic cells in the blood may occur, the presence or absence of neoplastic cells cannot be accurately determined unless blood is examined repeatedly.

If neoplastic cells occur in the blood, they may do so in extremely large numbers, sometimes exceeding 200,000/μl, or they may be present in a small number in a cat with an absolute lymphopenia. A confirmatory diagnosis of lymphocytic leukemia is indicated by the presence of lymphoblasts in the blood accompanied by an absolute lymphocytosis of more than 14,000 μl or more than 15 per cent lymphocytes in the marrow.

Neoplastic lymphocytes in the blood are usually prolymphocytes and lymphoblasts. These are large cells, 15 to 20 microns in diameter, with round or irregularly shaped, smooth, and homogeneous nuclei. The cytoplasm is usually abundant and stains basophilically. Blast cells, as with all immature forms, are characterized by nucleoli that stain lighter than other nuclear material. Occasionally cats can be found in which all of the lymphocytes appear to be typical mature cells. It is more common to find mixtures of cells from mature to blast forms occurring in cats with lymphocytic leukemia.

The hematologic feature of reticuloendotheliosis is the presence of immature, undifferentiated cells in blood and bone marrow. Total leukocyte counts are usually in the normal range but have an average of about 20 per cent reticuloendothelial (undifferentiated) cells. They also constitute more than 15 per cent of the nucleated cells in the marrow of affected cats.

Reticuloendothelial cells are round, have an average diameter of about 14 microns, and have a large, round, reddish-purple–staining nucleus. In contrast to findings in immature lymphocytes, the cytoplasm is not abundant, stains a medium dull blue, and has a finely stippled appearance. Nuclei of most cells are located eccentrically and have a cytoplasmic perinuclear pallor.

In addition to the appearance of these abnormal cells in the peripheral circulation and marrow, the cats characteristically have a severe, persistent nonregenerative anemia.

Granulocytic leukemias include those of the neutrophilic, basophilic, and eosinophilic types. The usual hematologic feature of neutrophilic granulocytic leukemia is a persistent neutrophilic leukocytosis with morphologically abnormal and immature cells in both blood and marrow. Total leukocyte counts range from normal to more than 50,000/μl. The diagnostic feature is not the number of neutrophils but a peristently high proportion of immature and abnormal forms. Leukemic neutrophils in the blood may be as primitive as myeloblasts, progranulocytes, and myelocytes. Atypical neutrophils are often giant forms with oddly shaped nuclei or cells having a discrepancy between maturation of the cytoplasm and that of the nucleus.

The eosinophilic form of granulocytic leukemia is a rare variant characterized by a malignant proliferation of eosinophilic leukocytes. Anemia is usually severe and there a concomitant neutrophilic leukocytosis with a severe left shift.

The term *mast cell leukemia* is a misnomer, as it refers to a malignant proliferation of connective tissue cells rather than hematopoietic cells. However, in the systemic form of this disease, neoplastic mast cells can be found in blood and marrow, as can leukemic cells in other types of leukemia. Mast cells have often been confused with basophilic granulocytes. The diagnostic feature of the condition is the presence of mast cells in blood and marrow, usually accompanied by a leukocytosis, and the appearance of a few to more than 50 per cent mast cells in peripheral blood. Anemia is not usually as severe as in leukemias. Neoplastic mast cells are 10 to 20 microns in diameter and have a round, centrally placed nucleus. The cytoplasm is characterized by the presence of numerous, small, equal-sized, purple-staining granules that may tend to obscure the nucleus. Development of mastocytemia may be a sequel to cutaneous mastocytoma as the neoplasia becomes systemic.

Monocytic leukemia may be characterized by a normal total leukocyte count with a differential count that includes a high proportion (29 to 45 per cent) of monocytes.[39] In other cases the total leukocyte count may be very high with monocytes.

Predominating in the peripheral blood, most neoplastic cells are readily recognized as immature monocytes. Mild to severe nonregenerative anemia may occur and thrombocytopenia has been reported.[40]

Megakaryocytic myelosis has been reported[37] and was characterized by an abnormal prolifera-

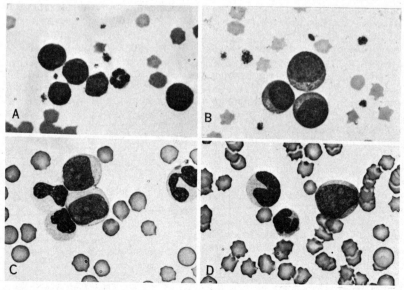

Figure 3–9. Myeloproliferative syndrome in cat. Note the large cells, many of which have distinct nucleoli. The precise cell line is difficult to establish.

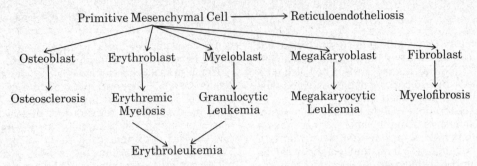

Figure 3–10. Cell lines and combination of cell types that may become involved in the myeloproliferative disease complex.

tion of megakaryocytes in the bone marrow and a severe nonregenerative anemia. Circulating thrombocytes were markedly increased, and giant and morphologically bizarre forms were present.

Myeloma has been reported.[36] Electrophoretic analysis of the serum proteins indicated a substantial increase in the gamma globulin level. The total leukocyte count ranged from normal to subnormal, but the differential count disclosed approximately 10 per cent large mononuclear cells.

Myeloproliferative diseases in cats have been classified as reticuloendotheliosis, erythremic myelosis, erythroleukemia, and atypical granulocytic leukemia.[41]

Cytologic characteristics of blood and bone marrow in myeloproliferative diseases are exceedingly variable.

A diagram to help visualize cell lines and combinations of cell types that may become involved in the myeloproliferative disease complex has been developed (Fig. 3–10).[42]

In erythremic myelosis and myelofibrosis, bone marrow is almost entirely devoid of cells of the granulocytic maturation series. The majority of the cells are undifferentiated, but cells that had early nuclear differentiation characteristics of prorubricytes and basophilic rubricytes with an occasional cell having cytoplasmic characteristics of hemoglobin synthesis may be observed.

Erythremic myelosis should be suspected when there is a severe anemia and a marked anisocytosis of erythrocytes with no accompanying polychromasia. Some cats may have an increase in nucleated erythrocytes in all stages of development, but this is not accompanied by the presence of reticulocytes. Megaloblastoid erythrocytes may appear that show asynchrony between the cytoplasm and the nucleus. These cells are much larger than the usual nucleated erythrocytes and appear to be somewhat deficient in chromatin. Erythroblasts with typical nucleoli may appear in the peripheral circulation.

Giant forms of neutrophils with bizarre nuclei may be seen in cats of all ages that have histories that include anorexia and pyrexia in which there is a leukopenia with a left shift. As similar cells may be seen in granulocytic leukemia, especially when there is an accompanying leukopenia, the clinician must be wary of such counts and their

interpretations. Differentiation can best be accomplished by repeated blood sampling, as in nonleukemic diseases these giant forms of neutrophils are rapidly replaced by normal cells as the cat begins to recover. Such changes can take place within 24 to 48 hours.

Equine. Neoplasia of the hematopoietic tissue of the horse appears to be relatively rare. Malignant lesions involving lymphocytic cells have been reported.[1] The blood picture in these animals included a moderate leukocytosis with a neutrophilia. In two animals, monocytoid cells were present in the peripheral blood.

Myelomatosis has been recorded in the literature.[43] This condition was observed in a patient admitted with a history of lameness and weakness of two days' duration. Examination of the blood revealed a severe macrocytic anemia. The horse recovered from the original condition, but three months later a partial paralysis developed, and the animal was unable to rise. Two examinations of peripheral blood were made prior to euthanasia, and bone marrow was aspirated from the tuber coxae. Anemia was more severe than at first treatment and was of the macrocytic normochromic type. The leukocyte picture at the time of the second examination was one of leukopenia with relative neutrophilia. Bone marrow findings were diagnostic, as myeloma plasma cells accounted for 65 per cent of the nucleated cells in the bone marrow.

Porcine. Lymphocytic involvement seems to be the most common type of neoplasia occurring in the hematopoietic tissue of swine. It is, however, rather unusual to find this condition. One case of lymphocytic leukemia in a hog that received ionizing radiation has been described.[44] There is, however, little information on the blood findings associated with this type of neoplasia in swine.

REFERENCES

1. Schalm, O. W., Jain, N. C., and Carroll, E. J.: *Veterinary Hematology*, 3rd ed., Lea & Febiger, Philadelphia, 1975.
2. Bulgin, M. S., Munn, S. L., and Gee, W.: Hematologic changes to 4½ years of age in clinically normal beagles. J.A.V.M.A., *157*:1064, 1970.

3. Schalm, O. W.: Notes and comments on feline hematology. Calif. Vet., *22*(1):24, 1968.
4. Heller, V. G., and Paul, H.: Changes in cell volume produced by varying concentrations of different anticoagulants. J. Lab. Clin. Med., *19*:777, 1934.
5. Schalm, O. W., and Murray, R.: Estimation of blood leukocyte numbers by means of a DNA viscosity test. J.A.V.M.A., *145*:1177, 1964.
6. Gossett, K. A., and Carakostas, M. C.: Effect of EDTA on morphology of neutrophils of healthy dogs and dogs with inflammation. Vet. Clin. Pathol., *XIII(II)*:22, 1984.
7. Weiss, D. J.: Uniform evaluation and semiquantitative reporting of hematologic data in veterinary laboratories. Vet. Clin. Pathol., *XIII(II)*:27, 1984.
8. Prasse, K. W.: White blood cell disorders. In *Textbook of Veterinary Internal Medicine. Diseases of the dog and cat*, 2nd ed. Edited by Ettinger, S. J., W. B. Saunders Company, Philadelphia, 1983.
9. Bowles, C. A., Alsaker, R. D. and Wolfle, T. L.: Studies of the Pelger-Huet anomaly in foxhounds. Am. J. Pathol., *96*:237, 1979.
10. Feldman, B. F., and Romans, A. U.: The Pelger-Huet anomaly of granulocytic leukocytes in the dog. Canine Pract., *3*(5):22, 1976.
11. Pace, E. M.: Pelger-Huet anomaly transmission. Canine Pract., *4*(3):33, 1977.
12. Weber, S. E., Evans, D. A. and Feldman, B. F.: Pelger-Huet anomaly of granulocytic leukocytes in two feline littermates. Feline Pract., *11*(1):44, 1981.
13. Weiden, P. L., Robinett, B., Graham, T. C. Adamson, I., and Storb, R.: Canine cyclic neutropenia: A stem cell defect. J. Clin. Invest., *53*:950, 1974.
14. Lund, J. E., Padgett, G. A., and Ott, R. L.: Cyclic neutropenia in grey collie dogs. Blood, *29*:452, 1967.
15. Cheville, N. F.: The grey collie syndrome. J.A.V.M.A., *152*:620, 1968.
16. Renshaw, H. W., Catburn, C., Bryan, G. M., Bartsch, R. C., and Davis, W. C.: Canine granulocytopathy syndrome: Neutrophil dysfunction in a dog with recurrent infections. J.A.V.M.A., *166*:443, 1975.
17. Renshaw, H. W. and Davis, W. C.: Canine granulocytopathy syndrome. Am. J. Pathol., *95*:731, 1979.
18. Renshaw, H. W., Davis, W. C., and Renshaw, S. J.: Canine granulocytopathy syndrome: Defective bactericidal capacity of neutrophils from a dog with recurrent infections. Clin. Immunol. Immunopathol., *8*:385, 1977.
19. Kramer, J. W., Davis, W. C., and Prieur, D. J.: The Chédiak-Higashi syndrome of cats. Lab Invest., *36*:554, 1977.
20. Kramer, J. W., Davis, W. C., Prieur, D. J., Baxter, J. and Norsworthy, G. D.: An inherited disorder of Persian cats with intracytoplasmic inclusions in neutrophils. J.A.V.M.A., *166*:1103, 1975.
21. Schalm, O. W.: Mucopolysaccharidosis. Canine Pract., *4*(6):29, 1977.
22. Crowell, K. R., Jezyk, P. F., Haskins, M. E. and Patterson, D. F.: Mucopolysaccharidosis in a cat. J.A.V.M.A., *169*:334, 1976.
23. Langweiler, M., Haskins, M. E., and Jezyk, P. F.: Mucopolysaccharidosis in a litter of cats. J.A.A.H.A., *14*:748, 1978.
23a. Hirsch, V. M., and Cunningham, T. A.: Hereditary anomaly of neutrophil granulation in Birman cats. Am. J. Vet. Res., *45*:2170, 1984.
23b. Leifer, C. E., Matus, R. E., Patnaik, A. K., and MacEwen, E. G.: Chronic myelogenous leukemia in the dog. J.A.V.M.A., *183*:686, 1983.
24. Ragan, H. A., Hackett, P. L., and Dagle, G. E.: Acute myelomonocytic leukemia manifested as myelophthisic anemia in a dog. J.A.V.M.A., *169*:421, 1976.
25. Green, R. A., and Barton, C. L.: Acute myelomonocytic leukemia in a dog. J.A.A.H.A., *13*:708, 1977.
26. Linnabary, R. D., Holscher, M. A., Glick, A. D., Powell, H. S., and McCallum, H. M.: Acute myelomonocytic leukemia in a dog. J.A.A.H.A., *14*:71, 1978.
27. Medway, W., Weber, W. T., O'Brien, J. A., and Krawitz, L.: Multiple myeloma in a dog. J.A.V.M.A., *150*:386, 1967.
28. Osborne, C. A., Perman, V., Sautter, J. H., Stevens, J. B., and Hanlon, G. F.: Multiple myeloma in the dog. J.A.V.M.A., *153*:1300, 1968.
29. Shepard, V. J., Dodds-Laffin, W. J. and Laffin, R. J.: Gamma A myeloma in a dog with defective hemostasis. J.A.V.M.A., *160*:1121, 1972.
30. Liu, S., and Carb, A. V.: Erythroblastic leukemia in a dog. J.A.V.M.A., *152*:1511, 1968.
31. Hartziolos, B. C.: Lymphoblastic lymphoma in a bovine fetus. J.A.V.M.A., *136*:368, 1960.
32. Goetze, R., Rosenberger, G., and Ziegenhagen, G.: Uber Ursachen und Bekampfung der Rinderleukose. V. Ubertragungswege und Bekampfungvorschlog. Deutsche Tierartzl. Wchnschr., *63*:112, 1956.
33. Bendixen, H. J.: Studies on leukosis in cattle. 3. Control of leukosis herds using hematological examination. Nord. Vet. Med., *11*:733, 1959.
34. Dungworth, C. L., Theilen, G. H., and Lengyel, J.: Bovine lymphosarcoma in California. Pathol. Vet., *1*:323, 1964.
35. Hyde, J. L., King, J. M., and Bentinck-Smith, J.: A case of bovine myelogenous leukemia. Cornell Vet., *48*:269, 1958.
36. Holzworth, J., and Meier, H.: Reticulum cell myeloma in a cat. Cornell Vet. *47*:303, 1957.
37. Michel, R. L., O'Handley, P., and Dade, W.: Megakaryocytic myelosis in a cat. J.A.V.M.A., *168*:1021, 1976.
38. Gilmore, C. E., and Holzworth, J.: Naturally occurring feline leukemia: Clinical, pathologic and differential diagnostic features. J.A.V.M.A., *158*:1013, 1971.
39. Holzworth, J.: Leukemia and related neoplasms in the cat. II. Malignancies other than lymphoid. J.A.V.M.A., *136*:107, 1960.
40. Henness, A. M., Crow, S. E., and Anderson, B. C.: Monocytic leukemia in three cats. J.A.V.M.A., *170*:1325, 1977.
41. Schalm, O. W. P: Comments on feline leukemia: Clinical and pathologic features. J.A.V.M.A. *158*:1025, 1971.
42. Sodikoff, D. H., and Schalm, O. W.: Primary bone marrow disease in the cat. III. Erythremic myelosis and myelofibrosis. A myeloproliferative disorder. Calif. Vet., *22*(6):16, 1968.
43. Cornelius, C. E., Goodbary, R. F., and Kennedy, P. C.: Plasma cell myelomatosis in a horse. Cornell Vet., *49*:478, 1959.
44. Trum B. F., and Carll, W. T.: Lymphatic leukemia in a hog following atomic exposure to gamma radiation. J.A.V.M.A., *131*:448, 1957.

CHAPTER

4

BONE MARROW

In the embryo, blood is formed essentially in the mesenchyme, endothelium, liver, spleen, thymus, and lymph nodes; but as bone marrow develops, the formation of blood cells is transferred to this organ.

In the young animal, bone marrow is cellular. As the animal ages, cellular marrow decreases in quantity, particularly in the more distal bones of the body, and is replaced by yellow marrow. Cellular marrow continues to exist in flat bones, including the sternum, ribs, bones of the pelvis, and vertebrae. In the mature animal, there is little active marrow in long bones, except for the humerus and femur. Although there is a limited quantity of actively regenerating marrow in a mature individual, primitive cells remain that are capable of multiplication and production of mature blood cells.

The majority of blood cells in the mature animal are formed by mitosis of already differentiated cells that produce progeny cells in a similar stage of development. In this manner, a neutrophilic myelocyte produces two neutrophilic myelocytes, which may either mature from that point without any further division or redivide at the same level of maturity then redivide again at a more mature level. This kind of cellular division may occur with any type of cell produced in marrow. Bone marrow is capable of producing erythrocytes, thrombocytes (platelets), eosinophils, basophils, monocytes, and neutrophils. In addition, it is a minor site of production of lymphocytes and plasmacytes.

BONE MARROW EXAMINATION

In the differential diagnosis of diseases characterized by alterations in the peripheral blood, examination of the bone marrow may be a valuable diagnostic tool. Such an examination is especially indicated in diseases associated either with a decrease or increase in cellular elements or with the appearance of abnormal cellular forms. When a peripheral blood count indicates the presence of leukopenia, nonregenerative anemia, or thrombocytopenia, or if abnormal cell types appear, a bone marrow examination should be considered. Bone marrow study may be of value in confirming a diagnosis of leukemia and in differentiating it from a leukemoid reaction. Although some leukemias can be specifically identified by alterations present in peripheral blood, bone marrow examination may be necessary when neoplasia is suspected but cannot be confirmed by examination of peripheral blood.

Refractory anemias are often difficult to diagnose, and use of a bone marrow examination may be of great assistance. Megaloblastic anemia can be accurately differentiated from normoblastic anemia only by bone marrow examination. Nutritional anemias, such as those occurring with vitamin B_{12}, folic acid, and vitamin B_6 deficiencies, can be readily differentiated by means of a bone marrow examination. The only accurate method for diagnosing erythroleukemia is examination of bone marrow.

Bone marrow examinations may be contraindicated if the animal has a severe coagulation defect. Such an examination may, however, be of some value in determining the status of thrombocyte production in animals having a thrombocytopenia.

LIMITATIONS OF BONE MARROW EXAMINATION

Theoretically, it should be possible to determine by bone marrow examination the exact state of production of formed elements of blood and to accurately evaluate alterations. However, difficulties may be encountered in the interpretation of the results of bone marrow examination.

Representative samples of bone marrow may be somewhat difficult to obtain from domestic animals, but with care adequate specimens can be secured. With a bone marrow biopsy it is difficult to obtain a sample that is not contaminated with peripheral blood. Such contamination may occur as a result of the surgical procedure required or by entrance into a sinusoid in the marrow and aspiration of peripheral blood. Although there is some experimental evidence to indicate that the concentrations of cellular elements in the marrow may differ in bones from different parts of the skeleton of many species of animals, there is evidence suggesting that in the dog, these differences are not of any great interpretative significance.[1]

It is almost impossible to make a quantitative evaluation of cellular elements in bone marrow, as no reproducible technique for a total count of the nucleated cells in bone marrow has been described. Thus, results are recorded on a relative basis, making interpretation of differential counts more difficult and less reliable than it would be if absolute numbers could be accurately recorded. Interpretation of bone marrow examination is enhanced and reliable only if reference is made to peripheral blood values.

Accurate interpretation of bone marrow examination is dependent upon the experience and ability of the individual examining the smear. Since normal marrow is generally quite cellular, the individual examining the slide must be familiar with the stages of development of the formed elements of blood. Particularly difficult is the differentiation between nucleated forms of erythrocytes and other mononuclear cells.

Normal values for different cell types in various species of domestic animals are presented in Table 4–1. Although these percentages are based on a limited number of surveys, they are relatively accurate and may be used as a guide for interpretation of results.

TECHNIQUE OF BONE MARROW EXAMINATION

Although some difficulty may be encountered in aspirating adequate marrow samples, aspiration can be successfully accomplished in most animal species. Since the possibility of infection exists, care should be taken to use aseptic techniques. Skin over the selected site should be shaved, washed twice with a good soap or detergent, and finally treated by application of a skin disinfectant. All equipment used should be sterilized by hot air or autoclaving. The operator should wear rubber gloves. Infection at the op-

TABLE 4–1. Normal Values for Bone Marrow Examinations in Various Species of Domestic Animals (Species Variations Reported in Literature)

ANIMAL	Cells (Per Cent)													
	MYB.	PRO-GRAN.	PREMYL.	NEUT. MYEL.	META-MYEL.	BAND	NEUT. SEG.	EOS.	BASO.	MONO.	LYM.	NUCL. RBC	MEGA.	M:E RATIO
Dog	0.6		1.6	6.0	3.4	11.7	30.1	2.0		0.2	0.9	42.2	0.5	1:1
Male	1.4	1.5		9.3	5.3	27.8	12.0	3.7	0	—	7.9	24.1	1.1	2.7:1
Fem.	1.1	1.4		8.5	5.6	24.6	8.2	4.6	0	—	7.7	32.3		1.68:1
Cat	1.1	2.8		5.9	15.0	14.7	14.0	2.1	0	—	5.1	38.4	—	1.6:1
Cat	0.82			5.22	7.96	30.6	22.5	2.81			9.05	20.1	—	3.5:1
	0.34	1.11		6.13	16.01	32.51		2.9	0.26	0.56	3.51	40.7	—	1.46:1
	1.74	0.88		9.76	7.32	25.8	9.24	3.8	0.002	—	7.63	25.88	—	2.47
Cow			1.51	19.39			5.73	8.61	0.34	2.64	6.68	51.95		0.676
Cow			0.79	2.90	4.14	8.2	11.46	7.76	0.19	0.16	10.69	50.24	0.05	0.79
Cow	2.3	1.5		6.5		9.7	6.2	8.3	0.3	0.4	7.2	51.6	0.1	0.71
Goat	0.58		0.79	2.69	8.25	8.88	9.98	1.79	0.06	0.02	7.49	56.33		0.69
Horse			1.83	38.06			13.31	0.60	0.60	2.46	3.91	35.25		1.64
Horse	0.237		0.50	17.94	21.80		14.70	6.09	0.05		9.71	26.16		2.43
Sheep	0.47		0.24	4.60	4.33	16.38	4.58	18.49	1.0	0.26	1.73	46.03		1.09:1.0
Sheep	0.42	0.52		2.23	4.22	9.07	6.61	8.77	0.42	2.24	3.64	60.83	—	0.5

Myb. = myeloblast, Progran. = progranulocyte, Premyl. = premyelocyte, Neut. Myel. = neutrophilic myelocyte, Neut. Seg. = neutrophilic segmenter, Eos. = eosinophil, Baso. = basophil, Mono. = monocyte, Lym. = lymphocyte, Nucl. RBC = nucleated erythrocytes, Mega. = megakaryocyte, M:E ratio = myeloid:erythroid ratio.

erative site is difficult to explain to a client, and a death following infection in the marrow even more difficult. Utilization of an aseptic surgical technique should assist the operator in avoiding these possibilities.

In some animal species it is necessary to make a skin incision. Experience in this laboratory indicates that use of a local anesthetic containing epinephrine has some advantage, as it assists in the control of hemorrhage. If hemorrhage occurs, vessels should be clamped and the area carefully sponged in order to avoid contamination of the sample with peripheral blood.

Equipment and supplies necessary for obtaining a sample of bone marrow will vary according to the species of animal being examined and the collection site. There are, however, several items of equipment and some supplies that are common to all bone marrow examinations. Equipment recommended for the sterile bone marrow tray includes:

1. Twenty-ml syringe with metal tip.
2. Two 20-ml syringes with metal tip.
3. Two or three hemostats.
4. Six or more cotton sponges.
5. Knife handle and blades.
6. Two bone marrow needles. (The size and length of the needles will depend upon the species of animal.) (Fig. 4–1)
7. Two 20-gauge hypodermic needles, each 1 inch long.
8. Suture needles of appropriate size.
9. Suture material (nylon or other nonirritating material.

This bone marrow tray should be covered and sterilized by autoclaving. In some species of animals, additional equipment may be necessary. If a sample is to be removed from the femur of a dog, the equipment should include an intramedullary pin drill, intramedullary pins of the appropriate

size, a split Silverman needle, a Silverman biopsy needle with stylet, and a Jacobs chuck wrench. In aspiration of bone marrow from the rib of a cow, it is advisable to include a hand drill with drill bits of appropriate size and a muscle spreader.

Equipment not enclosed in the sterile tray but accompanying it should include:

1. Sterile rubber gloves and shroud.
2. Procaine or other suitable local anesthetic.
3. A skin disinfectant.
4. Several clean new glass slides. (Slides can be stored in alcohol and dried prior to use with a lintless soft cloth.)
5. A small bottle containing 10 per cent buffered formalin.
6. A test tube containing a small quantity of ethylenediaminetetraacetic acid (EDTA) or other suitable anticoagulant.

Methods of Collection. A number of different techniques for collection of marrow are described below.

Dog and Cat. The best source of marrow for the dog and cat is the humerus. Collection is relatively simple and it is easy to obtain representative samples.

The site is located on the anterolateral part of the humerus. The collection point is located by palpating the scapulohumeral joint and locating the ridge on the lateral part of the upper humerus. The ridge is followed downward for about a third of its length and the flat area just medial to the ridge is anesthetized with a local anesthetic, being sure to include anesthesia of the periosteum. A small skin incision is made over the flat spot and a Jamshidi bone marrow needle, with stylet in place, is placed against the bone. The hand not used for handling the needle is placed on the inside of the humerus and with constant pressure and a twisting motion the needle is introduced

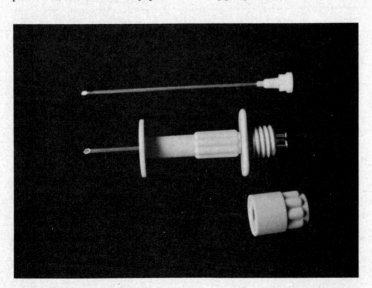

Figure 4–1. The Jamshidi bone marrow needle is preferred for collections from the humerus and crest of the ilium of dogs and cats. The needle should be introduced into the marrow cavity with the stylet in place.

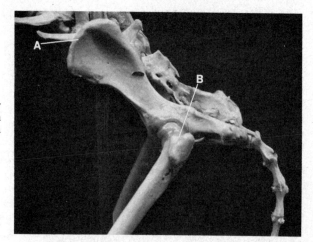

Figure 4–2. Anatomical sites for bone marrow sampling. *A*, Crest of ilium. *B*, The trochanteric fossa can be used in the dog and is the preferred site in the cat.

into the marrow cavity. The stylet is removed, a 10 to 20 ml syringe is attached, and with a quick sudden movement the plunger is withdrawn. If the marrow cavity has been entered and the lumen of the needle is free of bone, a small amount of marrow will appear in the syringe. If no marrow is aspirated, the stylet should be replaced and the needle moved slightly; the stylet is removed and the syringe re-attached. If no marrow appears in the syringe, withdraw the bone marrow needle without its stylet. Push any material out of the marrow needle by introducing the stylet while holding the needle over a microscope slide. Spicules of marrow can sometimes be collected in this manner that can be used for making slides or for histologic sectioning.

Dog. Bone marrow samples are readily obtained from the iliac crest of the dog (Fig. 4–2). Although a specimen can be taken without anesthetic, use of procaine or other suitable anesthetic has proved advantageous. In excitable dogs use of a tranquilizer may be indicated. The iliac crest is outlined with the fingers and the surface prepared for aseptic surgery. A short skin incision is made to facilitate penetration. The dog may be in a standing position, but if the animal resists, it should be placed on its side with the hind legs extended or in a sitting position with the hind legs held tightly under the abdomen.

A sterile aspiration needle, such as a Turkel or Jamshidi bone marrow needle or a 2-inch, 14- to 16-gauge needle with a stylet in place is passed through the skin and muscle over the anterior dorsal angle of the iliac crest. When the periosteum is reached, the needle is forced into the bone by steady pressure accompanied by rotation. When the needle becomes firmly embedded, it has usually penetrated the medullary cavity. The stylet is removed and a dry, 10- to 20-ml glass syringe is fitted to the needle. The plunger should be pulled out quickly to establish a vacuum and withdraw marrow fluid. Only a small amount of fluid (0.5 to 1.0 ml) should be aspirated. As soon as fluid

appears, vacuum should be discontinued, as further negative pressure may result in rupture of a sinusoid and contamination with peripheral blood. This technique is useful in most large breeds of dogs. However, it may be difficult to enter the marrow cavity of the iliac crest of small breeds. Difficulty may also be encountered in older dogs, as bone of the iliac crest is hard and may be difficult to penetrate.

The sternum may also be utilized for obtaining bone marrow specimens. The dog is placed in dorsal recumbency, and a bone marrow biopsy needle is inserted vertically into the first or second sternebra. When the sternum is used, care should be taken to ensure that the guard plate on the bone marrow needle is in position about ½ inch from the end. This is done to avoid the possibility of creating cardiac tamponade as a consequence of penetration of the thoracic cavity and entrance into the pericardium. Occasionally, the needle will tend to roll off the sternum, since this structure is somewhat narrow and sharp in the dog.

Bone marrow can be obtained from a rib. The dog is placed in left lateral recumbency. The junction of the upper and middle third of the seventh rib is utilized as the site. A needle is inserted near the anterior border of the rib in a posteromedial direction approximately 65 degrees to the vertical. When the bone marrow needle is firmly fixed in the rib, a syringe can be applied and a small specimen of marrow obtained. This is a difficult site to enter, since the rounded edge of the rib and the pressure required to penetrate the bone make risk of pleural puncture a distinct possibility.

The femur may also be used. Preoperative technique for a femoral puncture is similar to that for the iliac crest except that it is wise to employ general anesthesia. A Kirschner intramedullary pin drill, or other suitable drill, is used to introduce an intramedullary pin through the skin incision and muscles and into the proximal portion of the femur medial to the summit of the trochanter major. When the pin is introduced into the med-

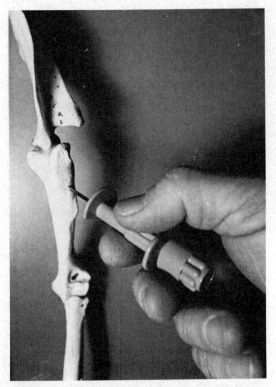

Figure 4–3. The easiest way to collect bone marrow from a dog or cat is from the humerus. The preferred site is on the anterolateral part of the humerus, as shown. A Jamshidi bone marrow needle, with stylet in place, is introduced into the marrow cavity using a twisting motion while applying pressure. When the marrow cavity is entered the stylet is removed, a 10 to 20 ml syringe is attached and with a quick sudden movement the plunger is withdrawn. If the marrow cavity has been entered a small quantity of marrow will enter the syringe.

ullary cavity, a distinct "give" may be felt. Do not allow the pin to penetrate deeply into the cavity. The pin is removed from the cavity and an aspirating needle with stylet in place are introduced through the same tract. The stylet is removed and a 10-ml syringe attached. With gentle suction a marrow sample is obtained. It is important to have the needle in either the proximal or distal third of the femur, as it is almost impossible to obtain a representative sample of cellular marrow from the middle third of the marrow cavity.

Cat. Because of the small size of the iliac crest, sternum, and rib, the femur is the preferred site for bone marrow aspiration in the cat. The cat is anesthetized, an area over the trochanteric fossa (Fig. 4–2) is prepared for surgery, and a small skin incision is made. An intramedullary pin of approximately 15 gauge is directed through the skin incision until it contacts bone of the fossa. The shaft of the pin is aligned with the shaft of the

femur, and a slight drilling motion is utilized to open the medullary cavity. The pin is removed and replaced with a 16-gauge needle with stylet. A 16-gauge Rosenthal needle (Becton-Dickinson, East Rutherford, New Jersey) may be used in place of the pin. A 2 ml syringe is attached and slight suction is applied to the syringe and discontinued as soon as marrow appears. The syringe and needle are withdrawn, and the contents expressed onto clean glass slides. Marrow collected in this fashion appears as soft, reddish-gray clumps and is free of excessive quantities of peripheral blood. Excessive drilling with the medullary pin as well as excessive suction with the syringe should be avoided. If these precautions are not followed, marrow samples may become contaminated with peripheral blood. If contamination occurs, the sample can be concentrated by centrifugation, and the smear can be prepared from the buffy coat.

The crest of the ilium can be used for obtaining marrow specimens. The cat is placed on a table and gently restrained in sternal position by an assistant. The anterodorsal margin of the ilium is located by palpation, and the area is prepared for surgery. A local anesthetic is utilized to infiltrate under the skin and against the bony margin of the ilium at its most prominent point. After sufficient time has elapsed (three to five minutes), a small incision is made through the skin over the iliac crest. A sterile aspiration needle such as an 18-gauge, ¾-inch needle with a large-hub Luer attachment and a seated stylet is most acceptable. This needle is positioned perpendicular to the bone between the medial and lateral margins of the iliac crest at its most prominent point. Moderate pressure is applied, and the needle is rotated alternately in short clockwise and counterclockwise movements until firmly seated in the bone. The stylet is withdrawn, and a 10-ml syringe is attached to the needle. The plunger is withdrawn to about the 3-ml mark and immediately released. The stylet is replaced in the needle and immediately withdrawn. A film of marrow on the stylet suggests that the needle is properly positioned. If no marrow is seen on the stylet, the needle should be redirected or introduced more deeply into the cavity. When marrow is seen on the stylet, the syringe is reattached and the plunger withdrawn until marrow enters the syringe. The plunger is released, and the syringe and needle are gently withdrawn by mild rotation. Small drops of marrow from the needle can be placed on one or more clean glass slides, and smears can be prepared. Occasionally, no marrow will enter the syringe. Under these circumstances, the vacuum should be held and the needle gently and slowly rotated. With this technique, adequate quantities of marrow are often introduced into the needle, and smears may be made from this specimen.

Cow. The two most common sites for obtaining a bone marrow specimen from the bovine species are the sternum and rib.

Sternal collection is most easily accomplished by first restraining the animal in a chute and selecting a site for biopsy. This site may be anywhere along the sternum near the center of one of the sternebrae. This site should be carefully cleansed, disinfected, and anesthetized. This procedure can be completed without anesthesia, but less restraint is necessary if anesthesia is used. A 1½- to 2-inch Turkel bone marrow biopsy needle is carefully introduced through the skin to the periosteum. When the periosteum has been reached, continual upward pressure is applied while the needle is rotated until it penetrates the marrow cavity. A quick, hard blow with a wooden mallet may be necessary in order to enter the marrow cavity. The stylet is removed, a syringe is attached, and marrow fluid is aspirated by creating a gentle vacuum within the syringe. This method of collection works well in young animals, but in older ones difficulty may be encountered in entering the marrow cavity.

Since difficulty is sometimes encountered in penetrating the marrow cavity of the sternebrae, bone marrow may be obtained from a rib. For this technique, the animal is confined in a stock or restrained against the side of the stall. The back and side should be thoroughly scrubbed, and the rib with the least amount of tissue covering, usually the eleventh or twelfth, should be located by palpation. The operative site, about 2 inches below the costovertebral articulation, is prepared for aseptic surgery. Anesthesia is obtained by injecting 5 to 10 ml of a suitable local anesthetic containing epinephrine. Care should be taken to ensure that the periosteum is anesthetized. An incision approximately 2 inches long is made through the skin and fascia, avoiding the latissimus dorsi and serratus dorsalis posterior muscles. A muscle spreader may be employed to allow the operator more freedom. A hand drill equipped with a straight shank $\frac{3}{32}$-inch jobber's drill is used to bore into the marrow cavity. A point midway between the anterior and posterior borders of the rib is chosen for insertion of the drill. When the medullary cavity is entered there is a tendency for the drill to "give" slightly. Following removal of the drill, a 12-gauge blunted needle with a shaft 0.75 cm long is inserted. This needle has the same outside diameter as the opening in the bone. An airtight 10-ml syringe is attached to aspirate the marrow. If a biopsy is preferred, a 14-gauge needle with a shaft 3 cm long and a blunt end may be inserted through the 12-gauge needle, and a plug of marrow may be obtained. Throughout this procedure hemorrhage should be controlled, as contamination with peripheral blood is a frequent problem. The incision is sutured with a nonabsorbable material. Bone marrow obtained in this manner is usually adequate; however, it may be contaminated with sinusoidal blood if too much vacuum is created in the syringe.

Other Species. Bone marrow specimens from other species of domestic animals are obtained in a similar manner. The site of choice for the horse is the rib or sternum and for the sheep, the sternum.

Preparation of Aspirated Material for Examination. **Bone Marrow Smear.** Delay in preparation of a smear for examination, no matter how brief, should be avoided. If small amounts of liquid material are obtained, films can be made in a manner similar to that used in preparation of films of peripheral blood. A few drops of marrow are placed on the end of a slide and excess blood is aspirated back into the syringe. If tissue fragments are aspirated, a "squash" preparation is made by placing a second slide firmly down on top of the marrow particles and very carefully drawing the two slides apart. Slides should be waved in the air for rapid drying. If desired, some aspirated marrow may be placed into a tube containing anticoagulant for later examination. It is preferable, however, to make smears from differential counting immediately following collection.

Properly collected marrow specimens can be quite cellular and the concentration of cells so great that individual cell identification is difficult. This problem can be avoided if aspirated marrow that has been collected in a small quantity of EDTA is immediately added to an equal amount of homologous plasma. Such a procedure reduces cell concentration, and a slide can be made directly from the diluted marrow. Cells are most widely distributed and cell identification is easier. This technique is particularly useful if numerous slides are to be prepared.

If small particles of bone from the medullary cavity are aspirated, these may be utilized for making a smear as follows. The particles are picked up with either a capillary pipette or the broken end of a wooden applicator or toothpick, transferred immediately to a slide, and made to stick to the slide by a gentle smearing motion. These slides should be rapidly air dried. In some animals, particularly the bovine, utilization of such particles of marrow has resulted in preparation of excellent smears for differential examination. A smear may be prepared by picking up a small amount of marrow on a fine camel's-hair brush and gently brushing the material on a slide. In such preparations cells are free of distortion and evenly distributed over the slide.

If one prefers, a coverslip can be utilized for preparing the smear in a manner similar to that described in Chapter Three for making a blood smear. Excellent preparations are made with this technique.

Bone Marrow Sections. It is often advantageous to prepare both smears and sections from a bone marrow biopsy. Identification of cells is best made from a smear, but the frequency and distribution of cells are better observed in the normal marrow architecture as seen in sections. One method for preparation of sections is to remove the amount of marrow required for preparation of smears and permit the remainder of the aspirate to clot in the syringe. This clot is placed in a fixative for sectioning. An alternative technique is to collect the marrow aspirate in an anticoagulant such as EDTA. With this technique, the biopsy specimen is placed on a slide, the slide is tilted, and excess blood is removed from the edge of the slide with gauze or absorbent paper. Marrow granules left on the slide are relatively free of blood and can be utilized for preparation of the smear or placed in a fixative for centrifugation and later sectioning.

Core biopsies from the dog and cat can be made by use of a pediatric Jamshidi bone marrow biopsy-aspiration needle. In small dogs and cats an 18-gauge bleeding needle and stylet can be used. The needle is introduced into the marrow of the iliac crest or humerus, the stylet is removed and the needle advanced more deeply into the marrow cavity. The needle is twisted and redirected to detach the marrow plug. A 20-ml syringe is attached and vacuum applied by quickly withdrawing the plunger of the syringe. While gentle vacuum is maintained, the needle is withdrawn. The plug is removed by reinsertion of the stylet, and the core is placed in 10 per cent formalin and processed as a tissue section.

An agar gel method for preparation of bone marrow sections has been described.[2] In this technique, marrow is aspirated into the anticoagulant. Smears are made for detailed examination of cytology, and the remainder of the aspirate is discharged onto a fine screen that retains marrow granules but permits sinusoidal blood to pass through. The remaining granules are washed free of blood with saline, and 2 per cent agar at 55°C is placed over the granules and allowed to solidify. This agar with the marrow embedded in it is removed from the screen and placed in a fixative. Since the marrow is on the surface of the agar, fixation is practically instantaneous, and cytologic details of the marrow are retained. The agar retains its shape throughout fixation, dehydration, and embedding and takes up very little stain. This technique has an advantage over the routine method of collecting specimens for preparation of sections for histologic examination. Use of this technique makes it possible to perform serial aspirations on the same animal. However, serial aspirations are not feasible if exceedingly large-sized instruments are utilized.

Staining. Any polychrome stain, such as Wright's, Wright-Giemsa, or May-Grünwald-Giemsa, may be utilized. Bone marrow smears should be exposed to stain for a longer period of time than is necessary for peripheral blood smears. (For details of polychrome staining methods, see Appendix, p. 000.)

Occasionally supravital signs may be indicated. Supravital staining techniques for bone marrow are similar to those for peripheral blood.

EXAMINATION OF MARROW FILM

Ability to accurately interpret marrow cytology is gained only by experience. In general, there are two ways in which a marrow film is examined. The first method entails scanning the slide under the low power of the microscope, then under the high dry objective, and, finally, under oil immersion magnification. On the basis of previous experience, it is possible for an operator to formulate impressions concerning the number and distribution of cells, in a manner similar to that utilized by a pathologist in reading sections of tissue. The second method entails making a differential count and calculating the percentage of each cell type. In making a differential count on bone marrow, a minimum of 500 cells should be examined, and it is preferable to count 1000 cells.

A painstaking differential count is used to confirm impressions gained in the original examination. Such differential counts afford an objective record against which future alterations may be measured. Ability to recognize cell types, particularly the various stages of cell development, tends to vary from one laboratory to another and from one technician to another (Plate 4–1). No normal value, or even range of values, can be accepted as universal. The most valid base line must be established in each laboratory and by each individual. With practice and experience, laboratory workers achieve a high degree of reproducibility in marrow counts.

Cell Identification. All cells that develop in bone marrow alter morphologically as they progress from primitive to mature types (Plate 4–1).

Primitive cells are usually larger than mature cells, and the nuclei of these young cells are relatively large in relation to the amount of cytoplasm contained in the cell. As cells develop through various stages of maturation, nuclei become smaller, and in erythrocytes they disappear completely. Another nuclear alteration that takes place is a change in shape. In primitive granulocytic cells, nuclei are round or oval or may have a slight indentation. As granulocytes mature, the nuclei lose this shape, become more deeply indented, and eventually are segmented. Color changes in the nucleus also become apparent as the cell matures. In young cells, nuclei are rich in deoxyribonucleic acid (DNA), and standard polychrome-stained films may have a red or reddish-purple tinge. As the nucleus begins to differentiate, it becomes predominantly blue and stains more darkly.

Alterations in nuclear chromatin also occur during cell maturation. In immature cells, chromatin strands have a fine, delicate structure. In the aging and degenerative process, there is a coarsening and irregular arrangement of the chromatin network. In some cells, the chromatin becomes dense and the nucleus a structureless pyknotic mass.

The presence of nucleoli is an indication of cellular immaturity. Nucleoli, which are signs of metabolic activity, are, in all probability, portions of cytoplasm in the process of formation. Nucleoli are usually visible as structureless masses within the nucleus that are light blue with Romanowsky-type stains. They are composed of ribonucleic acid (RNA). After the cell divides nucleoli lose their blue color and remain as structureless rings.

In addition to these nuclear changes, the cytoplasm is also altered in its staining characteristics. Primitive cells contain cytoplasm rich in RNA, which stains predominantly blue. The cytoplasm in developing cells becomes paler blue and is reddish as it begins to mature.

Since the nuclear, granular, and cytoplasmic changes do not take place at the same rate of speed, rapidly developing primitive cells may be small, whereas cells lacking essential maturation requirements may grow without dividing and become abnormally large. If maturation sequences that are out of phase with each other are observed in a bone marrow smear, this may be an indication of abnormality.

Since all developmental alterations from one cell type to another do not occur as a single step but as a gradual process, cells may be observed that are morphologically on the borderline between one stage of development and the next. Identification of such cells may prove to be difficult, but the best rule to follow is to "name the cell by the company it keeps." In other words, cells should be classified according to the most frequently occurring cell, which is usually the more mature form.

Occasionally, in specimens of abnormal marrow, cells will be seen that do not fall into any classification but closely resemble one another. These cells should be tallied separately, the characteristic morphology noted, and the total number of such cells recorded.

Stem Cells. When examining bone marrow or body fluid, one may encounter primitive cells that have no features that can be used to positively identify them as belonging to a particular cell series. For these undifferentiated mesenchymal cells the term *stem cell* is used. These primitive cells have morphologic characteristics similar to immature developmental forms of all cell types. These characteristics include a relatively large, round nucleus with fine chromatin that takes a reddish stain; the presence of fine nucleoli; and cytoplasm that takes a blue stain. The intensity of cytoplasmic basophilia may vary widely. The cytoplasm frequently has a foamy or mottled appearance and is likely to be less intensely stained in the area immediately surrounding the nucleus. Stem cells may be either large or the size of small leukocytes, depending upon the frequency of cellular division and the length of the period of growth between cell divisions. Margins of stem cells are often torn or jagged and contain protoplasmic projections.

Primitive cells, if associated with large numbers of identifiable cells or surrounded by differentiated cells that can be positively identified, are named by adding a specific prefix indicating the family of cells to the suffix *blast*. Thus, if such a primitive cell is observed in a bone marrow smear containing large numbers of lymphocytes, it is identified as a lymphoblast; whereas, if there is marked hyperplasia of the erythrocytic series, it is probably a rubriblast.

Granulocytic Series. The developmental stages (from immature to mature) of the granulocyte are: myeloblast → progranulocyte → myelocyte → metamyelocyte → band cell → segmented granulocyte.

MYELOBLAST. This cell has a fine chromatin structure and does not contain cytoplasmic granules. Nucleoli are usually visible, and the cytoplasm is distinctly basophilic. Cells with this morphology found in association with an increase in identifiable cells of the granulocytic series should be tentatively classified as myeloblasts.

PROGRANULOCYTE. This cell has a nuclear structure denser than that of the blast cell and has darkly stained azurophilic cytoplasmic granules. These are referred to as nonspecific, or primary, granules and may be present in varying numbers. Nucleoli are usually visible but are fewer in number than in less mature cells. The cytoplasm stains a less intense blue, and the nuclear:cytoplasmic ratio is altered, as the cytoplasm is more abundant than in less mature blast forms.

MYELOCYTE. This cell contains specific granules that are identified by their staining properties as neutrophilic, eosinophilic, or basophilic. The myelocyte is distinguished from the progranulocyte by the presence of these specific granules. Primary, azurophilic-staining granules similar to those observed in the progranulocyte may be present in small numbers. The nucleus is round or oval, and the chromatin is coarser than the chromatin of the progranulocyte. Nucleoli are not usually visible in this stage of development. Frequently, there are so many specific granules present that the structure and outline of the nucleus are hazy, but in most instances its round or oval shape and the coarseness of its chromatin can be distinguished. At this stage of development the cytoplasm has lost most of its basophilic properties and stains a faint grayish-pink.

A wide variation in the shape, size, and concentration of granules occurs in eosinophilic cells from various species of domestic animals. Eosinophilic granules in cells from the dog vary in size and stain lightly. In the cat, eosinophil granules are rod-shaped and stain a grayish-orange. In the cow, the granules are small and round and stain an intense red. Eosinophilic granules of sheep cells are easily stained and ovoid. The eosinophilic granules in horse cells are characteristic, as

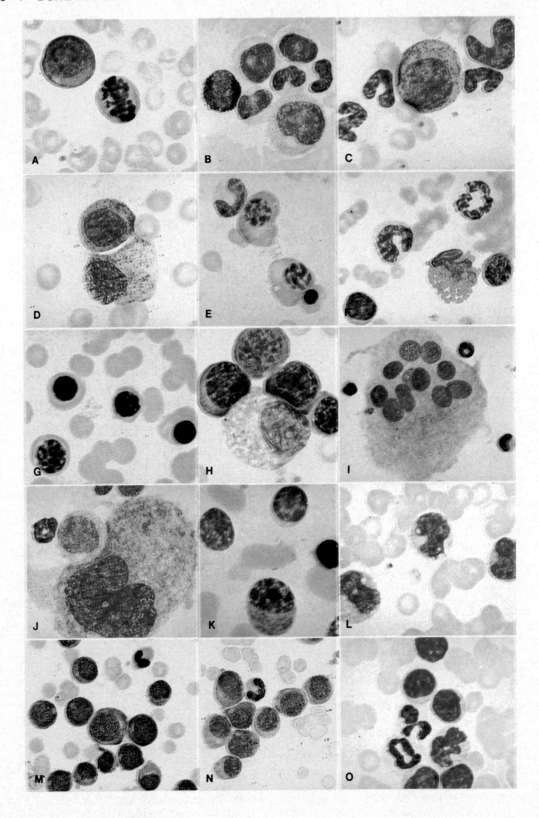

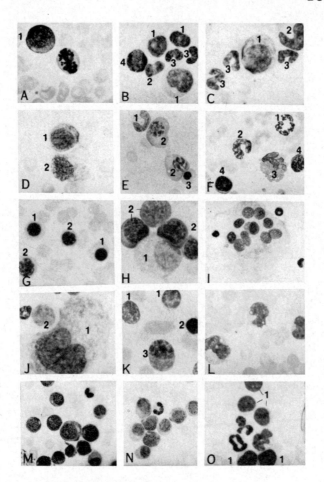

Plate 4–1   Key

A. Canine marrow with blast cell (1) and cell in mitosis. (500×)

B. Porcine marrow with neutrophilic myelocytes (1), a metamyelocyte (2), band neutrophils (3), and a basophil (4). (500×)

C. Canine marrow with a progranulocyte (1), a large band neutrophil (2), and usual-sized band neutrophils (3). (500×)

D. Canine marrow with an early progranulocyte (1) and a granular histiocyte (2). (500×)

E. Equine marrow with a band neutrophil (1), plasma cells (2), and a metarubricyte (3). (500×)

F. Equine marrow with a segmented neutrophil (1), a band neutrophil (2), an eosinophil (3), and rubricytes (4). (500×)

G. Equine marrow with metarubricytes (1) and polychromatic rubricytes (2). (500×)

H. Canine marrow with a vacuolated early neutrophilic myelocyte (1) and basophilic rubricytes (2). (670×)

I. Canine marrow with a multinucleated osteoclast. (200×)

J. Canine marrow with a megakaryocyte (1), a neutrophilic myelocyte (2), and a band neutrophil.

K. Equine marrow with lymphocytes (1), a late rubricyte (2), and a plasma cell (3). (670×)

L. Canine peripheral blood with three monocytes. Note the vacuolated cytoplasm. (500×)

M. Peripheral blood from a cat with myeloproliferative disease. Note the immature mononuclear cells with a basophilic cytoplasm. (330×)

N. Bone marrow from the same cat (M), with similar immature mononuclear cells. (330×)

O. Peripheral blood from a dog with lymphosarcoma characterized by the presence of many large lymphocytes (1).

they are large and stain a dull red-orange. In the pig, these granules are pale pink-orange to light red and are ovoid.

The basophilic myelocyte is also distinct in appearance, and the tendency for the granules to obscure the nucleus is even greater than with the eosinophil. These granules stain a dark blue to black and often vary in size within a single cell. Cat and dog basophils have granules that vary in size and staining quality. A few are large, round, and black, but the majority are smaller, round, and pinkish-gray. Both types of granules may be present in a single cell.

Granulation in the neutrophil is not obvious in cells from various species of domestic animals. Granulation is often indicated only by a granular appearance of the cytoplasm without the presence of definite granules. The myelocyte and cells in all subsequent stages of development of the granulocytic series are characterized by the staining properties of granules within the cytoplasm.

METAMYELOCYTE. This cell closely resembles the myelocyte but has a slightly indented nucleus. This indentation occupies less than half the width of the nucleus, and the portions of the nucleus on either side of the indentation are not parallel. The nucleus often resembles a kidney bean. The nuclear chromatin is coarser than that in younger cells. Cytoplasmic granules (eosinophilic, basophilic, or neutrophilic) are present. The cytoplasm is rarely basophilic if maturation is proceeding normally.

BAND CELL. This cell of the granulocytic series has a nucleus that resembles a curved or coiled band. The band cell may be differentiated from the metamyelocyte by the lengthening of the nucleus and a tendency for the sides to become parallel. In examination of blood from domestic animals, it is important to distinguish between the true band neutrophil and the mature neutrophil that contains only a single lobe. Membrane irregularity and narrowing of the nucleus at a single point indicate maturity, and such a cell should be classified as a segmented granulocyte. If this differentiation is not carefully made, the value of a differential leukocyte count may be affected. Typical cytoplasmic granules (eosinophilic, basophilic, or neutrophilic) are present.

SEGMENTED GRANULOCYTE. This cell may be eosinophilic, neutrophilic, or basophilic, depending upon the staining properties of the cytoplasmic granules. The nucleus is lobated, and the lobes of the nucleus are connected by filaments. If the nucleus is monolobed, the nuclear membrane is ragged in appearance. If lobes overlie each other, it may be difficult to ascertain the true character of the cell. If the identification of a cell as a mature segmented neutrophil or a band cell is uncertain, the former category should be chosen, as these cells occur with much greater frequency than do the more immature band forms.

Lymphocytic Series. Lymphocytes are formed in lymphoid tissue in many parts of the body, including the spleen, thymus, tonsils, lymph glands, and Peyer's patches. A few lymphocytes are formed in the marrow, but they are not normally present in this organ in large numbers.

LYMPHOBLAST. It is difficult to differentiate this cell from other blast forms, as it has characteristics similar to those of the myeloblast. These cells are identified by "the company they keep."

PROLYMPHOCYTE. The morphologic characteristics of the prolymphocyte are intermediate between those of the lymphoblast and those of the mature lymphocyte. It has a coarser chromatin structure than the lymphoblast, and yet the chromatin structure is too fine for the cell to be classified as a lymphocyte. The nuclei usually contain indistinct nucleoli and are somewhat larger in diameter than the nuclei of mature cells. The cytoplasm stains a shade of blue that is intermediate between the dark blue of the lymphoblast and the light blue of the mature lymphocyte.

LYMPHOCYTE. The nucleus of a mature lymphocyte has a coarser chromatin structure and is usually located eccentrically. Azurophilic granules may be observed in the cytoplasm of lymphocytes; they occur most frequently in the bovine and ovine species. The small quantity of cytoplasm stains light blue. Occasionally, the nucleus has a slight indentation.

Erythrocytic Series. The developmental stages (from immature to mature) of the erythrocyte are: rubriblast → prorubricyte → rubricyte (basophilic → polychromatophilic → normochromic) → metarubricyte → reticulocyte → erythrocyte.

RUBRIBLAST. Rubriblasts have characteristics of other blast cells. In young rubriblasts, the cytoplasm stains a light blue, but in more mature forms, there is a superimposed reddish tint that gives the cytoplasm a peculiar dark purplish-blue color. The nucleus usually contains nucleoli and is round. The chromatin pattern is delicate but has a tendency to be stippled and has a slightly red coloration.

PRORUBRICYTE. The prorubricyte is smaller than the rubriblast, and the nuclear chromatin is less delicate. Nucleoli are indefinite or absent. The cytoplasm is predominantly blue or basophilic. A reddish tint may appear in the cytoplasm, or spots of reddish material may be present because of the beginning development of hemoglobin. The nucleus is commonly located in the center of the cell surrounded by a narrow zone of blue cytoplasm.

RUBRICYTE. The rubricyte is smaller than the prorubricyte and may have a nuclear chromatin arrangement in a pattern suggesting the spokes of a wheel. This nuclear arrangement is due to the appearance of darkly stained portions of nuclear chromatin separated by light streaks. The cytoplasm is bluish red or polychromic. This variation in cytoplasmic staining permits classification of the cell as a basophilic, polychromatophilic, or normochromic rubricyte, depending on the degree of hemoglobination.

METARUBRICYTE. The cytoplasm in this cell is predominantly red, but there may be a slight residual basophilia. In some cells, the cytoplasm stains the same way as do nonnucleated erythrocytes found in the same field. The nucleus of this cell is pyknotic and appears as a blue-black mass with no distinguishable chromatin strands.

RETICULOCYTE. This is a nonnucleated cell of the erythrocytic series that when stained by a supravital technique has one or more granules present or, more commonly, has a diffuse network of fibrils. In routinely stained blood smears reticulocytes are larger than mature cells and are usually polychromatophilic.

ERYTHROCYTE. These are the mature cells of the series and stain buff or reddish. Crenation and slight irregularities of the surface are considered to be normal variants and may occur in any smear of peripheral blood or bone marrow. The number of such cells in a smear is dependent, to a large degree, upon the manner in which the slide was prepared.

Thrombocytic Series. MEGAKARYOBLAST. Megakaryoblasts resemble other undifferentiated stem cells. The cytoplasm stains a light blue with outer layers tending to be differentiated as a darker blue, vacuolated zone. Cytoplasmic masses appear to be breaking off at the margin of the cell. The nucleus is relatively large, red-staining, and round with a fine chromatin pattern and nucleoli. Frequently the cell is binucleate.

PROMEGAKARYOCYTE. The nucleus of the promegakaryocyte has a chromatin structure similar to that of an immature cell, but the nucleus is multilobed or indented. The cytoplasm stains blue and contains a variable number of granules that stain bluish. Projections on the cytoplasm, sometimes referred to as cytoplasmic buds, are present.

MEGAKARYOCYTE. This is the largest cell present in bone marrow, often being more than 100 microns in diameter. The cytoplasm is plentiful and has coarse granules. Some cytoplasmic granules are aggregated as well-defined masses or as small, ill-defined clumps. The well-defined massed are thrombocytes and are most numerous at the cell periphery. The nucleus of a mature megakaryocyte is lobulated or indented, no nucleoli are present, and the chromatin pattern is similar to that of any mature cell. Anuclear cytoplasmic masses may be present, and, occasionally, a nucleus devoid of cytoplasm is observed.

THROMBOCYTE. The thrombocyte is the non-nucleated fragment of megakaryocyte cytoplasm that contains azurophilic granules similar to those seen in the megakaryocyte.

Monocytic Series. Young forms of monocytes, particularly monoblasts, may be difficult to differentiate from other immature cells in marrow.

The monoblast is often larger than the corresponding blast cell of the neutrophilic and erythrocytic series. Nucleoli are usually prominent, and the cytoplasm is finely granular and basophilic.

As the monocyte matures it begins to assume the characteristics of the cell commonly seen in peripheral blood. The nucleus becomes indented, and a fine nuclear chromatin pattern develops. This chromatin is evenly stained, and pale reddish-purple strands appear in a flowing pattern often described as a lacy network. Occasionally, the chromatin may be more darkly stained and compact near the edges of the nucleus. The relatively large nucleus is irregularly shaped and sometimes folded upon itself in the mature monocyte.

Some monocytes in the marrow may show signs of increased activity. Such cells have a vacuolated cytoplasm, many contain remnants of erythrocyte nuclei, and a few may have hemosiderin. Hemosiderin may appear as dark golden granules, but if the granules are extremely dense they will be black. Hemosiderin is most easily identified by use of an iron-specific stain such as Prussian blue.

Other Cells. RETICULUM CELLS. The reticulum cell, often thought to be the basic stem cell for production of all formed elements of peripheral blood, is a relatively large, oval to irregularly shaped cell. The nucleus is also oval to irregularly shaped. The cytoplasm constitutes approximately one-third of the total cell volume, is somewhat pale-staining, and has an indistinct border. The cytoplasm stains a lilac-gray and contains small nonspecific polychromatic granules. These granules are often indistinct and difficult to see. The nucleus contains two to four nucleoli, and its chromatin arrangement is fine and usually linear. These cells are sometimes seen in small groups on a marrow film, although they are present in limited numbers, usually less than 1 per cent of all cells. Nuclei devoid of cytoplasm are not uncommon in bone marrow smears.

PLASMA CELLS. The plasma cell is oval or elongated with a round, relatively small, eccentrically placed nucleus. The cytoplasm stains a dark purplish-blue, and there is a clear, relatively unstained area immediately next to the nucleus. The cytoplasm of these cells may contain unstained globules that give these cells a foamy appearance (Russell bodies). Only a few plasma cells are present in bone marrow preparations, but are increased in plasmacytoma or following antigenic stimulation.

TISSUE EOSINOPHILS. These cells are similar to the eosinophils in circulating blood. Tissue eosinophils, however, are usually larger than those in the peripheral circulation. They have an irregular shape, and cytoplasmic projections are obvious. The nucleus of the tissue eosinophil is usually round or oval and has a coarse nuclear chromatin. As these are tissue cells and are found only when damage has occurred to fixed cells in the marrow, the cytoplasmic membrane is often ruptured and eosinophilic granules will be found freed from the cell.

TISSUE BASOPHILS. These cells have numerous deep-staining basophilic granules that are round and fairly uniform in size and may be present in such large numbers as to almost obscure the nucleus. These cells vary in shape, usually having a stellate appearance. They may or may not be related to free basophils in circulating blood. Evidence furnished by special staining procedures suggests that the free basophil is closely related to the tissue basophil, the primary difference between the two being in the lack of motility of the latter.

OSTEOBLASTS. The osteoblast is a fixed tissue cell that is present in all normal marrow but is aspirated during routine procedures only with difficulty. These are seldom seen in marrow smears but may be seen in sections made from bone marrow. These cells closely resemble plasma cells, as they are oval with an intense blue cytoplasm and an uneven granular appearance. Pale zones may be present in the cytoplasm, usually some distance from the nucleus. In bone marrow smears or sections they are usually observed in clumps.

OSTEOCLASTS. The osteoclast is a multinuclear cell. Several small, round nuclei may be seen in a reddish-purple, unevenly stained, finely granular cytoplasm. It can be differentiated from the megakaryocyte by the nuclei, which are not connected but separate and distinct.

INTERPRETATION OF BONE MARROW EXAMINATION

An accurate interpretation of bone marrow examination can be made only in light of the peripheral blood findings. A blood sample should be collected near the time of a marrow aspirate. Serious errors in interpretation may occur unless the results from both examinations are available.

In interpreting the results of a marrow examination one should evaluate the following: (1) degree of cellularity; (2) presence of all cell series; (3) presence of morphologic abnormalities; (4) sequence of development of each cell type; (5) approximate myeloid erythroid ratio; and (6) presence or absence of abnormal cells.

DEGREE OF CELLULARITY. The degree of cellularity is difficult to determine unless spicules of marrow are present. Some fluid samples are not representative of the amount of cellularity and unless a spicule is examined an erroneous impression can be obtained. If spicules are not present a core biopsy is required in order to accurately evaluate the degree of cellularity.

PRESENCE OF ALL CELL SERIES. In a normal marrow each cell series is well represented. If a cell series is absent or greatly reduced in relationship to other cell types, one must note this finding and compare it to peripheral blood values.

MORPHOLOGIC ABNORMALITIES. Any abnormal cell morphology, including size, staining characteristics, nuclear characteristics, presence or absence of phagocytosed particles or cells, and any other morphologic abnormality, should be recorded.

SEQUENCE OF DEVELOPMENT. All cell series in normal bone marrow develop in a sequential fashion with the number of mature forms exceeding that of the immature cell types. For example, there are more segmented neutrophils than bands, more bands than metamyelocytes, and more metamyelocytes than myelocytes. Deviations from this pyramidal type of cell maturation suggest an alteration in marrow activity.

M:E RATIO. In normal animals the ratio between myeloid and erythroid elements is approximately 1:1. Determining an exact M:E ratio can be a laborious and time-consuming activity. However, M:E estimates can be made by scanning the marrow film and obtaining an impression of the relationship between these cell series. A more accurate estimation can be made by doing a quick count of granulocytes and nucleated erythrocytes. At least 500 cells should be enumerated and identified as belonging to either the myeloid or erythroid series. No attempt is made to identify the individual cells within the series and only the total number of erythrocytic and granulocytic cells are recorded. The ratio is calculated by dividing the total number of granulocytes by the number of nucleated erythrocytes.

ABNORMAL CELLS. Clumps of neoplastic cells are occasionally present in marrow and their presence is of significance. As these are frequently immature cells, one should attempt to determine to which cell series they belong. The characteristics of the cells should be noted and a written description prepared.

HYPOPLASIA. A reduction in marrow cellularity may involve all cell types or it may be specific for a single series. Generalized marrow hypoplasia is usually accompanied by a decrease in the number of all cell types in the peripheral blood (pancytopenia). Such conditions are frequently idiopathic. Ehrlichiosis in the canine, feline leukemia virus infections, and panleukopenia virus all produce a hypoplastic marrow. In hypoplastic marrow all cell types may be present and distribution between the various stages of development may be normal, as is the M:E ratio. Confirmation of hypocellularity may, as previously indicated, depend upon examination of a core biopsy.

In addition to overall hypoactivity, an animal may have erythroid hypoplasia with relatively normal or increased myeloid activity. Conditions producing such changes include chronic renal disease, chronic inflammation, hypothyroidism in the dog, panleukopenia in the cat, feline leukemia virus infections, and trichostrongyloid parasitism in cattle and sheep. The myeloid elements in the marrow are frequently within normal range or might be increased if there is inflammation. With some conditions they may be reduced. Because of the decrease in erythroid elements, the M:E ratio is usually increased. In some cases there may be evidence of erythroid activity, but if it is insufficient to provide the regeneration necessary to correct the anemia it is referred to as an inappropriate response.

APLASIA. The term aplasia suggests complete lack of cell production. Under such conditions bone marrow taps are frequently almost completely devoid of myeloid and erythroid elements. Final confirmation is dependent upon a core biopsy and histologic evaluation. This condition has been associated with the use of toxic drugs, viral infections, exposure to high doses of radiation, and plant toxins.

The prognosis for animals with marrow hypoplasia or aplasia is poor. However, some animals will recover. Early in the stages of recovery blast cells predominate, and examination of a smear at this time is difficult to interpret. One might confuse this reaction with a neoplastic process. However, it can be differentiated from neoplasia as there is still marrow hypoplasia, while with neoplasia hyperplasia is present. If recovery continues, sequential marrow examinations will reveal increased maturity of the cell lines.

HYPERPLASIA. Marrow hyperplasia seldom occurs simultaneously in all cell compartments. If there is a peripheral demand for erythrocytes accompanying or following an anemia, erythroid hyperplasia will prevail. Inflammatory processes result in granulocytic hyperplasia while thrombocytopenia is followed by megakaryocytic hyperplasia. If tissue destruction has been considerable and a demand exists for tissue macrophages, monocytic hyperplasia may occur.

With erythroid hyperplasia an increase occurs in nucleated erythrocytes, which reduces the M:E ratio. The amount of erythroid activity depends on the severity of the anemia. An erythroid response should always be interpreted in relationship to the status of erythrocytes in the peripheral blood. If erythroid hyperplasia is present and there are few or no peripheral blood values that support the presence of anemia, such activity may indicate an inappropriate erythroid response and should be judged accordingly. The type of response seen in various anemias will be discussed later.

An increase in the production of granulocytes in the marrow occurs in response to peripheral demands for leukocytes. If the marrow reserve pool has been depleted, a bone marrow examination may suggest granulocytic hypoplasia. This is quickly followed by an increase in myeloid activity that begins with the increased production of myelocytes. Unless peripheral demands exceed production this is followed by an increase in more mature granulocytes. In chronic inflammation the marrow typically has an increase in mature segmented neutrophils and the erythroid series may be decreased on a relative basis. In some chronic inflammations there is an absolute decrease in erythrocyte production. Such erythroid hypoplasia is thought to be associated with interference in iron metabolism.

Megakaryocytic hyperplasia occurs when there has been consumption, destruction, or sequestration of thrombocytes. Occasionally there may be an increase in megakaryocytes in association with erythroid hyperplasia. Megakaryocytes are readily observed in marrow films but normally constitute only about 0.5 per cent of the nucleated cells. With hyperplasia there is a dramatic increase in the number of megakaryocytes, and immature megakaryocytes may be present. Clusters of megakaryocytes are sometimes present.

BONE MARROW FINDINGS IN DISEASE

Anemia. Regenerative anemias are accompanied by an increase in immature erythrocytes in the bone marrow. This increase causes a decrease in the M:E ratio if the total neutrophil count is within normal range.

Increased erythropoiesis and punctate basophilia of metarubricytes are associated with symptomatic hemolytic anemia in the dog. In iron deficiency anemia due to chronic blood loss, bone marrow has a predominance of metarubricytes, and the M:E ratio indicates erythroid hyperplasia. Lead poisoning in the dog produces an alteration in bone marrow erythrogenesis as it interferes with normal heme synthesis, and delays nuclear expulsion and metarubricytes accumulate. Bone marrow in dogs with autoimmune hemolytic anemia is hypercellular. This hypercellularity may be accompanied by an absence of thrombocytes in the peripheral circulation, but the number of bone marrow megakaryocytes is sometimes adequate. Occasionally canine autohemolytic anemia is accompanied by erythroid depression, as indicated by an increased M:E ratio. Such animals may be thrombocytopenic.

A bone marrow dyscrasia involving erythrocytes has been described in the poodle.[3] This condition is characterized by the presence of macrocytic erythrocytes in the peripheral blood of nonanemic poodles. Abnormal nucleated erythrocytes characterized by an incomplete separation of daughter cells in the metarubricytes are present in the marrow. These cells are larger than normal metarubricytes and frequently contain fragmented nuclei. Occasionally, hypersegmented or bizarre neutrophils are observed.

In a cat with severe hemorrhagic or hemolytic anemia, prorubricytes and basophilic rubricytes become more prominent, and there is a marked increase in the number of polychromatophilic rubricytes.[4] The bone marrow picture in cats recovering from feline infectious anemia is characterized by intensified erythrogenesis with an M:E ratio commonly less than 0.5.

Megaloblastic erythropoiesis may occur in cats deficient in vitamin B_{12} and folic acid. There is maturation arrest at the prorubricyte and basophilic rubricyte stages that results in the appearance of cells with a chromatin-deficient nucleus characterized by condensation of the chromatin into clumps. In addition, the rubricytes are larger than those found in normal cats. Hemoglobin synthesis proceeds normally, the nucleus is extruded, and large macrocytic erythrocytes are released into peripheral blood. Because of defective nucleoprotein synthesis, a few large, hypersegmented neutrophils may be present in the marrow and peripheral blood. This condition may be difficult to differentiate from myeloproliferative disorders affecting erythrocytes.[3]

Anemias in the horse are not accompanied by typical peripheral blood signs of regeneration. Consequently it may be necessary to resort to a bone marrow examination in order to evaluate erythropoietic response in this species. If the anemia is regenerative, the M:E ratio is decreased, often falling below 0.5. Polychromatophilic and basophilic rubricytes are usually increased. In lead poisoning in the horse there is maturation arrest at the metarubricyte stage. Such an occurrence can be interpreted as ineffective erythropoiesis.

Bovine congenital porphyria is accompanied by a megaloblastic marrow. Nucleated erythrocytes in marrow are typically large with a basophilic cytoplasm and the M:E ratio is reduced.[3]

Experimental bleeding of sheep resulted in bone marrow regeneration, which was apparent following the first bleeding but later became more pronounced, peaking on day 9 when 65 to 90 per cent of the cells were of the erythrocytic series.[5]

The bone marrow picture in aplastic anemia is somewhat different from that in responding anemias. A relative lymphocytosis is usually present with 60 to 100 per cent of the nucleated cells in marrow being lymphocytes. This is accompanied by a striking immaturity of the erythrocytes and leukocytes. These findings are a consequence of marked depression of marrow production of erythrocytes, granulocytes, and thrombocytes.

Not all anemic conditions are accompanied by increases in erythroid elements in bone marrow. Animals may have clinical anemias readily identified by physical signs and confirmed by examination of peripheral blood with none of the bone marrow alterations typical of anemia. In such cases there is a diminution of erythroid production that suggests a nonresponding anemia. This lack of bone marrow response warrants an unfavorable prognosis unless subsequent bone marrow examination indicates a recovery of ability to produce erythrocytes.

Inflammation. Inflammatory processes stimulate granulopoiesis in the marrow. In acute inflammation there is usually a marrow left shift as mature neutrophils have been released into the peripheral circulation. This is accompanied by a slight decrease in the M:E ratio. Twenty-four to 48 hours following an initial depletion the total number of myeloid elements increase and the M:E ratio may reflect this change. At this time there is also an increase in immature neutrophils. If a toxic condition exists, granulocytes begin to show morphologic alterations. Neutrophil toxicity is reflected by a persistence of cytoplasmic basophilia. If toxicity is severe, vacuolization of the cytoplasm may also occur. If toxicity persists cell death occurs in dividing granulocytes and macrophage activity is increased. At this time the macrophages will contain cellular debris. Such a finding is an unfavorable sign as it is an indication of a severe toxic condition.

With chronic inflammatory processes, granulopoiesis expands and neutrophil hyperplasia becomes more pronounced. If the marrow has expanded to meet peripheral demands the left shift that was apparent early in the process disappears and segmented neutrophils predominate. If there is considerable toxicity there will be an accumulation of active macrophages containing cellular debris.

As chronic inflammatory processes interfere with normal iron metabolism, there may be an accumulation of hemosiderin in marrow macrophages. This may be accompanied by a diminution of erythropoiesis. In many chronic inflammations antigenic stimulation occurs, and there may be an increase in plasma cells.

Neoplasia. Lymphosarcoma. Canine lymphosarcoma is not always characterized by distinct alterations in bone marrow. Scattered nodules of lymphoma cells are often present in affected dogs. Surrounding these nodules are many megakaryocytes, a few erythroid cells, and extensive hyperplasia of myeloid cells. It is possible to obtain biopsy specimens that miss these lymphoid nodules. Conversely, it is possible to insert the needle directly into one of these nodules so that numerous neoplastic cells are aspirated and a high lymphocyte count obtained. The typical finding in the bone marrow of most dogs having lymphosarcoma is hyperplasia of myeloid cells accompanied by a variable decrease in immature erythrocytes.

In the bovine, an increase of marrow lymphocytes to more than 30 per cent may, in connection with an examination of peripheral blood, support a diagnosis of lymphosarcoma. Bone marrow of almost all cattle with lymphosarcoma is sometimes deficient in granulocytes with segmented nuclei; myelocytes may dominate the field, and a marked eosinophilia frequently occurs.[6] In one study of marrow in cows with lymphosarcoma,[7] lymphocyte percentages ranged from a low of 32 to a high of 51. The mean percentage of lymphocytes was 45, as compared with a normal lymphocyte percentage of 5 to 16. Calves with lymphosarcoma have a neoplastic infiltration of marrow that was accompanied by anemia.[8]

Many animals with lymphoid malignancies have a normal bone marrow. Typical increases in lymphocytes may be seen in the terminal stages of lymphosarcoma and in some animals the malignancy may originate in the marrow. In such cases there is a marked increase in lymphocytes in the peripheral blood, anemia is frequently severe and nonregenerative, and there is thrombocytopenia. Lymphoblasts predominate in the marrow.

Myeloproliferative Disorders. A complex of disease conditions that results from proliferation and only partial differentiation of a primitive mesenchymal cell of the bone marrow, spleen, lymph nodes, and liver is called myeloproliferative disorders. Included in these disorders in cats are granulocytic leukemia, megakaryocytic leukemia, polycythemia vera, erythremic myelosis, and erythroleukemia.[9]

In erythremic myelosis, almost no cells of the granulocytic series are found in the bone marrow. Clusters of undifferentiated cells having characteristics of prorubricytes and basophilic rubricytes predominate. Occasionally these cells show some cytoplasmic evidence of hemoglobin formation.

The most common bone marrow finding in erythremic myelosis of the cat is a maturation defect leading to production of megaloblastoid rubricytes characterized by asynchronism in maturation of nucleus and cytoplasm.[4] The granulocytic maturation series may be normal or suppressed. If it is suppressed, vacuolation of the nucleus and cytoplasm of metamyelocytes, band cells, and mature neutrophils may be observed.

Cells of the erythrocytic series predominate in the bone marrow of a cat with a myeloproliferative disease that has characteristics of erythroleukemia. Early forms of granulocytes are absent, but a few metamyelocytes and mature neutrophils may be observed as well as some mature lymphocytes.

Bone marrow in reticuloendotheliosis is characterized by the presence of a large number of reticular or reticuloendothelial cells. These cells vary in morphology among different individuals and to some extent in different samples from the same individual. Morphologic and staining characteristics are inconsistent and suggestive of early erythrocytic, granulocytic, monocytic, or plasmacytic cells. There is no evidence of progressive maturation in any of these cell types. The cells are round and vary in size from 12 to 16 microns in diameter. Nuclei are large and round and usually stain a medium red-purple. The chromatin has a fine woven mesh pattern with infrequent clumping. A single large nucleolus is usually visible. Nuclei are located eccentrically and are often accompanied by a pale perinuclear area in the cytoplasm. The cytoplasm stains a rather dense dull blue, has a finely stippled pattern, and is seldom abundant. A varying number of fine azurophilic granules are seen either in a clump or scattered diffusely throughout the cytoplasm. M:E ratios are variable and not quantitatively related to the leukocyte count, number of reticulum cells, or degree of anemia. Most ratios are near normal. Cats with severe deficiency of erythrocyte cells have a high M:E ratio.

Myelofibrosis may result from proliferation of fibrous tissue by these reticulum cells.[12] These fibrous deposits gradually replace normal marrow, causing myelophthisis. Bone marrow taps are usually nonproductive; diagnosis is confirmed by a core biopsy that reveals varying degrees of fibrosis. Peripherally there is an anemia and nucleated erythrocytes are abundant. Poikilocytosis is marked, as is polychromasia. Extramedullary hematopoiesis in the liver and spleen is common. This is accompanied by splenomegaly and hepatomegly. Progranulocytes and blast cells may be seen as they are inappropriately released from the sites of extramedullary granulopoiesis. The erythrocyte and leukocyte alterations in the peripheral blood are characteristic of an inappropriate hematopoietic response.

In feline eosinophilic leukemia, the cat is anemic and eosinophils predominate in bone marrow.

In cats with lymphocytic leukemia, as evidenced by an increase in the number of abnormal lymphocytes in the peripheral circulation, there is usually more than 15 per cent lymphocytes in the marrow.[11]

In granulocytic leukemia giant forms of neutrophils having oddly shaped nuclei or cells with sharp discrepancies between cytoplasmic and nuclear maturation are present in the peripheral circulation as well as the bone marrow.[11]

In granulocytic leukemia in cats, the bone marrow is exceedingly cellular and has an intense, diffuse proliferation of myeloid forms, among which myeloblasts and myelocytes predominate. Mitotic forms are often numerous. Hyperactivity of marrow is often reflected by the presence of increased numbers of megakaryocytes. Although anemia is severe, there is frequently a tremendous activity of surviving erythrocytic elements.[13]

Granulocytic leukemia in the bovine is rare; however, a single case has been reported.[13] This occurred in a four-month-old female Angus-Holstein crossbreed that died on the ninth day of illness. At necropsy, bone marrow impressions were made, and 70 per cent of the cells were the infiltrative blast type. The differential leukocyte count in the blood revealed the presence of large numbers of immature forms of the granulocytic series.

Granulocytic leukemia in the canine is also characterized by marked bone marrow hyperplasia. The cells most characteristically observed in this hyperplastic marrow include myeloblasts, promyelocytes, myelocytes, and metamyelocytes. There is a relative decrease in segmented neutrophils. Myeloid hyperplasia is accompanied by a decrease in the percentage of erythroid elements.

Multiple myeloma is a neoplastic disease primarily affecting bone and characterized by a marked increase in the number of plasma cells in the marrow. Although a relatively rare condition, it has been reported in the horse, cat, rabbit, pig, calf, and dog.[15]

The majority of the cases of multiple myeloma have been diagnosed by the demonstration of typical cells in tissues of the animal body. Bone marrow characteristically has an increased number of plasma cells. These cells are frequently observed in clusters and are spherical or oval and contain eccentrically located nuclei that are slightly larger than normal. The nuclear chromatin of most cells has a relatively fine net-like background with irregularly spaced, dense chromatin aggregates. Most plasma cells have a well-defined clear zone in the cytoplasm beside the nucleus, and the cytoplasm is vacuolated. Some plasma cells contain large confluent, or smaller individual, homogeneous pink-staining masses in the cytoplasm.

Other Leukemias. In feline monocytic leukemia the bone marrow has an increase in immature and mature monocytic types of cells. Blast cells with a basophilic cytolasm and a round leptochromatic nucleus with a variable number of nucleoli are frequent. Granulocytes are rare, and their development may be arrested at the band cell stage.[13]

Mast cell invasion of the bone marrow may occur in the dog and cat. These are usually metastatic lesions. Mast cells can be differentiated from blood basophils by their nuclear and cytoplasmic characteristics. Mast cell nuclei are round to oval and do not have the lobulation seen in most blood basophils. The granules usually stain intensely and are sometimes so numerous that the nucleus is obscured. If mast cells are very immature the granules are less intensely basophilic and may have a pink tint. In such cells there are also more mature deeply staining granules. The presence of these immature forms suggests a rapidly proliferating neoplasm.

Occasionally other metastatic malignancies may be encountered in a marrow smear or biopsy.

Other Diseases. Bovine. Bone marrow changes associated with mastitis in cattle have been studied.[16] The M:E ratio was generally greater than 1.0 in mastitic cows. The reserve of mature neutrophils in the marrow was greatly reduced in response to experimentally induced or naturally acquired mastitis due to *Streptococcus*

agalactiae. The introduction of *Escherichia coli* endotoxin produced similar results. Along with the depletion of the marrow reserves, a neutropenia and left shift developed in the peripheral blood, and there was an increase in immature granulocytes in the marrow. Marrow reserves returned to normal or above normal within four to five days.

Canine. Peripheral blood findings in pyometra are characterized by a pronounced neutrophilic leukocytosis, a decided shift to the left, and toxic changes in the neutrophilic cells. Bone marrow changes in pyometra include a marked hyperplasia, particularly of neutrophilic forms; increased numbers of megakaryocytes; and widespread toxic changes accompanied by differences in the maturation time of neutrophilic cells.

A marked alteration in the M:E ratio in chronic kidney disease has been reported.[3] In one case, the M:E ratio was 6.85 as compared with a normal value of 1.15. There was also an increase in the percentage of band and mature neutrophils. The most dramatic alteration, however, was a decrease in the number of erythroid elements. In this case only 9 per cent of the cells were of the erythroid series as compared with a normal finding of approximately 46 per cent. There was also an increase in lymphocytes and monocytes.

Estrogen compounds have been observed, both clinically and experimentally, to have a toxic effect on dog marrow. This estrogen effect appears to be specific for the dog, as other species are not affected. Excess estrogens produce an initial leukocytosis that progresses to severe leukopenia, thrombocytopenia, nonregenerative anemia, and possibly death. Bone marrow examination reveals an aplasia if the animal has survived the initial thrombocytopenic episode.[17]

In immune-mediated diseases there may be some bone marrow changes. Plasma cells are frequently increased. In autoimmune hemolytic anemia erythrophagocytosis may be present in marrow neutrophils and macrophages. Similar cells can be seen in hemolytic anemias caused by erythrocyte parasites such as *Haemobartonella* and *Babesia*. In cases of immune-mediated thrombocytopenia, platelet phagocytosis by neutrophils has also been reported.[18] In cases of systemic lupus erythematosus, LE cells are sometimes present in the marrow.

REFERENCES

1. Penny, R. H. C., and Carlisle, C. H.: The bone marrow of the dog: A comparative study of material obtained from the iliac crest, rib, and sternum. J. Small Anim. Pract., 11:727, 1970.
2. Valli, V. E., McSherry, B. J., and Hulland, T. J.: A review of bone marrow handling techniques and description of a new method. Can. J. Comp. Med., 33:68, 1969.

3. Schalm, O. W., Jain, N. E., and Carroll, E. J.: *Veterinary Hematology*, 3rd ed., Lea and Febiger, Philadelphia, 1975.

4. Schalm, O. W.: Interpretations in feline bone marrow cytology. J.A.V.M.A., *161*:1418, 1972.

5. Winter, H.: Myelogram of sheep in post hemorrhagic anemia. Am. J. Vet. Res., *28*:1389, 1967.

6. Koehler, H.: Untersuchungen am Knockenmark bei der Leukose des Rindes. D.T.W., *64*:132, 1957.

7. Griffing, W. J.: The significance of bone marrow examination in certain diseases of the bovine and canine. M.S. Thesis. Kansas State University, Manhattan, KS, 1960.

8. Theilen, G. W., and Dungworth, D. L.: Bovine lymphosarcoma in California. III. The calf form. Am. J. Vet. Res., *26*:696, 1965.

9. Sodikoff, D. H., and Schalm, O. W.: Primary bone disease in the cat. III. Erythremic myelosis and myelofibrosis. A myeloproliferative disorder. Calif. Vet., *22*(6):16, 1968.

10. Simon, N., and Holzworth, J.: Eosinophilic leukemia in a cat. Cornell Vet., *57*:579, 1967.

11. Gilmore, C. E., and Holzworth, J.: Naturally occurring feline leukemia: Clinical, pathologic, and differential diagnostic features J.A.V.M.A., *158*:1013, 1971.

12. Feldman, B. F., and Zinkl, J. G.: Diseases of the lymph nodes and spleen. In *Textbook of Veterinary Internal Medicine, Diseases of the Dog and Cat*, edited by Ettinger, S. J., W. B. Saunders Company, Philadelphia, 1983.

13. Holzworth, J.: Leukemia and related neoplasms in the cat. I. Lymphoid malignancies. J.A.V.M.A., *136*:47, 1960; II. Malignancies other than lymphoid. J.A.V.M.A., *136*:107, 1960.

14. Hyde, S. L., King, J. M., and Bentinck-Smith, J.: A case of bovine myelogenous leukemia. Cornell Vet., *48*:269, 1958.

15. Squire, R. A.: Hematopoietic tumors of domestic animals. Cornell Vet., *54*:97, 1964.

16. Schalm, O. W., and Lasmanis, J.: Cytologic features of bone marrow in normal and mastitic cows. Am. J. Vet. Res., *37*:359, 1976.

17. Legendre, A. M.: Estrogen-induced bone marrow hypoplasia in a dog. J.A.V.M.A., *42*:525, 1976.

18. Lewis, H. B., and Rebar, A. H.: *Bone Marrow Evaluation in Veterinary Medicine*, Ralston Purina Company, St. Louis, 1979.

5

HEMOSTASIS AND COAGULATION OF BLOOD

Induced or spontaneous hemorrhage is halted by the process of hemostasis. Three principal factors are involved in hemostasis: (1) vascular factors, e.g., integrity of blood vessel walls, (2) thrombocytes, and (3) clotting mechanism, i.e., blood coagulation. Knowledge of the details of the hemostatic mechanism has increased considerably in the past several years, and this information has assisted in the recognition, management, and treatment of coagulation defects. The veterinarian must depend upon a normal hemostatic mechanism for ultimate success during major surgery. Occasionally, the veterinarian will encounter diseases in which the clotting mechanism fails to function properly. Methods for detecting such failure and an understanding of the various factors involved in hemostasis will permit an accurate diagnosis and treatment.

FACTORS INVOLVED IN HEMOSTASIS

Vascular Factors

The vascular component of hemostasis depends upon blood vessels that are functionally and structurally normal. Unfortunately, procedures to evaluate the integrity of blood vessels are not well known in veterinary medicine, and those employed in human medicine are not adaptable for use by the veterinarian. Vascular abnormalities are often suspected when there is clinical evidence of a bleeding tendency but all laboratory measurements are within the normal range.

Restoration of vascular integrity is obviously a requirement in traumatic wounds resulting in lacerations of major arteries. Coagulation of blood is effective only after such a defect of the artery has been repaired by surgical intervention. With injury to smaller vessels, however, the action of platelets and plasma coagulation factors promptly stops blood flow. When a blood vessel is injured or severed, vasoconstriction occurs almost immediately, and it may be sufficient to reduce the escape of blood if the injury is minor.

In addition to producing vasoconstriction, injury may also damage the vessel wall, exposing collagen fibers. Thrombocytes (see following section) adhere to these collagen fibers, initiating hemostasis.

Thrombocytes

Thrombocytes (blood platelets) are small cytoplasmic fragments from megakaryocytes and are found in circulating blood. Thrombocytes are produced principally from megakaryocytes of bone marrow. The lung and spleen are also sites of megakaryocyte development. Total thrombocyte counts in various animal species range from 175,000 to 500,000/μl.

In spite of its seemingly simple morphology, the platelet has a number of important physiologic activities related to hemostasis. In addition to its role in aggregating to form a hemostatic plug, it also serves as a catalyst to assist in initiating the coagulation cascade and plays an important role in clot retraction.

As platelets adhere to an injured vessel wall and to each other, active substances are released. These include serotonin, histamines, and ADP. The release of ADP causes adherence and aggregation of additional platelets that, along with fibrinogen and calcium, assist in forming the plug in a damaged vessel. ADP also makes the platelet phospholipoprotein, platelet factor 3 (PF3), available for its thromboplastic activity. Release of PF3 serves an important function in activation of the coagulation cascade.

Serotonin and histamines released by disintegrating platelets act as vasoconstrictors and contribute to the overall hemostatic reaction.

Platelets are also active in the synthesis of proteins, carbohydrates, nucleotides, and lipids. Platelets have the ability to generate metabolic activity, to phagocytize some particles, to synthesize and release some major components of the factor VIII complex, and, via the prostaglandin pathway, to assist in maintaining thromboresistance of intact endothelium.

Platelets also play an important role in clot retraction. If whole blood is allowed to clot and is observed over a period of time, the clot decreases in size, and serum is expressed. Clot retraction is, in part, dependent upon the presence and action of thrombocytes. It may also be affected by the nature of the surface on which the clot has formed. The effect of the surface on clot retraction can be most readily demonstrated by permitting clot formation to take place in a test tube. Retraction will occur only where blood has been in contact with the glass. There is a quantitative relationship between the number of platelets and clot retraction. If blood is deficient in platelets, clot retraction is usually poor, although fibrinogen concentration may also be a factor. Low fibrinogen levels are associated with poor retraction in the presence of a normal platelet count. The platelet substance responsible for clot retraction is a contractile protein termed thrombosthenin.

THE CLOTTING MECHANISM

Grossly, blood coagulation appears as a simple action, namely, the conversion of a liquid into a solid state. However, behind the clot that forms after a cut or scratch lies a highly complex mechanism. Complicated reactions of various factors functioning in a normal sequence are required to produce clotting. The clotting mechanism can be compared to the foundation of a building: if the foundation is weak, eventually a situation that creates an additional weight or pressure could cause the structure to collapse.

When an animal whose clotting mechanism is adequate for everyday functioning is submitted to a surgical procedure or other traumatic experience, it may develop a hemorrhage that is difficult to control. Such uncontrolled bleeding may be the

TABLE 5–1. International Nomenclature of Blood Clotting Factors

Factor	Synonym
I	Fibrinogen
II	Prothrombin
III	Tissue thromboplastin
IV	Calcium
V	Labile factor, Ac-globulin, proaccelerin
VII	Proconvertin, stable factor
VIII	Antihemolytic factor (AHF), thromboplastinogen
IX	Plasma thromboplastin component (PTC), Christmas factor
X	Stuart-Prower factor, Stuart factor
XI	Plasma thromboplastin antecedent (PTA)
XII	Hageman factor, glass activation factor
XIII	Fibrin stabilizing factor (FSF), Fibrinase, Laki-Lorand factor

result of a deficiency in a single specific factor required for coagulation, or it may be caused by a combination of other deficiencies contributing to the lack of the specific factor. The international nomenclature of blood clotting factors is presented in Table 5–1.

The mechanism for blood coagulation consists of an intrinsic, or intravascular, system and an extrinsic, or extravascular, system (Fig. 5–1). The intrinsic system consists of factors essential for clot formation, including factors XII, XI, IX, and VIII. A sequential activation of these factors in the presence of platelet phospholipid and calcium ions will result in the formation of intrinsic thromboplastin. The extrinsic system for enhancement of blood coagulation consists of factors VII and III. Factor VII is activated by tissue thromboplastin (factor III). In the presence of calcium ions, this activation results in the production of extrinsic thromboplastin. Intrinsic, extrinsic, or both types of thromboplastin then react with factors in the common system (factors X and V) and in the presence of platelets and calcium form prothrombin-activating principle. This prothrombin-activating principle converts the inactive prothrombin to an active enzyme called thrombin. Activated thrombin converts fibrinogen to a monomer, and in the presence of factor XIII and calcium converts it to the insoluble fibrin clot. This coagulation mechanism is summarized in Figure 5–1.

The diagram does not show the system of inhibitors that destroy each molecule of any activated factor soon after its appearance. Without these inhibitors, either the intrinsic or the extrinsic system could be stimulated to create massive thrombosis by a very small activating stimulus.

The coagulation system, which culminates in the formation of a clot in response to a damaged blood vessel, must be reversed and the clot removed. This is accomplished by a fibrinolytic en-

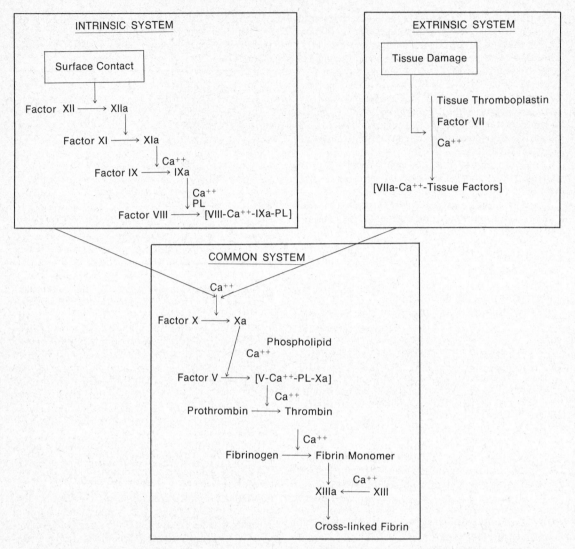

Figure 5–1. Blood coagulation scheme (a = activated factor; PL = phospholipid). Complexes are indicated by square brackets.

zyme system consisting of the inactive precursor plasminogen (profibrinolysin) and the active component plasmin (fibrinolysin).

Plasmin is a proteolytic enzyme that is active at a neutral pH and is capable of digesting fibrin into a number of soluble fragments. It also has the capacity to digest fibrinogen and to attack a number of other coagulation factors. For protective purposes, body fluids contain large amounts of antiplasmin. Antiplasmin can be found in plasma globulin and in platelets.

An activator system for converting plasminogen to plasmin exists in tissues and has been demonstrated in urine, seminal fluid, milk, tears, and secretions of various epithelia. Plasminogen activator can be demonstrated in the walls of blood vessels, particularly veins, which appear to be a major site for this substance. Bacterial plasmi-

nogen activators have been identified and originate from bacterial cells. The most important of these is probably streptokinase, which is produced by streptococci. Activator activity has also been associated with staphylococci, clostrida, and pseudomonades.

Nonenzymatic agents have also been shown to increase fibrinolytic activity in vivo. Included are testosterone, anderolone, corticosteroids, tolbutamide, and chlorpropamide. Vasoactive substances such as epinephrine, acetylcholine, vasopressin, and nicotinic acid also induce intense but transient fibrinolytic activity, possibly by causing an increase in plasma activator levels.

Fibrinolytic activity, normally kept under control by the naturally existing plasmin inhibitors of the body, may be increased. Such increases in fibrinolytic activity are known to occur in domestic animals as a consequence of snakebite; incompatible blood transfusions; neoplasia; obstetric complications; surgery; and a variety of miscellaneous diseases including endotoxemia, gastric torsion, heartworm disease, severe hepatic necrosis, diaphragmatic hernia, pancreatitis, hemorrhagic enteritis, polycythemia, and others. This entity is known as disseminated intravascular coagulation (DIC), consumption coagulopathy, or intravascular coagulation-fibrinolysis syndrome. DIC does not occur as a primary condition but is always secondary to a primary abnormality.

Mechanistically, DIC is a paradox, as there is both hypercoagulation and increased fibrinolytic activity. The simultaneous activation of these two systems results first in intravascular formation of fibrin, which, in turn, results in thrombus formation in small blood vessels throughout the body. This immediately activates the fibrinolytic system to remove the thrombi. With hypercoagulation there is massive consumption of thrombocytes and coagulation factors. As fibrin and fibrinogen are removed by the fibrinolytic activity, the split products resulting from this activity begin to circulate. These split products may serve as anticoagulants and in combination with the decrease in platelets and coagulation factors produce a severe hemorrhagic diathesis.

Patients with such a syndrome exhibit clinical signs that include petechial and ecchymotic hemorrhages, abnormal bleeding following venipuncture, epistaxis, bleeding from the gums, gastrointestinal hemorrhages, and hematuria. The disease is frequently quite severe and if untreated usually culminates in death.

LABORATORY TESTS FOR COAGULATION DEFECTS— GENERAL TECHNIQUES

CARE OF GLASSWARE AND EQUIPMENT

In order to maintain consistency and avoid variables, all glassware used in coagulation testing should be kept separate from glassware used in other laboratory procedures. This glassware must be chemically clean. Cleaning is best accomplished by thorough washing with fresh chromic acid solution or with soap and water with repeated rinsing, first with tap water and finally with distilled water. All glassware should be completely dry before being used. Any glassware that has become etched, scratched, or cracked should be discarded. Plastic or siliconized syringes and glassware are preferred in order to avoid activation of factor XII and to reduce platelet aggregation.

For clean venipunctures, needles must be sharp and unclogged. A needle large enough to permit free flowing of blood at a steady rate is preferred. The syringe must be completely dry and fit so that no air bubbles form as the sample is drawn. Any pipettes used must be clean and dry and without chipped ends.

The temperature of the water bath must be constant during the performance of the tests, and the water should be checked with a thermometer to ascertain that the same temperature prevails throughout the bath.

SAMPLE COLLECTION

A poorly collected blood sample is useless for evaluating the activity of the coagulation mechanism. A blood sample that is improperly obtained and contaminated with tissue juices may fail to indicate the nature or presence of a defect. A good venipuncture is possible only when the animal is well restrained and a palpable blood vessel is visible. If the needle becomes dislodged during the venipuncture, it will introduce tissue juices, and the sample should be rejected. The blood should be drawn without excessive pressure to avoid formation of air bubbles. If the blood is to be mixed with an anticoagulant, exact measurement of both anticoagulant and blood must be made. Vacutainers (Becton-Dickinson, Rutherford, New Jersey) containing the proper anticoagulant are available and are recommended. Trisodium citrate is the best anticoagulant. It is used as one part of a 3.8 per cent solution to nine parts of blood. If a syringe is used, blood should be allowed to run into the test tube without being forced through the needle or tip of the syringe. Since animal blood coagulates rapidly, the anticoagulant should be in the syringe prior to sample collection so that blood is drawn directly into it. When plasma is needed, it should be separated from the red cells following centrifugation by using a medicine dropper. Harvested plasma should be placed in plastic or siliconized glass tubes. If the plasma is contaminated with erythrocytes, the specimen should be recentrifuged, as plasma must be completely free of erythrocytes. Any test for presence of a coagulation defect must be performed as soon as possible after collection, or else the sample should be frozen at $-20°$ C or lower.

If a sample is to be forwarded to an outside laboratory it should be divided into 1 ml aliquots in plastic tubes and rapidly frozen in alcohol and dry ice. The sample should be held at $-20°$ C or lower and should be packed with dry ice to maintain that temperature. Slow freezing of samples should be avoided as some coagulation factors may precipitate.

Coagulation determinations should always be run in duplicate, and a simultaneous test should be completed on a normal control sample. Some techniques utilize serum and others require plasma. If serum is used, blood is allowed to clot in acceptable tubes. The sample is then rimmed to detach it from the sides of the tube and centrifuged, and the serum is removed. As hemolysis interferes with some tests, every effort should be made to avoid erythrocyte destruction.

In order to provide the best diagnostic evaluation and to ensure test validity, appropriate reference and control plasmas should always be used. Such reagents include fresh-frozen pooled plasmas that are deficient in specific clotting factors and fresh-frozen pooled plasma from healthy animals of the species. Pooled plasmas should be obtained from at least eight animals and be age-matched whenever possible with the patient sample.[1] Deficient substrate plasmas do not need to be from the same species as the reference standard or test samples, because heterologous substrates can be used.

LABORATORY TESTS FOR COAGULATION DEFECTS—SPECIFIC TECHNIQUES

COAGULATION TIME

The whole blood clotting time can be determined by several techniques. As with other more critical techniques, care must be taken in obtaining blood specimens for determination of whole blood clotting time, as contamination with tissue juices will alter results. This test is of no value in slight deficiencies of various factors, as only a small amount of thrombin is required to form a fibrin clot. It is even less likely to reveal defects in later stages of clotting, such as those occurring with deficiencies in factor V, factor X, or prothrombin, as these steps are rapid in comparison with the earlier thromboplastin generation stages. Since only a small number of normal thrombocytes are required for clotting, clotting time is usually normal in thrombocytopenic purpura. If whole blood clotting time is prolonged, further investigations of disturbances in coagulation should always be initiated. Because of difficulties in standardization of coagulation times and the variable results, most of these tests are of little diagnostic value except for detection of severe problems.

Lee-White Coagulation Time. To collect blood for a Lee-White coagulation time, rinse a sterile syringe and needle with sterile physiologic saline solution. The saline should be carefully expelled so that the dead space in the end of the barrel and needle remains filled. More than 3 ml of blood should be collected and the blood clotting time should be recorded from the moment that blood first appears in the syringe. Every attempt should be made to avoid introduction of air into the syringe, as air will hasten coagulation. The needle

is removed from the syringe and 1 ml of blood is placed into each of three tubes having an inside diameter of 13 mm and a length of 75 mm. These tubes should be chemically clean and rinsed with physiologic saline solution just before use. Before the addition of blood, the tubes should be placed into a container of water that is maintained at 37° C. The tubes are tilted at 30-second intervals, starting with tube 1; when this clots, proceed to tubes 2 and 3, respectively. Be careful not to allow the tubes to cool or to agitate the blood to excess until coagulation has occurred. Clotting time is recorded when the tube can be inverted without spilling the contents. The endpoint is reached when the blood in tube three has coagulated, and coagulation time is measured from the moment the blood sample is obtained until coagulation is completed in tube three. Normal values for Lee-White coagulation time are presented in Table 5-2.

An alternative method for studying clotting time employs four 10 × 75 mm test tubes, two of which are glass and two of which are silicone-coated glass or plastic. One milliliter of blood, collected as just described, is placed in each of the four tubes, and coagulation is timed. Clotting time in plastic or siliconized tubes is approximately twice as long as it is in glass tubes.

Capillary Tube Method. A simple technique for determining whole blood coagulation time is the capillary tube method.

A capillary tube approximately 15 cm long and 1 to 1.5 mm in diameter is used. The skin is punctured, the first drop of blood is wiped away, and the capillary tube is filled with blood. It is important to note the time when blood first appears in the capillary tube. Unfortunately, it is extremely difficult to obtain whole blood in this

TABLE 5–2. Normal Values of Whole Blood Clotting Time in Various Species of Domestic Animals (Lee-White Method)

Species		Time in Minutes
Bovine	glass	4–15
	glass	10–15
Ovine	glass	4–8
	glass	5–15
	plastic	5–27
Equine:	glass	20–32
	silicone	57–86
Equine	glass	4–15
	glass	8–17.5
	silicone	13–25
Porcine	glass	6.2
Canine:	glass	6–7.5
	silicone	28–40
	glass	3–13
	silicone	15–45
		6–8
Feline	glass	9.2 ± 0.3

TABLE 5–3. Normal Values of Whole Blood Clotting Time in Various Species of Domestic Animals (Capillary Tube Method)

Species	Time in Minutes
Bovine	3–15
	2.5–11.5
Ovine	1–6 (2.5)
Caprine	2.5–11.5
Equine	3.5–11
	3–15
Porcine	2.5
Porcine	4
Canine	4
	3
Feline	5.2 ± 0.2

fects or a severe hypofibrinogenemia.[2] As with other coagulation tests, a sample from a normal animal of the same species should be run in parallel with the patient sample.

Interpretation of Coagulation Time. Prolonged whole blood clotting time is seen in a variety of coagulopathies in domestic animals. Included are the following conditions: (1) fibronogen (factor I) deficiency, (2) hemophilia A (factor VIII deficiency), (3) hemophilia B (factor IX deficiency), (4) von Willebrand's disease (clotting time may also be normal in this disorder), (5) severe liver disease, (6) vitamin K deficiency, (7) thrombocytopenia (if test conducted in siliconized or plastic tubes), (8) advanced stages of DIC, (9) the presence of circulating anticoagulants, and (10) uremia (occasionally).

fashion without also contaminating the specimen with excessive quantities of tissue juices. When this occurs, the blood will coagulate rapidly (frequently within one to two minutes). Such contamination can be avoided by filling the capillary tube with blood collected by venipuncture. Timing is begun when blood is first collected and terminates when a fibrin strand appears.

Holding the tube between the thumb and index finger of both hands, gently break off small pieces every 30 seconds until a strand of fibrin is seen extending across the gap between the two broken ends of the tube. The interval between the appearance of blood and the appearance of a fibrin strand is the coagulation time. This technique is simpler to perform and less time consuming than the Lee-White method, but the results are subject to question because of the possible addition of excess quantities of tissue fluids. The normal values for clotting time as determined by the capillary tube method are presented in Table 5–3.

Variations occurring in normal coagulation times undoubtedly represent variations in technique, temperature, and endpoint interpretation. As with all other tests, a normal control sample should be examined at the same time blood from a patient is under study.

Activated Coagulation Time A more sensitive test for coagulation is the activated coagulation time (ACT). This technique utilizes diatomaceous earth as a surface-activating agent. The coagulation time is considerably shortened and this produces an increase in sensitivity. In this test 2 ml of whole blood is placed in the ACT tube, mixed, and incubated at 37° C for one minute. The tube is examined at five-second intervals for the first evidence of clotting. This test can be recommended for presurgical or prebiopsy screening of patients. Although normal values in the dog have been reported to range from 60 to 90 seconds, values should be established for each laboratory. Intrinsic factor defects produce an abnormal ACT as does thrombocytopenia; abnormal ACT is also seen if there are qualitative platelet function defects or a severe hypofibrinogenemia.

BLEEDING TIME

Determination of bleeding time is a simple and sometimes useful tool for evaluating the efficiency of the capillary-platelet aspect of hemostasis. This technique is necessarily somewhat imprecise. To determine bleeding time, make a small, deep puncture in clean, dry skin with a lancet or No. 11 Bard-Parker blade. An area relatively devoid of hair should be selected. The time when blood first appears should be noted. As drops of blood accumulate, they should be removed with filter paper every 30 seconds, the operator being careful not to touch the skin. When blood no longer appears from the puncture site, the endpoint has been reached, and the time should be noted. In domestic animals the normal value is from two to five minutes.

The reliability of the bleeding time test depends in large part upon the area selected, the care taken not to disturb the wound by permitting the filter paper to come in contact with the skin, and the depth of the cuts.

Interpretation of Bleeding Time. The normal bleeding time of one to five minutes may be prolonged in the following conditions: (1) defects in the blood vessel wall, (2) platelet defects resulting from thrombocytopenia or the presence of abnormal platelets, (3) severe liver disease, (4) uremia, (5) administration of large doses of anticoagulants, and (6) von Willebrand's disease.

PLATELET COUNTING AND EVALUATION

In any study of hemostasis, evaluation of the platelets must be included.

Counting. The total number of thrombocytes in peripheral blood can be determined directly by a counting method or indirectly by an estimation made by examination of a stained blood film.

The platelet count is performed in the same manner as is the erythrocyte count, except that a different diluting fluid is utilized—Rees-Ecker, ethylenediaminetetraacetic acid (EDTA), or ammonium oxalate. The procedure is as follows: (1) Rinse an erythrocyte-diluting pipette with diluting fluid. (2) Draw blood to the 0.5 mark. (3) Draw diluting fluid to the 101 mark. (4) Shake the pipette for several minutes. (5) Discard several drops. (6) Fill both sides of the counting chamber. (7) Place the hemocytometer in a moist chamber, such as a petri dish, containing a piece of wet filter paper and allow to stand for 10 to 20 minutes. (8) Count platelets in the entire central ruled area on each side of the counting chamber. Platelets are identified as rod- or oval-shaped bodies approximately one-half the diameter of erythrocytes. (9) Multiply the number of thrombocytes in the ruled area by 1000 to give total thrombocytes/μl.

Diluting fluids commonly used include: (1) a 1 per cent solution of EDTA dissolved in saline to which brilliant cresyl blue has been added to a concentration of 0.05 to 0.25 per cent; (2) one per cent ammonium oxalate solution in distilled water; or (3) Rees-Ecker diluting fluid containing sodium citrate, formaldehyde, and brilliant cresyl blue (formula in Appendix). A standardized diluent and capillary pipette unit is available for use in making thrombocyte counts (Unopette, Becton-Dickinson, Rutherford, New Jersey), and reproducible results have been obtained in our laboratory with the Unopette. Total platelet counts can also be completed using an electronic counter.

Less accurate, but perhaps more practicable, is an indirect method for estimating the number of platelets. This screening test may be performed from a stained blood film such as that prepared for routine hematologic examination. Note the number of platelets per field under the oil immersion of objective. Finding three or less per field suggests thrombocytopenia. If the total leukocyte count is known, the number of platelets may be compared with the number of white blood cells (WBC) in the smear. Record the number of platelets observed in tallying 100 leukocytes. This relative number can be converted into an absolute number by the following formula:

$$\frac{\text{Number of platelets}}{100 \text{ WBC}} \times \text{Total WBC count}$$
$$= \text{Number of platelets}$$

A similar comparison can be made using the total red blood cell (RBC) count. Record the number of platelets observed in counting 1000 erythrocytes. Calculate platelet count by the following formula:

$$\frac{\text{Platelets counted} \times \text{RBC}/\mu l}{1000} = \text{Platelets}/\mu l$$

If counts obtained by this estimation are borderline, confirmation by a more sensitive method should be completed.

Platelet numbers can be estimated by scanning the monolayer area of a blood film and counting the number of platelets per field under 1000 × magnification. A monolayer area is that part of the blood film where the erythrocytes are close together with about half of them touching each other. Platelet estimations should be based on the average number per field in at least 10 fields. Platelets are reported as normal, decreased, increased, or clumped. Normal for most species is 10 to 25 platelets per field, decreased is less than 10 per field, and increased is 26 or more per field.[3] Horses should have more than six per field, and an increase should be reported if there are more than 20 per field. An average of 10 platelets per oil-immersion field represents a total count of 150,000 to 180,000/μl.[3] Accurate estimates are difficult if the platelets are clumped. Clumping often accompanies the formation of small clots in the blood sample. Excessive platelet clumping may artificially increase total erythrocytes if counted electronically. These counters detect cells by their volume and thrombocyte clumps may have the same volume as some small erythrocytes.

Platelet morphology should also be reported. They are evaluated as to size, granularity, and shape. Platelets are round to oval in EDTA blood. Although ruminants and horses have smaller platelets than dogs and cats, size will vary according to method of slide preparation and their location within the smear. They will appear much smaller in the thicker portion of the film. The appearance of immature platelets that are larger than normal suggests increased platelet turnover. This finding occurs more frequently in the dog than in other species.

Granularity is marked in Romanowsky-stained blood films from cats, less intense in dogs and ruminants, and often absent in horse platelets. Horse platelets may be difficult to identify because of their lack of granularity. The absence of granules in cats, dogs, and ruminants is abnormal and may indicate degranulation.[3] Bizarre-shaped thrombocytes in an animal with thrombocytopenia suggests platelet destruction or consumption.

Interpretation of Platelet Counts. The normal thrombocyte count in domestic animals ranges from 175,000/μl to 500,000/μl and in most animals less than 100,000/μl is considered clinically significant, although prolonged bleeding rarely is observed until the total count is below 50,000/μl. In all probability, many of the clinically identifiable hemostatic defects in domestic animals are related to a deficiency in number or function of blood platelets. Hemorrhage that results from thrombocytopenia takes the form of petechiation or ecchymoses of mucous membranes and skin, although severe bleeding episodes can occur.

As the megakaryocyte is the precursor cell for the thrombocyte and its site of formation is in the bone marrow, any disease condition affecting bone marrow may result in thrombocytopenia. Thrombocytopenia may occur secondarily in association with some bacterial and viral diseases and frequently accompanies autoimmune diseases such as autoimmune hemolytic anemia and systemic lupus erythematosus. In some animals, no specific cause for the thrombocytopenia can be detected, and these disorders are described as being idiopathic. DIC is also accompanied by thrombocytopenia.

Some animals with coagulopathies not related to a decrease in or abnormal function of thrombocytes may have a decrease in circulating platelets. Immediately following severe hemorrhage the platelet number may be temporarily reduced.

Thrombocytosis may occur transiently as a response to disease or following trauma.

It must be recognized that the number of platelets may be normal, but if platelet function is abnormal, coagulation problems may occur. Terms utilized to describe conditions in which there is abnormal function are *thrombocytopathia* and *thrombasthenia*. These platelets may be morphologically normal or abnormal and may be defective in blood coagulation, clot retraction, or adhesive or aggregation capabilities. Platelet function defects have been described in dogs, cattle, and cats.[4]

Clot Retraction. As mentioned previously, if blood is permitted to clot in a clean, dry test tube, it will separate from the wall. Obvious abnormalities in clot retraction can be observed by placing a tube of blood (with no anticoagulant added) in an incubator at 37° C. A normal clot will retract markedly within two to four hours and by the end of 24 hours will be a compact mass. A more quantitative measure of clot retraction may be obtained by placing 5 ml of fresh blood into a conical glass centrifuge tube and fitting the tube with a rubber stopper to which a coiled copper wire is attached. The clot should be easily lifted at 24 hours when the stopper is removed.

A more sensitive method for evaluation of clot retraction utilizes blood diluted 1:10 with cold buffered saline. One-half milliliter of fresh whole blood is drawn into a plastic syringe and added to 4.5 ml of saline. Two milliliters of this mixture is added, in duplicate, to two small glass test tubes, each containing one unit of bovine thrombin, and the sample is mixed by inversion. Tubes are kept in a refrigerator for 30 minutes and then transferred to a 37° C water bath. These tubes are examined every 30 minutes to detect retraction. This is continued for two hours, and in most animals the samples are retracted by one to two hours, at which time the clot begins to lyse.[1]

Interpretation of Clot Retraction. Retraction of a formed clot is influenced by the number and function of platelets, the fibrinogen content of the plasma, and other chemical and enzymatic factors as well as the container. Thus, clot retraction is impaired in afibrinogenemia, in thrombocytopenia when platelet counts are less than 100,000/µl, and in some coagulation defects. Clot retraction can also be influenced by the presence of fibrinolysins. In such conditions, the clot will dissolve during the 24-hour incubation period following formation. Clot retraction may be reduced in anemia and prolonged in polycythemia. Clot retraction is not widely used because better tests exist for evaluating thrombocytes.

Other Tests of Platelet Function. A rather sensitive test for determining platelet aggregation has been described.[5] In this technique, approximately 6 ml of freshly citrated blood is drawn from a patient and from a normal control. Platelet-rich plasma for the test is prepared from the blood by slow spinning of the sample in polycarbonate or other plastic test tubes. For the assay, 0.4 ml of the platelet-rich plasma is placed in a plain glass test tube, and thrombin (0.1 ml of a 10 unit/ml solution) is added. The tube is gently tilted back and forth under a lamp until platelet aggregation begins. This will require approximately 30 seconds and produces a snowflake effect in the sample. Following platelet aggregation, coagulation will occur, and incubation for one hour at 37° C will permit retraction. The retraction should be recorded as 1 to 4 +. There is a good correlation between degree of aggregation and subsequent clot retraction. Abnormal results occur if the number or function of platelets is reduced. Other tests of platelet aggregation should be conducted in specialized coagulation laboratories.

Platelet function can also be assayed by the Russell's viper-venom test (RVVT), which depends upon phospholipid release from cells in the test plasma, usually thrombocytes. The results of this test are also abnormal if the sample is deficient in factor V, factor X, or prothrombin.

Although not a commonly used test, the RVVT can be used as a measurement of factors involved in the extrinsic coagulation system. This venom has thromboplastic activity in high dilutions and is used in the place of thromboplastin in performance of a one-stage prothrombin time test.

Normal RVVT is 10 to 14 seconds. If this time is prolonged, the sample is deficient in factor V, factor X, or prothrombin, or a thrombocytopenia is present.

FIBRINOGEN

Of all of the clotting factors, only fibrinogen can be directly assayed. A relatively accurate simple technique for completing a fibrinogen assay takes advantage of the hand refractometer routinely used for determining urine specific gravity and total protein content of plasma. Two microhematocrit tubes filled with blood containing EDTA as the anticoagulant are centrifuged for five minutes as for determining packed cell volume. The plasma protein concentration from one tube is determined by breaking the tube just above the junction of plasma and erythrocytes and placing the plasma on the chamber of a hand refractometer and recording the quantity of plasma protein. The second tube is placed in a water bath at 56° C for three minutes. This will precipitate fibrinogen, which is removed from the plasma by further centrifuging for five minutes. Total plasma protein of the sample in the heated tube is determined with the refractometer. Fibrinogen concentration is calculated by subtracting the protein value of the plasma in the heated tube from that of unheated normal plasma. Decreases in fibrinogen may be associated with advanced liver disease, although such decreases may be congenital in the dog. The concentration of fibrinogen may be of critical significance in assays involving measurement of some of the extrinsic factors. Fibrinogen levels of 60 to 100 mg/μl or less may delay or prevent clot formation in some determinations.

ONE-STAGE PROTHROMBIN TIME TEST

The one-stage prothrombin time (OSPT) test measures the extrinsic system of blood coagulation. It is carried out by adding tissue thromboplastin to plasma and then recalcifying the mixture. The exact details of the method will depend upon the commercial reagents used, and directions should be carefully followed. Normal values for the OSPT should be established in each laboratory according to the reagents used.

Plasma for use in the OSPT test must be carefully collected, using the correct ratio of blood to anticoagulant. Exactly 0.5 ml of 0.1 M sodium oxalate or sodium citrate is used for exactly 4.5 ml of blood. The equipment required for this determination is minimal. Provision must be made for a water bath at 37° C, and a stop watch is required, as are proper-sized test tubes. In laboratories not having a thermostatically controlled water bath, the proper temperature can be achieved by adjusting the water tap in such a manner that the water temperature is 37° C. This water is allowed to run continuously into a small beaker or pan that will remain constantly at the temperature of the running water. If such an arrangement is utilized, care must be exercised to prevent contamination of the sample tube with tap water. Test accuracy can be improved by use of a fibrometer to measure clot formation.

A lack of factor V, factor VII, factor X, fibrinogen, or prothrombin may produce a delay in this reaction. Thus, any time longer than is normal for this test indicates that one or more of these factors may be deficient. A control should always be used in a one-step prothrombin test, and the value obtained for this control should be reported along with the normal prothrombin time for the control and the prothrombin time of the sample being tested. A OSPT that is 30 to 50 per cent greater than the control should be considered abnormal. Hypoprothrombinemia may occur in any of the following conditions: (1) dietary deficiency of vitamin K; (2) inadequate absorption of vitamin K; (3) impaired formation of prothrombin by the liver, such as that occurring in infectious canine hepatitis, and administration of an anticoagulant such as dicumarol, or accidental consumption of an anticoagulant. It must be remembered that a decrease in plasma fibrinogen will also interfere with a normal prothrombin test, since clot formation may be delayed or not occur in animals with fibrinogen levels of 60 to 100 mg/μl or less.

TESTS FOR MEASURING INTRINSIC SYSTEM FACTORS

ACTIVATED PARTIAL THROMBOPLASTIN TIME

Several tests are available for determining defects in the intrinsic system, but the most practical for the routine veterinary laboratory is determination of the activated partial thromboplastin time (APTT).

The APTT test is conducted by using a partial thromboplastin, such as purified brain thromboplastin, that has been activated by kaolin or ellagic acid. This substance is added to plasma, the mixture is incubated, and clotting time is recorded following the addition of $CaCl_2$. Several commercial reagents are available for this test, and, as the normal values will vary according to the type of incomplete thromboplastin utilized, each test should be conducted along with a plasma sample from a normal animal. An APTT 30 to 50 per cent greater than the control is considered abnormal.

If the APTT is abnormal, it can be assumed that there is a defect involving a deficiency of one of the following thromboplastic factors: VIII, IX, X, XI, or XII. If prothrombin time with tissue thromboplastin is normal, factor X deficiency can be ruled out, since this deficiency is characterized by both a prolonged APTT and a prolonged prothrombin time.

If identification of the specific factor is required, additional tests using the APTT can be completed by mixing plasma with a known deficiency and plasma from the patient. Failure to correct APTT to a normal value utilizing plasma with a specific deficiency suggests a deficiency in that factor.

PROTHROMBIN CONSUMPTION

The prothrombin consumption test, although not routine, has been found to aid in detecting deficiencies in the formation of thromboplastin. Although more specific tests have been devised, they are complex and require special equipment and reagents. Because of its simplicity and the availability of the required reagents, the prothrombin consumption test can be performed in any laboratory equipped to do routine prothrombin time studies.

When prothrombin conversion is impaired, prothrombin is not converted to thrombin and prothrombin is not consumed. The amount of prothrombin converted to thrombin in the formation of a clot is proportional to the amount of prothrombin conversion factor formed; however, when there is an abnormality in the formation of plasma thromboplastin, prothrombin is not fully consumed in clotting, and there is a significant concentration of prothrombin remaining in serum after clot formation.

The prothrombin consumption test is performed on clarified serum that has been stored no longer than two hours prior to testing. If storage is necessary it should be at 5° C. The technique for this test is similar to that for a one-stage prothrombin time, except that serum is used instead of plasma.

In the presence of adequate quantities of prothrombin but inadequate quantities of plasma thromboplastin, serum will clot rapidly, and in dogs a result of less than 13 seconds is considered abnormal.

Prothrombin consumption is abnormal in a number of conditions including hemophilia A, hemophilia B, thrombocytopenia, thrombocytopathias, or any defect in the intrinsic pathway.

The prothrombin consumption test is of little value in an animal in which the prothrombin time is prolonged, since the quantity of prothrombin present is probably abnormal. Therefore, this test is of value in an animal in which the prothrombin time is normal but there is a hemostatic problem. Prothrombin consumption time will also be abnormal when platelets are significantly reduced in number or their thromboplastic function is insufficient.

OTHER ASSAYS

FUNCTIONAL ACTIVITY. Techniques are available for assaying intrinsic clotting factor activity. These tests should be completed in experienced coagulation laboratories. Factors VIII, IX, XI, and XII can be measured with methods based on either the APTT or the thromboplastin generation time. Specific clotting factor activity is measured in dilutions of test plasma mixed with standard quantities of a substrate plasma specifically deficient in that factor.

Extrinsic clotting factor activity (V, VII, X) can also be done in coagulation laboratories. The OSPT or the RVVT test, or both, are used.

IMMUNOLOGIC ASSAYS. Factor VIII-related antigen is measured utilizing an immunologic method. As with specific factor assays it is run only in experimental coagulation laboratories in which adequate methods and controls have been developed. Similar assays are available for antigens related to factors V, VII, IX, X, XII, and XIII as well as prothrombin and fibrinogen. Information relative to the utilization of these tests in animal patients is limited.[1]

FIBRIN-FIBRINOGEN DEGRADATION PRODUCTS. A test for the presence of fibrin-fibrinogen products (FDP) is commercially available (Thrombo-Wellcotest, Burroughs Wellcome Co., Research Triangle Park, North Carolina). This test utilizes antibodies to human fibrinogen that are adsorbed to latex particles. Blood is collected in special tubes furnished as a part of the kit. The harvested serum is diluted and added to the latex particles on a glass plate. If fibrin-fibrinogen degradation products are present in the serum, agglutination will occur.

FIBRINOLYSIS ASSAY. The simplest method for evaluating fibrinolysis is the clot lysis time. After a clot retraction test is completed the tube is allowed to stand until lysis occurs. If clot retraction is poor, lysis will be retarded. Another method for determining clot lysis is to permit blood to clot in glass tubes and incubate them at 37° C. Most animals will have lysis of the clot between eight and 20 hours. If it is accelerated lysis will begin within three to five hours after the clot has formed.

PLASMA RECALCIFICATION TIME. Plasma collected in citrate will form a clot after the addition of calcium chloride. This assay measures the intrinsic system. Nine parts of citrated blood are collected and centrifuged at 2000 g to obtain a platelet-poor plasma. Mix 0.1 ml of this plasma and 0.1 ml of 0.145 M sodium chloride in a 13 × 100 mm test tube and warm the mixture to 37° C. Add 0.1 ml of 0.025 M calcium chloride to the plasma and start a stopwatch. Allow the reaction mixture to stand undisturbed for 90 seconds, then gently tilt the tube every 30 seconds and observe for a clot. Normal values should be established in each laboratory. The number of platelets remaining in the plasma and the length of time blood is exposed to glass surfaces will affect test results.

THROMBIN TIME. Thrombin time is measured by determining the length of time required for a fibrin clot to form following the addition of bovine thrombin to citrated plasma. A stock thrombin solution is commercially available. Mix equal volumes (0.2 ml) of the stock solution with platelet-poor plasma that has been warmed to 37° C. Start the stopwatch and record the time necessary for formation of a fibrin clot. A normal plasma should be run along with the patient plasma. A thrombin time greater than 1.3 times the normal control value should be considered abnormal. Thrombin time measures the speed of conversion of fibrinogen to fibrin but is independent of other intrinsic or extrinsic factor activities. It is prolonged in animals with hypofibrinogenemia or dysfibrinogenemia, or if fibrin degradation products are elevated or heparin is present. In humans thrombin time is increased in individuals with macroglobulinemia.

LABORATORY FINDINGS IN HEMORRHAGIC DISORDERS

HEREDITARY COAGULATION DEFECTS

Deficiency of Factor VIII (Hemophilia A).
Most of the work on hemorrhagic disorders has used disease in the dog as a model. The best known coagulation disorder is probably hemophilia, and there is little doubt that forms of hemophilia exist in all species of animals and only require recognition and diagnosis. Hemophilia has been reported in thoroughbred horses and in cats. The following breeds of dogs are also affected: Shetland sheepdogs, beagles, English and Irish setters, Labrador retrievers, German shepherds, collies, greyhounds, Weimaraners, Chihuahuas, Samoyeds, Vizslas, English bulldogs, miniature poodles, miniature schnauzers, Saint Bernards, and mixed breeds.[4]

In hemophilia A there is a distinct abnormality in the intrinsic system of blood coagulation. This defect is a lack of factor VIII activity. In such animals, clotting time is prolonged and prothrombin consumption is deficient, although prothrombin time is normal. The platelet count is within the normal range, but the platelet clumping time is prolonged (Table 5–4). In dogs, this defect appears to be similar pathologically to classic hemophilia in humans and is inherited as an X-linked characteristic.

Laboratory findings in hemophilia A are compatible with a defect in the intrinsic clotting mechanism. Whole blood clotting times, plasma clotting times, and activated partial thromboplastin times are prolonged. Factor VIII activity is greatly reduced but factor VIII-related antigen levels are normal or elevated. The results of tests for the extrinsic system (OSPT, RVVT) and platelet function are normal. Initial bleeding time is usually normal. However, there is frequently rebleeding in animals with hemophilia A, as the original clot is unstable, and secondary bleeding time is prolonged.

Hemophilia A is an X chromosome–linked recessive trait in which affected males are hemizygous, carrier females are heterozygous, and affected females are homozygous. The severity of the condition ranges from mild to marked in the

TABLE 5–4. Laboratory Diagnosis of Hereditary Coagulation Defects in Dogs and Cats

Defect	Bleeding Time	Coagulation Time	ACT	OSPT	APTT	Specific Tests
Factor I (fibrinogen)	P	V	P	P	P	Decreased fibrinogen level
Factor II	P	V	N	P	N	Low prothrombin, abnormal RVVT
Factor VII	N	N	N	P	N	Low FVII activity, normal Stypven time OSPT corrected with normal serum
Factor VIII	N	P	P	N	P	Low FVIII activity, normal to increased FVIII-related antigen, APTT not corrected by addition of normal serum
Factor IX	N	P	P	N	P	Low FIX activity, APTT is corrected by addition of normal serum
Factor X	N	V	P	P	P	Low FX activity, abnormal RVVT
Factor XI	N	V	P	N	P	Low FXI activity, prolonged recalcification
Factor XII		P	P	N	P	Low FXII activity, prolonged recalcification
Von Willebrand's	P	V	V	N	V	Low FVIII activity, low factor VIII-related antigen
Thrombasthenic thrombopathia	P	V	V	N	N	Poor clot retraction, low prothrombin consumption, defective platelet aggregation, low PF3 availability

ACT = Activated coagulation time, OSPT = One-stage prothrombin time, APTT = Activated partial thromboplastin time, RVVT = Russell's viper-venom time, N = Normal, P = Prolonged, V = Variable.

dog, is quite mild in the cat and is marked in the horse.

Deficiency of Factor IX (Hemophilia B). This condition, also known as Christmas disease, is an X chromosome–linked recessive trait. It occurs with less frequency than hemophilia A but has been reported in several breeds of dogs including Cairn terriers, American cocker spaniels, Labrador retrievers, French bulldogs, black-and-tan coonhounds, Saint Bernards, Alaskan malamutes, Scottish terriers, Old English sheepdogs, Shetland sheepdogs, Bichon frises, Airedale terriers, and a family of British shorthair cats. Some affected animals have a severe coagulation problem. The most severe bleeding problems occur in the larger breeds; bleeding is mild to moderate in small breeds. Hemophilia B can be differentiated from hemophilia A by the addition of fresh normal serum to plasma and completion of an intrinsic coagulation factor test such as the APTT. Fresh serum contains factor IX but not factor VIII. If there is a factor IX deficiency, serum will correct the prolonged APTT of patient plasma.

Factor VII Deficiency. A third coagulation disorder in dogs was classified as a factor VII deficiency. The animals discovered to have this impairment were an inbred strain of beagles. The deficiency has also been reported in Alaskan malamutes, boxers, miniature Schnauzers, and bulldogs. Affected animals have normal clotting time, platelet count, prothrombin consumption test results, and platelet clumping time; however, the prothrombin time is prolonged. The prolonged prothrombin time of plasma from affected dogs is shortened to normal by the addition of 10 per cent normal canine or human serum but not by normal aluminum hydroxide-treated canine or human plasma or plasma from patients receiving dicumarol therapy. Factor V assays are normal in affected dogs. The thromboplastin generation test results are normal. Russell viper-venom (Stypven) times are normal. The defect is inherited as an autosomal dominant trait. Heterozygotes are asymptomatic and have 35 to 65 per cent factor VII, whereas homozygotes have 1 to 5 per cent factor VII. There is a prolonged OSPT in both forms of the disease. Affected animals do not usually have serious bleeding tendencies but excessive bleeding can occur during surgery. Some affected dogs bruise easily and others have a predisposition to systemic demodicosis. As factor VII is a vitamin K-dependent product of the liver and has a very short half-life, it may be deficient in advanced liver disease or with vitamin K deficiency such as that associated with warfarin toxicity.

Factor XI Deficiency. Factor XI (plasma thromboplastin antecedent) deficiency was detected in cattle[5] and in dogs.[6]

The defect in dogs was characterized by autosomal inheritance, minor bleeding episodes, severe protracted bleeding following surgical procedures, abnormal prothrombin consumption, prolonged partial thromboplastin and recalcification times, and an abnormal factor XI assay using human or bovine factor XI-deficient plasma.[6] Heterozygotes have 40 to 60 per cent factor XI activity while homozygotes have less than 20 per cent activity. Platelet function and other coagulation tests, including specific assays for factors V, VII, VIII, IX, X, XII, and XIII, are normal. This deficiency has been diagnosed in springer spaniels, Great Pyrenees, Kerry blue terriers, and Weimaraners. It is unlikely that this deficiency occurs with any frequency as a clinical problem.

In affected cattle the disease is mild and problems occur in association with surgical procedures. Abnormal laboratory tests include prolonged APTT and a marked reduction in factor XI activity.

von Willebrand's Disease. A canine pseudo-hemophilia that mimicks von Willebrand's disease of humans has been described.[7] This disorder has also been reported in pigs.[8] The condition is characterized by prolonged bleeding time, decreased platelet adhesiveness, and a variable reduction in the level of factor VIII.

There are two forms of VWD: An autosomal incompletely dominant disease and an autosomal recessive disease. In the autosomal incompletely dominant disease both homozygotes and heterozygotes can manifest a bleeding tendency. In the autosomal recessive disease, affected individuals are homozygous for the VWD gene and have two asymptomatic, heterozygote parents (carriers).

The incompletely dominant disease has been recognized in many breeds including Doberman pinschers, standard Manchester terriers, German shepherds, golden retrievers, miniature schnauzers, Scottish terriers, Pembroke Welsh corgis, English springer spaniels, English cocker spaniels, Labrador retrievers, Cairn terriers, Lakeland terriers, Great Danes, basset hounds, boxers, Afghan hounds, rottweilers, Irish setters, standard and miniature poodles, standard and miniature dachsunds, Shetland sheepdogs, Airedale terriers, Lhasa apsos, papillons, toy Manchester terriors, soft-coated Wheaten terriers, and Tibetan terriers.

The recessive disease has been recognized in Scottish terriers, Chesapeake Bay retrievers, and Poland China swine.

Most screening tests for intrinsic clotting are normal except in severely affected individuals. Classically there is a variable reduction in factor VIII activity and a parallel reduction in factor VIII–related antigens. Dogs with the recessive disease are homozygotes and have no factor VIII–related antigen and their parents have 15 to 60 per cent of normal. Animals with the incompletely dominant disease have 7 to 60 per cent factor VIII–related antigen. In some breeds in which VWD is a problem, special screening procedures have been instituted to detect carriers.

In addition to the deficiency in factor VIII activity or concentration of factor VIII–related antigen, platelet defects can be detected. There is reduced platelet retention as measured by adhesiveness to glass beads and abnormal ristocetin-induced platelet aggregation.

Clinical signs include excessive bleeding following even minor surgical procedures; recurrent epistaxis; gingival, penile, and vaginal bleeding; gastrointestinal bleeding with or without diarrhea; hematuria; prolonged postpartum or estral bleeding; hematoma formation; lameness; prolonged bleeding from the umbilical cord at birth; and stillbirths or neonatal deaths with necropsy evidence of hemorrhage.

Individuals with VWD can synthesize their own factor VIII activity for about 24 hours following transfusion with substances such as fresh-frozen plasma, cryoprecipitates, and special concentrates containing factor VIII. Such transfusions correct the factor VIII deficiency, but bleeding time and platelet retention are only temporarily corrected.

Factor X Deficiency. A factor X deficiency has been described in a family of cocker spaniels.[4] In mature dogs, this deficiency does not produce severe episodes of clinical hemorrhage unless the dog is subjected to surgery. However, in newborn and young dogs, hemorrhagic problems may be serious and include massive hemorrhage into the thoracic or abdominal cavity and, in the newborn, umbilical hemorrhage. Many of the puppies are stillborn or die soon after birth. Some puppies may live for one or two weeks, then suddenly fade and die. In young adults, hematuria, hemorrhage of the gums, prolonged bleeding during estrus, and intrathoracic hemorrhages have been reported.

Laboratory findings include a slight prolongation of prothrombin time and RVVT with a concomitant increase in the partial thromboplastin time, whereas other platelet function and clotting assays are normal. Specific assays for factor X always show a reduction in activity.

Fibrinogen Deficiency (Factor I). A congenital deficiency of fibrinogen in dogs has been reported, and an afibrinogenemia has been discovered in a family of Saanen goats.[9] Deficiencies in fibrinogen are characterized by a severe bleeding tendency, and minor trauma may result in protracted and sometimes lethal hemorrhage. In the laboratory, severe deficiencies are characterized by marked prolongation of all clotting tests, as fibrinogen is required for clot formation. Fibrinogen measurements are abnormal, and the erythrocyte sedimentation rate (ESR) is greatly reduced.

Prothrombin Deficiency (Factor II). This is a rare coagulation deficiency which has been reported in a family of boxer dogs in Texas and a cocker spaniel in Iowa. Affected animals have epistaxis, and there are umbilical bleeding in newborn puppies and a mild mucosal surface bleeding in young adults.[1] Prothrombin time and RVVT are prolonged, whereas the APTT and other intrinsic coagulation factor tests are normal. This appears to be a dysprothrombinemia because prothrombin levels are normal but prothrombin activity is reduced.

Factor XII Deficiency. A factor XII deficiency has been reported in cats[1] and was discovered accidentally while screening animals for intrinsic clotting factor defects. It has also been reported in a standard poodle and a German shorthair pointer. Affected animals do not have any clinical signs of a coagulation problem. The APTT, whole blood coagulation time in glass, and recalcification times are all prolonged; bleeding time, platelet count, thrombin time, fibrinogen level, and OSPT are normal. Heterozygotes have a reduced level of factor XII.

Platelet Function Defects. A thrombasthenic thrombopathia has been described in otterhounds and basset hounds, and isolated cases have been reported in a Scottish terrier and a foxhound.[4] The hemorrhagic diathesis in these animals is moderate in homozygotes with only minor problems with heterozygotes. Surgical procedures and trauma aggravate the problem. Bleeding from surface abrasions and hemarthroses are common.

As might be expected, these animals have a prolonged bleeding time with normal to slightly reduced platelet counts and a reduction in platelet adhesiveness. There are various defects in platelet aggregation, clot retraction, whole blood and serum clotting times, and RVVT. Affected otterhounds also have an abnormal platelet survival, a defective release of platelet thromboplastic phospholipids, and reduced platelet fibrinogen. Serum clotting times are short and the RVVT is long. One half to two thirds of the thrombocytes are very large macrothrombocytes.

A thrombopathia with abnormal platelet retention, prolonged bleeding time and platelet aggregation defects has been reported in a family of Simmental cattle.

The conditions just discussed constitute the hereditary defects identified in animals as of this writing. Defects known to occur in humans but not yet identified in animals are factor XIII deficiency, factor V deficiency, and familial thrombocytopenia.

ACQUIRED COAGULATION DEFECTS

Problems in hemostasis encountered by the veterinarian are more likely to be due to an acquired defect than to a congenital condition. The laboratory findings that can be anticipated in acquired defects are listed in Table 5–5.

Liver Disease. As mentioned previously, liver deficiencies may result in the development of a hemorrhagic tendency.

TABLE 5–5. Laboratory Diagnosis of Acquired Coagulation Defects in Dogs and Cats

Cause	Bleeding Time	Coagulation Time	ACT	OSPT	APTT	Other Test Results
Advanced liver disease	N-P	N-P	N-P[1]	N-P[2]	P	Decreased FVII, FXI activities; increased FVIII-related antigen in some; in very advanced disease FII levels decrease
Coumarin poisoning	N-P	N-P[3]	P	P	P	Responds to vitamin K-1 therapy
Vitamin K deficiency	N-P	P[3]	P	P	P	Also responds to K-1 therapy
DIC	V	P	P	P	P	Decreased platelet count, increased FDP, decreased fibrinogen
Thrombocytopenia	V	V	V	N	N	Platelet count below 50,000/μl before petechiae appear

ACT = activated coagulation time, OSPT = one-stage prothrombin time, APTT = activated partial thromboplastin time, N = Normal, P = Prolonged, V = variable.
[1] May be prolonged earlier than APTT, as factor VII has a shorter half-life.
[2] May be prolonged later as other intrinsic factors become deficient.
[3] Prolonged if there is considerable platelet loss.

Hemostatic defects associated with liver disease result from diminished synthesis of proteins, metabolic abnormalities, and diminished clearance mechanisms. Severe bleeding problems are not common but can occur.

The liver is the major site of production of plasma coagulation factors I, II, V, VII, VIII, IX, X, XI, and XII. It has been estimated that the OSPT or APTT screening tests may be abnormally long in is many as two thirds of dogs with hepatic disease.[11] Because of the short half-life of many of the factors, particularly V, VII, IX and X, a lack of production associated with hepatic disease may be detected with the appropriate tests.

In a recent study of 28 dogs[12] with naturally occurring hepatic disease 93 per cent had at least one abnormal coagulation test value. Hepatic degeneration was characterized by a decrease in factor XI; hepatic inflammation with an increase in factor VIII–related antigen; hepatic cirrhosis by a shortened thrombin clot time, a decrease in factors IX, X, XI, and an increase in factor VIII related antigen; and in hepatic neoplasia there was a decrease in factor VIII procoagulant activity and an increased factor VIII–related antigen.

With very advanced severe liver disease, fibrinogen decreases may occur. If this is sufficient to affect coagulation test results, it is an unfavorable prognostic sign.

Decreased plasma prothrombin activity (factor II) has also been associated with hepatic disease. This is a consequence of (1) lack of production in the presence of adequate metabolites or (2) biliary obstruction and the resultant decrease in absorption of fat-soluble vitamin K because of decreased bile in the intestine. In advanced severe hepatic disease, both mechanisms may be involved. In less severe disease, there is usually sufficient functional liver parenchyma to synthesize pro-thrombin in quantities adequate to prevent abnormal hemostasis. If hypoprothrombinemia is the result of biliary obstruction, the injection of vitamin K may correct the prothrombin deficiency.

Thrombocytopenia may occur in association with advanced liver disease if there is abnormal hepatic metabolism. If hepatic disease is accompanied by DIC, a consumptive thrombocytopenia will be present. In addition, the fibrin-fibrinogen degradation products associated with DIC are normally cleared by the liver, but if there is hepatic dysfunction they will continue to increase and interfere with platelet function.

Interpretation of laboratory tests may be complicated by very low levels of plasma fibrinogen, which occur rarely in animals. Under such circumstances there is complete failure to clot in any of the routine tests.

Chemicals. Chemicals interfering with hemostasis must also be considered when the veterinarian is faced with diagnosing and treating an animal with a hemostatic problem. It is well known that coumarin derivatives and various chemical analogs are utilized as poisons for rodents and occasionally are accidentally consumed by another animal. These substances interfere with vitamin K metabolism and therefore will prevent synthesis of those coagulation factors dependent upon vitamin K. Included in this group are prothrombin and factors VII, IX, and X. Deficiencies of these factors are most easily detected by the prothrombin time test. A vitamin K deficiency may also result from the ingestion of moldy sweet clover by cattle.

Other drugs have been discovered that will predispose to hemorrhagic tendencies. Most of these interfere with hemostasis by inhibiting the second phase of blood platelet aggregation. Included in this group are aspirin, phenothiazine derivatives, and phenylbutazone. Therefore, the veterinarian should be cautioned against administering such drugs in patients with advanced liver disease, hereditary hemophilia, or coumarin poisoning.

Occasionally vitamin K deficiencies will develop in animals having a malabsorptive syndrome. Such deficiencies can be corrected by the administration of small doses of vitamin K parenterally. If, however, the prothrombin deficiency is the result of parenchymal liver disease, parenteral administration of vitamin K will not correct the deficiency, and the prothrombin time will remain prolonged.

Thrombocytopenia. As previously suggested, the vast majority of hemostatic problems occurring in a veterinary practice are related to a thrombocytopenia or a defect in the function of thrombocytes. The first procedure that should be adopted with an animal having a problem in hemostasis is to estimate the number and activity of blood platelets in the peripheral circulation. If a thrombocytopenia or thrombocytopathia can be ruled out as the cause of the problem, a more intensified search for a definitive diagnosis must be made.

Thrombocytopenia is identified by a reduction in total platelet count, abnormal clot retraction, prolonged bleeding time, and an increase in RVVT. Whole blood clotting time is usually normal in glass tubes but may be prolonged in plastic or siliconized glass tubes. In patients with a recurrent thrombocytopenia, circulating platelet antibodies can sometimes be demonstrated following an acute thrombocytopenia.

Occasionally, a primary or idiopathic thrombocytopenia occurs in which the etiology is not established. Thrombocytopenia is more likely to occur as a secondary condition following, or in association with, viral and bacterial septicemias, autoimmune hemolytic anemias, leukemias, and systemic lupus erythematosus (SLE).

A generalized pancytopenia and reduction in thrombocytes may be caused by certain drugs or by infection with *Ehrlichia canis*. Neoplastic infiltration of the marrow may reduce platelet formation and result in a clinically identifiable problem. Thrombocytes are greatly reduced in DIC, as they are consumed because of extensive thrombus formation.

Platelets may be destroyed in large numbers following antigen-antibody reactions on the platelet surface membrane. This probably causes the majority of the so-called idiopathic thrombocytopenias in domestic animals. The best test for detecting the presence of an immune-mediated thrombocytopenia is the platelet factor 3 release assay. This test is based on the fact that antiplatelet antibodies will trigger release of PF3 and shorten clotting time. Such tests are usually conducted in a laboratory experienced in specialized coagulation studies. The test sytem uses globulins

from a normal control and globulins from the patient. Normal dog platelets are incubated with these globulins and calcium chloride is added to the mixture and the clotting time determined. If antiplatelet antibodies are present, they will damage the normal platelets causing release of PF3. Times that are 10 seconds less than the normal control indicate the presence of antiplatelet antibodies. False-negative tests have been reported in patients that have been treated with corticosteroids for two or three days. Not all patients with an immune-mediated thrombocytopenia have positive results. As immune-mediated thrombocytopenia may accompany other autoimmune diseases such as AIHA and lupus, appropriate tests for these conditions should be conducted.

Other drugs may cause an immune-mediated thrombocytopenia, and in the dog certain antibiotics, sulfonamides, digitoxin, quinidines, phenytoin, phenylbutazone, thiazides and their derivatives, and dinitrophenol have been incriminated.[10] Drug therapy used for the treatment of leukemia will also cause thrombocytopenia.

Disseminated Intravascular Coagulation (DIC). DIC occurs secondarily in a variety of disease conditions in animals, including infections, neoplasia, obstetric complications, and with a variety of other conditions as shock, heartworm disease, heat stroke, burns, trauma, and liver disease.

Viral infections that cause DIC include canine hepatitis, hog cholera, fowl plague, equine viral arteritis, and epizootic hemorrhagic disease of deer. Bacterial infections may also cause DIC. Endotoxins associated with gram-negative bacterial infections produce the Shwartzman reaction and its characteristic DIC in humans as well as animals (horse, dog, rabbit, guinea pig, and rat).

DIC may occur as a acute, subacute, or chronic condition. In the early stages of this syndrome clinical signs may be absent; it is not until the reduction in coagulation factors and platelets becomes marked that coagulation problems become evident. If the platelet count is less than 50,000/µl, petechiae and ecchymoses may develop on mucous membranes. Hematuria, epistaxis, and excessive bleeding following venipuncture may occur in the terminal stages of DIC. As there is deposition of fibrin in the microvasculature, ischemia may occur, particularly in the kidney and lungs. When this occurs there is other clinical evidence of organ failure. The predominant clinical signs are those associated with the primary disease condition that initiated DIC.

Laboratory findings in DIC vary depending upon the stage in which the animal is first seen. Initially, DIC is manifested by hypercoagulability, then the condition progresses to a secondary phase characterized by consumption coagulopathy. The veterinarian seldom sees the animal in the early phase of DIC but is more likely to be faced with an animal in the consumptive phase.

The consumptive phase is characterized by

thrombocytopenia, abnormal partial thromboplastin time, increased prothrombin time, hypofibrinogenemia, and increased levels of fibrinolytic split products in the plasma. Fragmented erythrocytes (schistocytes) are frequently encountered on blood films prepared from animals with DIC.

Fibrinolytic split products can be detected utilizing a latex agglutination test. Such material is available for detection of human fibrinolytic split products and has been found useful in detecting these breakdown products in animal blood.

REFERENCES

1. Dodds, W. J.: Hemostasis and coagulation. In: *Clinical Biochemistry of Domestic Animals*, edited by Kaneko, J. J., 3rd ed., Academic Press, New York, 1980.
2. Green, R. A.: Bleeding disorders. In: *Textbook of Veterinary Internal Medicine: Diseases of the Dog and Cat*, edited by Ettinger, S. J., 2nd ed., W. B. Saunders Company, Philadelphia, 1983.
3. Weiss, D. J.: Uniform evaluation and semiquantitative reporting of hematologic data in veterinary laboratories. Vet. Clin Pathol., *XIII(II)*:27, 1984.
4. Dodds, W. J.: Bleeding disorders. In: *Textbook of Veterinary Internal Medicine: Diseases of the Dog and Cat*, Vol. 2, edited by Ettinger, S. J., W. B. Saunders Company, Philadelphia, 1975.
5. Dodds, W. J., and Kaneko, J. J.: Hemostasis and blood coagulation. In: *Clinical Biochemistry of Domestic Animals*, Vol. II, edited by Kaneko, J. J. and Cornelius, C. E., 2nd ed., Academic Press, New York, 1971.
6. Dodds, W. J., and Kull, J. E.: Canine factor XI (plasma thromboplastin antecedent) deficiency. J. Lab. Clin. Med., *78*:746, 1971.
7. Dodds, W. J.: Canine von Willebrand's disease. J. Lab. Clin. Med., *71*:713, 1970.
8. Muhrer, M. E., Hogan, A. C., and Bogart, R.: A defect in the coagulation mechanism of swine blood. Am. J. Physiol., *136*:355, 1942.
9. Breukink, H. J., Hart, H. C., Arkel, C., Veldon, N. A., and Watering, C. C.: Congenital afibrinogenemia in goats. Zentrabl. Veterinaermed.[A], *19*:661, 1972.
10. Wilkins, R. J.: Thrombocytopenic purpura. In: *Current Veterinary Therapy. VI Small Animal Practice*, edited by Kirk, R. W., W. B. Saunders Company, Philadelphia, 1977.
11. Badylak, S. F., and Van Vleet, J. F.: Alterations of prothrombin time and activated partial thromboplastin time in dogs with hepatic disease. Am. J. Vet. Res., *42*:2053, 1981.
12. Badylak, S. F., Dodds, W. J., and Van Vleet, J. F.: Plasma coagulation factor abnormalities in dogs with naturally occurring hepatic disease. Am. J. Vet. Res., *44*:2336, 1983.

CLINICAL CHEMISTRY

Measurement of the chemical constituents of various body fluids is another portion of a comprehensive examination designed to disclose the nature of a disease process. When such analyses are combined with other laboratory procedures, complete physical examination, and history of the patient, they may assist the veterinarian in arriving at a final diagnosis, evaluating the prognosis, and following the efficacy of the therapy. Chemical studies should not be requested indiscriminately or substituted for a thorough physical examination. Information received from such analyses is of value only if the proper studies have been requested and the clinician has the ability to interpret the results.

The purpose of this chapter is to discuss the principles of clinical chemistry with respect to basic laboratory procedures, equipment utilized in chemical analyses, quality control in the clinical laboratory, clinical enzymology, and biochemical profiling. Discussions of specific chemical analyses and their indications and interpretation are included in the appropriate chapters elsewhere in this book.

Clinicians must have knowledge of the normal values with respect to the species, age, and sex of the patient and must be aware of variations that may be associated with the analytical procedure. They should also be cognizant of the alterations encountered in various disease states. A practitioner must have some understanding of the precision attainable for a particular determination in order to adequately interpret results. It must be emphasized that the values for the various chemical components found in the body fluids vary from species to species, sometimes according to

the age of the animal, and frequently from one laboratory to another.

BASIC PROCEDURES

Accurate and reproducible results from chemical analyses are dependent upon the care with which the sample is collected and procedures are conducted. The use of incorrect quantities or concentrations of the various chemicals incorporated in these precise techniques may influence results, as may the use of dirty glassware. Therefore, before describing the principles involved in, indications for, normal values of, and techniques for testing, it may be useful to consider some of the basic concepts of laboratory procedures that are important in chemical analyses.

SPECIMEN COLLECTION AND HANDLING

In order to achieve accuracy and reproducibility, standardized techniques should be adopted for collection and processing of blood and other body fluids. The clinical specimen most frequently examined chemically in the laboratory is blood. As other body fluids and their methods of collection are discussed in the following chapters, it seems appropriate to give special consideration here to blood and blood collection.

Blood samples obtained for clinical chemistry should be taken as carefully as possible in order to minimize trauma, either physical or psychological. As with hematologic examination, excitement, apprehension, and physical exercise influence the values obtained in clinical chemistry. Therefore, the veterinarian should attempt to reduce these effects. Time spent in soothing the animal, and sometimes its owner, is well worthwhile if by doing so one can avoid collecting a sample from an animal that is hyperadrenalized as a consequence of fear, excitement, or muscular exercise.

Blood is most frequently collected by venipuncture, although arterial blood is occasionally required. In young animals, particularly puppies and kittens, venipuncture may prove difficult. On these occasions blood from a capillary bed may be used. Details for methods of collecting blood from various animals have been previously discussed. In obtaining a specimen care must always be taken in order to avoid contaminating the blood or the patient. Sterile equipment should always be utilized and the skin cleansed and disinfected prior to collection.

The most acceptable specimens for clinical chemistry are obtained by using plastic disposable syringes and needles or by using a commercially available evacuated blood collecting apparatus such as the Vacutainer (Becton-Dickinson, Rutherford, New Jersey). Vacutainers are available either with or without anticoagulants and in sizes suitable for most animals. This system has the advantage of providing the laboratory with a constant sample size and, if required, a standard quantity of the anticoagulant of choice. It also assures the practitioner of always having the available equipment required for obtaining blood samples, including a sharp, disposable needle. Special Vacutainers are also available for collecting blood for culture.

Techniques for collecting arterial blood are discussed in the chapter on serum electrolytes and acid-base balance (Chapter 10).

If blood is drawn with a syringe and needle, the needle should be removed before blood is discharged into a sample tube. Failure to do so and forcing blood through a small-gauge needle may disrupt erythrocytes and result in abnormal values for some chemical determinations. The blood sample, regardless of the method of collection, should always be handled gently. Overenthusiasm in mixing blood may disrupt erythrocytes and influence results of chemical analysis.

Processing of blood following collection is just as important as the method of collection, if not more important. Chemical analyses should commence as soon as practicable after withdrawal in order to prevent alterations in the constituents to be quantitated. Ideally, measurements should be performed within one hour following collection. If this is not practical, or if the blood is to be forwarded to a commercial laboratory for analysis, the sample should be properly stored. If whole blood is to be analyzed, it should be refrigerated immediately and kept under refrigeration until

sample processing is begun. Serum is preferred for most determinations and it should be separated as quickly as possible. Serum can be readily separated from a clot if the sample is permitted to coagulate at room temperature for approximately 30 minutes. The clot is gently removed from the sides of the tube by rimming it with a wooden applicator stick or thin glass rod. The sample should be centrifuged and serum collected into a chemically clean tube. Plasma can be separated immediately by centrifugation. Care should be taken not to overcentrifuge the blood or to centrifuge it at a high speed. Serum or plasma is refrigerated or frozen (if freezing does not destroy test validity) until analysis can be completed.

Failure to heed these precautions can result in abnormal values that are not representative of the physiologic status of the animal. For example, if blood is allowed to stand in a warm room, as much as 20 mg/dl of glucose may be lost per hour, and in most animal species hemolysis will alter the electrolyte levels of either serum or plasma.

Other changes that may occur include breakdown of nitrogenous constituents, alterations in electrolyte composition of the serum resulting from a change in erythrocyte permeability, increase in organic phosphate at the expense of erythrocyte organic phosphate, and changes in enzyme levels.

Plasma or serum is preferred to whole blood for most determinations of chemical constituents. The three media—whole blood, plasma, and serum—are not equally desirable or interchangeable, as blood chemical constituents are unequally divided among them. Whole blood provides a less sensitive medium than either plasma or serum, and changes taking place are often obscured by the effect of erythrocytes. If plasma is used, heparin is generally the anticoagulant of choice. Samples to be processed in an automated analyzer should be permitted to clot and the serum submitted for analysis. The majority of normal chemical values presented in succeeding chapters are for either plasma or serum.

Blood samples acceptable for most chemical analyses can be obtained if the following precautions are taken:

1. Avoid hemolysis by:
   A. Care in collection. This means a quiet animal, sharp needle, and dry, chemically clean syringe or, preferably, a Vacutainer.
   B. Careful transfer of blood if a syringe is used. This is not a significant factor if the Vacutainer system is used.
   C. Use of caution in blood separation, i.e., careful rimming of the clotted specimen and slow-speed, brief centrifugation of the clotted or unclotted blood sample.
2. Avoid volume changes due to dilution or evaporation.

A. Wet syringes should be avoided.
B. Do not use liquid anticoagulants, as they may cause significant dilution.
C. Do not allow blood to stand in open containers for long periods of time, and avoid centrifugation in open containers. Evaporation can occur under either circumstance.
3. Avoid composition changes resulting from bacterial or enzymatic effect, loss of volatile constituents, and cell-liquid interchanges.
    A. Bacterial or enzymatic alterations can be minimized by the use of sterile equipment, prompt separation of liquid from cells, and rapid cooling or freezing of plasma or serum.
    B. Blood gas changes can be reduced by filling the chamber nearly to capacity and keeping it tightly closed.
    C. Cell-liquid interchange is minimal if separation is completed as quickly as possible and hemolysis is avoided.

RECORDS AND RESULTS

Complete and accurate identification of blood specimens for submission to the laboratory is an essential part of clinical chemistry just as it is for any other clinical laboratory determination.

All samples submitted to a clinical laboratory should have complete identification including the owner's name and the case or accession number. These identifications are not only of value to the laboratory personnel responsible for handling the specimen but also provide the clinician with two means of positive identification when results are returned. An identification system that provides an indelible mark on the tube or container should be adopted. Each specimen should be accompanied by a request form indicating what tests are required. Any sample presented to a laboratory without positive identification and indication of test requirements should not be examined.

Veterinarians who have their own laboratories will undoubtedly choose to devise their own reporting system or adopt one that has already been successfully utilized in other practices.

A daily log should be maintained in the clinical laboratory. This log is an invaluable tool for both laboratory and practice. The log should include date, specimen number (assigned laboratory number), patient identification (name and number), tests required, and results obtained. Such a log serves as a source of data that can be utilized in the laboratory quality control program and provides a reference for retrieval of information from a particular patient on a specific date. If large numbers of specimens are analyzed, a laboratory work sheet for use by the technologist is recommended. It should provide space for recording sample identification number; data observed, such as per cent transmission or optical density (absorbance); calculations made; and values for patient, standard, and control samples.

The orderly handling of a specimen in a clinical laboratory begins with (1) a properly identified sample and its request sheet and proceeds to (2) the log sheet where preliminary information is entered, then to (3) the work sheet where the final results are recorded along with details of the analysis, next returns to (4) the log sheet, and finally culminates in (5) the laboratory report submitted to the veterinarian for inclusion with case records.

If circumstances do not warrant maintaining a clinical laboratory in the confines of the veterinary practice, the majority of the samples for clinical chemistry evaluations should be forwarded to a commercial laboratory for processing. If a reference laboratory is used, the veterinarian will undoubtedly be provided with request forms. In addition, the veterinarian should maintain a log book that includes the date, patient identification (name and number), tests requested, and a column for results. This provides the practitioner with a readily available record of samples submitted and results obtained. Result sheets from the commerical laboratory should be filed with the case record.

PREPARATION OF SOLUTIONS

Carefully prepared solutions are required if accurate and reproducible results are to be expected. Since most veterinary hospitals are not equipped with precise analytic balances, it is more practical to purchase reagent solutions that have been prepared for use in a specific analysis. These commercially prepared reagents are manufactured in large quantities and their accuracy is determined by the manufacturer. Most reagents are available from a variety of commercial sources. However, one must take care to ensure that these solutions retain their activity and chemical composition, as solutions deteriorate with age and are no longer usable in chemical analyses. Commercially manufactured reagents should be stored according to the manufacturer's directions and should be discarded when outdated.

The development of precalibrated spectrophotometric systems for clinical chemistry assays has been accompanied by development of kits that include all chemical reagents needed for a specific determination as well as standardized capillary micropipettes. These kits are generally adequate, although problems have been encountered with some techniques that were developed for use in analysis of human blood and are not acceptable for chemical determinations using specimens from animals. Although more costly than reagents purchased in bulk, kits provide a readily available source of precalibrated and quantitated reagents for routine laboratory use. They are particularly useful in the smaller clinical laboratory where the demand for tests is limited. Care must be taken in purchasing to avoid overstocking supplies that might deteriorate before being used.

FILTRATION AND CENTRIFUGATION

Both filtration and centrifugation are utilized to separate solids from liquids, a procedure commonly employed in chemical analyses of blood. Usually, paper is used for filtration, but sometimes cloth, cotton, or glass wool may be preferable, particularly if rapid filtration is desired. The filter medium utilized should depend on the size and character of the solid particles being removed and on the chemical activity of the liquid in which these solid particles are suspended. Filter paper is available in many types and degrees of porosity and with low mineral or ash content.

Centrifugation is usually more satisfactory than filtration for separating solids from liquids. This is particularly true in the case of protein-free extracts. Use of centrifugation avoids contamination by paper and almost always yields a larger volume than does filtration. Unfortunately, centrifugation does not always produce a clear solution. However, centrifugation can be supplemented by subsequent filtration, which is more rapid after centrifugation because most solid material has already been removed.

A great variety of centrifuges are available commercially. The effectiveness of a centrifuge depends on the speed of rotation, the distance of the sample from the center of rotation, and the length of time the material is centrifuged. In purchasing a centrifuge, one must be aware of the factors influencing equipment efficiency. Basically, effectiveness is dependent upon the extent of centrifugal force developed. For example, at a speed of 2000 revolutions per minute, and a distance of 4 inches from the center of the axis, a tube with its contents develops a force 454 times that of gravity, whereas at double the distance (8 inches), the force will be doubled (908 times that of gravity). Centrifugal force increases in direct proportion to the distance from the center of rotation but increases at the square of the speed. Therefore, doubling the speed of a centrifuge is far more effective than doubling its size. This factor must be taken into consideration when equipment is purchased for the laboratory. Another factor that must be taken into account is whether the centrifuge allows the tubes to swing out horizontally as they spin or maintains them at a fixed angle. A centrifuge whose buckets swing out horizontally will leave a flat upper surface in the sedimented layer, whereas an angle-head centrifuge leaves the solid surface at an angle. However, an angle centrifuge has less air resistance and will develop more speed for the same motor power.

Since the force developed in a centrifuge is relatively great, all rotating parts must be carefully balanced to prevent vibration, which may damage the instrument. Excessive vibration may also be a hazard to laboratory personnel, as it may cause breakage. Cups or tubes should always be placed opposite one another in a centrifuge, and tubes should be paired for equal weight. Do not put a nearly empty tube opposite a nearly full one. If necessary, put in extra tubes filled with a liquid comparable in specific gravity to the material being centrifuged (water is usually acceptable). Adequate balance can usually be obtained by visually matching the quantity of fluid in tubes to be placed opposite one another. Weighing of tubes is usually unnecessary unless extremely high speeds are used.

The tube carrier should always be equipped with a rubber cushion of appropriate size. If glass tubes are centrifuged, they should be free of defects such as cracks, chips, or other obvious flaws. If centrifugation is lengthy, the tubes should be capped or stoppered to prevent evaporation.

Care should be taken in centrifugation to avoid resuspension of sedimented material. Centrifuges are usually permitted to come to rest without the use of a braking system that would slow the speed sufficiently to agitate the contents.

One should not allow curiosity to get the better of good sense by opening a centrifuge that is in operation and braking it with a hand. The sudden breakage of a tube in a closed centrifuge is not a catastrophe, but if a tube breaks when the centrifuge is open, a laboratory accident is inevitable.

MEASUREMENT OF VOLUME

Measurement of volume is the most frequent manipulation in clinical chemistry, and inaccuracy in such measurements is a major cause of error. Attempting to reduce expenses by purchasing cheap glassware for use in measuring quantities of specimens or reagents is counterproductive.

Volumetric glassware is available in several grades based on the accuracy of the calibration. The most precise equipment conforms to specifications of the National Bureau of Standards, but other glassware can be accurate although not certified by the National Bureau of Standards. Before glassware is purchased for use in chemical analysis, the manufacturer's specifications should be closely examined, and the best grade possible should be purchased.

Pipettes. Considerable confusion exists in the minds of some laboratory workers concerning measuring pipettes and their use. Pipettes may be graduated at one point or many, and they may be calibrated either to contain (TC) or to deliver (TD). In addition, they may be calibrated to deliver by drainage or by having the last drop blown out;

pipettes may also be calibrated to deliver to the tip or to another point above the tip.

Measuring pipettes that are graduated to the tip are usually calibrated for blowout, and manufacturers mark such pipettes with either two etched rings or a sanded band ring near the upper end of the pipette. Transfer or volumetric pipettes are calibrated to deliver only one volume and have a single calibration mark above a bulb in the pipette. This type of pipette is preferred in making measurements for chemical determinations, as volume can be determined more accurately with these than with pipettes having several calibrations. These volumetric pipettes are calibrated to deliver by drainage with the tip of the pipette touching the side of a receiving vessel. Utilization of this procedure will leave a small quantity of fluid in the pipette, but this quantity remains constant each time a pipette is used. These pipettes are calibrated to deliver a specific quantity provided they are completely clean. Retention of a small quantity of material, such as protein, on the inside bore of the pipette may interfere with proper and complete delivery.

Pipettes that are calibrated to contain are accurate only when the material is completely rinsed from the interior of the pipette. Most TC pipettes are of small volume, and rinsing will increase the accuracy of their delivery, especially of blood or other viscous liquids.

With the development of micro techniques for clinical chemistry, micropipettes that deliver very small quantities of fluid have become available. The majority of these are of the TC variety and must be washed out into the diluting fluid. Automatic pipetters with disposable tips are now available and provide excellent accuracy for many analytical procedures (Fig. 6–1).

Accuracy in clinical chemistry assays is dependent upon development of a good technique in handling pipettes. The following points should be remembered:

1. Hold the stem of the pipette between the thumb and second finger, leaving the index finger free.

2. Place the pipette tip deeply enough into the fluid to permit removal of the required volume without drawing air. With micropipettes it is advantageous to utilize a rubber tube equipped with a mouthpiece.

3. Using gentle suction, draw fluid past the calibration mark and close the mouthpiece with the index finger, or, if using a rubber tube with mouthpiece, open your lips.

4. Remove excess fluid from the outside of the pipette with a piece of clean tissue.

5. Remove excess fluid that is above the calibration mark by placing the pipette tip against the original container and gently but easily rolling the index finger over the mouthpiece until the meniscus reaches the calibration mark. Do not remove the finger, as complete removal makes volume control impossible.

6. Hold the pipette tip to the wall of the receiving vessel.

7. Remove the index finger and permit the pipette to drain. If using a volumetric pipette or any pipette calibrated to deliver, do not blow out the remaining drop in the tip unless the pipette has

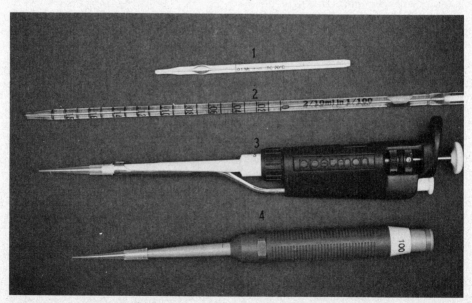

Figure 6–1. Pipettes used in clinical chemistry include (1) the micropipette, (2) serological pipette, (3) variable volume automatic micropipettor, and (4) standard volume automatic micropipettor.

an etched band on the mouthpiece. If a TC pipette is being used, it should be carefully rinsed into the diluent, the operator making sure that all of the sample is removed.

By following these precautions, the accuracy and reproducibility of clinical examinations can be improved. Similar techniques must be followed in measuring all reagents.

Veterinarians who utilize reagents containing materials that are either corrosive or poisonous should invest in a rubber bulb or other type of automatic pipetting instrument.

The use of automatic pipetters reduces measurement errors, but accuracy is still dependent on care in their use. Directions provided with these instruments should be carefully followed, as minor deviations in quantity will drastically alter results.

Volumetric Flasks. Volumetric flasks are precise measuring instruments and should be employed in preparing reagents to be used in chemical analyses. Since many commercially prepared reagents are available in tablet or premeasured powder form, accuracy can be achieved only if solvent volume is measured in a volumetric flask. To mix reagents in the volumetric flask, carefully add the powder or tablet to the flask, then, using a beaker, add the solvent, making sure that all reagent goes to the bottom of the flask. Do not fill the flask completely to the etched line at this time, but allow the material to dissolve and then bring it to its final volume. If water is permitted to fill the neck of the flask before the reagent is completely dissolved, it will be difficult to completely mix the reagent.

Care must be taken in reading the fluid meniscus. If the solution is clear and the line readily observed, the bottom of the meniscus should always be read. With highly colored solutions, it is necessary to read the top of the fluid column. In order to avoid parallax, all readings on pipettes and volumetric flasks should be made at eye level. Most glassware utilized for measuring is calibrated at a specific temperature (usually 20° C), and the liquid temperature should be at or near the calibration temperature. For most analyses, the allowable limits are ±10° C.

Burets. The buret is a graduated pipette equipped with a stopcock near its tip. The stopcock facilitates flow control. Burets are available in almost any size from microburets to those capable of holding large quantities of fluid. The same precautions utilized in measuring with pipettes or volumetric flasks also apply to the use of the buret.

Graduated Cylinders. Graduated cylinders should be utilized for measurement only when a high degree of accuracy is not essential. They are rarely utilized in making fluid measurements for preparing clinical chemical solutions or dissolving repackaged tablets or powders.

CLEANING AND HANDLING GLASSWARE

Glassware for use in clinical chemistry determinations must be free from all contaminating substances. The presence of even small quantities of residual specimen or chemical reagent can interfere with accuracy. Residues in pipettes and test tubes can be avoided if these instruments are placed in a container of tap water immediately after use so that serum, blood, and chemical solutions do not dry in them. Pipettes are usually washed by being rinsed several times in tap water and then in distilled water. If an automatic pipette washer is available, it should be adjusted to permit eight to 10 water replacements per hour. Pipettes should be washed for three or four hours.

It is easiest to wash test tubes by placing them in a solution of washing powder and boiling them for 25 minutes, then cooling them with tap water and thoroughly rinsing them. This rinse should be followed with two distilled water rinses, and the tubes should be drained and allowed to dry in a hot-air oven.

It is occasionally necessary to place glassware in a dichromate cleaning solution. This solution will remove stain or residual matter that has accumulated. Dichromate cleaning solution is made by slowly adding 250 ml of concentrated sulfuric acid to 500 ml of water. This mixture is cooled, and 100 gm of potassium dichromate is added and dissolved. When the dichromate is completely dissolved, increase the volume to 1 liter. Glassware should be soaked overnight in this solution and rinsed in several changes of tap water and two or three changes of distilled water.

Because of the problems of maintaining and cleaning special glassware for chemical determinations, many laboratories use disposable glass tubes and pipettes. This type of glassware is inexpensive and suitable for most chemical determinations.

COLORIMETRY

The most useful of the various quantitative analysis techniques in clinical chemistry is colorimetry. The value of colorimetry lies in its simplicity and sensitivity. If a given constituent of a body fluid such as serum can be converted into a colored solution by the addition of various chemical reagents, it is possible to estimate the quantity of that constituent by the intensity of color.

Comparison Colorimetry. The simplest form of colorimetry is comparison colorimetry. A series of standard solutions containing a known amount of a specific chemical is prepared in concentrations either comparable to or less than that of any sample to be analyzed. The specimen is treated to develop the color, which is then compared with that of the standards and, if necessary, diluted until the color is comparable. The chemical concentration of the specimen is estimated by relating the dilution factor to the amount of chemical in the standard that has a similar color intensity. Many of the screening tests utilized in veterinary medicine depend upon such a visual comparison. The disadvantage of this technique is the relative insensitiveness of the eye and its inability to discriminate between various shades and depths of color. In spite of this limitation, visual colorimetry has a place in veterinary medicine screening procedures.

The accuracy of color comparisons can be increased by use of a photoelectric colorimeter. Photoelectric colorimeters operate by measuring the amount of light that passes through a colored solution. In order to increase specificity, most colorimeters are equipped so that the wavelength of light passing through the colored solution can be varied.

The amount of light passing through a colored solution can be expressed in two ways. One is transmission, which represents that fraction of the light striking and coming through a colored solution. This fraction is multiplied by 100 to give the per cent transmission (% T). The second method of recording results is by absorbance, which records the amount of light *not* passing through a colored solution. This is a logarithmic value and is the same as optical density (OD). In general, the difference in the concentration of color of two solutions is the difference in absorbance.

Spectrophotometry. Spectrophotometry is the most widely used technique in the clinical chemistry laboratory and probably will remain so for some time to come. Excellent summaries of spectrophotometry and its principles are available in a variety of textbooks, so only a brief resume will be included here.

Basic requirements for any spectrophotometer include a power supply, a source of radiant energy, a monochromator, and a sample container (cuvette).

POWER SUPPLY. Since most sources of electricity have fluctuations of current and voltage, the electricity available at the wall plug is often not sufficiently stable for the peculiar demands of the spectrophotometer. Therefore, power sources capable of providing accurately regulated electrical energy are usually required. Power supplies specially designed for each type of spectrophotometer are available.

RADIANT ENERGY. A source of radiant energy that is able to provide a large number of wavelengths is a necessity. The tungsten lamp is a classic example of such an energy source. The average tungsten lamp will provide wavelengths from approximately 350 to 1000 mμ. Since this lamp serves as an important source of energy, deviations occurring as a consequence of aging should be obviated by frequent checking and replacement when needed.

MONOCHROMATOR. A monochromator is included in the instrument to remove unwanted radiant energies from the system. The simplest method for removal of these undesirable and unneeded wavelengths is the use of a filter. Filters used in spectrophotometers are normally made of glass in which a metal complex is suspended or dissolved. These are designed to limit passage of specific wavelengths. In this fashion, a filter permitting passage of only the desired wavelengths can be selected. Another type of filter is the interference filter, which is composed of a sandwich of half-

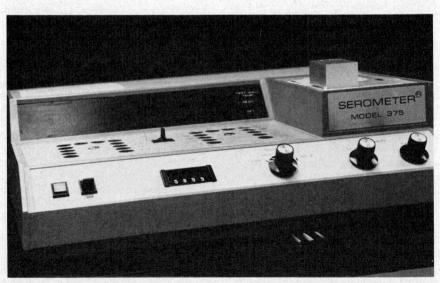

Figure 6–2. This spectrophotometer can be used for quantitating a great variety of substances in serum. Kits with pre-measured reagents are readily available.

silvered pieces of glass with a layer of controlled thickness dielectric material between the silvered layers. The thickness of the dielectric layer determines what wavelengths will pass through. Some instruments use diffraction gradings or prisms as monochromators. Wavelengths emitted by the source of radiant energy are separated by refraction or diffraction and presented as a spectrum from which desired wavelengths are selected.

CUVETTE. The sample container (cuvette) is an important part of any photometric system. The term *cuvette* is a fancy name for a test tube or other container in which a colored solution is placed in a colorimeter. In determinations of the absorbance or transmittance of light by a colored solution, the effect that the container might have must be considered. Anything placed in the light path, including scratches, dirt, fingerprints, or glass itself, will influence results. Cuvettes should be carefully cleaned and wiped routinely each time they are placed in the instrument. Flaws and variations in optical properties and thickness of the glass at various points on the cuvette mean that within the instrument, a single tube will not read the same in all possible positions. Consequently, the cuvette should be in the same position each time it is used. Most commercial cuvettes have an etched mark that can be used as a landmark and is always placed either directly away from or toward the operator of the instrument.

In practice, it is not necessary to have more than one cuvette. Usually, however, it is more convenient to have a series of matched cuvettes available. Optically matched cuvettes can be purchased, but their uniformity should not be assumed unless they are first checked. It is less expensive to select cuvettes from among ordinary test tubes. Test tubes must be chosen carefully, as they should fit the instrument easily and be small enough to fit into the holder without binding but large enough to fit the opening with little air space remaining.

When selecting tubes for an optical match, make sure that they are scratch-free and completely clean, both inside and out. In our laboratory, personnel are cautioned to wipe the test tube carefully with a piece of cheesecloth and check it for cleanliness immediately before inserting it in the instrument. It is particularly important to follow this procedure when attempting to match tubes for optical density. To match test tubes for use as cuvettes in an optical instrument of this type, fill the tubes with water and place them in the cuvette holder one at a time. Adjust the equipment to a wavelength of 540 mμ. The instrument should now be adjusted to an optical density of 0.1, or 80 per cent transmission. Care should be taken to put an identifying mark on the original test tube and to record its position in the machine. A series of similar test tubes is read in the same manner with the per cent transmission placed on each tube. When you have finished, decide whether you have enough tubes with the same per cent transmission to use as a matched set without correction or whether correction should be marked on each tube. To be used interchangeably, tubes should match within 0.004 OD (0.5% T). Rotation of the tubes within the cuvette holder may enable you to achieve a more nearly perfect match. Matched test tubes should be so marked and carefully handled to avoid any scratching or etching.

DETECTOR SYSTEM. A detector system must be included to detect transmitted radiant energy and convert it into electrical energy that can be measured. Such a conversion of one energy type to another is accomplished by means of a transducer. The most commonly used transducer in a spectrophotometer is the photocell. This may be either a photovoltaic or a photoemissive device.

READ-OUT DEVICES. Read-out devices are required to convert the energy reading into a numerical form. The most commonly used device is a meter calibrated so that current is recorded as per cent transmission or absorbance (optical density). Digital read-out mechanisms are available on some spectrophotometers. Electrical energy activates the digital read-out system, which records the result as a numeral and does not depend upon reading a needle that wavers over a scale. Spectrophotometers can be attached to recording devices that transfer electrical read-out energy into a special system that records results either on a print-out basis or as a tracing.

Flame Photometry. The flame photometer is similar to the spectrophotometer except that it is based upon the principle that solutions containing a metal ion will, when burned, release energy in the form of light. Light emitted in this fashion has a characteristic wavelength, and the amount of light emitted is proportional to the concentra-

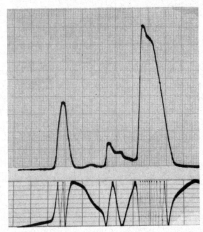

Figure 6–3. This is a densitometer scan of a cellulose acetate strip on which dog serum has been electrophoresed. The peak to the left is albumin and the high peak to the right represents globulins. This dog had an IgA myeloma.

tion of the metal ion. A flame photometer has the following basic components:

1. An atomizer by which a solution is sprayed into a flame.
2. A burner in which the flame is created. The burner is designed to accept a variety of gas mixtures that control the flame.
3. A monochromator, usually an interference filter, that removes unwanted radiation from elements other than the one being evaluated and from the flame itself.
4. A detector, which is usually a photocell.
5. A recording device.

The flame photometer is most frequently used for measuring sodium and potassium concentrations.

Atomic Absorption Spectrophotometry.
Atomic absorption spectrophotometry also utilizes a flame and is closely related to emission flame photometry. The basic technique is somewhat different, however, in that the light absorbed by ground state atoms is measured rather than the light emitted by atoms that have been excited in the flame. As the atoms of various elements absorb light at specific wavelengths, it is possible to measure the light absorbed by a particular element in much the same fashion as is the light absorbed by a colored solution. The light source utilized must be one that emits only the wavelengths absorbed by the element being measured. Thus, the tungsten lamp will not serve, as it emits a broad band of wavelengths. Specific wavelength emission is achieved with a hollow cathode discharge lamp that contains the element being assayed. Atomic absorption spectrophotometry permits accurate measurement of elements such as calcium, zinc, lead, copper, iron, and magnesium, some of which are present in small quantities in biological samples and for which few if any other satisfactory methods are available.

STANDARDIZATION

A common source of error in clinical chemistry is improper utilization of standards to check the accuracy of the equipment. Colorimeters should be utilized according to the manufacturer's directions, and standardization is a "must" for all chemical determinations. Unfortunately, some manufacturers of photoelectric colorimeters provide a precalibrated scale for various chemical determinations. Such precalibrations are accurate and reliable only if the technician follows exactly the same technique as and uses reagents equal to those of the manufacturer. Even then, results are accurate only if there has been no change in instrument response. Precalibrated values should not be used unless they are checked first. Standardization may be accomplished by preparing a solution containing a known quantity of the compound to be determined and running it through the analytic procedure. It is often difficult or impossible to obtain sufficient quantities of purified compounds for use as standards. This problem may be avoided by substituting an artificial standard in which a colored solution is prepared and its absorbance compared with that of a carefully prepared pure standard. From that time on, the artificial standard may be utilized in place of a natural one. Fortunately, most standards can be purchased from a reliable chemical supply dealer.

Another type of preparation that has become available is control serum. Basically, this is serum that has been predried and carefully analyzed. Each batch of control serum is accompanied by a chart of values for various chemicals. Such preparations are not usually utilized as standards but do enable the technician to determine whether correct results are being obtained. If analytical results on a control serum do not agree with the value furnished by the manufacturer, the procedure should be carefully analyzed to determine the possible source of error.

QUALITY CONTROL

Accuracy and trustworthiness of quantitative measurements in clinical chemistry are dependent upon the establishment of a good quality control program. Whether one's own laboratory or a commercial laboratory is used, one should be aware of the factors involved in a good quality control program. In choosing a commercial laboratory, the practitioner should always inquire concerning details of its quality control program. In addition, it is important to know what techniques are being utilized for specific chemical analyses, as some that are applicable to specimens obtained from humans may be inaccurate if conducted on specimens derived from animals.

Even the small laboratory that conducts only a few chemical analyses should have a system for checking the quality of the results obtained. Only by establishing a control system is it possible for the practitioner to rely on laboratory results.

The outline of a quality control program is presented by Bermes and Forman:[1] "The accuracy of an analytical result depends to a large extent on:

1. The ability to maintain proper analytical skill from start to finish.
2. The reduction of the number of manipulations to a minimum and the simplification of such manipulations, if this results in an increase in accuracy.
3. The ability to maintain the required quality of reagents.
4. The ability to maintain the desired performance of equipment.
5. The selection of the most accurate method

best suited for the needs of the particular clinical chemistry laboratory.

6. The routine use of primary standards, quality control, reference sera, and statistical methods to evaluate results obtained.

7. The availability of conscientious and well-trained technologists."

If these tenets are followed, any laboratory can provide excellent and reliable quantitative results.

The size and workload of a clinical chemistry laboratory will determine the extent of a quality control program. The following procedures provide the essentials for the most limited program.[2]

1. Standard deviations of routine procedures should be determined. If values obtained indicate poor precision, the methods of analysis should be re-evaluated. The average and standard deviation of a control serum should be calculated as follows for each method utilized.
   A. Analyze control serum (such as a pooled sample from several normal animals) daily for 15 to 25 days and record values obtained (column two in Table 6–1).
   B. Add values to determine total.
   C. Calculate average (av) of daily values.
   D. Record difference from average for each daily value (column three).
   E. Square the difference for each day and enter (column four).
   F. Add values of the squares of the differences from the average to obtain sum of the squared differences.

TABLE 6–1. Glucose Value of a Pooled Serum Sample Determined for 18 Days

Day	Value	Difference from Average	Square of Difference
1	98.2	.8	.64
2	99.7	.7	.49
3	97.3	1.7	2.89
4	100.4	1.4	1.96
5	97.0	2.0	4.00
6	99.8	.8	.64
7	97.6	1.4	1.96
8	99.9	.9	.81
9	98.7	.3	.09
10	100.1	1.1	1.21
11	99.3	.3	.09
12	98.9	.1	.01
13	98.8	.2	.04
14	99.6	.6	.36
15	100.4	1.4	1.96
16	99.7	.7	.49
17	97.2	1.8	3.24
18	100.4	1.4	1.96
	1783.0 (Average = 99.0)		22.84

G. Calculate standard deviation (SD) using the following formula:

$$SD = \sqrt{\frac{Sum\,of\,squared\,differences\,from\,average}{Number\,of\,measurements - 1}}$$

Calculations:

$$SD = \sqrt{\frac{22.84}{18 - 1}} = \sqrt{1.344}$$
$$= 1.16$$

If ± 3 SD from the average value is acceptable, the range is 99.0 ± 3.48 or 95.52 to 102.48 mg glucose/dl.

Modern hand calculators are frequently programmed to complete these calculations automatically.

2. Each batch or routine analysis should be accompanied by a pooled serum sample whose composition has been determined by careful replicate analyses. The standard sample should be treated in a manner identical to the way the unknown is treated. The value obtained should be plotted daily on a control chart that includes the accepted mean value and allowable limits of variation (usually ± 2 or 3 standard deviations). Practices having large volumes of clinical chemistry evaluations should provide the commercial laboratory with pooled serum samples from their own patients.

3. A commercial control serum whose values are unknown to the technologist should be analyzed at least once a week in the same manner as the routine test samples. This can be done easily, making small changes in the amount of water used to reconstitute serum or by mixing two different lots of serum in varying proportions.

Procedural problems in a clinical chemistry laboratory can be detected by observing changes occurring in values obtained for specific tests. The most common sign of development of a problem is a continual rise or fall in results obtained or the appearance of increasing variability. When such trends occur, laboratory personnel should be so advised in order that they can correct the problem before results become so variable as to be worthless to the clinician.

Dr. William E. Moore, Head of the Department of Laboratory Medicine at Kansas State University, developed the following guidelines for minimizing laboratory errors.[3]

1. Sampling.
   A. Anticoagulants
      (1) Use none or those that do not interfere with method

      (2) Use minimum quantity acceptable to avoid hemolysis, dilution and reaction inhibition

  B. Use care in obtaining sample
      (1) Avoid exciting animal
      (2) Use sharp needle
      (3) Use chemically clean, dry equipment
  C. Techniques of handling specimen
      (1) Avoid hemolysis—handle carefully
      (2) Separate cells from plasma or serum as soon as possible

2. Laboratory glassware and reagents.
  A. Use of disposable glassware will eliminate errors associated with contamination of tubes, pipettes, flasks, and so forth
  B. Prepackaged reagents or kits should be used whenever possible
  C. If reusable glassware is utilized, be sure it is completely free of contaminating substances (chemically clean)
  D. Never put contaminated pipettes into bulk reagent bottles
  E. Avoid opening or storing reagent bottles near volatile chemicals such as ammonia, bleach, and so forth

3. Equipment malfunction.
  A. Spectrophotometer
      (1) Check wavelength setting before use
      (2) Re-evaluate standards frequently, especially with precalibrated instruments. Aging particularly affects light source and phototube
      (3) Check zero and blank readings frequently
      (4) Check accuracy of wavelength setting by use of standards available from the manufacturer
  B. Water baths, incubators, and heating blocks
      (1) Check accuracy frequently using thermometer, as many reactions are temperature dependent
  C. Automatic samplers and dilutors
      (1) Check accuracy frequently—leaky dilutors cause serious problems
      (2) Keep clean

4. Human technical errors—impossible to completely avoid but can be minimized.
  A. Pipetting errors—consequence of sloppy technique
      (1) Wipe excess reagent or sample from outside of pipette before adjusting final volume—extremely important with micro-methods
      (2) Select proper-sized pipette for volume required. Should use smallest volume pipette consistent with technique
      (3) Fill pipettes properly and consistently

      (4) Use pipettes properly:
        a. TC (to contain) pipettes—deliver sample into reagent mixture (diluent) and then rinse
        b. TD (to deliver) pipettes—deliver sample into reaction tube and touch side of tube with tip of pipette to remove last drop—DO NOT BLOW OUT
        c. TD pipettes with etched ring near mouthpiece end—use as just described but blow out last drop (only last drop) with delivery tip on side of tube

  B. Errors of methodology
      (1) Timing errors—significant, as many reactions, particularly of enzymes, are time-temperature dependent
      (2) Reagent errors — add in proper sequence
      (3) Dilution errors (usually of sample)—check calculations for making dilution
      (4) Recording errors — either misreading of instrument or identifying reading with wrong specimen
      (5) Identification errors — confusion of specimen identification is unforgivable but does occur unless care is taken
      (6) Calculation errors—avoid by double checking results before reporting
      (7) *When all else fails, read directions*

5. Clinical chemistry quality control.
  A. Check standards frequently
  B. Use quality control serum—pooled sample or commercially prepared standard
      (1) Check value exactly as though it were a patient's sample and compare results, taking into consideration allowable limits
      (2) Detectable errors include:
        a. Inconsistent or poor technique
        b. Equipment malfunction
        c. Reagent contamination or degeneration
        d. Dishonesty—only if *you* alone know expected values
      (3) Undetectable errors include random errors in sample handling or pipetting, calculation and recording errors
  C. Interpretation of quality control data
      (1) Trend analysis—a trend is formed by the values of control that continue either to increase or to decrease over a period of six consecutive days. This may be result of deterioration of a reagent(s), change in standard, incomplete protein precipitation, and so forth

(2) A shift (increase or decrease) occurs if control values are distributed on one side of a mean value line but maintain a constant level

   a. Upward—may be due to: standard deterioration or shift in reagent sensitivity or preparation and use of a new standard at lower concentration; use of a faulty timer, resulting in prolonged color development, particularly if a precalibrated scale panel is used; use of a faulty indicator that has lost sensitivity thereby prolonging end-point reading in titration reactions

   b. Downward—generally opposite of causes for upward

(3) If the value obtained for the standard deviates significantly, *do not* make assumptions about what "might have happened," but recheck all facets of analysis, determine the cause of error, and repeat all determinations.

CLINICAL ENZYMOLOGY

Enzymology has been the most rapidly developing field in clinical chemistry. Demonstration that specific serum enzyme activity increases with disease stimulated investigators to evaluate a number of enzyme systems in search of those that are organ or tissue specific. The veterinarian soon became aware of these studies and realized that clinical enzymology could play an important role in diagnosis and prognosis of animal disease.

Unfortunately, an aura of mystery surrounded enzymology, and techniques for enzyme determination were thought to be difficult, time consuming, and impossible to run in any but the most sophisticated laboratory. Nothing could be further from the truth, as most enzyme determinations of value in veterinary medicine can be conducted in any laboratory equipped with a spectrophotometer and having an adequate quality control program.

General Properties of Enzymes

Enzymes are protein catalysts synthesized by all living organisms. As catalysts their only biologic activity is to alter the rate at which an equilibrium is established between reactants and their products. In the living animal they are constantly and rapidly degraded, and the supply is replenished by new synthesis. The rate of an enzyme reaction is subject to a number of factors including hydrogen ion concentration (pH), substrate concentration, temperature, enzyme concentration, presence of activators and inhibitors, and the nature and concentration of the products of the reaction. All of these factors are taken into consideration in methodology developed for enzyme analysis.

Enzyme nomenclature is now based on the concept of providing two names for each enzyme. The systematic name describes the nature of the reaction catalyzed and has a numerical code designation associated with it. The second name, and the one most likely to be encountered by a clinician, is the working or practical name, which is often either identical with the systematic name or slightly modified. It has become a common practice to use capital letters to designate certain enzymes, such as ALT (formerly GPT) for alanine-aminotransferase, LDH for lactate dehydrogenase, AST (formerly GOT) for aspartate aminotransferase, and so on. As this is a well established method of designating enzymes, it will be utilized hereafter in this text, but only after the meaning of the abbreviation has been indicated.

As clinical identification and quantitation of enzymes is difficult, the method for designating enzyme levels is based on activity units present in a given mass or volume of specimen. Several different units of enzyme activity for similar or identical enzymes have been introduced as each investigator defined a unit according to his own wishes. A classic example is encountered in the units used to measure phosphatase activity. At least four different unit designations have been made depending upon pH of the analysis, substrate used, and final product being measured. The same is true for unit activity designations of other enzymes.

In order to alleviate confusion, the Commission on Enzymes proposed that a unit of enzyme activity should be defined as that quantity of enzyme that will catalyze the reaction of one micromole of substrate per minute and that this be called the international unit (IU). Therefore, the activity of an enzyme is expressed as micromoles of substrate transformed per minute by a given quantity of serum or other fluid under specified conditions of time, temperature, pH, substrate concentration, presence of activators, and ionic concentration. This designation for enzyme activity has created confusion, as some laboratories have accepted the international unit while others continue to report units of activity using empirical unit values. In interpreting enzyme analyses, the clinician must be aware of the types of units being reported and relate this to known normal values for the laboratory.

Blood Serum Enzymes. Plasma (serum) enzymes can be placed into two distinct classes. The first consists of the plasma-specific enzymes, which are those that have a definite and specific function in plasma. Their normal site of action is in the plasma, and they are present in higher levels in plasma than in most tissue cells. Analysis for these enzymes is seldom done in veterinary medicine.

The second class consists of the nonplasma-specific enzymes, which have no known physiologic function in plasma and are present in concentrations much lower than their concentration in certain tissues. This group is divided into two subclasses: (1) enzymes associated with cellular metabolism and (2) enzymes of secretion. Enzymes of cellular metabolism are located within tissue cells and are present there in high concentrations. As long as the cell remains healthy and the membrane is intact, these enzymes are contained within cell walls. The level of these enzymes in extracellular fluid and plasma is low.

Included among the enzymes of secretion are amylase, phosphatases, and lipase. Secretory enzymes are rapidly disposed of through excretory channels such as the intestinal tract, urine, and bile and by inactivation and degradation. Their normal plasma levels are relatively low and are constant.

Elevations in serum enzyme activity occur by one or more of the following mechanisms: (1) increase in cell membrane permeability, (2) cell death, (3) increased enzyme production, (4) obstruction of normal excretory route, and (5) impaired circulation.

Cell membrane permeability may be increased by the effect of infectious agents, which can cause functional damage to the cell membrane, permitting intracellular enzymes to escape into the extracellular compartment and then into blood. A disturbance of cell respiration (anoxia) may result in membrane dysfunction and permit the escape of enzymes. It has also been suggested that alterations in intracellular fluids may be accompanied by damage and release of enzymes. This may account for increased serum enzyme activity in animals in which there is no demonstrable cell or membrane destruction. Enzymes of low molecular weight are more likely to diffuse through a damaged cell membrane.

Cell death and rupture of the membrane result in a marked increase in serum enzyme activity that is greater than the increase seen with altered membrane permeability. This is particularly true of those enzymes associated with subcellular particulate organelles.

Increased enzyme production does not occur frequently but can be seen when there is accelerated cellular growth, particularly with hyperplasia, some types of neoplasia, increased metabolic rates, and accelerated growth in young animals, and during regeneration of diseased tissue.

Obstruction of the normal removal of enzymes will increase serum enzyme activity. Enzymes are eliminated from extracellular and vascular compartments by excretion through the urine or biliary systems or by inactivation and degradation within the body. Some enzymes may be reabsorbed into cells. If damage occurs to the normal routes of degradation or excretion, serum enzyme activity will increase. Examples include the increased levels of liver-origin alkaline phosphatase (AP) in biliary obstruction and increased serum amylase activity associated with renal failure.

Circulatory impairment may delay removal of serum enzymes and increase activity. This is a consequence of decreased serum enzyme removal or increased leakage due to cell anoxia.

The usefulness of serum enzyme activity as an aid to diagnosis is dependent upon the organ specificity of a particular enzyme. A diagnostic utopia could be reached if each organ of the body had but one enzyme not found in other organs. Unfortunately, this situation does not exist except in a few organs, and the search for organ-specific enzymes continues.

As only a few enzymes are organ specific, a comparison of levels of several different enzymes may be of value, since enzymes are present in different tissues in different ratios. Another characteristic of enzymes that may prove to be of value in improving organ specificity is the existence of enzymes in multiple forms called isoenzymes. The term *isoenzyme* is used to describe enzymatically active proteins catalyzing the same reaction and occurring in the same animal species but differing in certain physiochemical properties. Enzyme systems with isoenzymes are numerous and include lactate dehydrogenase, malate dehydrogenase, isocitric dehydrogenase, aspartate aminotransferase (AST), creatine kinase, acetylcholinesterase, alkaline phosphatase, acid phosphatase, and many others. The possibility exists that all enzymes occur in multiple isoenzyme form.

Isoenzyme characteristics that may be used for identification include electrophoretic mobility, heat stability, resistance to various chemical inhibitors, and affinity for substrates.

Enzymes of Clinical Significance. Evaluation of certain serum enzymes has assumed importance in veterinary medicine. One or more of the following conditions should be met before a particular enzyme determination becomes established in a medical practice:[4] (1) The assay method should be technically simple, reproducible, adequately precise, and not too time consuming. (2) Data obtained should be of diagnostic significance. The normal range should be well defined and reasonably narrow, with a minimal overlap between normal and abnormal values and with abnormal values consistently found in specific pathology. (3) The enzyme must be present in blood, urine, or some other readily available tissue fluid. (4) The assay procedure should not require complex instrumentation, although if the test is sufficiently useful, the purchase of required instruments might be justified.

Enzyme assays of value in veterinary medicine

are discussed in more detail in subsequent chapters.

BIOCHEMICAL PROFILING

Introduction of multiple channel autoanalyzers (Fig. 6–4) capable of performing a variety of chemical determinations on a small quantity of serum has opened an entirely new concept in veterinary clinical pathology. The use of these instruments in commercial laboratories patronized by veterinarians has provided information not previously available. It was not until the last few years that sufficient data accumulated to permit accurate interpretation of results.

Initially these units utilized analytic techniques and had capabilities compatible with determining chemical values in human blood. It was not until the veterinarian began to utilize the services of commercial laboratories that the biochemical differences between human and animal blood were appreciated. When it became obvious that biochemical profiling was useful to the veterinarian, test techniques were altered and equipment calibrated to accommodate normal values of domestic animals.

The biochemical profile provides a number of advantages to the veterinarian. Among these are: (1) A profile, because of its multiplicity of tests, will often reveal an abnormality that is unsuspected on the basis of clinical signs. (2) The use of a profile may eliminate the need for a specific determination to assess the physiologic status of a given organ system, as most profiles are designed to evaluate the physiologic status of all major organs. (3) Standardization of techniques and routine utilization of controls result in highly reproducible and accurate assessments of the various chemical components of serum. (4) The consistent use of profiling provides the veterinarian with an accurate data base that can be useful not only for detecting diseases in individual animals, but also as a method for identifying disorders in a group of animals. (5) Because of its simplicity, the biochemical profile is a readily accessible tool for the veterinarian in following the course of a disease. (6) A biochemical profile will sometimes reveal the presence of multiple system abnormalities that might have gone unrecognized had a clinician requested only those tests related to the specific organ malfunction suspected on the basis of clinical signs. (7) The total cost of a commercial biochemical profile is frequently less than the total cost of a single determination to assess the function of an organ.

In addition to these advantages of biochemical profiling there are also certain inherent disadvantages. Disadvantages include: (1) Unless the equipment is especially adapted for veterinary use, some of the analyses routinely utilized in human medicine have little clinical significance in veterinary medicine. (2) Since many of the instruments performing routine biochemical profiling are located in laboratories that devote most of their time and effort to evaluation of human serum, it may be difficult for the veterinarian to convince the laboratory to alter the equipment to accommodate the different values of animal serums. (3) There is sometimes a long delay between collection of the blood sample and its processing, which may influence laboratory values. (4) Because of the variability in techniques, the wide

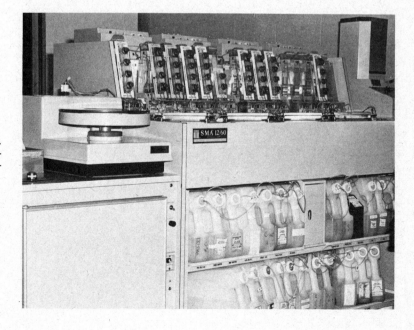

Figure 6–4. An autoanalyzer. Such multiple-channel automated analytical units are utilized in biochemical profiling.

range of animal species and age, and the variability in the capabilities of profiling units of different laboratories, normal values must be established for each laboratory serving the profession.

REFERENCES

1. Bermes, E. W., and Forman, D. T.: Basic laboratory principles and procedures. In: *Fundamentals of Clinical Chemistry*, edited by Tietz, N. W., W. B. Saunders Company, Philadelphia, 1976.

2. Lynch, M. J., Raphael, S. S., Mellor, L. D., Spare, P. D., and Inwood, M. J. H. *Medical Laboratory Technology and Clinical Pathology*, 2nd Ed., W. B. Saunders Company, Philadelphia, 1969.

3. Moore, W. E.: Interpretation and limitations of screening and organ profile testing in veterinary medicine. Proc. 39th Annual Meeting Am. Anim. Hosp. Assoc., p. 478, A.A.H.A., South Bend, IN, 1972.

4. Kachmar, S. F.: Enzymes. In: *Fundamentals of Clinical Chemistry*, edited by Tietz, N. W., W. B. Saunders Company, Philadelphia, 1976.

LIVER FUNCTION

The functional status of several organs—notably the liver, kidneys, and pancreas—can be evaluated by laboratory tests. Since the clinical manifestations of diseases of these organs are often not characteristic, it behooves the veterinarian to apply certain laboratory tests to detect the presence of disease. In other instances, clinical signs produced as a result of a diseased organ are characteristic, and laboratory techniques may then become a way of estimating the degree of organ damage and the response of the disease to therapy. The discussion of specific organ function tests in this and succeeding chapters is limited to those determinations that have been found to be the most practical in veterinary medicine and to those that may be of value in the future.

The liver is an organ of many diverse metabolic activities, and any assessment of its functional status is dependent upon its ability to perform a specific metabolic function. A number of tests have been devised for the detection of alterations in liver function. Of the more than 100 tests that have been developed, only a few have been found to be practicable in veterinary medicine.

No matter which test or technique is utilized, there are inherent difficulties in attempts to determine by laboratory methods whether a pathologic process has affected normal liver activity. Tests utilized for measuring the functional capacity of the liver are ultimately dependent on the combination of many integrated enzymatic activities that take place within hepatic cells. These enzymatic reactions are influenced by the intracellular supply of substrates, oxygen, and energy; the composition of the intracellular constituents; the activities of other organs; and the presence or absence of inhibitors or accelerators. Many factors may be altered qualitatively or quantitatively without histologic change in the organ. Consequently, direct correlation between the results of any given liver function test and the demonstration of morphologic alterations may be difficult. Estimation of the presence or absence of hepatic malfunction is further complicated by the tremendous functional reserve of the liver and its powers of regeneration. In animal experiments, it has been demonstrated that as much as 85 to 90 per cent of the liver can be removed before impaired function is detected by laboratory tests. Additional complications are encountered because the various functions of the liver may be altered unequally by hepatic disease.

Factors such as those just mentioned make it difficult to quantitate the amount of hepatic tissue involved in a disease or to differentiate diffuse damage from a localized process. As an example, diffuse but minimal involvement may result in a more marked depression of hepatic function as measured by laboratory determinations than will focal necrosis.

In spite of the complexities of liver physiology and the limitations of liver function tests, utilization of selected procedures may yield information that is of value clinically when a pathologic condition affecting the liver or biliary tract is present or suspected. Hepatic function tests may be used to: (1) differentiate types of jaundice, (2) establish the presence or absence of disease, and (3) attempt to determine, by serial performance of function tests, whether a disease process is remaining static, progressing or regressing. It must be emphasized that a pathologic process can exist and yet not be revealed by any hepatic function tests.

INDICATIONS FOR LIVER FUNCTION TESTS

A specific liver function test should be conducted whenever there is a suspicion that malfunction of the liver may be associated with the disease in question. Specifically, such tests should be conducted under the following circumstances: (1) As a method to assist in the differential diagnosis of icterus resulting either from a hemolytic crisis or from an extrahepatic or intrahepatic obstruction of the bile duct system. (2) In primary liver diseases that are present either with or without icterus, including conditions such as infectious hepatitis, suppurative hepatitis, hepatic fibrosis, acute toxic necrosis, leptospirosis, and neoplasia of the liver. (3) In secondary liver disorders such as the infiltrative and degenerative lipidoses that may accompany diabetes mellitus, pancreatic fibrosis and atrophy, starvation, and hypothyroidism; in association with chronic passive congestion, as may be seen in cardiac decompensation; as a manifestation of secondary amyloidosis; and in association with metastatic malignant lesions. (4) In the prognosis of hepatic disease, the evaluation of therapy, and the estimation of the degree of residual damage following recovery.

LIMITATIONS OF LIVER FUNCTION TESTS

Specific criticisms that have been leveled against liver function tests include: (1) extensive damage is required before tests show impaired function because of the great reserve power of the liver; (2) the tests are lacking sensitivity or are too sensitive; (3) there are so many functions of the liver that testing one does not indicate the functional status of the entire organ; and (4) specific hepatic functions are greatly affected by a wide variety of pathologic conditions of extrahepatic origin.

Although many of these criticisms of liver function tests are no doubt applicable, there is, nevertheless, a place in veterinary medicine for the use of these procedures in the determination of hepatic function. Although a great reserve power does exist, since the liver is able to function after removal of a large portion of the organ, pathologic conditions affecting all hepatic cells may produce effects rapidly. Because of the rapid regenerative ability of the liver, interpretations of function tests must be viewed in terms of short-term intervals. Since there are many hepatic functions

that can be measured, the clinician may select specific functions that are disturbed early. Based on the severity of their change from normal, the veterinarian may then be able to obtain quantitative indices of liver cell damage.

Criticism concerning the sensitivity of tests usually arises when results appear normal even though liver damage is great. As each test is different, its procedure, the factors it depends upon, and possible laboratory inaccuracies must be understood. Criticism concerning the hypersensitivity of tests often is the consequence of an attempt either to correlate abnormal hepatic function test results to subsequent autopsy findings of a regenerated liver or to substantiate a clinical diagnosis.

It must be recognized that the liver can be affected secondarily to a variety of primary conditions. This observation is of considerable interest in itself, even if it does, at times, confuse the diagnostician. However, unless an animal shows unequivocal signs of liver pathosis, the diagnosis of a latent primary pathologic disorder is still largely dependent upon a liver function test or biopsy. Additional criticisms as to the sensitivity of the test might be refuted by the fact that it is known that a cell's functions may be altered and result in an abnormal value for a specific liver function test even though histologic changes may not be obvious. In view of these facts, it remains for the clinician and clinical pathologist to correlate clinical findings with laboratory results in an overall view of the disease as it exists at a given time in a specific animal. Correlation of necropsy findings made on an animal 10 days or two weeks following a liver function test may prove disappointing. It must be emphasized that tests of liver function indicate the functional status of that organ at the time the test is made and may not be a reflection of what did or will happen prior or subsequent to the determination.

CLASSIFICATION OF LIVER FUNCTION TESTS

All liver function tests may be classified according to the type of hepatic function examined. Liver function tests may be categorized as follows:

1. Tests dependent primarily on hepatic secretion and excretion.
   A. Bile pigments
   B. Clearance of foreign substances
2. Tests dependent upon specific biochemical functions.
   A. Protein metabolism tests
   B. Carbohydrate metabolism tests
   C. Lipid metabolism tests
3. Tests dependent upon the measurement of serum enzyme activity.

A. Transaminases
B. Alkaline phosphatase
C. Other enzymes

In addition, although not in essence a liver function test, liver biopsy will be considered.

TESTS BASED ON HEPATIC SECRETIONS AND EXCRETIONS

Bile Pigments

Serum Bilirubin

The chief bile pigment found in the serum of domestic animals is bilirubin. Bilirubin is derived from hemoglobin; a schematic outline of the degradation of hemoglobin is presented in Figure 7–1. As will be noted in this figure, bilirubin may exist in two forms—as a protein-bound substance in plasma and as a conjugate known as bilirubin glucuronide. Normal values for the two types of serum bilirubin in domestic animals are presented in Table 7–1.

The determination of total bilirubin and conjugated bilirubin in serum is based on the van den Bergh reaction. This test is based on the ability of bilirubin to couple with diazobenzosulfochloride (diazo reagent) to form a characteristic red-violet pigment. Since unconjugated bilirubin is insoluble in water and the diazo reagent is in an aqueous solution, the detection of unconjugated bilirubin requires the use of a substance in which both bi-

lirubin and the diazo reagent are mutually soluble, e.g., alcohol. The reaction requiring the addition of alcohol to the serum reagent mixture is termed the "indirect" reaction and is a specific test for unconjugated bilirubin. The addition of alcohol is not required for the coupling of the conjugated bilirubin to the diazo reagent since they are both soluble in water. This constitutes the "direct" reaction.

The accepted method for the van den Bergh test requires the addition of alcohol to a mixture of diazo reagent and serum in order to measure total serum bilirubin. One minute following this, the pigment of direct-reacting bilirubin is measured. The difference between the values for total and direct-reacting pigments is the indirect-reacting bilirubin value.

INDICATIONS FOR SERUM BILIRUBIN DETERMINATION. Serum bilirubin determinations are of value in classifying icterus in a diseased animal and may also be used, if performed in a serial manner, to measure the response of the liver to therapy and thus assist in making an accurate prognosis. Comparison of results of the direct and indirect van den Bergh tests is often significant in assisting the clinician to classify icterus.

TECHNIQUES FOR SERUM BILIRUBIN DETERMINATION. As indicated previously, the van den Bergh reaction depends upon the use of a diazo reagent either alone or mixed with alcohol. The details for determining the van den Bergh reaction are given in the Appendix, pp. 439–440. The development of tablets containing chemicals required

TABLE 7–1. Normal Values of Serum Bilirubin in Domestic Animals

Species	Total Bilirubin Mg/dl		Direct-Reacting Bilirubin Mg/dl	
	MEAN	RANGE	MEAN	RANGE
Cow	0.31	0–14		
	0.21	0.01–0.47	0.18	0.04–0.44
	0.19	0.0–0.41		
Calf	0.70		0.40	
		0.5–1.9		
Sheep	0.19	0.0–0.39	0.12	0.0–0.27
	0.10	0.0–0.18		
Goat		0.0–1.0		
Pig	0.09	0.0–0.18		
	0.20		0.10	
	0.34	0.2–0.70		
Horse	1.25	0.81–2.07	0.37	0.18–0.72
	0.99	0.50–1.5	0.15	0.02–0.40
	2.70	0.20–6.20	0.10	0.0–0.40
	1.68	0.68–3.28	0.49	0.19–0.85
Dog	0.10		0.0	
	0.10	0.0–0.30	0.07	0.0–0.14
	0.25	0.07–0.61	0.14	
Cat		0.15–0.20		

for preparation of the diazo reagent has simplified the procedure.

INTERPRETATION OF THE VAN DEN BERGH REACTION. DOG. Interpretation of the results of a van den Bergh reaction conducted on canine serum resembles the interpretation of results with human serum more nearly than the analysis of findings with serum of other animals. The percentage of conjugated or unconjugated bilirubin is more important in interpretation of results than is the total concentration of each form. High levels, less than 20 per cent conjugated, of unconjugated (free) bilirubin are indicative of hemolytic disease of the dog, whereas if more than 40 per cent of the total bilirubin is of the conjugated type, hepatocellular disease is probably present. Conjugated bilirubin levels that are 25 to 35 per cent of the total may occur when there is hemolysis plus hepatocellular disease. Obstruction of the bile duct system (cholestasis) results in a greater increase of conjugated bilirubin in the serum (55 to 90 per cent), and this, in turn, is associated with the presence of a small quantity of free bilirubin.

Interpretation of total serum bilirubin must be tempered by the fact that the dog has a low renal threshold for bilirubin conjugates, and, consequently, slight elevations in concentration are indicative of cellular damage. Since the renal threshold is low, urine bilirubin determinations may be of value and will be discussed later. An additional factor that must be considered in interpretation of bilirubin levels is the functional status of the kidney. In the presence of renal parenchymal disease the bilirubin level may be affected. Bilirubin values in most hepatocellular diseases are less than 4 mg/dl of serum, although levels as high as 19 mg/dl have been reported to occur in prolonged extrahepatic obstruction or intrahepatic cholestasis. Estimations of total and direct bilirubin should always be accompanied by other tests for liver function.

HORSE. Interpretation of the values for free and conjugated serum bilirubin in the horse is quite different. The greatest portion of serum bilirubin found in horses with either hemolytic or hepatic icterus is unconjugated. Unconjugated bilirubin levels of up to 25 mg/dl of serum may occur in liver disease in the equine with less than 2 mg/dl of direct-reacting bilirubin.

Increases in unconjugated bilirubin are observed in a variety of conditions in the horse that are unrelated to primary liver disease. Elevation of the unconjugated serum bilirubin level has been reported in cardiac insufficiency, constipation, gangrenous pneumonia, hemolytic diseases, and primary hepatic disorders. In the constipation-and-colic syndrome of horses, free serum bilirubin is markedly elevated. An elevation in unconjugated serum bilirubin as high as 80 mg/dl was observed in a case of equine hemolytic anemia. Serum bilirubin levels between 25 and 75 mg/dl are associated with equine infectious anemia.

Fasting may also increase bilirubin levels. Plasma bilirubin levels increased within 12 hours of the last feeding and in two to four days increased to levels as high as eight times those of prestarvation values. The increase was principally in unconjugated bilirubin; conjugated bilirubin increased only slightly during the period of starvation. The bilirubin increase is due to decreased removal of bilirubin by hepatocellular transport.[1]

Clinical experience would suggest that if more than 25 per cent of the total serum bilirubin is of the conjugated (direct-reacting) type, one should suspect hepatocellular damage, and if conjugated bilirubin is greater than 30 per cent of total serum bilirubin, cholestasis should be suspected. As with the dog, the percentage distribution between conjugated and unconjugated bilirubin is more significant than total bilirubin concentration.

Cow. In severe hepatic disease in the cow, serum bilirubin levels are only slightly increased. This test may occasionally be of assistance in helping one to arrive at a diagnosis and prognosis of liver disease, but it cannot be considered a sensitive indicator of hepatic dysfunction in the bovine. Most hyperbilirubinemias in cattle result from excessive destruction of erythrocytes (hemolysis). There is an increase in conjugated bilirubin in cattle with biliary obstruction.

OTHER ANIMALS. Interpretation of the quantitative van den Bergh test in sheep, goats, and swine is similar to that in cattle. Any significant elevation in total bilirubin is usually found in association with a hemolytic crisis. The presence of increased concentrations of serum bilirubin conjugates indicates either severe hepatic involvement or extrahepatic obstruction.

Bile Pigments in Urine

URINARY UROBILINOGEN. This pigment in urine represents a group of substances rather than a single chemical entity. The term urobilinogen refers to all substances reacting positively with Ehrlich's reagent. These pigments are produced by bacterial reduction of bilirubin conjugates in the intestine where they are partly absorbed into the total circulation and partly recycled. The remaining portion of this pigment is present in the feces as stercobilin.

A small portion of the urobilinogen reabsorbed from the intestine passes unchanged through the liver and enters the general circulation where it is excreted via urine. The presence of urobilinogen in urine signifies that the bile duct is open and also indicates that there is enterohepatic circulation of bile pigment. The absence of this pigment from urine at a single sampling does not necessarily reflect complete closure of the bile duct.

Urobilinogen may be absent from urine of normal dogs and dogs poisoned with carbon tetrachloride. The absence of urobilinogen should be considered significant only if continued for several days. Decreased bacterial action on bilirubin in the intestine as a consequence of antibiotic therapy may also reduce levels of urinary urobilinogen. Diuresis associated with chronic renal disease may dilute the urobilinogen below the sensitivity of the test commonly used in urinalysis.

In animals with liver cell damage, a defect of re-excretion of urobilinogen into the bile may result in the escape of a higher percentage of these pigments into the circulation and consequently into the urine. Urine urobilinogen may be increased in association with hemolytic or hepatic diseases.

Most studies utilizing 24-hour urine specimens indicated that an absolute increase in urinary urobilinogen occurs in domestic animals with hepatopathy. The difficulty of obtaining 24-hour urine specimens in veterinary medicine and the fact that urobilinogen is rapidly oxidized to urobilin if samples are exposed to light limits the value of a 24-hour sample. This is particularly true since urobilin does not react in the Ehrlich test.

The most common method for determination of urinary urobilinogen in 24-hour samples is Watson's quantitative method, which depends upon the reduction of all urobilin to urobilinogen utilizing ferrous hydroxide. Fresh urine may be tested for urobilinogen using Ehrlich's aldehyde reagent. The technique for this determination is detailed in the Appendix, p. 440.

BILIRUBIN CONJUGATES. Only conjugated bilirubin complexes are detected in the urine, as unconjugated bilirubin does not normally pass the glomerular filter. Bilirubin conjugates are not found normally in urine of the cat, pig, sheep, and horse. The urine of the dog and occasionally of the cat may contain small amounts of conjugated bilirubin. Twenty to 60 per cent of normal dogs may excrete conjugated bilirubin in their urine. This phenomenon is probably due to the low renal threshold for conjugated bilirubin in the dog. Bilirubinuria is uncommon in cats, but when present is usually associated with liver disease.

The low renal threshold for conjugated bilirubin in the dog permits the use of a urine bilirubin test as a sensitive method for the early detection of hepatocellular changes and as an indicator of bile duct obstruction. Because of the dog's extremely low renal threshold for bilirubin, one must exercise a certain degree of caution in interpreting the presence of bilirubin in canine urine, as it may be present in small quantities in any febrile state. The presence of a 1 + reaction in a test utilizing a commercial diazo tablet is common in many febrile diseases. In cases of hepatocellular damage or obstruction in the dog, a 2 to 3 + reaction is considered to be of diagnostic significance when the specific gravity of the urine is between 1.020 and 1.035. The concentration of this bile pigment in the urine is directly proportional to the degree of biliary obstruction whether intrahepatic or extrahepatic.

Interpretation of bilirubinuria in cattle requires careful evaluation, as it has been reported that as many as 25 per cent of normal cattle have traces of bilirubin in the urine. The presence of bilirubin in the urine must be closely correlated with a careful clinical examination and other liver function tests.

Although the renal threshold for bilirubin in the horse has not been experimentally established, it appears that this species may have a low threshold for bilirubin conjugates. However, cases of equine hemolytic anemia with unconjugated serum bilirubin levels as high as 180 mg/dl have been observed without the presence of bilirubin in the urine. Chronic hemolytic diseases accompanied by hepatic hemosiderosis or hepatic necrosis result in bilirubinuria.

Detection of urine bilirubin conjugates is relatively simple. The most easily conducted screening examination is the foam test. Freshly voided urine is placed in a bottle, which is then vigorously shaken. In normal urine, a white foam appears, whereas in urine containing bilirubin conjugates, the foam will be yellowish green or brown. If there is a marked increase in urinary urobilinogen, a false positive foam test may appear. A rapid and sensitive test is based on the use of a stable diazonium compound. The reaction of bilirubin in the urine with the diazo compound (Ictotest, Ames Co., Elkhart, Indiana) produces a blue or purple color. It is advantageous, particularly in the dog, to dilute urine 1:5 or 1:10 before completion of the test. The dip strip technique is less sensitive than the Ictotest and does not require dilution of the urine. Details for conducting this test are in the Appendix, p. 440.

Fecal Bile Pigments

Fecal bilirubin appears in conditions that prevent the reduction of bilirubin to urobilinogen. This occurs (1) in diarrhea, (2) as a result of the suppression of bacterial action, or (3) in the newborn receiving milk. Under these circumstances, little bilirubin is reabsorbed from the intestinal mass. Clinically, either Harrison's or Gmelin's test may be used as a qualitative measure of the presence of bilirubin. The clinical value of the fecal bilirubin test is limited, and this assay is not routinely performed in veterinary medicine.

Urobilinoid pigments similar to those observed in the urine are normally present in feces. The predominant pigment is stercobilin. These pigments are increased in a hemolytic process and markedly decreased in bile obstruction. Visual inspection of the color of a stool from an icteric patient is important, as urobilinoid pigments give feces their characteristic color. If there is an obstruction of the bile duct the feces are often clay colored. This color change is probably due to a lack of bile pigments plus an increase in the amount of fat present in the feces. In hemolytic disease the feces are frequently orange. Quantitative examination of the feces for stercobilin is not recommended for routine practice, as reproducible techniques are complicated and should be used only in cases in which the cause of icterus is obscure.

Serum Bile Acids

The level of serum bile acids has not been extensively investigated because of the difficult analytic procedures. Development of a direct spectrometric determination for serum bile acids in the dog and cat[2] and a radioimmunoassay[3] will make this determination more readily available.

In the normal animal bile acids are synthesized in the liver, secreted into bile, and are important in the digestion of dietary fats in the small intestine. Serum levels of bile acids are low in the fasted animal with a normal enterohepatic recirculation. If there is disease that alters enterohepatic circulation or interferes with the normal hepatobiliary system, serum levels of bile acid increase.

Experimental studies have supported this fact. However, very few clinical studies have been conducted. In one study[3] serum bile acids were determined in dogs and cats with hepatobiliary disease. High fasting serum bile acid levels were observed in all patients with extrahepatic biliary obstruction, cholangiohepatitis, portasystemic shunt, biliary cirrhosis, hepatic lipidosis, and in a dog with Bedlington copper hepatopathy. These results suggest that an assay for serum bile acids may prove to be a valuable test for detecting liver disease. Additional studies comparing this test with other, more established tests used for evaluating the liver need to be completed before the assay of serum bile acids can be recommended as part of a routine evaluation of liver function.

Clearance of Foreign Dyes from the Serum

The clearance of a foreign dye from the serum following parenteral injection is a measure of both biochemical integrity and blood flow in the liver. Delay in removal of such a dye from the blood may be an indication of hepatic necrosis or fibrosis that has resulted in a reduced parenchymal mass, reduced hepatic blood flow, or both. Dyes that have been used in veterinary medicine include sulfobromophthalein (Bromsulphalein [BSP]), rose bengal, indocyanine green (ICG) and phenoltetrachlorophthalein. Today only BSP and ICG are routinely used. These dyes compete for hepatic uptake with bilirubin, and the presence of a large quantity of bilirubin may delay dye clearance from the plasma. Consequently, these tests are not indicated if there is icterus and a high level of serum bilirubin.

Sulfobromophthalein (BSP)

The BSP clearance test is a widely used index of hepatic function in domestic animals. When injected intravenously, this dye is taken up rapidly, concentrated by the liver, and excreted into the bile. BSP excretion involves the following steps: (1) transfer of the dye from blood to hepatic parenchymal cells, (2) brief storage bound to ligand and Z protein, (3) conjugation with glutathione, and (4) active excretion of conjugated dye into bile. A small fraction may be excreted in an unconjugated form.

BSP CLEARANCE IN THE DOG. The BSP retention test can be valuable in assessing the functional capacity of the liver in the dog. The rate of BSP disappearance and the percentage of retention in the dog are independent of dosage between 5 and 20 mg BSP/kg of body weight. The generally accepted dosage is 5 mg/kg of body weight.

The technique for BSP clearance in the dog is as follows: (1) Weigh the dog and divide the weight in pounds by 22. This will provide the number of milliliters of BSP solution to be injected in order to assure a dosage of 5 mg/kg of body weight. (2) Inject the dye solution intravenously, being careful to avoid perivascular infiltration. (3) Thirty minutes after injection, remove 5 ml of blood, using heparin as the anticoagulant. This sample should be removed from a vein other than the one in which the injection was given. (4) Centrifuge the blood and place 0.5 ml of unhemolyzed plasma into each of two cuvettes. (5) Add 2.5 ml of distilled water to each tube. (6) Add 3 ml of 0.1 N NaOH to one tube to produce maximum BSP color. Add 3 ml of 0.1 N HCl to the other tube. (7) Read the tube containing NaOH against the tube containing HCl at 555 mμ on a standard curve. (8) Per cent retention can be calculated by multiplying the 30-minute concentration (mg/dl) by 10.

INTERPRETATION OF BSP CLEARANCE IN DOMESTIC ANIMALS

DOG. In the dog, less than 5 per cent BSP retention at 30 minutes has been accepted as normal. However, up to 10 per cent retention 30 minutes following injection can occasionally be demonstrated in dogs having no apparent hepatic damage. Prolonged BSP retention in dogs has been reported to occur in a variety of diseases producing liver damage. Included in the list of conditions capable of causing prolongation of BSP retention are hepatic lipidoses with centrilobular necrosis, periportal fibrosis, focal hepatitis, carbon tetrachloride poisoning, and infectious hepatitis. Other diseases producing liver damage and causing prolongation of BSP retention include diabetes mellitus with hepatic lipidosis and degeneration, leukemia with hepatic metastasis, diffuse hepatic fibrosis, secondary hepatic degeneration associated with ascites, ulcerative duodenitis, gastroenteritis, coccidial hemorrhagic enteritis, thallium and tetrachloroethylene intoxication, and leptospirosis. Delayed BSP retention may also be observed in conditions that reduce hepatic blood flow. Such conditions include cardiac decompensation, severe dehydration, and shock.

As BSP is bound to albumin, a reduction in the amount of circulating albumin may affect results. Normally only unbound BSP is cleared by the liver. In animals with hypoalbuminemia there is more unbound BSP available for removal and therefore BSP retention may be falsely lowered in patients with hepatic disease and hypoalbuminemia.[4] It has been reported that phenobarbital increases the rate of removal of BSP.

HORSE. A clearance method rather than a retention method for evaluation of liver function in the horse has been recommended. Advantages of the BSP clearance method reported include: Sampling can be completed within 12 minutes after injection; plasma samples can be taken at any time between five and 12 minutes after injection; plasma volume can be calculated; and quantitative assessment of liver function can be made in terms of the kinetics of BSP disappearance from the plasma. The disadvantages of the retention technique are: The animal must be weighed; the influences of plasma volume and estimated hepatic blood flow are not accessible; and plasma must be taken at one critical time only. The retention technique does not permit estimation of hepatic blood flow, and it is impossible to assess the influence of plasma volume.

This dye is available in 1-gm ampules for use in large domestic animals. In the horse, 1 gm of dye is injected intravenously. After a period of approximately five minutes and before 12 minutes have elapsed, two heparinized blood samples are taken, preferably about four minutes apart (five and nine or six and 10 minutes post injection). The BSP concentration of a sample is determined spectrophotometrically, and plotted on semilog paper. The half-life ($T_{\frac{1}{2}}$) for BSP clearance is the time required for BSP concentration to be halved in the plasma. Average $T_{\frac{1}{2}}$ for normal mature horses is 2.8 ± 0.5 minutes with a range of 2.0 to 3.7 minutes.

Delayed BSP excretion in the horse occurs in hepatic hemosiderosis, extensive lipidosis, and carbon tetrachloride intoxication. BSP clearance tests are useful in horses, as mild icterus often accompanies a variety of clinical entities, and liver pathosis can be eliminated or established as the cause. These clearance tests are rather specifically diagnostic in horses with symptoms of hepatoencephalopathy. Hepatic involvement can be distinguished from equine encephalomyelitis or "wobbles" if excessive dehydration is not present.

COW. The BSP clearance technique is sufficiently sensitive to detect the presence of hepatic necrosis or fibrosis in cattle. This clearance test can be performed on cattle in exactly the same way as on horses, by intravenous injection of 1 gm of BSP or 1 mg BSP/lb of body weight. Blood samples should be obtained periodically between five and 20 minutes after injection and the concentration plotted on semilog paper at each sampling time. The average $T_{\frac{1}{2}}$ value for mature, nonlactating dairy cows during the first 20 minutes after injection is 3.3 ± 0.5 minutes with a range of 2.4 to 4.1 minutes.

Low BSP clearance as indicated by an increased $T_{\frac{1}{2}}$ was observed in cows with suppurative hepatitis following acute coliform mastitis, extensive fascioliasis with hepatic fibrosis, and hepatic abscesses.[5,6] Cows with the fatty liver syndrome also have a delayed BSP clearance. The BSP $T_{\frac{1}{2}}$ is frequently greater than seven minutes.[7]

SHEEP. In sheep, the percentage retention method is preferable, as BSP is cleared from the plasma quite rapidly, and the $T_{\frac{1}{2}}$ is difficult to calculate. BSP retention in the serum of normal mature sheep 10 minutes following injection is approximately 6 ± 2 per cent.[5] Ewes with ketosis had BSP retentions between 13 and 64 per cent at 15 minutes after the injection of 2 mg of BSP/kg of body weight. This slow clearance of BSP by sheep with clinical signs of ketosis is probably the result of biochemical lesions associated with cellular necrosis and of an impediment to hepatic blood flow resulting from extensive lipidosis.[5]

There is little evidence to indicate that either BSP clearance or retention tests are of notable value in the diagnosis or prognosis of liver diseases of other domestic animals.

Although BSP clearance is a reliable test for residual liver function, it must be remembered that BSP clearance is altered only when there is a severe reduction in liver mass. It has been estimated that the functional capacity of the liver must be reduced more than 50 per cent before clearance is altered. An abnormal BSP clearance is not absolute evidence of hepatocellular failure, as reductions in blood flow and competition from bilirubin also interfere with hepatic uptake and clearance of BSP. Thus, hyperbilirubinemia associated with a hemolytic crisis usually results in abnormal BSP clearance. With cholestasis, BSP is excreted via the usual route but may be reabsorbed, just as is bilirubin, and returned to blood, giving the appearance of prolonged retention.

Indocyanine Green (ICG)

Indocyanine green has been recommended for use in the dog to determine the functional status of the liver. The removal rate of this dye is exponential for the first 15 minutes following injection.

The rate of dye disappearance from the plasma of seven normal dogs was determined.[8] Animals were administered 1 mg of indocyanine green/kg of body weight, and venous blood was sampled at five-minute intervals for 15 to 30 minutes. The average disappearance rate of dye from plasma was 7.6 per cent/minute, with a range of 5.5 to 9.8 per cent/minute. This removal rate was continuously and consistently exponential for a minimum of 15 minutes in all animals tested. In the same studies, biliary obstruction produced by clamping the fistula tube in three dogs caused a slowing of the plasma disappearance rate. In the period immediately after obstruction, the plasma disappearance rate was 4.8 per cent/minute following a dose of 1 mg of dye/kg of body weight. Carbon tetrachloride in a single oral dose of 2.5 mg/kg of body weight given to one dog reduced plasma disappearance to 1.5 per cent/minute by the third day with a gradual return to normal in 20 days.

Indocyanine green clearance was studied in 22 clinically normal dogs and the average $T_{\frac{1}{2}}$ was 8.4 ± 2.3 minutes with a range of 4.7 to 12.0 minutes.[9] Indocyanine green clearance was measured in five dogs with centrilobular necrosis of the liver produced by oral administration of carbon tetrachloride. The $T_{\frac{1}{2}}$ in these animals ranged from 9.1 minutes to 27.6 minutes. The serum alanine amino transferase (SGPT) level was markedly increased with values of 900 to 15,000 units/dl being observed. The $T_{\frac{1}{2}}$ for indocyanine green in a dog with diffuse hepatic fibrosis was 100.4 minutes. Lymphosarcoma that infiltrated the liver resulted in an ICG $T_{\frac{1}{2}}$ clearance of 26.7 minutes; the ICG $T_{\frac{1}{2}}$ clearance was 38.0 minutes in a second dog with a similar condition. These authors concluded that the indocyanine green clearance test was superior to the BSP clearance assay for detection of liver pathosis in the canine.

In another experiment[11] ICG clearances were determined by the injection of 0.5 mg of dye/kg of body weight and the normal $T_{\frac{1}{2}}$ was 24.9 ± 8.0 minutes. This was extended to over 100 minutes by a 60 per cent hepatectomy, but dogs with a surgically induced portacaval shunt had an ICG $T_{\frac{1}{2}}$ of 18.7 ± 11.9 minutes. The authors concluded that, at the dosage used, ICG clearance in clinical portasystemic shunt would not be expected to be abnormal until a critical degree of atrophy had occurred.

Clinical experiences with ICG clearance are so limited that interpretation is difficult. As BSP is rarely used today in human medicine the manufacturer of this dye has, in the past, threatened to discontinue it. If this happens, ICG may be the only choice that the veterinarian has for evaluating hepatic blood flow and excretory capacity.

The BSP determination has a practical advantage in that colorimetric standards are commercially available and results can be read in a standard spectrophotometer.

The method for indocyanine green clearance has been detailed.[10]

In addition to providing the value for removal rate of the dye by action of the liver, the ICG test can be used to determine the plasma volume and an estimated hepatic blood flow. Thus, there are many advantages to using this test for studying hepatic problems in the dog. The greatest disadvantage, however, is that it requires a spectrophotometer with wavelengths in the infrared range.

TESTS BASED ON SPECIFIC BIOCHEMICAL FUNCTIONS

Plasma Proteins

A protein is a compound of high molecular weight consisting primarily of chains of amino acids united in a peptide linkage. Until late in the nineteenth century it was assumed that plasma was composed of a single protein. With various salt precipitation methods two proteins were recovered from serum and identified according to their characteristic solubilities as albumin and globulin. Additional research revealed that globulin could be further divided, and the terms euglobulin and pseudoglobulin were introduced into the scientific literature. The identification of these fractions was based primarily on the relative solubilities of these compounds in ammonium sulfate solutions and in water. Further study utilizing the principles of electrophoresis has ultimately resulted in the identification of at least 22 distinct plasma proteins.

Although considerable information has been available on the chemical properties of plasma proteins, only in the last 15 to 20 years have these properties and functions been related to possible significance in disease conditions. A separate discussion of the plasma proteins is justified by two considerations. First, the plasma proteins occupy a central and dominant position in the metabolism of protein because of their intimate relation to metabolism in the liver and their interactions with other tissues throughout the body. The second, and perhaps more practical, consideration is that plasma proteins happen to be the most readily obtainable sample of protein available in the animal body. Because of the very close relationship between proteins of plasma and those of tissues, a considerable amount of information can be gleaned concerning the general status of the body's protein metabolism from examination of the plasma proteins.

Identity and Properties

Plasma proteins represent a heterogeneous group of chemical compounds. This heterogeneity is readily demonstrable in the ultracentrifuge.

Evaluation of the molecular weights of the various components of plasma proteins lends further support to their heterogeneous characteristics. Albumin, which is the smallest, has a molecular weight of approximately 69,000; alpha (α) globulins, 200,000 to 300,000; beta (β) globulins, 150,000 to 350,000; gamma (γ) globulins, 150,000 to 300,000; and fibrinogen, 400,000. Since osmotic pressure is a function of the number of molecules in solution, albumin has considerably more influence on osmotic pressure than do the other plasma proteins. Being the smallest of the molecules, it is also the first to escape from the bloodstream if the permeability of the capillary walls is increased in conditions such as inflammation.

Perhaps the most accurate method for determining the relative values for plasma proteins is electrophoresis. In addition to identifying specifically the albumin and globulin fractions of the plasma proteins, this technique will resolve the globulins into the four main groups: alpha 1, alpha 2, beta, and gamma.

ALBUMIN. In plasma from normal animals, albumin constitutes 40 to 60 per cent of the total serum protein concentration; however, the mean concentration of albumin will depend upon the species of animal and other factors that will be discussed later. In addition to affecting osmotic pressure, albumin may act as the primary source of reserve amino acids for tissue proteins. Albumin also has certain capabilities of binding with a variety of substances. These capabilities prevent rapid excretion of drugs and are of assistance in detoxification and inactivation of materials that may be toxic to the animal body. Albumin also plays an important role in fatty acid transportation.

GLOBULINS. The globulins represent a group of proteins that are insoluble in water but may be dissolved in dilute acid, bases, and salt solutions of low concentration. These globulins are identified as alpha, beta, and gamma globulins according to their mobility in an electrical field. Each of these globulins has been further subdivided. However, the separation of these subfractions depends upon the characteristics of the species and the conditions employed to complete a laboratory separation.

The *alpha* and *beta globulins* vary in concentration depending upon the species of animal. The primary function of alpha and beta globulins is to serve as carriers of various lipids, lipid-soluble hormones and vitamins, and other lipid-like substances. These lipids are not free in the plasma during transportation but are bound to the globulins and called lipoproteins.

The alpha globulins also include a glycoprotein component that has been termed ceruloplasmin. This substance is the carrier of copper. Also included in the alpha globulins is haptoglobin, which binds hemoglobin and consequently serves

as a transport mechanism for this compound in plasma.

Transportation of iron may be related to the beta globulins. The glycoprotein responsible for this binding of iron has been called transferrin or siderophilin. Transportation occurs primarily from the site of absorption of iron in the intestinal tract to the storage areas of the body, including the liver and spleen.

Gamma globulins have been primarily associated with antibodies. In general, an increase in concentration of gamma globulin accompanies a rise in antibody titer. However, this does not always occur.

FIBRINOGEN. This plasma protein, which acts primarily in the clotting of blood, is also a globulin and is so classified because of its solubility characteristics. Fibrinogen is synthesized in the liver where it is produced by microsomes of the hepatocytes. Fibrinogen is stored in hepatic parenchymal cells until required by the body. There is a more rapid turnover of fibrinogen than of other plasma proteins. Such a turnover may be required to supply new fibrinogen coatings, which protect the vascular endothelium. It is also possible that fibrinogen may be utilized in some metabolic processes, although experimental evidence does not support this view.

GLYCOPROTEINS. Although a variety of terms have been applied to the carbohydrates bound with plasma proteins, the term glycoprotein is most widely accepted. These compounds, primarily protein in nature, contain a considerable quantity of bound carbohydrate components, such as hexoses, hexosamines, sialic acid, and a small quantity of fucose. Intimately bound carbohydrate components are found in all the plasma proteins; however, the alpha globulins contain the majority.

Glycoproteins are apparently produced in the liver, although evidence confirming this organ as their sole site of production is not available. It has been suggested by some workers that these substances may be released directly into the circulation from tissues that have been altered. There is also a possibility that the plasma glycoproteins may be synthesized as a response of tissue to injury in the form of a proliferative process. Another hypothesis is that such proliferating tissue utilizes the proteins low in carbohydrate content; thus, the carbohydrate-containing proteins remain.

LIPOPROTEINS. A considerable portion of the lipids present in plasma are in the form of lipoproteins. Two lipoprotein fractions, an alpha 1 and a beta 1 globulin, have been isolated. There is some evidence that a larger number of such lipid-protein combinations may be present in the plasma. These compounds function as carriers of steroid hormones, fat soluble vitamins, glycerides, cholesterol and its esters, phospholipids, and other fat-soluble substances.

Metabolism

Gamma globulins are synthesized by lymphoid cells of the lymph nodes, spleen, and bone marrow, whereas albumin, fibrinogen, and prothrombin are thought to be formed solely in the liver, which is also the primary site of formation of the alpha and beta globulins.

The nutritional status of an animal has a marked effect on the synthesis of plasma proteins. The direct effect is in provision of raw materials for synthesis; indirectly, protein deficiency may have a deleterious effect on the liver. Lack of dietary protein has its most marked effect on the levels of plasma gamma globulins and albumin. An excessive decrease in plasma albumin may lead to edema. A decrease in gamma globulins may result in impaired resistance to infectious agents.

In normal dogs depleted of plasma proteins, it has been found that 90 per cent of the total plasma protein may be regenerated weekly. Under optimum conditions, including an adequate protein supply and stimulus to synthesis, plasma proteins can be manufactured in a relatively short period of time.

In addition to the functions discussed previously, plasma proteins also serve as a source of nutrition for tissues. A dynamic equilibrium exists between the proteins of plasma and those of tissue. In this equilibrium state each group sustains the other when such a need arises. In protein deprivation, the level of plasma proteins is more stable, since tissue proteins are often degraded to provide for maintenance of plasma protein levels. Consequently, a considerable loss of tissue protein may occur with only minor changes in the concentration of plasma proteins. In human hypoproteinemia due solely to protein deprivation, it has been calculated that a decrease in total circulating plasma protein of 1 gm represents a concomitant loss of 30 gm of tissue protein.

Observations in experimental animals indicate that there is a continual passage of plasma proteins from the plasma and other extracellular fluids into the lymph and back again. It has been estimated that in the dog approximately 50 per cent of the total plasma protein traverses the thoracic duct daily. Experimental evidence also indicates that intravascular plasma protein is in a state of dynamic equilibrium with extravascular plasma protein. That is, a decrease in the plasma protein of one compartment results in a movement toward that area from the compartment containing more plasma protein.

Indications for Determining Plasma Protein

Plasma protein alterations are not usually specific for a particular disease condition. However, certain alterations in the total concentration or a variation in the components comprising the total plasma protein may be of significance both diagnostically and prognostically. Any abnormality in plasma proteins indicates that some pathologic, physiologic, or other induced factor is responsible.

The water balance status of an animal can be evaluated utilizing estimation of total plasma protein. This test, along with determination of packed cell volume or hemoglobin or both is of great value in ascertaining the presence or absence and degree of dehydration.

An estimation of the total quantity of plasma proteins (expressed in grams per deciliter) may be utilized as an estimation of the nutritional state of the animal. The nutritional state may depend on the proper and adequate intake of protein materials or protein-building materials. It may also reflect alterations in metabolism. Alterations in plasma protein concentration may be indicative of disease.

Of particular significance in respect to the internal metabolism of proteins is the functional state of the liver and kidneys. Drastic alterations in plasma protein values may be observed in association with both kidney and liver diseases, and an estimation of the plasma proteins may be of value both diagnostically and prognostically.

As is true with many other laboratory estimations, plasma protein analyses are useful in diagnosis when these values, as well as other factors, can be associated with the case history. Plasma protein values may also be utilized prognostically if sequential specimens are examined and the trends of absolute or relative alterations in these components can be estimated over a relatively long period of time. Perhaps the most significant change occurring in disease is a decrease in the albumin fraction. Such a decrease may be due to a defect resulting in an inhibition of the synthesis of albumin or an increase in the concentration of globulins, or it may indicate a rapid breakdown or loss of albumin. Alterations in gamma globulin usually reflect a response of the reticuloendothelial system to antigenic stimulation. Infections accompanied by invasion of the body by foreign material—whether it be of bacterial, viral, protozoal, or parasitic origin—usually result in an increase in the concentration of gamma globulins.

Estimation of total protein values following shock, dehydration, or hemorrhage is of value as a guide in the administration of fluids during an emergency. The total level of protein may vary in these conditions. Both shock and dehydration result in an increase in the total plasma protein, whereas hemorrhage may result in a decrease in total plasma protein if water balance between the intravascular and extravascular compartments has been reestablished.

Generally speaking, more information can be gained from an estimation of total serum albumin and total globulin than can be obtained from a determination of total protein. If abnormalities in the albumin or globulin fractions or both are apparent, then protein fractionation may reveal the basis for this alteration.

Normal Values

There is a wide discrepancy in normal values for the various components of the plasma proteins. This has occurred primarily because of the wide variation in techniques for estimating normal value. Different techniques, including electrophoresis, refractive index, and salt precipitation, have all been utilized and may give different results on an identical specimen of plasma. The disagreement in values that occurs with the various techniques is dependent upon the particular property of the protein that is being determined. These variations are accentuated when specimens obtained from diseased animals are assayed.

Normal values obtained by various researchers for both total plasma proteins and the various plasma protein components are presented in Table 7–2.

Analytical Procedures

Before deciding which analytical method might be employed in studying plasma proteins, one should determine what property is of primary interest. This decision not only will affect the analytical procedure utilized, but may also directly affect the type of sample that is to be obtained for analysis.

Analyses of total plasma protein and of the concentrations of the various components use either serum or plasma. Only clear, nonhemolyzed samples of serum or plasma should be employed. Total protein and electrophoretic analysis requires a minimum of 3 ml of serum or plasma.

Serum is preferable for use in electrophoretic analysis. If plasma is used in electrophoretic analysis, fibrinogen will interfere with the proper determination of gamma globulin.

Although there is little alteration in the concentration of the various plasma protein components associated with aging of the specimen, it is wise to complete the analysis as soon as possible after the serum or plasma is collected. If the examination must be delayed for some period of time, the serum may be frozen.

Determination of Total Serum Proteins

Total serum or plasma proteins may be conveniently determined in the laboratory by two methods.

REFRACTOMETRIC METHOD. The availability in recent years of refractometric instruments has made routine determination of total proteins an easy task for the technician. Use of the refractometer is simple and does not require the preparation or accurate measurement of reagents. An instrument commonly used for such determinations is the hand refractometer (TS meter). The concentration of protein is recorded in grams per deciliter by a direct reading from the refractometer (see Chapter 2 for a discussion of the method).

In our laboratory comparable results were obtained when this technique was compared with a quantitative chemical analysis for total serum proteins. The convenience and reproducibility that are characteristic of analyses using such equipment make this technique adaptable for any laboratory. It must be remembered, however, that the presence of substances that increase the concentration of total solids will affect results. Electrolytes and nonelectrolytes, if present in greater than normal concentrations, will increase total protein concentration as determined by the refractometer. Lipemic plasma is not suitable for the refractometric measurement of protein.

BIURET METHOD. The biuret technique for determination of total serum or plasma protein concentration is the simplest chemical quantitative analytical method. The biuret reaction utilizes an alkaline copper sulfate reagent and depends upon the peptide links that characterize protein. It is only slightly affected by qualitative changes in the protein.

Biuret reagent may be purchased in the form of a tablet, which is diluted in a given quantity of distilled water. Once prepared and stored in a polyethylene bottle, it is stable for several months at room temperature. Often a slight sediment will

TABLE 7–2. Normal Values for Plasma Proteins in Absolute Concentrations

Species	Sex	Age	Absolute Concentrations Gm/dl				
			TP*	ALBUMIN	ALPHA	BETA	GAMMA
Bovine	M	18–30 mo	6.97 ± 0.53	3.2	0.98	0.61	2.18
Bovine	F	5–9 yr	7.56 ± 0.5	3.4	0.85	1.08	2.16
Ovine	—	122 day	5.81	2.96	1.10	0.45	1.30
Caprine	M, F	7–9 mo	6.25	3.95	0.42	1.24	0.97
Equine	—	—	6.72	2.60	2.63	0.81	0.68
Porcine	—	5–6 mo	7.40	3.40	1.50	1.10	1.40
Canine	—	—	6.1–7.8	3.1–4.0	1.20	1.3	0.8

* TP = total protein

appear, but it does not impair the usefulness of this reagent. Details of the biuret technique for determination of total serum protein are presented in the Appendix, p. 441.

In addition to being useful as a technique for determination of total serum protein, this method may be utilized for estimation of the quantity of both albumin and globulin (Appendix, pp. 442–443).

Determination of Protein Fractions

Although not a routine procedure in most veterinary practices, the quantity of the various serum protein fractions can be estimated by means of electrophoresis. Electrophoresis has replaced salt fractionation procedures as the method of choice for quantitation of the various serum protein fractions. Separation is based on the fact that these fractions differ in their isoelectric points; therefore the components of a mixture of proteins migrate at different velocities in an electrical field. If the pH is adjusted by use of the proper buffer so that it is alkaline, the proteins all carry a negative charge, but each has a different magnitude of charge. The passage of an electrical current through a solution of proteins will then cause them to migrate toward the positively charged electrode at characteristically different rates.

Introduction of electrophoretic techniques in an immobilized medium, such as paper, cellulose acetate, or acrylamide gel, has simplified electrophoresis. This type of analysis (zone electrophoresis) has enabled the clinician to rapidly and economically determine the status of the proteins in a patient. Cellulose acetate is a popular and efficient medium, and many instruments using this medium have been marketed.

Strips on which the analysis is to be completed are placed in a rack that is in contact with the buffer solution and submerged therein. The strips are soaked in the proper buffer, and after a period of stabilization, the plasma or serum is added by means of a special applicator. Electricity is allowed to pass through the buffer, and the protein fractions migrate for a given period of time at a given electrical force. After this period of migration, the strips are removed and, depending upon the material utilized, are stained. The results are analyzed either by means of a specialized scanning spectrophotometer or by elution of the stained areas followed by colorimetric evaluation. Details of the technique are contained in the instructions supplied with each piece of equipment.

Interpretation of Results

Interpretations of alterations in plasma proteins depend on an understanding of the various physiologic and pathologic or induced factors that might cause such alterations. Analysis of variations in plasma components depends on the type of assay completed, its accuracy, and its reproducibility. Often, interpretations of variations in plasma components are based on percentage values. Just as with interpretation of differential leukocyte counts, a more accurate interpretation is possible if the amounts of the various plasma proteins are calculated as absolute values. Absolute values are determined by multiplying the total protein concentration by the per cent values for plasma protein fractions.

TOTAL PROTEINS. Alteration in the total plasma protein is most often due to a decrease in the quantity of albumin. A decrease in total albumin is often accompanied by a relative hyperglobulinemia. However, such a hyperglobulinemia is not usually sufficient to maintain the total plasma protein concentration, and hypoproteinemia results.

Since the majority of the decreases in total protein are a direct reflection of hypoalbuminemia, they will be discussed in relation to albumin deficiencies.

Hyperproteinemia occurs with less frequency and is most commonly associated with shock, dehydration, and certain types of neoplasms such as lymphosarcoma and plasmacytoma.

FIBRINOGEN. The value of a fibrinogen determination as a reflection of inflammation and necrosis has been discussed in Chapter 2. Although fibrinogen increases are nonspecific, they can be of value in following the course of disease and in assessing the severity of inflammation and tissue destruction. Calculation of the plasma protein:fibrinogen (PP:F) ratio is useful in the interpretation of disease in the presence of dehydration.

Decreased plasma fibrinogen levels are associated with congenital afibrinogenemia, hepatic insufficiency, and acute hypofibrinogenemia, which may occur in shock, severe burns, neoplasia, and as a complication associated with major abdominal or pulmonary operations. Many of these conditions induce disseminated intravascular coagulation (DIC), and the hypofibrinogenemia may be associated with this syndrome.

ALBUMIN. Hyperalbuminemia is rarely seen except in the presence of acute dehydration and shock. Increases in albumin are usually masked by increases in total plasma volume. The increase in plasma volume is related to the relatively low molecular weight of albumin and its rather high concentration in the bloodstream. Because of its high oncotic properties, albumin exerts more influence on plasma volume than any of the other plasma proteins. Thus, when there is an absolute increase in albumin, total plasma volume is also increased.

Distinct causes for decreased albumin concentrations are not always identifiable, since homeostatic processes operate to minimize alterations in the plasma concentration of this protein fraction. A decrease in total serum albumin may result from (1) deficient intake of protein, (2) deficient synthesis of albumin, (3) excessive protein breakdown, or (4) loss of albumin.

Lowered serum albumin concentrations are present in starvation and malnutrition and in chronic gastrointestinal diseases in which there is interference with protein digestion and absorption. There may also be a decrease in albumin in conditions that impose an extra demand for protein if the dietary intake of protein is insufficient. Animals placed on a protein-deficient diet, particularly in certain areas of the United States during the winter, will have a low serum albumin level.

Deficient synthesis of albumin occurs commonly in association with chronic hepatic disease. A decrease in the concentration of albumin has been reported to occur in hepatitis and liver cirrhosis in the dog.

Hypoalbuminemia develops as a result of excessive protein breakdown, which occurs in prolonged fever, uncontrolled diabetes mellitus, and trauma. In humans, hypoalbuminemia may accompany thyrotoxicosis. Alterations in total protein due to excessive catabolism are usually not severe but may provide an indication of some change in the oncotic pressure in the plasma proteins.

Albumin loss is a common cause of hypoalbuminemia in domestic animals. Loss of this protein component may be excessive in nephritis and nephrosis in which a longstanding albuminuria exists. This loss is particularly significant in acute nephritis and nephrosis or disease of the glomerulus. However, there is little or no proteinuria in the more chronic forms of nephritis in domestic animals. Although protein lost through the urine may be significant, in all probability it does not account for the complete depression of albumin. Rather, there is probably an accompanying defect in albumin synthesis, an increase in utilization, or both.

Excessive enteric loss of protein or a malabsorption syndrome may result in marked hypoproteinemia. In dogs, gastrointestinal diseases causing a hypoproteinemia include nontropical sprue, chronic enteritis, colitis, neoplasia of the intestinal wall, chronic granulomatous enteritis, and intestinal lymphangiectasia. Similar conditions may occur in other animals but are not well documented. Johne's disease of cattle results in intestinal protein loss and accompanying hypoproteinemia.

Parasitized animals often have a decrease in serum albumin. In sheep parasitized by *Haemonchus* organisms there is a decrease in the concentration of albumin and an increase in the concentration of globulin.

The catabolic rate and intravascular pool of serum albumin in cattle suffering from Type II ostertagiasis has been measured.[12] Infected cattle became hypoalbuminemic and had an increased fractional catabolic rate for albumin. The authors suggested that the hypoalbuminemia might be due to abnormal leakage of plasma proteins into the gastrointestinal tract.

In certain cases of massive ascites, a diminished albumin may be observed, since ascitic fluid contains a large amount of protein. In addition, large quantities of albumin may be lost following extensive burns and severe hemorrhage.

GLOBULINS. Although decreases in concentrations of individual globulin fractions may be encountered, there is seldom a decrease in total globulin concentration. This is primarily due to the fact that other globulins may be simultaneously increased to compensate for the decreased component. An exception may be encountered in agammaglobulinemia. Hypogammaglobulinemia and hypoglobulinemia will occur in animals deprived of colostrum.

ALPHA GLOBULINS. Decreases in this complex, heterogeneous component of the plasma are seldom observed in diseases of domestic animals. However, increases occur in a variety of inflammatory reactions. In particular, the alpha 2 component of this protein is markedly increased in both bacterial and viral infections. The mechanism underlying this increase is not completely understood, but the fact that glycoproteins are contained in this fraction may be of some significance. Electrophoretic analysis of serum from dogs with mastocytoma revealed an increase in alpha 2 globulins.[13] These authors suggested that such serum protein changes may have occurred as a consequence of histamine elaboration by the mast cells of the tumor.

BETA GLOBULINS. Decreases in beta globulins seldom occur in disease conditions; however, elevated levels may be associated with an increase in the beta lipoprotein, such as that occurring in hyperlipemia.

IMMUNOGLOBULINS (GAMMA GLOBULINS). Immunoglobulins vary in size, weight, site of production, and function. These globulins include immunoglobulins G, M, E, and A (IgG, IgM, IgE, IgA). These, among all of the globulins, are most likely to vary in concentration. Elevations occur in gamma globulins in bacterial infections, viral infections, parasitism, and liver diseases. Increases have also been associated with certain types of neoplasms, notably lymphosarcoma and plasmacytoma.

Abnormalities in the immunoglobulins, which are predominantly in the beta and gamma globulin regions on an electrophoretic separation, are termed gammopathies. Increased levels of immunoglobulins can be either monoclonal (homogenous) or polyclonal (heterogenous).

Monoclonal gammopathies in domestic animals are most frequently associated with neoplasia involving the immunoglobulin-forming cells. These abnormalities are identified electrophoretically by the appearance of a narrow, sharp globulin spike. In contrast, with polyclonal gammopathies there is an overall increase in gamma globulins resulting in a broad peak. Myeloma frequently has an associated monoclonal gammopathy. The type of immunoglobulin varies according to the molecular structure of the globulin produced by the neoplastic cell. In the dog, IgG, IgA, and IgM myelomas have been reported.

A macroglobulinemia similar to Waldenström's macroglobulinemia in humans was reported in a dog.[14] Clinically, this animal was anemic and had an increased serum viscosity and hemorrhagic diathesis. The total serum protein was high and approximately 60 per cent of it consisted of a macroglobulin that was considered gamma M.

Multiple myeloma characterized by increased IgA and serum hyperviscosity syndrome has been reported in the dog.[15] These authors emphasized that serum hyperviscosity is not consistent in all patients with multiple myeloma, as serum viscosity is dependent upon the concentration and chemicophysical properties of serum proteins. Hyperviscosity is more commonly associated with IgM myelomas because of the large molecular size. This syndrome is uncommon in patients with IgG myelomas. A similar hyperviscosity syndrome has been reported in three dogs with lymphocytic leukemia.[16] In two dogs the immunoglobulin increased was IgM, and in the third it was IgA.

Occasionally, a monoclonal globulin spike is detected in the electrophoretic pattern of a specimen from a normal individual.[17] This condition has been designated "essential benign monoclonal gammopathy." Hurvitz cautions that a substantial number of these benign gammopathies may convert to symptomatic conditions. An idiopathic monoclonal (IgA) gammopathy has been reported in one dog.[18]

Polyclonal gammopathies usually represent nonspecific immunoglobulin increases, which may occur in a variety of diseases including systemic lupus erythematosus, rheumatoid arthritis, and myasthenia gravis; in infections such as trypanosomiasis and chronic bacterial infections; and in conditions in which extensive liver damage has occurred. Nonspecific increases have also been reported in chronic infections such as pyometra, feline infectious peritonitis, pyoderma, and granulomatous diseases. Parasitism may also have an associated increase in immunoglobulins. Polyclonal gammopathies have been reported in *Ehrlichia* infection,[19] heart-worm disease,[20] and liver fluke disease of sheep,[21] as well as in ascariasis and ancylostomiasis.[17]

The most common cause of a deficiency in serum immunoglobulins occurs in neonates deprived of colostrum. Placental transfer of immunoglobulins is minimal in domestic animals, and all newborns are hypogammaglobulinemic at birth. An animal that fails to obtain immunoglobulins from colostrum is susceptible to a variety of infections. Septicemia and diarrhea are common

in such animals. Immunoglobulin-deficient newborn animals can be identified early by an estimation of the concentrations of albumin and globulin in the plasma. A rapid field test for determining the immune status of neonatal calves has been developed.[22] This test is conducted as follows: (1) Prepare three solutions (14, 16, and 18 per cent) from anhydrous sodium sulfite and distilled water. (2) Dispense 1.9 ml of each sodium sulfite concentration into individual test tubes. (3) Add 0.1 ml of serum to each of the three sodium sulfite solutions. (4) Mix the samples and allow them to stand at room temperature for one hour to permit precipitation. (5) The results are interpreted according to Table 7–3.

This technique has been found to be acceptable in calves but is not reliable in foals.[23] These workers found that the sodium sulfite test in foals indicated low concentrations of immunoglobulin, but concentrations in many animals with middle and high values were misinterpreted as being low. The zinc sulfate turbidity test is probably a more accurate method for estimating immunoglobulin levels in neonates. Details of this technique are included in the Appendix, p. 442.

A latex agglutination test for estimating the blood or serum concentration of immunoglobulins in the equine is now available commercially (Bayvet). Measured quantities of blood or serum are incubated in a premeasured diluent at room temperature. One, two, or three drops from a special pipette are placed within the ring of a glass plate and one drop of latex bead coated with antibodies to equine globulin is added to each ring. The plate is rotated and the presence or absence of agglutination is noted. Immunoglobulin concentration is estimated according to the presence or absence of agglutination in each of the three rings.

A rapid screening test was developed to detect hypogammaglobulinemia in neonatal calves, using a 10 per cent glutaraldehyde reagent.[24] The glutaraldehyde reagent was prepared by diluting a 25 per cent solution to a final concentration of 10 per cent. A 0.5-ml aliquot of serum is transferred to a 13-mm by 100-mm glass tube and 50

TABLE 7–3. Interpretation of Results of Field Test for Determining Immune Status of Neonatal Calves

IG Concentration Range	Sodium Sulfite Concentration (%)		
	14	16	18
<500 mg/dl	−*	−	+
500–1000 mg/dl	−	+	+
>1500 mg/dl	+	+	+

* − = no precipitation in one hour, + = flakes of precipitation in one hour.

μl of the reagent added. Serum and reagent are mixed immediately, and the tube is examined at intervals up to one hour for evidence of coagulation. A positive reaction occurs when a firm "button" develops in the bottom of the tube. An incomplete reaction is characterized by the presence of a semisolid gel. When the serum gamma globulin concentration was >0.6 gm/dl, addition of the reagent resulted in complete coagulation. There was no alteration in serum viscosity from calves with gamma globulin concentrations of <0.4 gm/dl. The authors indicated that this test would have practical application in identification of calves with hypogammaglobulinemia.

Hypogammaglobulinemia may also occur as a congenital immunodeficiency. This immunodeficiency has been most extensively studied in Arabian foals in which three forms have been identified. With a combined immunodeficiency there is an absence of both T and B cells resulting in lymphopenia and agammaglobulinemia. With the primary agammaglobulinemia the lymphocyte count is normal but the gamma globulin level is greatly reduced. A selective IgM deficiency has also been identified. The type of immunoglobulin deficiency can be differentiated only by careful evaluation of the concentrations of IgG and IgM. Similar deficiencies may occur in other domestic animals but have not been well documented.

Acquired immunoglobulin deficiencies may occur under conditions of clinical immunosuppression. These disorders may or may not have an associated hypogammaglobulinemia.

Protein Metabolism Tests of Liver Function

Although the liver plays an important role in protein metabolism, alterations in serum proteins are not specific for liver damage. However, detection of alterations in the various fractions of plasma proteins may be of some value. The combination of an absolute low value for serum albumin and a high gamma globulin level or either of these alone is typical of liver damage. In addition to studies of plasma proteins, evaluation of coagulation and ammonia may have some significance.

Serum Albumin and Globulins

The absolute fall in serum albumin concentration resulting from a disturbance of normal synthesis by the liver is not an early biochemical alteration. Such a fall is found more commonly in chronic liver diseases such as subacute hepatitis or diffuse fibrosis. In portal fibrosis, there is a characteristic decrease in serum albumin and an elevation in gamma globulin. In acute hepatitis, changes in albumin are less significant, but an elevation in gamma globulin occurs rather consistently. Decreased albumin levels are not only associated with liver disease, but comparable alterations may be seen in animals with circulatory diseases, deficient protein digestion due to disease or lack of protein intake, nephritis, nephrosis, and a variety of chronic diseases accompanied by cachexia.

The serum globulin level is increased in both diffuse fibrosis and hepatitis. This absolute increase in globulin is difficult to explain, although it may be a response of the antibody-producing mechanism. In addition to liver diseases, many other conditions may result in elevation of gamma globulin.

Coagulation Factors

Since the liver is the major site for production of coagulation factors, advanced liver disease may affect some coagulation test results. Factors with a short half-life (V, VII, IX, X) are affected first. If the liver disease progresses, factors I, II, and XII may also decrease. As factor VIII is produced by the endothelial cells, it is not reduced by hepatocellular disease but may be increased. If DIC ensues, the increased catabolism will result in a decrease of factors I, V, and VIII.

Although few dogs with hepatic disease have a clinical bleeding problem, a number of screening tests such as the prothrombin time and activated partial thromboplastin time may be high. Severe bleeding problems are more likely to occur in animals with acute severe hepatic failure than in animals with chronic liver disease.

The prothrombin time may be affected as a consequence of the inability of the liver to synthesize prothrombin even if adequate metabolites are present, or as a failure to synthesize prothrombin because of inadequate bile-fat soluble vitamin K. If the lengthened prothrombin time is due to a lack of production of prothrombin, the administration of vitamin K will not correct the condition. If, however, there is an impaired bile release into the intestine, vitamin K will not be absorbed. In such cases the administration of vitamin K will return prothrombin levels to normal, usually within 48 hours.[4]

In a study of plasma coagulation factor abnormalities in dogs with naturally occurring hepatic disease,[25] plasma coagulation factor values and screening tests were consistently abnormal in more than half of the dogs with each type of hepatic disease. With hepatic degeneration there was a decrease in factor XII; with inflammation, an increase in factor VIII–related antigen; in cirrhosis, a decrease in factors IX, X, XI with an increase in factor VIII–related antigen and a shortened thrombin clot time. With neoplasia the thrombin clot time was decreased, there was decreased factor VIII activity, and an increase in factor VIII–related antigen. These authors reported that selected individual coagulation factors were more sensitive than serum chemistry values for the detection of certain types of hepatic disease.

They found that an increased plasma factor VIII–related antigen occurred more commonly in dogs with hepatic inflammation than did an increase in serum ALT or ALP. Decreased activity of plasma factors IX and/or X occurred in dogs with hepatic cirrhosis but not in dogs with other types of hepatic disease. They cautioned that extrahepatic disease should be ruled out before ascribing coagulation factor abnormalities to a specific type of hepatic disease as they did not study the specificity of abnormal coagulation factors values for hepatic as opposed to extrahepatic disease. Another sequela to liver inflammation may be the onset of DIC. Damaged liver cells may release a thromboplastin-like substance or may fail to clear clot-promoting factors from the plasma. The presence of DIC can be confirmed by demonstrating, in addition to the abnormal coagulation screening test results, the presence of FDP in plasma and a concomitant low fibrinogen level.

Amino Acid Tolerance Test

Although amino acid tolerance tests based on the rate of deamination of injected amino acids have been used as liver function tests in animals, they have little application to veterinary practice, as the technique for determining various amino acid levels is difficult and time consuming. Amino acids used for this type of test include tyrosine, arginine, and hippuric acid. The hippuric acid test is not used in the canine, since any administered phenol derivative is conjugated primarily by the kidney.

Blood Ammonia

Samples for ammonia assay require special handling; before the test is requested the clinician should consult with the laboratory. Ammonia generally is derived from bacterial action in the gastrointestinal tract and reaches the liver through the portal circulation. If hepatic cellular damage has occurred or blood flow is greatly reduced, removal of ammonia is incomplete, and an increased serum value may ensue. Under such circumstances, the disease may be complicated by ingestion of large quantities of food high in nitrogen. An increase in blood ammonia may be an indication of impending hepatic coma. Blood ammonia is thought to be increased as a consequence of the "shunting" of portal blood past the liver or by the marked reduction of parenchymal function. Liver atrophy caused by portacaval shunting causes an increase in blood ammonia as does any decrease in hepatic mass. A decrease in urea nitrogen usually accompanies the ammonia increase.

In patients suspected of having a congenital or acquired portacaval shunt, an ammonia tolerance test may be of value. This test involves oral administration of ammonia salt and measurement of the amount of blood ammonia 30 minutes later.

The ammonium chloride enters the small bowel where ammonium is converted to ammonia and absorbed. If there is hepatocellular failure, significant portal blood shunting, or deficiencies of urea cycle enzymes, the blood ammonia concentration will be increased. The procedure is as follows:

1. Fast the patient for 12 hours.
2. Administer ammonium chloride orally at a dosage of 100 mg/kg body weight to a maximum of 3 gm. This salt should be diluted in 20 to 50 ml of water before oral administration.
3. Samples of heparinized blood are drawn at the time of administration and 30 minutes after the ammonium chloride is given. Normal values for the dog are 60 to 120 μg/dl on fasting samples and less than 200 μg/dl 30 minutes after the salt is given. In dogs with hepatic encephalopathy the blood ammonia level may be increased, but some dogs with severe hepatic failure will be normal so that a fasting blood ammonia alone may not be diagnostic. In such cases it has been recommended[4] that an ammonia tolerance test should be completed. In affected animals the 30-minute value will be considerably above 200 μg/dl. In one study[26] of six dogs, 30-minute venous blood ammonia was 1049 ± 256 μg/dl as compared with fasting levels of 236 ± 116 μg/dl. In young dogs with hepatic encephalopathy from inherited shunts, it is not at all uncommon to observe normal liver function tests except for BSP retention and altered ammonia tolerance tests.

Carbohydrate Metabolism Test

Because of the ability of the liver to participate in carbohydrate metabolism and its inherent ability to metabolize increased quantities of carbohydrates, several tests have been developed for the estimation of this metabolic function. None of these tests is extensively used in veterinary medicine, and they probably have their application primarily in research.

The galactose tolerance test has been studied most extensively, and experimental evidence suggests that it may be of some value in studying liver function in domestic animals. This test, however, is time consuming in both execution and analysis, and so has only limited value. It may be successful in detecting liver damage, because only the liver can utilize galactose in significant amounts.

The basic principle of the determination is the injection of galactose intravenously at the rate of 1 ml of a 50 per cent solution/kg of body weight. Blood samples are then removed at various intervals, and the concentration of galactose at these intervals is determined. The presence of galactose in a quantity greater than the anticipated value implies the presence of liver pathology. In the experimental work completed, the galactose tolerance determination was found to be inferior to the BSP test for the detection of early changes.

Lipid Metabolism Tests

The liver is involved in many phases of lipid metabolism including synthesis, esterification, and excretion of cholesterol. Only the determination of free and esterified cholesterol of the serum has been intensively applied to the study of hepatic diseases. In humans, low values for cholesterol esters have been observed with a variety of liver diseases. Such findings indicate that the esterification of cholesterol with fatty acids is principally a function of the liver parenchyma. Of considerable importance in the diagnosis of hepatocellular damage is the ratio of free cholesterol esters to total cholesterol in the serum. Esterification is significantly depressed with both chronic and acute hepatocellular disease and this results in a higher free cholesterol:cholesterol ester ratio.

Although only a limited amount of work has been done on the cholesterol values in liver diseases of animals, the data suggest that esterification is depressed in liver diseases. A per cent esterified cholesterol:per cent total cholesterol (CE/CT) ratio of more than 60 for normal animals has been reported.[27] Decreased CE/CT ratios were observed in dogs with leptospirosis, diabetes mellitus, advanced nephritis, and fatty degeneration of the liver. High total serum cholesterol levels (>300 mg/dl) were observed in dogs with leptospirosis, diabetes mellitus, or nephritis and in one dog with suspected liver neoplasia. Similar observations have been reported in cattle. Total cholesterol determinations are of limited value, as a variety of disease conditions other than those of the liver may result in an increase. If used as a liver function test, both the esterified and total cholesterol values should be determined.

TESTS BASED ON SERUM ENZYME ACTIVITY

Alterations in serum enzyme activity due to malfunctioning of the liver occur as a result of three processes: (1) An elevation of enzymes due to disruption of hepatic cells as a result of necrosis or as a consequence of altered membrane permeability. Included in this group are the enzymes alanine amino transferase (ALT) (formerly known as glutamic pyruvic transaminase [GPT]), aspartate amino transferase (AST) (formerly called glutamic oxalacetic transaminase [GOT]), triphosphopyridine nucleotide (TPN)–linked isocitric dehydrogenase (SIC-D), arginase, glutamic dehydrogenase (GD), iditol dehydrogenase (ID) (formerly known as sorbitol dehydrogenase [SD]), ornithine carbamyl transferase (OCT), and lactic dehydrogenase (LDH). (2) A decrease in concentration in the serum resulting from impaired synthesis by the liver (choline esterase). (3) An elevation in enzyme levels due to cholestasis. The enzymes affected include alkaline phosphatase (AP), γ-glutamyl transferase (γGT or GGT), and leucine aminopeptidase (LAP).

Enzymes that increase in concentration following hepatic necrosis (AST, ALT, GD, ID, OCT, and SIC-D) may be divided into those that are liver specific and those that exist in high concentration in organs other than the liver. Neither AST nor SIC-D is a liver-specific enzyme, but both are used diagnostically to measure the level of liver necrosis if no disease exists in other tissues in which these enzymes are found in high concentrations. Determinations of the so-called liver-specific enzymes (ALT in the dog, cat, and primate and arginase, OCT, GD, and ID in all animals) are sensitive and reliable tests utilized to detect the presence of hepatic necrosis, both mild and severe.

Transaminases (Amino Transferases)

Transaminases (amino transferases) function to catalyze the transfer of an amino group from an amino acid to a keto acid. The two clinically important amino transferases are alanine amino transferase and aspartate amino transferase. These enzymes have a wide distribution in animal tissues and are present in small quantities in the serum of all animals as a consequence of normal tissue destruction and subsequent enzyme release. Since these enzymes have their principal functions and greatest concentration within the cell, increases observed in the serum reflect cellular abnormalities.

Indications for Test

ALANINE AMINO TRANSFERASE (ALT). Tests for levels of serum ALT are of value in detecting liver diseases in the dog, cat, and primate. As this enzyme is present in large quantities in the hepatocyte cytoplasm of these animal species, ALT is increased in serum when cellular degeneration or destruction occurs in this organ. This determination is of no diagnostic value for liver disease in other animal species. Serum ALT activity should be determined when the attending veterinarian suspects the existence of a liver disease.

ASPARTATE AMINO TRANSFERASE (AST). Since AST is present in all tissues of the body, it is not an organ-specific test and consequently may be utilized to detect destruction in a wide variety of tissues. As this enzyme appears in extremely high concentrations in muscle, both skeletal and cardiac, it is of value in confirming a diagnosis of muscular degeneration. Serum AST levels may be increased with liver disease in all species but cannot be considered to be a specific test for liver damage.

Technique of Test

Determinations of serum ALT or AST activity depend upon the use of a spectrophotometer for detecting color intensity or alterations in optical density. A variety of kits containing all chemicals required for the determination are readily available, and results are expressed in units of activity. Either a colorimetric method or a reaction rate method, which requires a spectrophotometer having a light source in the ultraviolet range, may be used.

Normal Values

As methods for determining AST and ALT activity vary among laboratories, veterinarians are cautioned to establish normal values within their own practices.

Interpretation of Results

SERUM ALANINE AMINO TRANSFERASE (ALT). Increased ALT in the dog and cat is specific for hepatic disease. This is not true, however, of mature horses, sheep, pigs, or cattle, as their livers do not contain a significant level of ALT.

As the intracellular cytoplasmic level of ALT is several times that of extracellular fluid, whenever there is membrane damage, ALT will escape and the serum concentration will increase. The increase in serum activity of ALT is directly related to the amount of damage that has occurred to the hepatocytes. If the damage is minimal serum ALT activity will increase slightly, whereas with moderate damage there will be a three- to eightfold increase. With severe liver necrosis there will be a greater than eightfold increase in serum activity.

Although most of the increases in serum ALT activity are associated with hepatocellular damage, anything that will cause an overproduction of the enzyme may also result in an increase in serum activity.

The serum half-life of ALT is from two to five hours. If liver damage is acute and transitory, one would expect the serum levels to return to normal fairly rapidly. If, however, there is chronic or progressive liver disease, the serum level will remain high. If the values are reduced by half every one to two days, the prognosis should be good.

SERUM ASPARTATE AMINO TRANSFERASE (AST). Increased serum AST is associated with cell necrosis of many different tissues. Pathology involving either skeletal or cardiac muscle, or hepatic cells, or both, may allow for the escape of large quantities of this enzyme into the blood. Serum AST cannot be considered specific for liver necrosis. However, in animal species other than the dog, cat, and primate, AST levels may be dramatically increased with hepatocellular destruction. Care must be taken in interpreting the results to ascertain the normality of the heart and muscular system, as diseases in these tissues will also produce increased AST values. If liver cell damage has been ascertained previously by the use of another test, such as BSP clearance or serum and urine bilirubin determinations, then the AST test may be utilized prognostically for evaluating the degree of liver necrosis and its response to therapy.

In the dog, elevated serum AST activity has been reported in hepatic necrosis, myocardial infarction, and necrosis of skeletal muscle. In the cat, serum AST levels are elevated in hepatic necrosis and may be increased if a pathologic disorder of muscle is present. In the horse, elevated values are observed in azoturia, hepatitis, septicemia, and intestinal complications. In the bovine, increased enzyme activity has been reported in hepatic necrosis, white muscle disease, and starvation. In sheep and calves with white muscle disease, values of 400 to 4000 units of serum AST activity/dl of serum have been reported. Increased serum AST activity has been reported in calves that were depleted of vitamin E.

The serum activity of AST has been reported to be elevated in association with liver diseases in a variety of animal species. Elevated serum levels have been observed in cattle that have consumed contaminated herring meal and in postparturient cattle. Increased serum levels in the horse have been observed with halothane and chloroform anesthesia and carbon tetrachloride poisoning. In sheep, increased levels have been observed in animals infested with liver flukes and in those that have consumed contaminated herring meal. It has been suggested that an increased serum AST level is of value in predicting copper poisoning.

SERUM ARGINASE. Serum arginase determinations have been reported to be of value in testing for hepatic necrosis.

There is apparently a more rapid disappearance of plasma arginase than of ALT or AST activity in hepatic necrosis. The difference in behavior of arginase and transaminase activities in plasma may permit predictions concerning the nature of hepatic lesions. If both plasma arginase and transaminase activities are continuously elevated, a progressive hepatic necrosis is probably present. If normal plasma arginase and elevated transaminase activities are observed following significant elevations of both enzymes, the prognosis is favorable, as hepatic necrosis is subsiding. The determination of serum arginase activity is a liver-specific enzyme test for hepatic necrosis in horses, cattle, pigs, and sheep. As arginase is a mitochondria-bound enzyme, hepatocellular damage is usually great before there is an increase in serum activity. Other enzyme tests are more sensitive.

IDITOL DEHYDROGENASE (ID). Iditol dehydrogenase (formerly sorbitol dehydrogenase) is a liver-specific enzyme present in the liver in all animal species. Consequently, serum elevations of ID occur when the liver is damaged.

In horses and ponies poisoned with carbon tetrachloride, serum ID activity increased 400- to 600-fold.

Similar results have been reported in ponies[28] treated with aflatoxin B_1. In ruminants serum ID activity is increased in fascioliasis, hepatic lipidosis associated with the "fat cow syndrome," and other conditions with associated hepatocyte damage. Although assays for serum ID activity have not been extensively reported in dogs and cats, in those conditions in which it has been studied an increase in ID activity paralleled that of ALT.

SERUM ORNITHINE CARBAMYL TRANSFERASE (OCT). This enzyme is also liver specific and consequently can be of value in detecting diseases of that organ in all animal species. Elevations of serum OCT have been reported in a variety of liver disorders in cattle, horse, and swine.

LACTIC DEHYDROGENASE (LDH). Values for LDH are frequently included as part of an automated chemical profile. This enzyme has wide distribution in animal tissues and, as it is an intracellular enzyme, is released following cellular damage to the liver, lung, muscle, kidney, heart, and lymphoreticular tissue. It is also present in a high concentration in erythrocytes, and serum increases are frequently due to hemolysis or delayed separation of serum from a clot. Increases in LDH may also be observed in association with malignancies. Estimation of the isoenzymes of LDH is of value in humans, as isoenzyme distribution is rather specific for some cells or tissues. Comparable studies in domestic animals have not established such specific isoenzyme relationships. Serum LDH activity is greater in young than in mature dogs. As with other enzyme determinations, normal levels should be established for each practice situation.

Alkaline Phosphatase

Phosphatases are agents that hydrolyze phosphoric esters with the liberation of inorganic phosphate. Two principal types of phosphatases are found in blood. Alkaline phosphatase has a pH optimum between 9 and 10, whereas acid phosphatase has its optimum enzymatic activity at a pH of approximately 5.

Alkaline phosphatase is widely distributed in the body, and is found in high concentrations in bone (in the osteoblasts), intestinal mucosa, renal tubule cells, liver, and placenta.

Recent evidence indicates that each of these tissues has a distinctly different isoenzyme of alkaline phosphatase. An additional isoenzyme whose synthesis is induced by corticosteroids and possibly by other drugs has been reported.[29]

Indications for Test

Determinations of serum alkaline phosphatase (SAP) are frequently included as a part of routine biochemical profiles.

Normal Values

A great number of techniques for alkaline phosphatase determination have been developed. Normal values for domestic animals have been reported as Bodansky, King-Armstrong, Kind-King, or international units or as milliunits (mU)/ml of serum.

The veterinarian must be aware that serum alkaline phosphatase levels may normally be higher in the young animal. Normal values should be established for each practice situation.

Techniques for Test

Several colorimetric methods are available for estimation of the serum alkaline phosphatase level. Prepared kits containing all required chemicals are most commonly utilized. These techniques are usually based on the liberation of phenol or phosphorus.

Interpretation of Results

Serum alkaline phosphatase (SAP) activity in normal cattle and sheep presents such a wide range of values that its use as an indicator of liver insufficiency or obstructive icterus in these species is prohibited. In dogs, however, the serum alkaline phosphatase level is relatively narrow in range and may be utilized as an indicator of hepatic malfunction.

In an attempt to enhance interpretation of serum alkaline phosphatase levels in dogs, the disappearance rates of intravenously injected alkaline phosphatase isoenzymes were studied.[30] The isoenzymes were divided into two groups on the basis of half-life. Hepatic and steroid-induced alkaline phosphatases had half-lives of approximately three days, whereas isoenzymes from the placenta, kidney, and intestine had half-lives of less than six minutes. The authors did not study the half-life of the bone isoenzyme but suggested that it would be the same duration as that of hepatic and steroid-induced alkaline phosphatase isoenzymes.

The elevation of liver alkaline phosphatase in canine serum is associated with active pathology in that organ. The degree of elevation is dependent upon the nature of the lesion. Acute hepatocellular necrosis results in minimal increases in SAP, whereas the ALT and ID levels are dramatically increased in a comparable disease. In dogs that have traumatic lesions of the liver, or carbon tetrachloride intoxication, or that have been treated with sodium caparsolate, there was a two- to threefold increase in SAP with a concomitant 10- to 20-fold increase in ALT.[31]

Biliary obstruction results in a marked increase in SAP. Although complete biliary obstruction is rare in the dog, experimental bile duct ligation was followed by SAP increases as high as 70 times normal.[32] Cholestasis, regardless of cause, will produce large increases in SAP. Levels from 10 to 15 times normal are not uncommon. The interpretation of SAP increases must always take into consideration the possibility that the concentration of this enzyme is influenced by corticosteroids. Endogenous and exogenous steroids induce production of a specific alkaline phosphatase isoenzyme.[29] SAP activities of two dogs treated with prednisolone daily for 17 days were studied. The SAP activity increased 29- to 40-fold by day 17. There was a two- to fivefold increase in SAP by day three. In evaluations of increases in SAP, careful consideration must be given to the history and in particular to prior treatment with corticosteroids or adrenocorticotropic hormone (ACTH). Once induction of this isoenzyme has occurred the level of serum activity may remain high for several months even though the dog is no longer being treated. Phenobarbital will also increase SAP. Dogs with adrenocortical hyperplasia may have exceedingly high SAP levels (up to a 100-fold increase).

Early studies on alkaline phosphatase in the cat suggested that there was rapid excretion of this enzyme via the kidney. The disappearance of alkaline phosphatase in intact and nephrectomized cats was studied.[33] Investigators found that infusion of hepatic alkaline phosphatase into nephrectomized cats resulted in an enzyme half-life analogous to that of intact cats. This established that hepatic alkaline phosphatase is not excreted via the kidney but is removed from the circulation by some other, as yet undetermined, mechanism.

The mean half-life of feline hepatic alkaline phosphatase isoenzyme was found to be approximately 11 times less than for canine hepatic alkaline phosphatase. Such a short life for this isoenzyme might explain, in part, the reported failure of serum alkaline phosphatase levels to increase in cats following bile duct ligation.

Serum alkaline phosphatase determinations may be useful in the diagnosis of obstructive and degenerative hepatic disease in cats. Bile duct occlusion, both complete and partial, and carbon tetrachloride poisoning in cats were followed by significant increases in SAP.[34, 35] Four- to ninefold increases in SAP occurred in cats with common bile duct occlusion. Similar changes in serum leucine aminopeptidase (LAP) ALT and AST activity were observed. Although the increase in SAP associated with cholestasis in cats is not as spectacular as it is in dogs, the test is of value in cats. There is no evidence to support the presence of a steroid-induced isoenzyme of AP in the cat.

In addition to the consideration of SAP in relation to the liver, it must be remembered that increased activity of this enzyme can be associated with bone. Elevation of bone alkaline phosphatase is readily observed in animals with rapid bone formation. Elevations of bone AP are, however, of considerably less magnitude than those associated with liver AP. Increases in bone alkaline phosphatase are usually in the range of two to three times normal.

Gamma-Glutamyl Transferase

Gamma-glutamyl transferase (GGT) is an enzyme found in the cytosol associated with cell membranes, particularly those near the bile canaliculi. The enzyme is present in several organs but serum activity of this enzyme almost exclusively results from the GGT of hepatic origin. This would suggest that GGT might be more useful than SAP in the detection of cholestasis in the dog.

In a study of the effects of common bile duct ligation on SAP and GGT,[36] it was found that increases in serum GGT activity closely paralleled SAP. In glucocorticoid-induced hepatopathy in dogs[37] the GGT increase in serum activity was slower than that of SAP or ALT. The peak activity occurred at a later time and had a slower decrease. Serum GGT activity remained high for at least six weeks following prednisone administration and these investigators believed that it was the result of induction by prednisone. As there was no cholestasis observed in these dogs, it was thought that it was not a likely cause of the 23-fold increase observed. In view of these observations it would appear that GGT assay presents no distinct advantages over SAP assay. In cats serum GGT activity paralleled SAP activity following the disruption of bile flow but not following hepatic cell necrosis caused by carbon tetrachloride.[38] The magnitude of increase in serum GGT activity following extrahepatic cholestasis was greater than that of SAP. There was a sixfold increase in SAP as compared with an 18-fold increase in GGT. SAP also increased following the administration of carbon tetrachloride (fivefold increase) while there was no significant increase in GGT activity. These observations need to be confirmed in clinical cases of hepatic disease.

Serum GGT activity in the serum of ruminants has also been evaluated. Serum levels were increased with fascioliasis, but not with advanced hepatic fibrosis resulting from fluke infections. As the normal range of GGT activity in cattle and sheep is less than that seen with SAP, the GGT may be more easily interpreted in relation to the presence of cholestasis.

Additional work needs to be completed in order to confirm the experimental studies and establish the role that this enzyme may have in the diagnosis of hepatic disease in domestic animals.

LIVER BIOPSY

Although liver biopsy cannot be considered a liver function test, it would be remiss not to include it in a discussion concerning this organ. In spite of careful clinical examination and evaluation of a variety of liver function tests, the clinician may still be unable to make a diagnosis with-

TABLE 7–4. Laboratory Findings as Aids in Differential Diagnosis of Icterus

	Conjugated Bilirubin	Unconjugated Bilirubin	Urine Bilirubin	Urine Urobilinogen	Dye Retention	ALT or AST	Serum Albumin	Serum Globulin	Alkaline Phosphatase	GGT	Prothrombin Time
Prehepatic icterus, no liver pathology	N	↑	0	↑	N-↑[1]	N	N	N	N	N	N
Intrahepatic icterus, hepatocellular damage	↑[2]	N-↑[3]	↑	↑	↑	↑	N-↑	N	N-↑	N-↑	↑
Posthepatic icterus, bile duct obstruction	↑[4]	N-↓	↑	↓[5]	↑-N[6]	N	N	N-↑	↑	↑	N[7]

Key to symbols: ↑ = increased, ↓ = decreased, N = normal, 0 = none.

1. If serum bilirubin is elevated or animal has abnormal fat metabolism there may be competitive uptake resulting in increased retention and reduced clearance.
2. 25% of total in horse, 50% of total in dog and cat.
3. Always increased in horse, up to 40% of total in other animals.
4. 60 to 90% of total in dog and cat.
5. Absent only if obstruction is complete.
6. If obstruction has been present for several days the serum ALT or AST may be increased as a result of hepatocyte damage.
7. May be increased if obstruction is prolonged.

out the additional information that can be obtained from a histologic examination. Liver biopsies are usually of the needle type. Indications for such a biopsy include (1) malignant hepatic neoplasms; (2) suspected fibrosis when liver function tests are normal; (3) obscure liver disease; (4) metabolic diseases such as amyloidosis, lipidosis, and glycogen storage disease; (5) heavy metal intoxications by molybdenum, arsenic, or selenium. There is some danger associated with liver biopsy, and the complications that may ensue include hemorrhage as the result of rupture of a large vessel, hepatitis, or peritonitis resulting from bacterial contamination. Complications may also arise from a punctured gallbladder or dilated bile duct. If liver function is markedly reduced, synthesis of coagulation factors may be diminished, and control of bleeding may be a problem following biopsy.

The pathologist is handicapped in determining the histologic status of the liver because of the small quantity of tissue removed in the usual biopsy. Consequently, localized liver disease may be present and not be detected by microscopic examination of biopsy tissue, although it will usually be possible to detect lesions that are of a diffuse nature. Before attempting a liver biopsy, the clinician should be acquainted with the technique required for the animal species involved.

It must be remembered that an alteration in metabolic function may exist without an accompanying histologic change.

REFERENCES

1. Gronwall, R., Engelking, L. R., and Noonan, N.: Direct measurement of biliary bilirubin excretion in ponies during fasting. Am. J. Vet. Res., 41:125, 1980.
2. Center, S. A., Leveille, C. R., Baldwin, B. H., and Tennant, B. C.: Direct spectrometric determination of serum bile acids in the dog and cat. Am. J. Vet. Res. 45:2043, 1984.
3. Bunch, S. E., Center, S. A., Baldwin, B. H., Reimers, T. J., Balazs, T., and Tennant, B. C.: Radioimmunoassay of conjugated bile acids in canine and feline sera. Am. J. Vet. Res., 45:2051, 1984.
4. Hardy, R. M.: Diseases of the liver. In Textbook of Veterinary Internal Medicine. Diseases of the Dog and Cat, 2nd ed., edited by Ettinger, S. J., W. B. Saunders Company, Philadelphia, 1983.
5. Cornelius, C. E., Holm, L. W., and Jasper, D. E.: Bromsulphalein clearance in normal sheep and in pregnancy toxemia. Cornell Vet., 48:305, 1958.
6. Cornelius, C. E., Theilen, G. H., and Rhode, E. A.: Quantitative assessment of bovine liver function, using the sulfobromophthalein sodium clearance test. Am. J. Vet. Res., 19:560, 1958.
7. Morrow, D., Hillman, D., Dade, A. W., and Kitchen, H.: Clinical investigations of a dairy herd with the fat cow syndrome. J.A.V.M.A., 174:161, 1979.
8. Hunton, D. B., Bollman, J. L., and Hoffman, H. N., II: Hepatic removal of indocyanine green. Proc. Staff Meet. Mayo Clin., 35:752, 1960.
9. Bonasch, H., and Cornelius, C. E.: Indocyanine green clearance—liver function test for the dog. Am. J. Vet. Res., 25:254, 1964.
10. Ketterer, S. G., Wiegand, B. D., and Rapaport, E.: Hepatic uptake and biliary secretion of indocyanine green and its use in estimation of hepatic flow in dogs. Am. J. Physiol., 199:481, 1960.
11. Prasse, K. W., Bjorling, D. E., Holmes, R. A., and Cornelius, L. M.: Indocyanine green clearance and ammonia tolerance in partially hepatectomized and hepatic devascularized anesthetized dogs. Am. J. Vet. Res., 44:2320, 1983.
12. Halliday, G. J., and Mulligan, W.: Parasitic hypoalbuminaemia: Studies on type II ostertagiasis of cattle. Res. Vet. Sci., 9:224, 1968.
13. Howard, E. B., and Kenyon, A. J.: Canine mastocytoma: Altered alpha-globulin distribution. Am. J. Vet. Res., 26:1132, 1965.
14. Hurvitz, A. I., Haskins, S. C., and Fischer, A. A.: Macroglobulinemia with hyperviscosity syndrome in a dog. J.A.V.M.A., 157:455, 1970.
15. Shull, R. M., Osborne, C. A., Barrett, R. E., Schultz, R. D., Stevens, J. B., Hammer, R. F., and Hurvitz, A. I.: Serum hyperviscosity syndrome associated with IgA multiple myeloma in two dogs. J.A.A.H.A., 14:58, 1978.
16. MacEwen, E. G., Hurvitz, A. I., and Hayes, A.: Hyperviscosity syndrome with lymphocytic leukemia in three dogs. J.A.V.M.A., 170:1309, 1977.
17. Hurvitz, A. I.: Gammopathies. In Current Veterinary Therapy, 8. Small Animal Practice, edited by Kirk, R. W., W. B. Saunders Company, Philadelphia, 1983.
18. Dewhirst, M. W., Stamp, G. L., and Hurvitz, A. I.: Idiopathic monoclonal (IgA) gammopathy in a dog. J.A.V.M.A., 170:1313, 1977.
19. Burghen, G. A., Biesel, W. R., Walker, J. S., Nims, R. M., Huxsoll, D. L., and Hildebrandt, D. K.: Development of hypergammaglobulinemia in tropical canine pancytopenia. Am. J. Vet. Res., 32:749, 1971.
20. Barsanti, J. A., Kristenson, F., and Drumheller, F. B.: Analysis of serum proteins using agarose electrophoresis in normal dogs and dogs naturally infected with Dirofilaria immitis. Am. J. Vet. Res., 38:1055, 1977.
21. Kadhim, J. K.: Changes in serum protein values of sheep infected with Fasciola gigantica. Am. J. Vet. Res., 37:229, 1976.
22. Pfeiffer, N. E., and McGuire, T. C.: A sodium sulfite-precipitation test for assessment of colostral immunoglobulin transfer to calves. J.A.V.M.A., 170:809, 1977.
23. Rumbaugh, G. E., Ardans, A. A., Ginno, D., and Trommershausen-Smith, A.: Measurement of neonatal immunoglobulin for assessment of colostral immunoglobulin transfer. Comparison of single radial immuno-diffusion with the zinc sulfate turbidity test, serum electrophoresis, refractometry for total serum protein, and the sodium sulfite precipitation test. J.A.V.M.A., 172:321, 1978.
24. Tennant, B., Baldwin, B. H., Braun, R. K., Norcross, N. L., and Sandholm, M.: Use of the gluteraldehyde coagulation test for detection of hypogammaglobulinemia in neonatal calves. J.A.V.M.A., 174:848, 1979.
25. Bradylak, S. F., Dodds, W. J., and Van Vleet, J. F.: Plasma coagulation factor abnormalities in dogs

with naturally occurring hepatic disease. Am. J. Vet. Res., 44:2336, 1983.

26. Meyers, D. J., Strombeck, D. R., Stone, E. A., Zenoble, R. D., and Buss, D. D.: Ammonia tolerance test in normal dogs and in dogs with portasystemic shunts. J.A.V.M.A., 173:377, 1978.

27. Hoe, C. M., and Harvey, D. G.: An investigation into liver function in dogs. Part I. Serum transaminases. J. Small Ani. Pract., 2:22, 1961.

28. Asquith, R. L., Edds, G. T., Aller, W. W., and Bortell, R.: Plasma concentrations of iditol dehydrogenase (sorbitol dehydrogenase) in ponies treated with aflatoxin B_1. Am. J. Vet. Res., 41:925, 1980.

29. Dorner, J. L., Hoffmann, W. E., and Long, G.: Corticosteroid induction of an isoenzyme of alkaline phosphatase in the dog. Am. J. Vet. Res., 35:1457, 1974.

30. Hoffmann, W. E., and Dorner, J. L.: Disappearance rates of intravenously injected canine alkaline phosphatase isoenzymes. Am. J. Vet. Res., 38:1553, 1977.

31. Hoffmann, W. E.: Diagnostic value of canine serum alkaline phosphatase and alkaline phosphatase isoenzymes. J.A.A.H.A., 13:237, 1977.

32. Hoffmann, W. E., and Dorner, J. L.: Separation of canine alkaline phosphatase by cellulose acetate electrophoresis. J.A.A.H.A., 11:183, 1975.

33. Hoffmann, W. E., Renegar, W. E., and Dorner, J. L.: Serum half-life of intravenously injected intestinal and hepatic alkaline phosphatase in the cat. Am. J. Vet. Res., 38:1637, 1977.

34. Everett, R. M., Duncan, J. R., and Prasse, K. W.: Alkaline phosphatase, leucine aminopeptidase, and alanine aminotransferase activities with obstructive and toxic hepatic disease in cats. Am. J. Vet. Res., 38:963, 1977.

35. Center, S. A., Baldwin, B. H., King, J. M., and Tennant, B. C.: Hematologic and biochemical abnormalities associated with induced extrahepatic bile duct obstruction in the cat. Am. J. Vet. Res., 44:1822, 1983.

36. Shull, R. M., and Hornbuckle, W.: Diagnostic use of serum gamma-glutamyltransferase in canine liver disease. Am. J. Vet. Res., 40:1321, 1979.

37. Badylak, S. F., and Van Vleet, J. F.: Sequential morphologic and clinicopathologic alterations in dogs with experimentally induced glucocorticoid hepatopathy. Am. J. Vet. Res., 42:1310, 1981.

38. Meyer, D. J.: Serum gamma-glutamyltransferase as a liver test in cats with toxic and obstructive liver disease. J.A.A.H.A., 19:1023, 1983.

8

CARBOHYDRATE METABOLISM AND FUNCTION OF THE PANCREAS AND DIGESTIVE TRACT

CARBOHYDRATE METABOLISM

Carbohydrates function primarily as fuel, the degradation of which represents a major source of body energy. In addition, the products of carbohydrate metabolism aid in the breakdown of many foodstuffs, acting as catalysts or as oxidative reactants. Carbohydrates can also be used as starting material for the biological synthesis of other compounds, such as fatty acids and certain amino acids. Carbohydrates also play a role in the structure of biologically important compounds such as glycolipids, glycoproteins, heparin, nucleic acids, and other substances.

Digestion and absorption of carbohydrates begin with the initial contact of food with the enzymes of salivary secretion. Little digestion takes place in the stomach except for a small amount of acid hydrolysis. However, digestion is extensive in the small intestine, primarily as the result of the activity of carbohydrate-splitting enzymes. In the small intestine, starch and glycogen are hydrolyzed to glucose by amylase and maltase, lactose is hydrolyzed to glucose and galactose by lactase, and sucrose is hydrolyzed to glucose and fructose by the enzyme sucrase. The monosaccharides glucose, galactose, and fructose are the principal forms in which carbohydrates are absorbed. Absorption takes place through the mucosa of the small intestine by a mechanism of simple diffusion utilizing an active method.

The only sugar normally found in blood is glucose, which is stored in the form of its polymer, glycogen. Normally, glycogen is found only in the intracellular form, whereas glucose is found almost exclusively in extracellular fluids. The level of glucose in blood is maintained within a relatively narrow range and is controlled by several factors including (1) hepatic and renal uptake and release of glucose, (2) glucose removal by the peripheral tissue, (3) effects of hormonal influences on these processes, and (4) intestinal absorption of glucose, which has only a temporary effect on blood levels.

The liver, and to a lesser extent the kidneys, are the only endogenous sources of blood glucose. Both organs contain glucose-6-phosphatase, which is necessary for conversion of glucose-6-phosphate to glucose. The liver is the most important source, as it can both remove and contribute glucose to the blood as well as synthesize it from amino acids and fatty acid fragments. The blood sugar level may serve as a stimulus to the liver and is a factor in determining whether glycogenesis or glycogenolysis will predominate.

The principal hormone affecting the blood glucose level is insulin. Insulin acts to (1) accelerate glucose oxidation, (2) accelerate conversion of glucose to fat, (3) inhibit gluconeogenesis in the liver, (4) increase liver glycogen formation, inhibit hepatic glycogenolysis by other hormones, or both, and (5) inhibit excessive ketogenesis.

The activity of glucocorticoids has been studied principally in adrenalectomized animals. In such animals the principal alterations found are decrease in liver glycogen, decrease in muscle glycogen, hypoglycemia, and decreased intestinal absorption of glucose.

Hypophysectomized animals have been used for studies of anterior pituitary factors that influence carbohydrate metabolism. In such animals, there is a tendency to hypoglycemia on fasting, a decrease in liver and muscle glycogen on fasting, increased sensitivity to insulin, increased utilization of carbohydrates, and amelioration of diabetes in alloxanized or depancreatized animals.

Blood Glucose Determination. Blood glucose determinations should be completed in any animal suspected of having diabetes or pancreatitis, in any animal with unexplained comas or convulsions, in animals such as hunting dogs that tire easily and quickly, in sheep or cattle in which ketosis is suspected, and in young pigs suspected of having a hypoglycemia associated with starvation. In addition, a blood glucose determination may be included as a part of a routine physical examination of patients, particularly aged animals, as it will often reveal the existence of a disease entity not previously suspected. Glucose estimation is included in most biochemical profiles.

Limitations of Test. Some older techniques depend upon the ability of glucose to reduce an alkaline copper solution containing the cupric (Cu^{++}) copper to a cuprous (Cu^+) form. However, blood also contains some nonsaccharide reducing substances that may interfere with the results. Included in this group of reducing substances are creatine, creatinine, glutathione, uric acid, and ergothioneine. As a result of the presence of these nonsaccharide reducing substances, the type of test utilized will sometimes influence the results. The Folin and Wu method will give values approximately 20 to 30 per cent higher than other acceptable methods, since it depends on the reduction of an alkaline copper solution. The Nelson modification of the Somogyi method avoids some of the pitfalls of the Folin and Wu technique, as it eliminates much of the effect of nonsaccharide reducing activity. The principal limitation of this technique, however, is that it is not effective at extremely low levels. Glucose oxidase methods for determining levels of blood glucose have been developed, are the most accurate presently available, and have for the most part, replaced other methods.

The results of a blood glucose determination may be affected by the diet of the individual and, in particular, the length of time since the last feeding. A standard procedure must be utilized to minimize the influence that feeding and diet may have on blood glucose levels. In nonruminants and young ruminants, it is advisable to make blood glucose determinations using samples removed following a 12- to 24-hour fast. In older ruminants, there is little, if any, influence of diet, as it has been determined that carbohydrates given orally do not affect blood glucose levels.

Technique of Test. The handling of a sample of blood for glucose determination is important. Glucose breakdown in whole blood occurs at the approximate rate of 10 per cent per hour at room temperature and may be more rapid if the sample is contaminated with microorganisms. Consequently, filtrates and serum should be prepared as quickly as possible if there is to be any delay in completing the determination. If the testing procedure must be delayed, sodium fluoride should be used as an anticoagulant. Sodium fluoride at the rate of 10 mg/ml of blood acts both as an anticoagulant and as a glucose preservative. Refrigeration will preserve the glucose level in the specimen for a few hours.

Normal Values. Normal values for blood or plasma glucose in various species of domestic animals are presented in Table 8–1. These represent the results of several methods and can be used as a guideline for interpretation of laboratory results.

Plasma and serum glucose values are generally higher than those for whole blood. This occurs because adult erythrocytes contain less glucose than does plasma. This factor must be taken into consideration when interpreting results of laboratory estimations of glucose.

Interpretation of Results. HYPERGLYCEMIA. Increased blood glucose concentration results from either an imbalance between hepatic output of glucose and peripheral uptake of the sugar or disturbances in the endocrine regulatory influence upon these processes. Consequently, a hyperglycemia may result from (1) a normal hepatic output of glucose with a subnormal rate of peripheral removal, (2) an increase in hepatic production and release of glucose with normal removal rate by the peripheral tissues, or (3) a combination of these factors.

The most spectacular increase in blood glucose probably occurs in diabetes mellitus. In clinical cases of diabetes, blood glucose is generally above 200 mg/dl; however, levels as high as 1250 mg/dl have been reported. Although diabetes mellitus occurs most frequently in dogs and cats, it has also been reported in horses, cattle, sheep, and pigs. The incidence of diabetes has been estimated to be as high as 1:152 for dogs and 1:800 in cats. Such a relatively high incidence of diabetes is an indication of its importance as a clinical entity. Additional discussion of diabetes mellitus will be found in the section on diseases of the pancreas later in this chapter. The functional alteration in diabetes is an actual or relative lack of insulin that results in an inability of the body to utilize glucose.

Abnormal functioning of other hormone-producing organs may influence glucose levels. Increased activity of the anterior pituitary, the adrenal cortex, and, to a lesser degree, the thyroid may result in hyperglycemia. Hyperpituitarism in the early stages may produce hyperglycemia, as do endogenous or exogenous increases in glucocorticoids. The glucose increase is not usually great. Excessive quantities of thyroid hormone may increase blood glucose levels if the rate of peripheral utilization cannot keep pace with the increased hepatic output.

Anoxia may result in hyperglycemia, since liver glycogen is relatively unstable in the presence of

TABLE 8–1. Normal Values for Glucose in Blood, Plasma or Serum in Various Animal Species

Species	Specimen	Value	Method
Bovine	Plasma or serum	45–70	
	Plasma	39–52	Somogyi filtrate-glucose oxidase
	Blood	53.2 ± 8.3	Glucose oxidase
	Plasma	72.3 ± 6.9	Glucose oxidase
	Serum*	55–110	Glucose oxidase
Dairy cattle	Serum	65.5 ± 8.7	
Feedlot cattle	Serum	96.0 ± 14.6	
Ovine	Plasma or serum	50–80	
	Plasma	35–74	Somogyi filtrate-glucose oxidase
	Blood	45.9 ± 8.3	Glucose oxidase
	Plasma	54.5 ± 7.4	Glucose oxidase
Caprine	Blood	45–60	Somogyi
	Plasma or serum	50–75	
Porcine	Serum	64–122	
	Plasma or serum	85–150	
	Serum*	65–95	Glucose oxidase
Equine	Blood	66–100	Somogyi
	Blood	61.1 ± 6.7	Glucose oxidase
	Plasma	83.5 ± 4.7	Glucose oxidase
	Plasma or serum	75–115	
	Serum*	70–110	Glucose oxidase
Canine	Blood	53.7 ± 8.8	Glucose oxidase
	Plasma	75.0 ± 8	Glucose oxidase
	Plasma or serum	70–110	
	Serum*	60–100	
Feline	Blood	60–100	Somogyi
	Plasma or serum	50–75	
	Plasma or serum	64–118	
	Serum*	60–120	Glucose oxidase

* Values used in clinical pathology laboratory, Kansas State University, College of Veterinary Medicine.

a deficient oxygen supply. Convulsions associated with eclampsia, intracranial trauma, epilepsy, and tetany may cause an increase in glucose, probably due to a combination of anoxia and the secretion of epinephrine.

A transitory hyperglycemia may be associated with digestion, exposure to cold, and the administration of morphine or xylazine hydrochloride, or it may be found following general anesthesia or injections of epinephrine, and subsequent to glucose infusions or ingestion of large quantities of carbohydrate. A transitory hyperglycemia is common in cats, cows, and occasionally horses, particularly in those that are excited. Serum levels often approach values that suggest a diagnosis of diabetes mellitus. Since these transitory hyperglycemias occur following treatment or secondary to other conditions that may be readily assessed, one must consider all possible factors in interpreting the results of a blood glucose determination.

HYPOGLYCEMIA. A decrease in blood glucose values may result from (1) normal hepatic glucose output with increased peripheral uptake, (2) a decrease in hepatic gluconeogenesis combined with normal peripheral utilization of glucose, or (3) a combination of these two mechanisms.

Hyperinsulinism may result from a neoplasm of the pancreas that involves an increase in the number of functional cells in the islets of Langerhans or from an overdose of insulin in the treatment of diabetes mellitus. Neoplasia of the islets of Langerhans of the pancreas has been reported in the dog. This disease is characterized by a persistent hypoglycemia associated with periods of fainting and weakness and convulsions and coma during the hypoglycemic crisis. Establishment of the diagnosis depends upon the finding of a significant hypoglycemia, usually below 50 to 60 mg/dl at the time of occurrence of the signs. Clinical signs are usually relieved by the administration of glucose. In mild cases of neoplasm of the islets, a diagnostic hypoglycemia may be absent; however, it may be provoked by placing the animal on a low carbohydrate diet for one week, followed by a 24-hour fast, and finally by moderate exercise.[1] Blood glucose levels should be determined at the end of each step and the test terminated if hypoglycemia becomes evident.

Hepatogenic disorders may also result in a hypoglycemia. General hepatic dysfunction as a consequence of circulatory deficiency and cirrhosis may be accompanied by a decrease in plasma glucose. Glycogen storage disease, which is characterized by pathologic increases in liver glycogen, will result in a hypoglycemia. This is a rare disease in humans, and a similar syndrome has been reported in the dog.

Hypoglycemic states may be present following severe exertion, in stages of starvation, and in association with hormonal alterations accompanying hypothyroidism, and sometimes with adrenal cortical insufficiency, and hypopituitarism.

Hypoglycemia in hunting dogs has been described. The glucose decrease is transitory and usually occurs within one to two hours after the beginning of the hunt. Affected dogs become weak, stagger, and have grand mal seizures. They recover quickly but remain weak.

Hypoglycemia of baby pigs is a clinical entity that occurs during the first few days of life and is characterized by a blood glucose level usually below 40 mg/dl. This decrease in glucose is accompanied clinically by convulsions, weakness, coma, and finally death. At birth, the blood glucose level in the pig is high, being above 100 mg/dl, and unless the pig is fed, the glucose level drops rapidly within 24 to 36 hours. A similar syndrome is not observed in other domestic animals, as it has been found that newborn lambs, calves, and foals are able to resist a starvation hypoglycemia for more than a week.

Ketosis in ruminants is characterized by hypoglycemia. Carbohydrate metabolism in ruminants is considerably different from that in nonruminants. Energy metabolism in ruminants is related to the utilization of volatile fatty acids produced by rumen fermentation rather than by carbohydrates. Large quantities of indigestible carbohydrates ingested by ruminants are fermented by the rumen microorganisms. Digestible carbohydrate in the diet does not escape the same fermentation. Consequently, glucose absorption by the digestive tract provides for a minimal quantity of the daily glucose requirement of a ruminant. Blood glucose sources in the ruminant are derived principally from propionate, lactic acid, and, to a lesser extent, butyric acid. This mechanism of glucose conversion is a rather delicately balanced carbohydrate economy and undoubtedly plays an important role in the development of ketosis in both sheep and cattle. The mechanism by which imbalances occur has been studied extensively but as yet has not been fully elucidated.

Glucose Tolerance Tests. Glucose tolerance tests (GTT) are indicated as a confirmatory method for the diagnosis of deviations in normal glucose metabolism. Glucose tolerance is determined by evaluating the concentration of blood glucose at specific intervals before and after the oral or intravenous administration of a given quantity of glucose. Both oral and intravenous methods may be used in the dog; however, in ruminants the intravenous method must be used, since there is no blood glucose response to oral administration of carbohydrate.

Oral Glucose Tolerance Tests. If glucose is administered orally to a normal monogastric animal, a typical alteration in glucose concentration with time is observed. Three phases are seen. Phase one is the absorptive period, during which the rate of glucose absorption into the circulation exceeds that of removal, and the blood glucose concentration increases. As the level rises, hepatic glucose output is inhibited and the secretion of insulin stimulated. In one-half to one hour, the peak level is reached and the blood glucose concentration begins to fall. During this period of decreasing blood glucose (phase two), the rate of removal exceeds that of entry. This is followed by phase three in which the glucose level, having reached its original value, continues to fall to a minimal level and then returns to the pretest level.

To conduct the oral glucose tolerance test in the dog, first take a fasting blood sample then administer a test meal consisting of 4 gm of glucose per kilogram of body weight. Take blood samples at 30- to 60-minute intervals for a three- to four-hour period. In a diabetic animal, the fasting blood sugar level is usually more than 120 mg/dl of blood; the blood sugar level during the test is above 180 mg/dl and does not return to normal during the testing period. In a normal animal, the fasting blood sugar level is less than 120 mg/dl; this value does not exceed 160 mg/dl at the end of the first hour and returns to normal by the end of the second hour.

Intravenous Glucose Tolerance Tests. In the intravenous low-dose tolerance test, 0.5 gm of glucose per kilogram of body weight is injected intravenously as a 50 per cent solution. Before receiving the injection, animals (except adult ruminants) undergo a standard 24-hour fast. Care should be taken to administer the glucose slowly, over a period of at least five minutes for small animals and at the rate of 20 ml/minute for larger animals. As with the oral glucose tolerance test, a blood sample for analysis is taken prior to administration of glucose and at intervals for two to three hours. The essential difference between an oral and an intravenous glucose tolerance test is the lack of an absorptive phase in the latter test. However, phases two and three are similar to those described for the oral glucose tolerance test. Since phase one is eliminated, it must be remembered that the curve has been shortened and glucose will return to a normal level more quickly than it does in the oral test. The peak glucose level occurs at the end of the injection period. Although glucose tolerance tests are utilized principally in the diagnosis of diabetes, decreased tolerance may be observed, although with less consistency, in hyperpituitarism, severe liver disease, hyperadrenalism, and hyperthyroidism.

A high-dose intravenous glucose tolerance test (H-IVGTT) in which K values for glucose disappearance are calculated, has been used.[2] A blood sample is obtained at the beginning of the test (zero time), and glucose (as a 50 per cent glucose solution) injected intravenously within 30 seconds at a dosage level of 1 gm/kg body weight. Postinfusion blood samples are obtained at 5, 15, 30, 45, and 60 minutes from a vein other than the one used for glucose injection. Glucose values are estimated and the K value determined by the following formula:

$$K = \frac{69.3}{T_{1/2}}$$

The half-life ($T_{1/2}$) is calculated for either the time interval in which glucose falls from 500 to 250 mg/dl in dogs with a high plasma glucose value or from 300 to 150 md/dl in dogs with a normal plasma glucose.

Normal K values for glucose disappearance are in the range of 2.14 ± 0.19 to 3.01 ± 0.38. Acute pancreatitis significantly reduces mean K values (1.13 ± 0.44). The glucose tolerance curves for the H-IVGTT in normal animals showed that the plasma glucose concentration returned to the preinjection level 45 to 60 minutes following injection. If the return to preinjection levels is delayed beyond one hour, it suggests an altered tolerance curve. In dogs with hyperadrenocorticism, the plasma glucose level may remain high but K values are normal.

DISEASES OF THE PANCREAS

The mammalian pancreas possesses a dual function. The hormonal function is limited to the production of insulin, which is important in carbohydrate metabolism, and glucagon, which appears to have its activity confined to liver glycogen. The exocrine function of the pancreas is the production of digestive enzymes including amlyase, trypsin, and lipase.

In diseases of the pancreas, with the exception of diabetes mellitus, the principal alteration is in exocrine function. Diseases of the exocrine pancreas can be divided into the following categories:[3]

1. Acute pancreatitis
   A. Acute interstitial (edematous)
   B. Acute hemorrhagic (necrotic)
2. Chronic pancreatitis
   A. Relapsing
   B. Interstitial (persistent)
3. Exocrine pancreatic insufficiency
   A. Secondary to relapsing chronic pancreatitis; following acute pancreatitis; in protein-calorie malnutrition
   B. Pancreatic acinar atrophy
4. Neoplasia (ductile or acinar cell)

Acute pancreatic necrosis is characterized by sudden onset, severe abdominal pain, and some-times shock. This disease is usually observed in obese animals. If the animal survives for more than a few days, pancreatic acinar and insulin deficiencies may develop.

Chronic pancreatitis may represent the recovery phase of an acute attack of pancreatic necrosis. The onset of exocrine pancreatic insufficiency secondary to pancreatitis is usually gradual and may be observed in any age or breed of dog. The clinical signs include ravenous appetitie and voluminous stools that are characteristically gray and fatty and have a fetid odor. If the case is far advanced, the diabetic syndrome may be present.

Junveile acinar atropy, a rare disease in dogs, has similar clinical signs. Insulin deficiency does not usually occur, but the animal has characteristic voluminous, clay-colored, rancid stools and a ravenous appetite.

Neoplasia of the exocrine pancreas may result in clinical signs similar to those observed in diseases of the liver, stomach, and small intestine. These signs include epigastric pain, jaundice, chronic weight loss, vomiting, and diarrhea. Laboratory results are variable and may reflect metastasis to other organs. Although the amylase and lipase values may be increased, often they are within normal limits.[3] If the tumor is of the islet cells, clinical signs of hypoglycemia are present. Hypoglycemic signs can usually be induced by excessive exercise just prior to feeding and are evidenced by panting, trembling, a stiff-legged gait, and muscular twitching.

Abnormal function of the islets of Langerhans is most commonly associated with hypoinsulinism producing characteristic diabetes mellitus. This condition may occur as a primary entity or may be associated either with acute pancreatic necrosis, if the animal survives the acute attack, or with chronic pancreatitis. Hyperinsulinism is usually associated with neoplasia of the islet cells.

Indications for Pancreatic Function Tests. Tests for the functional status of the pancreas should be part of any complete examination when the clinician suspects that this organ may be involved either directly or indirectly as a cause of the disease in question. Diagnosis of pancreatic disease can be difficult, as the clinical signs may be atypical, and the only observable signs may be those characteristic of digestive disturbance. If such signs are present, laboratory tests of pancreatic function assume considerable importance as aids to diagnosis. The laboratory tests most commonly used for detection of pancreatic abnormalities are based on direct examination of pancreatic enzymes or on elevation of enzymes in the blood in association with necrotic lesions. Exocrine pancreatic disease assumes two forms: acinar damage or acinar deficiency. The history and clinical signs may assist in differentiation of these acinar diseases and laboratory determinations may be confirmatory. All tests for pancreatic function should be accompanied by tests for diabetes mellitus. Tests commonly used for pancreatic function include the following:

1. Microscopic examination of feces for detection of fat, undigested protein, or starch.
2. Examination of feces for presence of trypsin.
3. Serum lipase determinations.
4. Serum amylase determinations.
5. Blood glucose and glucose tolerance determinations.
6. Absorption tests.

Pancreatic disease is often accompanied by secondary involvement of other organ systems. These complications are most readily identified by clinical signs and completion of a biochemical profile.

Techniques for Pancreatic Function Tests

Examination of Feces. Examination of the feces is of value in chronic pancreatitis, pancreatic fibrosis, and pancreatic acinar atropy. Fecal examination will reveal gross and microscopic alterations suggestive of pancreatic disease. The results of testing the feces for proteolytic activity may also reflect diminished pancreatic exocrine function.

MICROSCOPIC EXAMINATION. In animals having exocrine pancreatic deficiency, little, if any, digestion of fat occurs. This lack of fat digestion is a direct result of a decrease in lipase in the pancreatic juices. Fat appears in the stool in the form of neutral fat globules. These fat globules can be detected microscopically by examining a diluted (approximately 1:1 with water) sample of feces that has been stained with Sudan III. Sudan III is prepared by mixing equal parts of 70 per cent alcohol and acetone with an excess of Sudan III stain. Fatty acids can be identified by heating a mixture of fecal smear with four drops of 36 per cent acetic acid and staining with Sudan III. The fatty acid soaps are transformed into free fatty acids and will stain with Sudan III. Fat globules are orange or red. If a pancreatic deficiency exists, large numbers of these globules can be demonstrated under low-power magnification of the microscope. Undigested starch can be demonstrated by staining a fecal smear with 2 per cent tincture of iodine. Undigested starch is blue. The presence of such blue particles suggests starch maldigestion; however, if the animal has been consuming poorly digestible carbohydrates (e.g., paper) a false-positive result can occur.

Feces may also be examined for the presence of striated muscle. Diluted feces are examined under the microscope, and muscle fibers appear light yellow. If fibers remain undigested because of a lack of trypsin, cross striations will be readily visible. This test is of little value unless the animal is being fed meat.

TEST FOR FECAL TRYPSIN. Two tests are routinely used for the detection of fecal trypsin activity. These tests are based on the incubation of gelation with feces to determine the proteolytic activity present in a fecal sample.

GELATIN TUBE TEST. This relatively simple test can be easily conducted in the laboratory, and all reagents can be purchased at the local supermarket. This test is based on the ability of trypsin to attack gelatin in such a manner that, following incubation of the enzyme and gelatin, the gelatin solution will no longer solidify. The procedure for this technique is as follows:

1. Bring 9 ml of water to a total volume of 10 ml by adding feces and mixing well. Samples from the patient and an apparently normal (control) individual should be tested.
2. Warm 2 ml of a 7.5 per cent gelatin solution (ordinary household gelatin) to 37° C, add 1 ml of 5 per cent sodium bicarbonate and 1 ml of the fecal dilution, and mix. Prepare a blank by placing 2 ml of gelatin, 1 ml of 5 per cent sodium bicarbonate, and 1 ml of distilled water in a second tube.
3. Incubate both tubes at 37° C for one hour or at room temperature for $2\frac{1}{2}$ hours.
4. Refrigerate the tubes for 20 minutes and read the results.

Failure of the sample to solidify indicates the presence of trypsin. The blank should gel readily at refrigeration temperature, whereas the control should remain liquid. Occassionally, solidification of the gel will not occur at 20 minutes and it will be necessary to prolong refrigeration. The test and control samples should not be read until the blank has solidified.

The gelatin tube test is conducted in our laboratory with 1:50 and 1:100 fecal dilutions in addition to the 1:10 dilution described earlier. If trypsin is present in normal concentration, the 1:50 and 1:100 dilutions do not solidify. The higher dilution reduces the contribution of proteolytic enzymes from intestinal bacterial flora as well as diluting any trypsin inhibitor that might be present in feces. It is advisable to dilute the normal fecal sample as an additional control.

Confirmation of trypsin deficiency is dependent on repeated demonstration of its absence. A single negative test (solidification of gelatin) should not be considered absolute evidence of an exocrine pancreatic deficiency.

FILM TEST. This procedure is based on the digestion of the gelatin present on exposed or fresh x-ray film and the identification of this action by clearing of the film.

1. Bring 9 ml of 5 per cent sodium bicarbonate solution to a total volume of 10 ml by the addition of feces, and mix.

2. Place a drop of diluted feces on a piece of x-ray film or place a strip of film in the diluted feces (the latter method is preferred). On a second strip, use 5 per cent sodium bicarbonate.

3. Incubate at room temperature for $2\frac{1}{2}$ hours or at 37° C for one hour.

4. Rinse off both pieces of film, being careful to avoid excessive pressure that might wash the emulsion from the film. When gelatin is wet for a long period of time, it has a tendency to separate from the film base. If this occurs, a false-positive test for trypsin will result.

5. Clearing of the test film where it has been soaked with the fecal mixture indicates the presence of trypsin and a functional pancreas. The second film soaked with the sodium bicarbonate solution should remain unchanged in appearance. The film test is a less sensitive technique for detecting the presence of fecal trypsin. False-negatives have been reported to be as high as 25 per cent. The tube test should be used for confirmation of samples negative for trypsin with the film test.

Total Fecal Fat. The qualitative assessment of fecal fat on the basis of microscopic examination using a specific fat stain can be difficult to interpret. Quantitative fecal fat and fecal trypsin determinations were completed in a series of dogs with a history of diarrhea.[4a] For this test 24-hour pooled collections of feces were obtained and the concentration of fat and trypsin determined in a sample from the pooled feces. Prior to testing, all dogs were weighed and fed a meat-based canned dog food at the rate of 50 gm/kg body weight for at least 72 hours. In order to standardize the results, total fecal fat and trypsin were expressed as gm/kg body weight/day. Normal values were 0.24 ± 0.01 for fecal fat and 4.96 ± 1.66 for fecal trypsin. In animals with pancreatic insufficiency total fecal fat was 2.08 ± 0.35 while fecal trypsin dropped to 0.49 ± 0.22 gm/kg body weight per day. Animals with intestinal malabsorption had 1.14 ± 0.11 gm/kg body weight per day of fecal fat while trypsin was 15.2 ± 1.94 gm/kg body weight per day. The authors indicated that total fecal fat could not be used to differentiate between exocrine pancreatic insufficiency and intestinal malabsorption. However, the marked decrease in trypsin in those with pancreatic insufficiency in comparison to the very high level of fecal trypsin in those with intestinal malabsorption permitted such a differentiation.

When results of other tests to differentiate intestinal malabsorption from exocrine pancreatic insufficiency are equivocal, the quantitative fecal fat and fecal trypsin tests may be of assistance.

Serum Lipase Determinations. Estimation of the quantity of lipase present in a serum sample is based upon the ability of this enzyme to hydrolyze a standard suspension (emulsion) of olive oil. Lipase activity is reflected by the release of fatty acids, which are titrated using a standard sodium hydroxide solution. Units of lipase activity are expressed as the number of milliliters of 0.1 N sodium hydroxide required to neutralize the fatty acids released per milliliter of serum. Reagents for this determination are commercially available from the Sigma Chemical Co., St. Louis, Missouri. Details for use of the Sigma Serum Lipase Kit are presented in the Appendix, p. 444. Serum lipase values in normal animals are 1 unit or less when this technique is used.

A one-hour method for determination of serum lipase has been described.[5] This method was used for estimating lipase activity in dog serum; the mean normal value was 5.6 Roe-Byler units with a normal range from 0.8 to 12.0 Roe-Byler units.[6] Details for this technique are presented in the Appendix, p. 445.

Spectrophotometric techniques for quantitation of lipase activity are now available. As with other enzyme determinations, normal values should be established in each laboratory.

Serum Amylase Determinations. Estimations of amylase activities in body fluids are generally based on determining the rate of appearance of the breakdown products of starch (saccharogenic technique) or the rate of disappearance of starch (amyloclastic method). A method for estimating amylase activity has been developed in which a dye is attached to a starch substrate (Amylochrome, Roche Diagnostics, Nutley, New Jersey). Amylase acting upon this substrate releases the dye, which can then be assayed photometrically.

Normal values for serum amylase activity are dependent upon the technique of the test utilized. Therefore, veterinarians should establish normal values for their own laboratories. Details of techniques for estimating amylase activity are presented in the Appendix, pp. 445–446. Amylase activity depends on the presence of calcium ions, and use of a chelating type of anticoagulant should be avoided. Serum is preferred to plasma as a sample for the amylase test.

Blood Glucose and Glucose Tolerance. As indicated previously, a glucose determination should be included as a part of any series of laboratory tests used for the diagnosis of pancreatic deficiencies. Methods for the determination of glucose levels and glucose tolerance have been discussed previously in this chapter.

Absorption Tests. The capacity of an animal to absorb dietary fats may be utilized as a method for measuring pancreatic deficiency or other malabsorption syndromes. Dietary fats must be hydrolyzed to fatty acids and glycerol in order to be absorbed. If pancreatic lipase is absent, little or no fat absorption occurs.

A simple absorption test is based on a comparison of plasma turbidity prior to and following a fatty meal. A heparinized blood sample is drawn from a fasted animal and centrifuged. Lipomul (Upjohn Co., Kalamazoo, Michigan) or corn oil is added at a rate of 3 ml/kg of body weight to a small quantity of food and fed to the patient. Two, three, and four hours following the fat meal, heparinized blood samples are drawn and centrifuged. The turbidities of the pre- and post-feeding samples are compared.

In the normal animal, the plasma in the postfeeding sample should be turbid, indicating development of lipemia from the breakdown and absorption of fat. If the plasma in the postfeeding sample remains clear, it can be assumed that there is a deficiency in exocrine pancreatic function or that the intestine is incapable of proper absorption. In order to differentiate between these two conditions, the test can be repeated at a later date with the addition of pancreatic enzymes to the feed. If the lack of fat absorption in the initial test was due to a lipase deficiency, hyperlipemia should develop. If the lack of postfeeding lipema was a consequence of malabsorption, the addition of pancreatic enzymes will not influence the results, and both the pre- and postfeeding plasmas will remain clear.

It has been suggested[3] that this absorption test is complicated by the delayed gastric emptying that accompanies a high fat meal. If a delay occurs, results may be false-negative if the post-meal sampling is discontinued too soon. Most normal animals will have a lipemia by three hours after feeding.

The vitamin A absorption test is based on the same principle as the fat absorption test. Vitamin A in an oil emulsion is administered orally, and absorption is determined by measurement of vitamin A levels in the blood. In the normal animal, an increase in serum vitamin A will occur. The absence of such an elevation indicates absorptive failure. This test has not been widely used because of difficulties in accurately determining serum vitamin A concentrations.

Tests based on absorption of ^{131}I oleic acid and ^{131}I triolein have been used to determine and differentiate intestinal absorption abnormalities. When these two assays are performed in sequence, it is possible to differentiate between steatorrhea caused by a deficiency of pancreatic enzymes and that caused by primary malabsorption.[4] If steatorrhea is due to a lack of pancreatic lipase, absorption of oleic acid will be normal, whereas that of triolein will be reduced. If the problem is malabsorption, absorption of both compounds will be reduced. Specific data regarding the utilization of these tests as routine measurements in clinical situations are not available.

A starch tolerance test has been used for detecting canine pancreatic malabsorption.[7] Soluble starch is made into a paste with 1.5 ml of cold water per gram of starch, then an additional 4 ml of hot water per gram of starch is added. This sus-

pension is well mixed to provide an almost clear liquid gel that can be administered to a dog by feeding or by stomach tube. The starch solution is fed at a rate of 3 gm/kg of body weight. A zero-time blood specimen is collected, and samples are collected at 30, 60, 90, 120, and 180 minutes following consumption of the starch solution.

Plasma reducing sugar levels were estimated, and in normal dogs a peak of 127 ± 19.2 mg glucose/dl of plasma was reached 60 minutes after the starch feeding. Dogs with pancreatic insufficiency had marginal peaks of 99.5 ± 6.9 and 100.5 ± 3.4 mg glucose/dl of plasma at 60 and 90 minutes, respectively, following starch consumption. The low plasma reducing sugar peaks found in dogs with pancreatic insufficiency after consumption of the starch solution readily distinguished them from healthy dogs in which there were substantial increases in plasma reducing sugar following administration of the starch solution. The animals in this study had extensive pancreatic damage. Dogs with less pancreatic insufficiency produce ambiguous test results.

A peptide, N-benzoyl-l-tyrosyl-p-aminobenzoic acid (BT-PABA), has been used in the diagnosis of exocrine pancreatic insufficiency in dogs. This peptide is cleaved by chymotrypsin from the pancreas but not to any great extent by pepsin or intestinal peptidases.[8] When cleavage occurs, p-aminobenzoic acid (PABA) is released, rapidly absorbed into the blood, and excreted by the kidneys. Following oral administration of the BT-PABA, urine or blood assays for PABA are completed and the level is an indication of the metabolism of the peptide and thus reflects chymotrypsin activity.

If chymotrypsin is present in normal amounts the six-hour PABA urine excretion has been reported to be 63.1 per cent ± 3.53 per cent.[8] In another study[9] a 73.6 per cent urine excretion was reported. PABA excretions less than 46 per cent have been considered abnormal. Dogs with PABA excretion greater than 20 per cent in six hours did not have problems that required pancreatic enzyme replacement therapy, although they probably had an enzyme deficiency. Because the test is dependent upon normal renal function, animals with renal disease are likely to have abnormal excretion of PABA. Dogs that are being treated with chloramphenicol, sulfonamides, pancreatic extracts, or diuretics within five days of the test should be excluded, because these substances may interfere with test results.[8]

In an attempt to differentiate between exocrine pancreatic insufficiency and intestinal malabsorption, the BT-PABA and xylose absorption tests were combined.[10,11] The test is conducted as follows:

1. The patient is fasted at least overnight and blood is collected in EDTA before administration of the chemicals.

2. The BT-PABA:xylose solution is prepared by dissolving BT-PABA (Adrin Laboratories, Columbus, Ohio) powder and D-xylose powder at a concentration of 1 gm/dl and 10 gm/dl, respectively.

3. The preparation is administered by stomach tube at a dosage of 5 ml/kg body weight.

4. Blood samples are collected in EDTA at 30, 60, and 90 minutes.

5. Plasma samples are analyzed for PABA[12] and xylose[13] (see Appendix, pp. 446–447).

In clinically normal dogs the 90-minute PABA values were 15.3 ± 5.2 µg/ml, in dogs with malabsorption they were 9.0 ± 3.4 µg/ml, and in dogs with pancreatic exocrine insufficiency they were 0.4 ± 0.4 µg/ml.[11] Xylose absorption was normal (a peak xylose level greater than 45 mg/dl at 60 to 90 minutes) in clinically normal dogs, was slightly decreased in dogs with pancreatic exocrine insufficiency, and was markedly decreased in those with malabsorption problems.

It appears that an absorption test combining BT-PABA and xylose would be of value in making a more definitive differentiation between exocrine pancreatic insufficiency and malabsorption syndromes.

LABORATORY FINDINGS IN PANCREATIC DISEASES

The laboratory findings in acute pancreatic necrosis, chronic pancreatitis, juvenile acinar atrophy, islet cell neoplasm, and diabetes mellitus are summarized in Table 8–2.

Acute Pancreatic Necrosis

Serum Amylase Determinations. Alpha amylase is an enzyme that acts on starch to liberate maltose. It is present in serum from normal animals. Amylase activity in serum increases in association with pancreatic diseases, although the mechanism of the entrance of pancreatic amylase into blood is not completely understood. The increase in serum amylase activity associated with acute pancreatitis probably results both from an escape of the enzyme into the peritoneal cavity, with increased absorption through lymphatics and veins, and from reabsorption of amylase from pancreatic interstitial tissue. Obstruction of the ductal system will also produce an elevation in serum amylase activity.

In experimentally induced pancreatitis in the dog,[14] maximum amylase activity was detected within 24 to 48 hours following induction of pancreatic damage. Peak activities of amylase varied from 800 to 8000 Caraway units/dl, with a mean increase of approximately eight times the preoperative value.

In naturally occurring cases of acute pancreatitis confirmed by histologic examination, mean serum amylase activity increased to about seven times the normal value.[15] In the same study, 22 dogs probably affected with acute pancreatitis had serum amylase activities approximately 2½ times greater than normal levels. The investigators were unable to demonstrate any significant increase in serum amylase in dogs with primary gastrointestinal disease. It was recommended that acute pancreatitis should be considered when serum amylase values exceed twice the normal value if no uremia is present.

Serum amylase levels increase in dogs with chronic primary renal failure.[16] Serum amylase activity two to four times normal may be seen in dogs with renal failure as indicated by tests for renal function. In one study, 59 per cent of the dogs with spontaneously occurring renal failure had hyperamylasemia.[16] There was no correlation between serum amylase activity and serum urea nitrogen concentrations. The authors believed that it was not possible to accurately predict changes in serum amylase activity on the basis of renal function parameters. This was true because of the wide baseline variations that occur in serum amylase activity in normal dogs. A two- to three-fold increase in serum amylase induced by reduction in renal function may produce widely varying serum amylase activities because the variation in baseline activity is apparently greater than the variation induced by different degrees of renal dysfunction.

Interpretation is further complicated because renal disease may occur secondarily to pancreatic disease. However, with acute pancreatitis, the level of serum amylase activity is usually more than four times normal.

Although stress has been reported to elevate serum amylase activity, this has not been proved. Dexamethasone treatment did not cause an increase in serum amylase activity.[17]

In acute necrotic pancreatitis, amylase activity is high in peritoneal fluid, and the activity in this fluid may be higher than that in plasma.

Serum Lipase Determinations. Because of the variability in normal values reported for amylase activity in serum and the reported nonspecific increases in amylase activity, it has been suggested that the serum lipase determination is preferable to the serum amylase assay in detecting pancreatic necrosis.

Hyperlipasemia usually occurs in animals with an acute necrotic pancreatitis. In acute pancreatitis that was experimentally induced by the injection of crude staphylococcic alpha toxin,[2] serum lipase values in six dogs increased from a preinjection mean value of 0.37 ± 0.109 units to 4.98 ± 0.967 units within 24 hours. Serum lipase values had returned to within normal limits (0.86 ± 0.402 units) in six days. Amylase activity followed the same general pattern. Similar observations were made following injection of carbon

TABLE 8–2. Laboratory Findings in Pancreatic Diseases

Disease	Character of Feces	Fecal Fat and Protein	Fecal Trypsin	Absorption Tests — FAT	Absorption Tests — BT-PABA	Absorption Tests — D-XYLOSE	Serum Amylase	Serum Lipase	Serume Glucose	Fasting Lipemia	Other Laboratory Tests
Acute pancreatitis	Blood-tinged after 1–2 days	Fat may be + if of 1–2 days' duration	Present	N-↓	N-↓	N	↑	↑	N-↑	Frequent	↑ Urine amylase, ↑ BUN & Cr, ↑ PCV, ↑ Cholesterol if lipemia: leukogram—stress + inflammation; ALT usually ↑ may be N; glucosuria if ↑ blood glucose
Chronic pancreatitis	Soft, pale, bulky, frothy, fetid	Fat + undigested protein + starch +	Absent 1:100, 1:50 and usually at 1:10	↓	↓	N	N-↑	N-↑	Often ↑	–	Glucosuria if ↑ blood glucose; leukocytosis if active inflammation —none if no inflammation; abnormal GTT if diabetic
Juvenile acinar atrophy	Massive, granular, soft, pale, frothy, fetid	Fat + undigested protein + starch +	Absent	↓	↓	N	N	N	N	–	
Islet cell neoplasm (functional)	N	Absent	Present	N	N	N	N	N	↓	–	Abnormal GTT; AIGR > 30
Diabetes mellitus	N	Absent	Present	N	N	N	N	N	↑	N-+	Glucosuria, ketonuria, ketonemia, ↑ cholesterol, abnormal GTT, ↑ ALT, ↑ BUN, ↑ SAP, acidosis, polyuria, polydipsia

↑ = Increased
↓ = Decreased
N = Normal
+ = Present
– = Absent

tetrachloride into the pancreatic parenchyma.[14] In these animals, maximum lipase activity was detected 24 to 48 hours after the pancreas was damaged. Maximum lipase activity varied from 18 to 260 Roe-Byler units per milliliter with a mean increase of five to seven times preinjection values.

It has been reported that in humans, serum lipase levels become elevated several hours after increases in serum amylase values and remain elevated for a longer period of time. Brobst et al.[14] were unable to duplicate these results, as they found that increases in serum lipase and amylase activity paralleled one another. In spite of this experimental evidence, reports from the field suggest that the serum lipase level may indeed remain elevated longer than the serum amylase level. Until sufficient data are obtained, we cannot assume that this prolonged serum lipase elevation does not occur in clinical cases of pancreatitis.

Serum lipase activity is also increased in dogs with renal failure.[16] In 41 dogs with spontaneously occurring primary renal failure, 37 per cent had increased serum amylase and lipase activities, 22 per cent had increased serum amylase activity with normal serum lipase activity, 12 per cent had increased serum lipase activity and normal serum amylase activity, and 29 per cent had normal serum and lipase activities. The following mechanisms were postulated to be responsible for the hyperamylasemia and hyperlipasemia in renal failure: (1) reduced renal excretion of pancreatic enzymes, (2) reduced renal degradation of pancreatic enzymes, and (3) functional or morphologic pancreatic alterations induced by uremia. In this series of dogs the authors were unable to demonstrate any relationship between the microscopic appearance of the pancreas and the increase in serum amylase or lipase activities. They concluded that the occurrence of chronic renal failure in dogs without acute pancreatitis would be expected to have an approximate increase in serum amylase activity of more than twofold and a two- to fourfold increase in serum lipase activity. Detection of any great increase in these enzymes in dogs with renal failure may suggest the presence of concurrent acute pancreatitis.

Dexamethasone injections produced a statistically significant increase in serum lipase activity.[17] In animals given a high dose of dexamethasone for seven days, the highest lipase activity occurred on day 8 and was 1.7 ± 0.4 Sigma-Tietz units/ml. Similar observations were made in a low dexamethasone dose (0.02 mg/kg TID for 21 days). The highest lipase activity was 1.8 ± 1.0 Sigma-Tietz unit/ml on day 22. Although these lipase increases represent a statistically significant deviation from the untreated control group, they are well below the lipase levels associated with acute pancreatitis that we see in our laboratory. These experiments do, however, emphasize the need for an individual evaluation of all laboratory results on the basis of treatment.

Hemogram. As with any other inflammatory condition, the leukocyte response in acute pancreatic necrosis is dependent upon the severity and duration of the condition. In early phases of acute pancreatitis, the leukocyte response is typical of stress, with lymphopenia and eosinopenia accompanied by neutrophilia. As the condition progresses, neutrophilia may increase and a left shift may appear. In the terminal stages, a degenerative left shift may develop.

Dehydration may occur in acute pancreatitis because of reduced fluid intake and prolonged vomiting, and in these animals the packed cell volume (PCV) is elevated. If dehydration is severe and flood flow reduced, renal impairment may occur, resulting in prerenal uremia. This is not a consistent finding, but occurs with enough regularity that blood urea nitrogen (BUN) levels should always be estimated in dehydrated animals with acute necrotic pancreatitis. An elevated UN value with a urine specific gravity greater than 1.030 will confirm prerenal uremia in dehydrated patients.

Hyperlipemia. A fasting hyperlipemia frequently occurs in dogs with acute pancreatic necrosis. The appearance of a "milky" plasma in an animal that has not eaten for some time is suggestive of lipemia, which can be confirmed by microscopic examination of the erythrocytes using new methylene blue stain. If plasma opacity is a result of increased lipid content, chylomicra can be observed surrounding the erythrocytes. Lipemia may also be associated with the nephrotic syndrome, hypothyroidism, diabetes mellitus, hepatic disease, and hyperadrenocorticism. Primary idiopathic hyperlipemia has been reported in the dog.

Other Laboratory Determinations. Blood glucose determinations may be of value in assessing acute necrotic pancreatitis, not as a diagnostic test, but to evaluate the simultaneous occurrence of diabetes mellitus. As diabetes is a frequent sequela to acute pancreatic necrosis, early evaluation of insulin productive capacity of the pancreas is indicated.

There may be a marked increase in blood cholesterol in hyperlipemic animals.

Hypocalcemia has been reported in association with acute pancreatitis in humans and may occur in acute pancreatitis of the dog. It is not, however, a consistent finding in dogs with an acute necrotic pancreatitis.

The serum alanine amino transferase (ALT) activity may be normal or increased in dogs with acute pancreatitis. An elevated ALT level is not a consistent finding and when present probably indicates liver damage that has occurred secondary to the primary pancreatic lesion.

If metabolic acidosis accompanies pancreatic

necrosis and shock, other biochemical alterations may be present (see Chapter 10).

If the patient is dehydrated, the UN level in serum may be increased. Occasionally, coagulation defects may be associated with acute pancreatitis and should be evaluated as previously discussed (Chapter 5).

Chronic Pancreatitis

Serum Amylase and Lipase Determinations. If the pancreas is inflamed or there is obstruction of the pancreatic excretory ducts, serum amylase and lipase activities may be elevated. If fibrosis has occurred and acinar tissue haas been replaced by connective tissue, serum enzyme activity will be normal. Serum enzyme determinations are valuable in chronic pancreatitis for assessing the presence or absence of continuing inflammatory and necrotic processes.

Glucose Levels. Chronic pancreatitis is often accompanied by destruction of the insulin-producing beta cells of the pancreas, which allows diabetes mellitus to develop. In one study[18] 50 per cent of the dogs with chronic pancreatitis were also diabetic. The mean blood glucose concentration of these animals was 352 mg/dl with a range of 252 to 420 mg/dl. As diabetes mellitus is a common sequela to chronic pancreatitis, blood or plasma glucose levels should always be determined when such a condition is suspected. Glucosuria will appear when the blood glucose value is above the renal threshold for glucose.

Fecal Examination. Examination of feces from an animal suspected of having a pancreatic insufficiency has value as a screening procedure. The examination should begin with visual observation of the feces. In pancreatic deficiencies, the fecal specimen is bulky, pale yellow to clay color, may glisten with undigested fat, and has a fetid odor.

Neutral fat may be detected microscopically by staining the specimen with Sudan III. If the animal is on a meat or meat-containing diet, undigested muscle fibers may be present.

The feces can be examined for the presence of trypsin as previously described. In chronic pancreatitis, fecal trypsin is usually absent at a fecal dilution of 1:50 and is not usually detected at a dilution of 1:10. This test must be interpreted with care, as bacterial enzymes capable of digesting protein may be present in sufficient concentration to give a positive test for trysin activity.

Absorption Tests. A number of absorption tests have been described. In interpreting the results of these tests it must be remembered that reduced ability to absorb fats may be a consequence of a pancreatic lipase deficiency or of the inability of the intestine to absorb digested fats. If the initial fat absorption test is negative, the test should be repeated utilizing commercially desiccated pancreatic enzymes either for predigestion of the test meal or for oral administration just prior to or simultaneously with the fat. The BT-BAPA absorption is also reduced, as is starch absorption.

Juvenile Acinar Atrophy. Laboratory findings in association with acinar atrophy of the juvenile type are essentially those consistent with a lack of pancreatic function without other sequelae. Fecal trypsin and lipase are absent; absorption tests are negative but return to positive with administration of pancreatic enzymes; and feces are characteristically bulky, fetid, and fat-containing.

As there is no inflammatory reaction, blood values for lipase and amylase are within normal limits. Diabetes does not usually occur and, therefore, blood glucose and glucose tolerance values are normal.

Pancreatic Neoplasia. Although pancreatic tumors are infrequent in domestic animals, they have been reported in the dog, cat, cow, and sheep. Anderson and Johnson[19] studied 14 dogs with pancreatic carcinoma. The clinical behavior of these carcinomas was similar to that of pancreatic carcinoma in humans, in that recognizable alterations in pancreatic function appeared late in the course of the disease. Total failure of exocrine function was not evident in any of the dogs in this study. The authors found rather extensive metastasis of the pancreatic carcinoma, with the liver being the organ most extensively involved. Laboratory tests supported this finding as evidence of inadequate liver function as reflected by sulfobromophthalein (BSP) retention; elevation of serum ALT was observed in some animals.

Functional islet cell tumors were reported in three dogs.[18] Blood glucose concentration in these animals was markedly reduced with a range of 30 to 40 mg/dl. This is characteristic for functional islet cell neoplasia of the pancreas.

Three cases of insulin-secreting islet cell carcinomas in dogs were described.[20] Clinically, the cases were characterized by convulsions and low fasting blood glucose levels of from 35 to 56 mg/dl. An intravenous glucose tolerance test of one dog showed a subnormal fasting blood sugar level with a peak of 114 mg/dl 30 minutes following glucose administration and a drop to subnormal levels within two hours. The low blood glucose level persisted for seven hours.

The glucose tolerance test as performed in the conventional manner is of limited value in hyperinsulinism.[1] The shape of the tolerance curve is influenced by the previous carbohydrate intake of the dog, since a high-carbohydrate diet favors a low peak in the tolerance curve and a low-carbohydrate diet a high peak. The glucose tolerance test curve is usually characteristic if the animal is placed on a high carbohydrate diet for three to four days, the intravenous test is used, and blood sampling is continued for six to eight hours. A prolongation of the hypoglycemic phase is the most significant portion of the curve. Although hypoglycemia is characteristic for hyperinsulinism in the dog, in mild cases the fasting glucose level may be normal. In these circumstances, a diagnostic hypoglycemia may be provoked by placing the animal on a low-carbohydrate diet for a week followed by a 24-hour fast and moderate exercising. If blood glucose levels are determined at the end of each step, a hypoglycemia will be evidenced in cases of mild hyperinsulinism.[1]

The development of radioimmunoassay for plasma insulin has made evaluation of the endocrine function of the pancreas much easier. For a dog suspected of having hyperinsulinism, it has been recommended[21] that a feeding be given at 7 AM and blood be drawn beginning at 9 AM every two to three hours until the glucose concentration has fallen below 60 mg/dl. Once this has occurred serum from that same sample is submitted to a laboratory for an insulin assay. The patient is then fed. Normally there is a direct relationship between serum concentration of glucose and insulin. As the serum glucose falls, serum insulin also falls. When the glucose concentration nears 30 mg/dl, serum insulin concentrations are near 0. An amended insulin-glucose ratio (AIGR) has been used based on these observations. The AIGR is obtained using the formula:

$$\frac{\text{Serum insulin } (\mu M/ml) \times 100}{\text{Serum glucose } (mg/dl) - 30} = \text{AIGR}$$

The normal AIGR has been reported to be 15.6 ± 4.14 in one study of four dogs, and in a review of 18 normal dogs the value was 13.9 ± 4.60.[22] Hyperinsulinism is confirmed by an AIGR level greater than 30. Borderline or unexpected normal values should be repeated.

Diabetes Mellitus. Diabetes mellitus is most frequently found in the dog and the cat, although it has been reported in horses, cattle, sheep, and pigs. Regardless of animal species, the fundamental defect in diabetes mellitus is an absolute or relative lack of insulin. As a result of this deficiency in insulin, the animal is unable to utilize glucose. Consequently, hyperglycemia is a constant finding in the diabetic animal. Clinical signs typically associated with diabetes include polydipsia, polyuria, increased appetite, and weight loss. These classic signs of diabetes are often followed by clinical signs of ketosis including anorexia, vomiting, weakness, lethargy, and an increased respiratory rate.

Hyperglycemia. A fasting hyperglycemia is probably the most important diagnostic criterion for diabetes mellitus. Glucose levels in clinical cases are generally above 200 mg/dl, but may be much higher. In early stages of diabetes, glucose levels may not be dramatically increased, and glucose levels of 125 to 180 mg/dl may be observed in animals with no clinical signs of disease.

Hyperglycemia in diabetic animals may tend to compensate in part for decreased peripheral utilization of glucose. This occurs partially as a mass action effect resulting in an inflow of glucose into tissues. Thus, in the absence of insulin, a diabetic animal may continue to utilize glucose at the expense of increased glucose production and hyperglycemia.

When the blood glucose level exceeds the renal threshold for glucose, glucosuria appears. Renal thresholds for glucose in domestic animals have been reported as follows:[1] bovine, 90 to 102 mg/dl; ovine, 160 to 200; caprine, 70 to 120; equine, 180 to 200; and canine, 175 to 220. It is obvious that renal threshold values for glucose are above the normal upper limits for plasma glucose. Thus, an animal may have an insulin deficiency without glucosuria. Glucosuria, even if glucose is present in only trace amounts, must be considered of significance, and further examinations must be completed to detect the cause.

The laboratory findings of survivors and nonsurvivors in 28 dogs with naturally occurring diabetes mellitus have been compared.[23] The mean blood glucose level in nonsurvivors was significantly greater than in those animals that survived (434 ± 65 mg/dl for nonsurvivors, 339 ± 76 mg/dl for survivors). The authors suggested that the stress of coexisting disorders in nonsurvivors might partially explain the significantly higher initial blood glucose level in nonsurvivors. They also mentioned that insulin resistance accompanying acidosis might have been a factor. Cotton et al. noted that the blood glucose concentration did not decrease significantly when nonsurvivors were being given insulin subcutaneously and suggested that intravenous administration of insulin might prove more beneficial, at least until an affected dog responded and danger of shock was over.

In animals in which the fasting blood glucose level is slightly or moderately elevated, a glucose tolerance test may be of value. Under no circumstances should a glucose tolerance test be administered to a frankly diabetic animal. The results of a glucose tolerance test in the diabetic animal are as indicated in Figures 8-1 and 8-2. The characteristic blood glucose curve shows a decreased tolerance for glucose, which is a direct reflection of the inability of the animal to dispose of the additional glucose presented to it.

Although polyuria and polydipsia are classically described as clinical signs of diabetes mellitus, it must be remembered that an appreciable polyuria probably does not occur until the blood glucose level approaches 250 mg/dl. As the blood glucose level continues to increase, diuresis becomes marked, and there is an increase in water intake when blood glucose levels surpass 300 mg/dl.

Lipemia and Ketonemia. As glucose utilization progressively diminishes in a diabetic animal, the metabolism rapidly turns to utilization of fatty acids for energy purposes. These fatty acids are obtained by mobilization from the body fat and are then utilized by the liver. Fat mobilization may become excessive, and frank lipemia is evidenced by the appearance of a cloudiness in the plasma of a fasted animal.

In addition to the appearance of neutral fat in the blood plasma, ketone bodies begin to accumulate in excess of the capacity of peripheral tissues to utilize them. When this occurs, the ketone bodies (acetoacetic acid, beta-hydroxybutyric acid, and acetone) appear in the urine. Ketonuria is frequently observed in advanced diabetic conditions. The appearance of ketone bodies in urine is an indication of developing acidosis. The presence or absence of ketone bodies in urine is frequently used as a method of evaluating the effectiveness of therapy.

Acidosis and Electrolyte Balance. Concentrations of ketone bodies in plasma may lead to vomiting and the loss of potassium, sodium, and chloride. Perhaps of more significance is the fact that acetoacetate and beta-hydroxybutyrate are strong acids. As a consequence, large amounts of sodium and especially potassium ions are lost in the renal excretion of acetoacetate and betahydroxybutyrate. These two acids also combine with fixed base in the plasma to reduce the alkali reserve, which is reflected by a bicarbonate deficiency and frequently a decrease in blood pH. As a compensatory mechanism, there is a hyperpnea that will decrease carbon dioxide partial pressure (P_{CO_2}).

There appears to be no relationship between the severity of the metabolic acidosis and the magnitude of the hyperglycemia.[24] Although the blood pH of a ketotic diabetic animal may be normal, a bicarbonate deficiency of as much as 50 per cent may be present. If there is a decrease in blood pH, the bicarbonate deficiency is almost always in excess of 50 per cent.

In spite of the loss of sodium and potassium, diabetic cats and dogs with ketoacidosis most frequently have near-normal serum levels of these two ions. Occasionally there may be a hyponatremia, since sodium may also be lost as a consequence of impaired kidney tubular reabsorption associated with the osmotic diuresis. Hypokalemia may be observed, although hyperkalemia occurs terminally owing to the severe acidosis. A severe hypokalemia may develop during intensive insulin therapy; therefore serum potassium should be monitored and replacement therapy initiated according to needs.

With the osmotic diuresis that accompanies diabetes mellitus there is a loss of water and electrolytes. Dehydration and acidosis may culminate in collapse and coma. This is of greater significance in individuals with renal insufficiency.

Because of the dehydration, one must always interpret serum electrolyte values in relation to total fluid volume. With reduced fluid volume, an animal may actually have hypokalemia even though the plasma potassium concentration is normal. This must always be taken into consideration in providing replacement fluids for diabetic acidotic animals. Administration of fluids without some potassium could effectively provide an increase in fluid volume but a subsequent hypokalemia.

Cholesterol Levels. Blood cholesterol levels are invariably increased in diabetic animals. Cholesterol levels are indicative of the chronicity and severity of the disease, with values ranging from 300 mg/dl in early cases to 900 mg/dl in more advanced cases.

Hemogram. There is little specific change in the hemogram in association with diabetes mellitus. Leukocytosis may occur. An increased leukocyte count in the diabetic dog dictates that the clinician search for coexisting disease that may require specific treatment. In one study,[23] nonsurvivor diabetic dogs had mean total leukocyte counts of 26,550 ± 1450 cells/μl as compared with a mean leukocyte count of 14,200 ± 550 cells/μl in animals that survived. Alterations in erythrocytes most frequently reflect the state of hydration of the individual. Hemolysis is generally present in significantly lipemic blood because the susceptibility of erythrocytes to hemolysis is increased when chylomicra are present in the plasma in large numbers. In addition to the hemoconcentration, there is usually a severe systemic stress, as indicated by lymphopenia and eosinopenia.

Serum Enzyme Activity. Although serum enzymes are not characteristically altered in primary diabetes mellitus, it is nevertheless beneficial to perform some serum enzyme determinations to detect the presence of coexisting disease.

Acute pancreatitis was a major factor in the deaths of five out of 10 dogs with naturally occurring diabetes mellitus.[23] This acute pancreatitis was characterized by an increase in serum amylase activity.

Serum ALT and serum alkaline phosphatase (SAP) levels are often elevated in association with the fatty metamorphosis that occurs in response to disturbed fat metabolism. Determination of serum ALT and SAP concentrations might be of value in monitoring the response of an animal to therapy. This is particularly true if other clinical signs of liver disease develop. If the condition progresses to a frank icterus, the prognosis is poor.

Blood Urea Nitrogen and Serum Creatinine Levels. Uremia is frequently seen with diabetes mellitus, although it is not a consistent finding. If the patient is dehydrated, prerenal uremia may exist. Blood urea nitrogen and serum creatinine levels were significantly increased in nonsurviving dogs with diabetes mellitus, whereas they were generally normal in animals that survived.[23] The mean UN value in 16 dogs that survived following treatment of diabetes mellitus was 23 ±

19 mg/dl, whereas in 11 patients that did not survive, the mean UN value was 58 ± 31 mg/dl. These authors cautioned that an initial increase in UN or creatinine values when a dog with diabetes mellitus is first presented should alert the clinician to a clinical entity that will complicate treatment of diabetes mellitus.

Urinalysis. As mentioned previously, glucosuria will occur when the blood glucose value exceeds the renal threshold for glucose. Renal glucosuria can be differentiated from diabetes mellitis by completion of a blood glucose determination.

Considerable information has been written about the specific gravity of urine in dogs and cats with diabetes mellitus. It is true that the addition of glucose to urine will increase its specific gravity. However, it must be remembered that glucose will increase urine specific gravity by only approximately 0.004 unit for each gram of glucose per deciliter of urine. Therefore, if glucose·is present even at a high concentration, its effect on specific gravity is minimal. Consideration must also be given to the amount of water intake and the functional capacity of the kidneys before evaluating specific gravity.

In advanced cases of diabetes mellitus, ketonuria is usually observed but is not necessarily diagnostic of diabetes, since starvation may also result in a ketonuria. In the mild diabetic, ketone bodies are often not detectable.

Proteinuria is frequently observed in association with diabetes in dogs. This is particularly true when diabetes is uncontrolled and changes in the renal basement membrane have occurred. Urine casts may be observed in animals with a proteinuria.

Anuria is frequent in seriously ill diabetic dogs. Urine production should be monitored by catheterization while an animal is being treated for diabetic ketoacidosis. Urine output, urine glucose, and ketones can be monitored.[24]

Diabetic patients that are on long-term insulin therapy should be monitored on a regular basis; the use of glycosylated hemoglobin has been recommended.[25] The rate of glycosolation of hemoglobin depends upon the nature and concentration of the carbohydrate in the erythrocyte over time. Because the erythrocyte is an insulin-independent cell, intracellular glucose increases as plasma glucose rises. Glycosylated hemoglobin is in low concentration of red cells of clinically normal animals and is found in increased amounts in patients with uncontrolled diabetes.

DIGESTIVE DISEASES

Although the manifestations of digestive tract diseases may be similar to those observed with diseases of the pancreas and liver, there are some alimentary system conditions that are not associated with malfunctioning of these organs.

DIGESTIVE DISEASES OF THE DOG AND CAT

Stomach. Laboratory findings in diseases involving only the stomach are not diagnostic. One common presenting sign of gastric disease is vomiting. The state of hydration should be assessed by evaluation of the PVC, hemoglobin, total protein and albumin. If dehydration is present and the animal is not anemic, both PCV and hemoglobin will be increased. Total protein, and particularly albumin, is increased because of a loss of body water. Estimation of total protein only can be misleading if the animal has a chronic inflammation and globulins are increased. Therefore, an increase in albumin is more reflective of water loss than is an increase in total protein.

A complete blood count usually reflects excess glucocorticoid activity. There is mature neutrophilia, lymphopenia, eosinopenia, and monocytosis in the dog. Monocyte increases are not constant in the cat with excess glucocorticoids. If the animal is dehydrated and vomiting, and there is no stress leukogram,* one might suspect hypoadrenocorticism. An increase in eosinophils suggests parasitism, allergy, or an eosinophilic gastritis. One should attempt to differentiate among these causes of eosinophilia. If there has been gastric hemorrhage, there is usually a regenerative anemia. If blood loss is chronic and iron is not reabsorbed, hypochromic microcytic erythrocytes may be present.

Biochemical profiles should be completed to rule out other organic disease and to obtain preliminary information on the acid-base status of the patient. The acid-base balance and electrolyte status should be evaluated in order to develop a protocol for electrolyte and fluid therapy. Estimates should include pH, P_{CO_2}, HCO_3 or total serum CO_2, sodium, potassium, and chloride. The changes in acid-base status and electrolytes will depend on the state of disease, the amount of fluid and electrolyte loss, and the duration of the disease. (See Chapter 10.)

A fecal examination should be done to rule out parasitism. Feces should be tested to detect melena. Occultest or Hemoccult tests can be used as long as one remembers that animals on a meat-protein diet will often have false-positive results. In order for positive tests for fecal blood or hemoglobin to be valid, the animal should be on a meat-free diet several days prior to the test.

Small Bowel. Dogs and cats with small bowel disease are usually presented for treatment of diarrhea. One must differentiate small bowel dis-

---

* One showing neutrophilia, monocytosis, lymphopenia, and eosinopenia.

ease from large bowel disease. Frequently this can be done by obtaining a complete history. With diseases of the small bowel the diarrhea is usually voluminous and fluid. With most diseases of the large bowel the amount of feces is not great but there is a history of frequent defecation. The feces are often mucus-covered and may contain blood. It has been recommended that the diagnosis of intestinal disease be approached in stages.[26] In stage 1, dietary problems, parasitism, and systemic disorders are excluded and the lesion is anatomically localized to the small or large bowel using history, physical examination, stool characteristics, and preliminary laboratory tests. In stage 2, small bowel diarrhea is characterized by determining whether digestive or absorptive functions are defective through studies that identify the steatorrhea of malassimilation and then differentiate maldigestion from malabsorption. In stage 3, a definitive etiologic or histopatholgic diagnosis is made by use of more sophisticated laboratory tests, radiographs, biopsies, and observation of response to therapy.

Preliminary laboratory tests should include CBC, total serum protein and albumin, and a fecal examination for the presence of parasites.

As with diseases of the stomach, increases in PCV and hemoglobin accompanied by an absolute increase in serum albumin and total protein reflect hemoconcentration. If the animal is anemic the PCV and hemoglobin may be within normal range but the albumin is increased unless there has been protein loss or protein maldigestion. Neutrophilia and regenerative left shift suggest the presence of infection, inflammation, or necrosis. The characteristics of the stress leukogram may or may not be seen. If a degenerative left shift and/or toxic neutrophils are present, there may be endotoxemia, septicemia, or bacterial peritonitis secondary to the primary disease. Anemia in the animal may have resulted from blood loss or decreased erythropoiesis. If the anemia is regenerative, blood loss should be suspected; if nonregenerative, it may be the result of chronic inflammation or other conditions that depress bone marrow activity. In such conditions the erythrocytes are normocytic and normochromic and there are no signs of regeneration (no reticulocytosis or polychromasia). Hypochromic microcytic anemia can occur if chronic blood loss has occurred at a point in the intestinal tract where iron cannot be absorbed or if there is deficient iron absorption. In severe panleukopenia with a degenerative left shift, parvovirus infection should be suspected.

Total protein and albumin estimations can be used to detect hypoproteinemia associated with protein-losing enteropathy. Since most of the loss is albumin, serum total protein and albumin levels should be determined. In this condition the serum albumin value is low and the quantity of globulin varies. In chronic inflammation, globulin

values may be normal to low normal but are frequently increased.

No evaluation of the small bowel is complete until the feces have been examined for parasites. This should begin with a gross observation for tapeworm proglottids and a fecal flotation for identification of parasite eggs. A direct smear should be done by suspending fresh feces in a few drops of saline and examining the specimen microscopically for protozoan parasites. Detailed methods for these examinations are included in Chapter 20.

Once a tentative diagnosis of small bowel disease is made, screening tests to characterize the malassimilation should begin. Feces should be tested for the presence of fat, protein, or starch as described previously. Examination of a fecal smear stained with new methylene blue or Wright's stain may reveal cytologic findings that will aid in diagnosis. If there is disruption of the colonic mucosa, neutrophils may be present in large numbers. With diseases of the upper intestinal tract very few leukocytes are seen in the feces and scrapings of the colonic mucosa are normal.

The total fecal fat content should be estimated. In addition to determination of the total fat content of feces, the output of fecal fat has been calculated as a percentage of assimilated ingested fat using a fat-balance procedure.[27] Net fat assimilation in normal dogs was greater than 94 to 96 per cent on a meat-based diet. Dogs with exocrine pancreatic insufficiency had assimilation of 41 to 78 per cent while dogs with malabsorption had 78 to 89 per cent assimilation.

The fat absorption test previously described is a simple method for identifying maldigestion or malabsorption. The feces should be examined for the presence of trypsin to rule out an exocrine pancreatic insufficiency. If trypsin is absent the fat absorption test should be repeated using fat that has been predigested for at least 30 minutes with a pancreatic enzyme preparation such as Viokase.

Absorption-digestion tests can also aid in diagnosis. The simplest is probably the oral glucose absorption test. Following a 12-hour fast, the animal is given 2 gm/kg of dextrose in a $12\frac{1}{2}$ per cent solution via stomach tube. Blood samples are taken at the time of dextrose administration and 15, 30, 60, 90, and 120 minutes later. In a normal animal with normal blood glucose there should be an increase in serum glucose 50 mg/dl above the resting level in 30 minutes and serum glucose should return to normal within two hours. With intestinal malabsorption a lower maximum and later peak is expected. However, there may be some overlap between normal and abnormal curves.[28]

A starch digestion test,[7] as previously described, can also be utilized.

The D-xylose absorption test is preferred to measure malabsorption. This pentose is absorbed by passive and active mechanisms and is eliminated, unaffected by insulin, via the kidney. After an overnight fast the patient is given 0.5 gm D-xylose/kg of body weight in a 5 to 10 per cent solution. Blood samples are drawn at the time of oral administration of xylose and at 30, 60, 90, and 120 minutes later. The blood samples are analyzed for pentose. In normal individuals a peak of greater than 45 mg/dl occurs 60 to 90 minutes after feeding. In dogs with malabsorption the level does not go above 45 mg/dl and the curve is much flatter than in normal dogs. This test can be falsely low if there is bacterial digestion of the xylose or if a delay occurs in gastric emptying. Because pentoses are eliminated by the kidneys, a reduction in GFR may produce a false high reading. Xylose can be combined with BT-PABA as previously described.

In addition to obtaining results for the tests discussed, the clinician should attempted to determine if an infection is present. This will necessitate a fecal culture for bacteria, viruses, or fungi or the use of serologic tests to determine the animal's experience with the agent. A positive test does not confirm that the problem is a specific infectious disease—it only tells us that the individual has had contact with the antigen. When possible, paired serum samples should be tested. An increasing or decreasing titer is better evidence for making a specific causal diagnosis.

Large Bowel. Animals presenting with diseases of the large bowel usually have clinical signs that assist the veterinarian in differentiating between diseases of the small and large bowel. The most frequent sign of large bowel disease is tenesmus.[29] The animal makes frequent attempts to defecate with only a small amount of fecal matter produced. The feces frequently contain large quantities of mucus and some intact erythrocytes.

Fecal examination for parasites, direct smears for protozoa, and cytologic examinations are all indicated. If the clinician suspects an infectious disease, fecal cultures for fungi and bacteria should be submitted. Examinations for fecal trypsin, fecal fat, fecal starch, and total fecal fat are not indicated in diseases of the large bowel. A cytologic examination of feces may be beneficial in diagnosing mucosal or transmural diseases of the colon. In mucosal diseases the feces often contains large numbers of leukocytes and some intact erythrocytes. Transmural diseases have erythrocytes but leukocytes are rarely seen.[30]

DIGESTIVE DISEASES OF FOOD ANIMALS

Diseases of the Ruminant Stomach. Although laboratory results are seldom definitive in diseases of the ruminant stomach, there are a few conditions in which laboratory results can aid diagnosis and therapy. Because many of the diseases of the ruminant stomach involve changes in acid-base and electrolyte balance, the primary findings will be discussed here; pathophysiology of the changes is discussed in the chapter on electrolytes and acid-base balance.

ACUTE RUMEN ENGORGEMENT. Most cases of acute ruminant engorgement occur when the animal consumes larger than normal quantities of highly fermentable carbohydrate. Such an overload abruptly changes normal fermentation patterns in the rumen and the principal fermentation end product becomes lactic acid. This alters rumen osmotic pressure and fluid is drawn into it from blood and body tissues. The rumen pH decreases; this produces stasis and much of the rumen microflora is killed. When the rumen pH reaches 4 to 5, clinical signs of acute rumen engorgement become severe.

Affected ruminants will be hemoconcentrated, causing an increase in PCV and serum total protein and albumin. The animal becomes acidotic; when this occurs, the urine pH becomes acid. If rumen ingesta can be aspirated, a check of the pH will reveal it to be 5 or below and frequently less than 4.

TRAUMATIC RETICULOPERITONITIS. Acute to subacute traumatic reticuloperitonitis is accompanied by an absolute increase in circulating neutrophils and a left shift. There is usually lymphopenia and eosinopenia characteristic of stress. If inflammation is significant, there will be an increase in fibrinogen and a decrease in the total protein:fibrinogen ratio. Although these hematologic findings are not pathognomonic for traumatic reticuloperitonitis, they may occur when any acute inflammatory or infectious process is present in the ruminant. However, use of the hemogram along with the clinical findings may enable the veterinarian to arrive at a correct diagnosis. In animals that develop diffuse peritonitis the total leukocyte count may decrease, often with a remarkable increase in immature neutrophils including metamyelocytes and occasionally myelocytes. Although cytologic examination of peritoneal fluid has been of benefit in some animals, the findings are not consistent. Serosanguineous fluid and large numbers of neutrophils may indicate penetration of a foreign object through the reticulum and the onset of peritonitis.

PERITONITIS. The hemogram in the early stages of peritonitis is much like that observed in traumatic reticuloperitonitis and leukopenia, with a marked left shift frequent as the disease progresses. Abdominal paracentesis can aid in establishing a diagnosis. The peritoneal fluid is serosanguineous or purulent. It contains large numbers of neutrophils and macrophages, many of which are degenerated and lytic (see Chapter 14). In some cases large numbers of bacteria are present and can be found in the cytoplasm of the neutrophils and macrophages. The total protein content is greatly increased. If peritonitis has developed following a rupture or penetration of the digestive tract, plant material is often present. If peritonitis has occurred secondary to rupture of the urinary bladder, peritoneal fluid will contain urine. Urine is most easily identified by warming the fluid and detecting the characteristic urine odor.

ABOMASAL DISORDERS. Right and left abomasal displacements and abomasal torsion are characterized by hypochloremia, hypokalemia, and metabolic alkalosis. The severity of these changes varies from one patient to the next. It depends, in part, on the nature of the displacement. Torsion of the abomasum produces the most severe alkalosis and the greatest hypochloremia. (The pathophysiology of these changes is discussed in Chapter 10.) Many cows with left displaced abomasum have metabolic alkalosis, although some may be normal and occasionally metabolic acidosis may be present if the condition has persisted for some time. There is usually hypochloremia but hypokalemia is less severe. Some affected cattle will have paradoxic aciduria. Hemograms obtained at the time of the displacement or torsion usually reflect an increase in endogenous corticosteroids. Hemoconcentration as a consequence of dehydration is seen in the late stages.

VAGUS INDIGESTION. If there is vagus nerve malfunction, the ingesta is not transported through the various levels of the ruminant forestomachs; this results in a decrease in the quantity of feces and in abdominal distension, weight loss, and dehydration. Hemoconcentration is almost always present. If dehydration has become severe enough to reduce renal perfusion, azotemia may develop. If there is functional pyloric stenosis, classic metabolic alkalosis and hypochloremia develop. Similar findings have been associated with abomasal impaction but do not occur as frequently as with vagal indigestion.

HEMORRHAGE INTO THE GASTROINTESTINAL TRACT. Several conditions (abomasal ulceration, abomasal torsion, foreign body trauma, parasitic infections, bacterial or viral enteritis, and poisoning) may cause gastrointestinal hemorrhage. If frank blood is present it can be detected by a microscopic examination of the feces. Occult blood can be detected by use of tests developed for the detection of blood in human feces. The most commonly used tests are the Hematest tablet (Ames Co., Elkhart, Indiana), the Hemoccult test (Smith Kline & French Laboratories, Philadelphia, Pennsylvania) or a dilute solution of guaiac. These tests have been compared[32] by introducing blood into the rumen of cattle through a rumen fistula and testing the feces for occult blood using the methods mentioned above. The most sensitive was the dilute guaiac test; however, occult blood was detected by all tests used. Details for the guaiac method are presented in the appendix. Multiple tests (reading of several slides) of the same fecal specimen ensures improved sensitivity and reliability of the tests.

REFERENCES

1. Kaneko, J. J.: Carbohydrate metabolism. In: *Clinical Biochemistry of Domestic Animals*, 2nd ed., edited by Kaneko, J. J. and Cornelius, C. E., Academic Press, New York, 1970.
2. Greve, T., Dayton, A. D., and Anderson, N. V.: Acute pancreatitis with coexistent diabetes mellitus: An experimental study in the dog. Am. J. Vet. Res., 34:939, 1973.
3. Rogers, W. A.: Diseases of the exocrine pancreas. in: *Textbook of Veterinary Internal Medicine. Diseases of the Dog and Cat*, 2nd ed., edited by Ettinger, S. J., W. B. Saunders Company, Philadelphia, 1983.
4. Kallfelz, F. A., Nordin, R. W., and Neal, T. M.: Intestinal absorption of oleic acid 131-I and triolein 131-I in the differential diagnosis of malabsorption syndrome and pancreatic dysfunction in the dog. J.A.V.M.A., 153:43, 1968.
4a. Burrows, C. F., Meritt, A. M., and Chiapella, A. M.: Determination of fecal fat and trypsin output in the evaluation of chronic canine diarrhea. J.A.V.M.A., 174:62, 1979.
5. Roe, J. H., and Byler, R. E.: Serum lipase determination using a one-hour period of hydrolysis. Anal. Biochem., 6:451, 1963.
6. Brobst, D., and Brester, J. E.: Serum lipase determinations in the dog using a one-hour test, J.A.V.M.A., 150:767, 1967.
7. Hill, F. W. G.: A starch tolerance test in canine pancreatic malabsorption. Vet. Rec., 91:169, 1972.
8. Imandi, A. P., Stradley, R. P., and Wolgemuth, R.: Synthetic peptides in the diagnosis of exocrine pancreatic insufficiency in animals. Gut, 13:726, 1972.
9. Strombeck, D. R.: New method for evaluation of chymotrypsin deficiency in dogs. J.A.V.M.A., 173:1319, 1978.
10. Stradley, R. P., Stern, R. J., and Heinhold, N. B.: A method for the simultaneous evaluation of exocrine pancreatic function and intestinal absorptive function in dogs. Am. J. Vet. Res., 40:1201, 1979.
11. Rogers, W. A., Stradley, R. P., Sherding, R. G., Powers, J., and Cole, C. R.: Simultaneous evaluation of pancreatic exocrine function and intestinal absorptive function in dogs with chronic diarrhea. J.A.V.M.A., 177:1128, 1980.
12. Smith, H. W., Finkelstein, N., Aliminosa, L., et al.: The renal clearances of substituted hippuric acid derivatives and other aromatic acids in dog and man. J. Clin. Invest., 24:388, 1945.
13. Roe, J. H., and Rice, E. W.: Photometric method for the determination of free pentoses in animal tissues. J. Biol. Chem., 173:507, 1948.
14. Brobst, D. F., Ferguson, A. B., and Carter, J. M.: Evaluation of serum amylase and lipase activity in experimentally induced pancreatitis in the dog. J.A.V.M.A., 157:1697, 1970.
15. Finco, D. R., and Stevens, J. B.: Clinical significance of serum amylase activity in the dog. J.A.V.M.A., 155:1686, 1969.
16. Polzin, D. J., Osborne, C. A., Stevens, J. B., and Hayden, D. W.: Serum amylase and lipase activities in dogs with chronic primary renal failure. Am. J. Vet. Res., 44:404, 1983.
17. Parent, J.: Effects of dexamethasone on pancreatic

tissue and on serum amylase and lipase activities in dogs. J.A.V.M.A., *180*:743, 1982.

18. Anderson, N. V., and Strafuss, A. C.: Pancreatic diseases in dogs and cats. J.A.V.M.A., *159*:885, 1971.

19. Anderson, M. V., and Johnson, K. H.: Pancreatic carcinoma in the dog. J.A.V.M.A., *150*:286, 1967.

20. Cello, R. M., and Kennedy, P. C.: Hyperinsulinism in dogs due to pancreatic islet cell carcinoma. Cornell Vet., *47*:538, 1957.

21. Feldman, E. C.: Disease of the endocrine pancreas. In: *Textbook of Veterinary Internal Medicine. Diseases of the Dog and Cat*, 2nd ed., edited by Ettinger, S. J., W. B. Saunders Company, Philadelphia, 1983.

22. Caywood, D. D., Wilson, J. W., Hardy, R. M., and Shull, R. M.: Pancreatic islet cell adenocarcinoma: Clinical and diagnostic features of 6 cases. J.A.V.M.A., *174*:714, 1979.

23. Cotton, R. B., Cornelius, L. M., and Theran, P.: Diabetes mellitus in the dog: A clinicopathologic study. J.A.V.M.A., *159*:863, 1971.

24. Schall, W. D.: Fluid and electrolyte therapy in diabetic ketoacidosis. J.A.A.H.A., *8*:206, 1972.

25. Wood, P. A., and Smith, J. E.: Glycosylated hemoglobin and canine diabetes mellitus. J.A.V.M.A., *176*:1267, 1980.

26. Sherding, R. G.: Diseases of the small bowel. In: *Textbook of Veterinary Internal Medicine. Diseases of the Dog and Cat*, 2nd ed., edited by Ettinger, S. J., W. B. Saunders Company, Philadelphia, 1983.

27. Hill, F. W. G.: Malabsorption syndrome in the dog. A study of 38 cases. J. Small Ani. Pract., *13*:575, 1972.

28. Hill, F. W. G., and Kidder, D. E.: The oral glucose tolerance test in pancreatic malabsorption. Br. Fet. J., *128*:207, 1972.

29. Lorenz, M. D.: Diseases of the large bowel. In *Textbook of Veterinary Internal Medicine. Diseases of the Dog and Cat*, 2nd ed., edited by Ettinger, S. J., W. B. Saunders Company, Philadelphia, 1983.

30. VanKruiningen, H. J.: Canine colitis comparable to regional enteritis and mucosal colitis of man. Gastroenterology, *62*:1128, 1972.

31. Wass, W. M., Thompson, J. R., Moss, E. W., Kunesh, J. P., and Eness, P. G.: Diseases of the ruminant stomach. In *Current Veterinary Therapy. Food Animal Practice*, edited by Howard, J. L., W. B. Saunders Company, Philadelphia, 1981.

32. Payton, A. J. and Glickman, L. T. Fecal occult blood tests in cattle. Am. J. Vet. Res., *141*:918, 1980.

KIDNEY FUNCTION

A basic understanding of the mechanism of kidney function is essential to an appreciation of the significance of urinary findings and renal function tests.

The kidneys are the chief organs regulating the internal environment of the body. Urine is a by-product of these regulatory activities. In maintaining a reasonable constancy of composition of the extracellular and, to a lesser extent, the intercellular fluids, kidneys become involved in: (1) Elimination of water formed in or introduced into the body in excess of the amount required for normal metabolic processes. (2) Elimination of inorganic elements according to the needs of the body. (3) Elimination of nonvolatile end products of metabolic activity. (4) Retention within the body of substances required for the maintenance of normal functions. Included in this group are amino acids, hormones, vitamins, plasma proteins, glucose, and so forth. (5) Elimination of certain foreign toxic substances. (6) Formation and excretion of substances such as hydrogen ions and ammonia. The kidneys, therefore, play an important role in the regulation of water balance, electrolyte balance, and acid and base balance. They also play an important role in the maintenance of osmotic pressures of body fluids and in removal of metabolic waste products as well as certain toxic substances.

The functional unit of the kidney is the nephron, which consists of two functionally distinct units: (1) the glomerulus, which is primarily a vascular channel or bed that serves as a filtration unit, and (2) the tubule, which is lined by epithelial cells.

The functional capabilities of the kidney are dependent upon the manner in which blood flows through it. After entering the kidney, the renal artery divides successively into interlobar, arcuate, and interlobular branches. The interlobular branches become the afferent glomerular arterioles, which become a set of capillary loops. Each loop is closely enveloped and bound to the external layer of Bowman's capsule. The attached walls of the capillaries of the glomerulus and Bowman's capsule form a semipermeable membrane across which substances pass from the blood plasma to the lumen of the tubule by means of simple filtration.

The glomerular arterioles unite to form the efferent glomerular arteriole, which has a diameter considerably smaller than the afferent arteriole. This difference in caliber of the vessels assists in maintenance of an effective filtration pressure in the glomerular capillaries. The efferent arterioles then pass to the tubules, forming a network of capillaries that lie in close approximation to the outer tubular lining. These capillaries eventually unite to form a venous plexus, which leads successively to the interlobular, arcuate, and interlobar veins, which unite to form the renal vein.

This tortuous route through which the blood must pass in the kidney has an important bearing on functional considerations. The greatest bulk of the blood that supplies the tubules first passes through the glomeruli. Any interference in blood flow through the glomeruli will affect total renal function and may be followed by degenerative changes in the tubules.

In passing through the glomeruli the blood loses an essentially protein-free plasma filtrate. As this filtrate passes through the tubules, it is modified by excretion, reabsorption, and other activities of the tubule epithelial cells. The end product of this complex of activities is urine.

Analysis of this end product of kidney function will often reveal alterations typical of diseases of that organ but in addition may provide information concerning alterations in other physiologic processes in the body.

URINALYSIS

A critical examination of urine is an important diagnostic procedure. This body fluid is easily obtained from most species of animals, and consequently urinalysis is a routine procedure. Unfortunately, many urinalyses are conducted without specific reference to the diagnostic problem encountered and too often without correct interpretation. Utilization of urinalysis as a routine procedure has tended to obviate its actual value. Therefore, urinalysis should be conducted on a somewhat selective basis and each test evaluated in terms of the clinical signs observed by the attending veterinarian.

Since urine is the end product of a complicated and delicately balanced physiologic process, many normal and pathologic mechanisms may influence the constituents. Urine is not only altered by diseases occurring in the kidneys, but many extrarenal conditions produce changes that may be of diagnostic significance.

COLLECTION AND PRESERVATION OF URINE SPECIMENS

Urine from most species of animals may be collected for analysis as the animal voids. If voided (midstream) samples are to be collected, the vulva or prepuce should be cleaned of all contamination. Addition of a small quantity of fecal or preputial material to a urine specimen will negate many results. Use of two containers, with the contents of the first used only if a second sample from midway through micturition cannot be collected, will minimize contamination. However, as it is difficult to obtain uncontaminated midstream specimens, catheterization or cystocentesis is preferred.

Containers used for urine specimens must be clean. Disposable plastic containers have proved to be acceptable in most laboratories.

Catheterization. Catheterization is employed in many species as a method of collecting urine specimens for analysis. Care must be taken to avoid contamination with substances that might interfere with urine analysis. Addition of a chemical sterilant or excessive quantities of petrolatum or other lubricant to a urine specimen may alter the sample sufficiently to change some of its chemical and physical characteristics. Because contamination of the lower urinary tract is almost always present, catheterization should be conducted as carefully as possible using sterile equipment. Every attempt should be made to avoid traumatizing the urethra or bladder. The smallest diameter catheter that will permit urine collection should be selected. Trauma can be minimized by lubricating the distal end of the catheter with a sterilized aqueous lubricant. In order to avoid traumatic damage, local anesthesia of the urethra can be induced using a topical anesthetic.

In order to maintain asepsis during catheterization, the periurethral area should be carefully cleansed with soap and water prior to passing the catheter. Care should be taken not to contaminate the catheter by permitting it to come into contact with nonsterile areas such as the clinician's hands or the patient's hair or skin. The catheter should be passed (1) by handling it through the sterile packing material in which it is contained, (2) by utilizing sterilized forceps, or (3) by wearing sterilized rubber gloves. If difficulty is encountered in inserting the catheter, it should be immediately withdrawn, relubricated, and reinserted with a slight rotating motion. It may be necessary to utilize a smaller catheter if difficulty is again encountered. After the catheter is gently introduced through the urethra, it should be placed so that the tip is located just beyond the junction of the neck of the bladder with the urethra. Urine may be collected by free-flow or by use of a syringe equipped with a two-way valve. All aspiration attempts should be made with as little suction as possible in order to prevent trauma to bladder mucosa by pulling it into the opening in the catheter.

The first portion of the urine should be discarded, as it is often contaminated with debris accumulated during catheterization.

Samples collected by catheterization often contain a few erythrocytes and this should not concern the clinician. Unless there has been severe trauma, hematuria is mild and should not interfere with results of most laboratory determinations.

Because of inherent risk of contaminating the lower urinary tract, repeated catheterizations should be avoided, unless absolutely essential. Catheterization is not a technique to be conducted indiscriminately, but one that may be required in order to obtain representative urine specimens for analysis and culture. If the clinician utilizes asepsis, the danger of contamination and subsequent urinary tract infection is minimized.

Cystocentesis. In the smaller domestic animals (dog and cat), urine can be obtained by cystocentesis (Fig. 9–1). This is specifically indicated to obtain urine specimens for bacterial culture as well as urinalysis. Cystocentesis is performed only when the bladder contains a sufficient volume of urine so that it is readily palpable and will permit needle puncture without risk of damage to

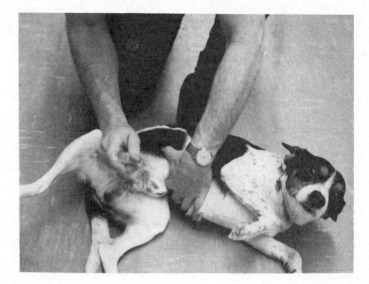

Figure 9–1. Urine can be readily obtained by means of bladder puncture in small domestic animals. The bladder should be held firmly while using a syringe and needle (1½ by 16 gauge) to tap the bladder.

the bladder or other structures. The skin should be cleansed and prepared aseptically. The bladder is located by abdominal palpation and manually immobilized. A syringe (5 to 20 ml) with a needle attached (20 to 24 gauge, 1½ to 2 inches long) is inserted through the abdominal wall and into the bladder. The needle should be inserted a few centimeters cranial to the neck of the bladder instead of into the vertex. The bladder decreases in size as urine is withdrawn and if the needle is located in the vertex, it may not remain in the lumen. The needle should be introduced into the bladder lumen at an angle, as this permits rapid sealing of the bladder wall wound when the needle is withdrawn. Gentle suction is used to remove as much urine as possible. If the bladder is distended, a two-way valve can be attached to the syringe to facilitate removal of most of the urine. If a large quantity of urine remains in the bladder, pressure may produce a leak that permits urine to escape into the abdominal cavity.

Cystocentesis should be attempted with caution in patients suspected of bladder atony as a result of a lengthy period of distention. If the cause of distention can be corrected, cystocentesis can safely be used as a therapeutic measure to relieve bladder pressure. In such circumstances, it is advisable to insert an indwelling catheter to relieve or prevent development of appreciable bladder pressure.

Manual Compression of Urinary Bladder. Urine specimens can sometimes be obtained by manual compression of the urinary bladder. In small animals, the bladder is outlined by abdominal palpation, and, with the patient in either a standing or a recumbent position, moderate digital pressure is utilized over a large area of the bladder. A steady continuous pressure is applied with the fingers and thumb of one hand or with the fingers of both hands. This pressure should be

continued until the sphincters of the urethra relax and urine is expelled. This may require several minutes of continuous gentle pressure. If the urinary bladder is greatly distended with urine, this procedure must be used with great caution in order to avoid rupture of the organ. In large animals, gentle but continuous pressure can be applied through the wall of the rectum. Specimens obtained in this fashion are often useful for urine analysis, but it must be remembered that the first portion of urine collected in this manner may be contaminated with material flushed from the genital tract or urethra. This technique is more successful in the female than the male dog because of the greater ease in overcoming urethral resistance in females.

An attempt should be made to collect as much urine as possible, although small quantities can be utilized for most of the analyses used in modern clinical pathology laboratories.

Storage. Urinalysis should be completed as quickly as possible following collection. Chemical and cytologic changes occur rapidly in urine, particularly if the specimen is held at room temperature. Bacteria, if present, multiply rapidly, and if the organism is capable of splitting urea, will increase the pH. If the urine is alkaline, casts tend to dissolve and may disappear completely in samples held for any length of time. Solutes may crystallize, changing the gross and microscopic appearance of the urine. Some cells undergo autolysis if urine is held prior to microscopic examination.

If it is impossible to complete an analysis on freshly collected urine, the specimen can be stored at refrigerator temperatures but should be warmed to room temperature prior to examination. Urine provides an excellent culture medium for a variety of microorganisms; bacterial growth and a concomitant alteration in urinary constituents begin quickly and proceed actively. If it is impossible to refrigerate a specimen, toluene, one of the better preservatives, can be added. A sufficient quantity of toluene should be added to form a layer on top of the urine. A crystal of thymol may also be used for preservation of specimens. If maintenance of the urinary sediments and in particular the structure of cells and casts is important, formalin at the proportion of one drop of 40 per cent formalin to 1 ounce of urine provides an effective agent. Formalin should not be added until chemical determinations are completed.

Urine specimens such as those discussed are adequate for qualitative analysis. However, if quantitative analyses are to be conducted, a 24-hour specimen should be collected. In the larger domestic animals, 24-hour specimens may be collected by means of a female collecting urinal, which is strapped onto the male animal. A collection cage can be utilized for obtaining 24-hour specimens of canine and feline urine. For collection of 24-hour specimens, a preservative should be added to the container in which the urine is to be collected. Either toluene or thymol has proved satisfactory.

GROSS EXAMINATION OF URINE SPECIMENS

Although the simplest of all procedures conducted on urine, this examination is the one most consistently overlooked. A considerable amount of information can be gained concerning urine if one takes time to observe and record volume, color, transparency, odor, and appearance of foam in the specimen.

Urine Volume. Urine volume is dependent upon several physiologic factors, including water and other fluid intake, environmental conditions, diet, and the size and activity of the animal. Normal urine production varies according to animal species: in the dog, production ranges from 12 to 30 ml/lb body wt/24 hours; in the cat, 4.5 to 9 ml/lb/24 hours; cattle, 8 to 20 ml/lb/24 hours; horse, 2 to 8 ml/lb/24 hours; swine, 2 to 14 ml/lb/24 hours; sheep and goat, 4.5 to 18 ml/lb/24 hours.[1]

In the normal animal, high urine volume is usually associated with low specific gravity and low urine volume with high specific gravity. High urine volume and low specific gravity are often, but not always, associated with renal disease.

Increases in urine volume (polyuria) may be present transiently owing to diuretic therapy or increased fluid intake and following parenteral administration of fluids or administration of adrenocorticotropic hormone (ACTH) or corticosteroids. Pathologic increases in urine volume are associated with chronic generalized nephritis, acute generalized nephritis, diabetes mellitus, diabetes insipidus, nephrogenic diabetes insipidus, diuretic phase of toxic nephrosis, primary renal glucosuria, pyometra, advanced renal amyloidosis, hyperadrenocorticism, generalized pyelonephritis, compulsive polydipsia, and some liver diseases.[2]

Urine volume will decrease (oliguria) with decreased fluid intake, high environmental temperature, and hyperventilation (dog). Oliguria is commonly associated with dehydration resulting from loss of body water, as in diarrhea and excessive vomiting, but may also occur with markedly decreased blood pressure, the oliguric phase of acute nephritis, prolonged fever, and circulatory dysfunction with edema as well as in terminal renal disease.

As renal failure may be associated with hypovolemic shock occurring with blood loss or sequestration of fluids, the early stages are characterized by decreased urine flow. Renal perfusion can be monitored by insertion of an indwelling catheter and observing the rate of urine flow. If renal perfusion is adequate, a flow rate of 0.5 to 1.0 ml/hour/lb body weight is expected. Development of anuria or oliguria is an indication that renal perfusion is decreased, and therapy should be instituted to restore it.

Color. The color of a urine specimen should be noted and recorded while the clinician is observing the specimen in a test tube or urinometer cylinder. The following color designations are used:

colorless	red
pale yellow	reddish-brown
yellow	brown
dark yellow	green
yellow-brown	blue
greenish-yellow	milky

The yellow color of urine depends on the concentration of urochromes. If urine is concentrated, the amount of urochrome per volume is increased, and urine appears darker than normal; whereas if urine volume is increased, urochromes are diluted, and the urine is pale.

Dark urine, due to the concentration of urochromes, occurs in association with dehydration, fever, decreased blood pressure, the oliguric phase of toxic nephrosis, terminal renal disease, circulatory dysfunction with edema, and reduced fluid intake. Pale urine, on the other hand, is seen in diabetes mellitus, diabetes insipidus, increased water intake, pyometra, the diuretic phase of toxic nephrosis, amyloidosis (advanced), primary renal glucosuria, hyperadrenocorticism, generalized pyelonephritis, and chronic and acute generalized nephritis. Urine may also be pale following administration of ACTH or corticosteroids or parenteral administration of fluids. In general, urine that is dark is high in specific gravity; conversely urine that is pale is usually of low specific gravity. However, exceptions may occur, as in circumstances in which polyuria exists and the urine contains a large quantity of an abnormal substance that will increase specific gravity.

Yellow-brown to greenish-yellow urine may be due to the presence of bile pigments in the specimen. Urine with a high concentration of bilirubin may turn green on standing as bilirubin is oxidized to biliverdin.

Hemoglobin produces a wine-red urine that changes to brownish as it is converted to alkaline or acid hematin depending upon the pH. Hematuria also results in a red to brown color but differs from hemoglobinuria in that with hematuria the urine is cloudy, whereas with hemoglobinuria it is more likely to be translucent.

Brown to black urine may be observed in normal horses. Horse urine is normally yellow when excreted but may turn deep brown upon standing, as a result of oxidation of pyrocatechin. Horse urine will be brown to black from the excretion of myoglobin, as occurs in azoturia.

In cases of congenital porphyria, a faint pink color may be observed in the urine, and when such urine is examined under Wood's light, an orange fluorescence is present.

Drugs may also produce alterations in urine color. A red color may result from the administration of phenothiazine, phenolphthalein, and azosulfamide. The administration of such drugs as methylene blue and dithiazanine iodide (Dizan) may impart a greenish to blue color to urine. Urine may be greenish following a dose of acriflavine. Phenolsulfonphthalein (PSP) and sulfobromophthalein impart a red to violet color to alkaline urine.

To be valid, interpretation of urine color must be associated with the physical condition of the animal, the history of drug dosage, and age of the specimen.

Transparency. The transparency of urine as observed in a test tube or urinometer cylinder should be recorded as clear, flocculent, or cloudy.

Urine excreted from most species of domestic animals is clear. The only exception occurs in the horse, in which it is normally thick and cloudy owing to the presence of calcium carbonate crystals and mucus. Normal urine from other species of animals, although clear on being voided, may become cloudy as it cools and precipitation of crystals occurs. Precipitation is most likely to occur in highly concentrated urine.

Pathologically, cloudy urine may be observed when any of the following are present: leukocytes, erythrocytes, epithelial cells, bacteria, mucus, fat, and crystals (if present when the urine is voided). The cause of cloudy urine can be accurately ascertained only by microscopic examination of the specimen. In general, however, crystals result in the appearance of a white sediment if they are due to the presence of amorphous phosphates, which occur principally in alkaline urine. Amorphous urates may result in the appearance of a white or pinkish cloud in acid urine that has been standing or is chilled. Leukocytes generally produce a white cloud and sediment that may be grossly in-distinguishable from those produced by amorphous phosphates. If erythrocytes are present, urine takes on a reddish brown or smoky color. Bacteria generally produce a uniform cloudiness or opalescence. Fat produces a cloudy, opaque urine if present in large quantities and can be positively identified by the addition of a fat solvent such as chloroform or ether, which causes the urine to become transparent. Centrifugation of urine specimens containing fat may also serve to identify this substance, as fat forms a layer on top of the specimen following centrifugation.

Odor. The odor of the urine is not diagnostic, although the urine of males of certain species (porcine, feline, and caprine) has an especially strong odor. The normal odor of urine is derived from the volatile organic acids present. An odor of ammonia may appear if urea is being converted to ammonia by bacterial action. Ketone bodies impart a characteristic sweetish, fruity odor and may be detected in urine in association with pregnancy disease, acetonemia, and diabetes mellitus.

Foam. When shaken after collection, normal urine produces a white foam that is limited in quantity. If there is proteinuria, the amount of foam produced is in excess and slow to disappear. If bile or bile pigments are present, the foam may be green, yellow, or yellow-brown. If hemoglobin is present, the foam is red to brown.

SPECIFIC GRAVITY

Specific gravity of urine is a measurement of the relative amount of solids in solution and is an indication of the degree of tubular reabsorption or concentration by the kidney. Under conditions of normal renal function and normal metabolism, the specific gravity or urine varies inversely with the volume of urine excreted. If large volumes of urine are excreted, the specific gravity is usually low, whereas if small quantities are being eliminated, the specific gravity is generally high.

Determination of the specific gravity of urine should be a routine procedure in any analysis. This is particularly true if a metabolic disease such as diabetes mellitus is suspected or clinical signs of kidney disease are observed. Specific gravity should be measured as a part of any examination in an animal with polyuria.

Normal Values. As urine specific gravity is related to urine volume, and urine volume, in turn, is related to water intake and body metabolism, it is difficult to ascribe specific values for the normal animal. In general, specific gravity for most animal species will be in the range of 1.015 to 1.045, but values as low as 1.001 and as high as 1.060 to 1.080 can occur. Randomly collected urine specimens may have a specific gravity from 1.001 to 1.080 in animals with normal kidney function. Thus, in interpretation, the clinician must take into consideration many factors influencing the amount of solute in urine. These will be discussed later.

Technique for Determining Specific Gravity

Specific gravity of urine is most readily determined by use of a refractometer (Fig. 9–2). This instrument provides a simple, reproducible, and accurate method for estimating urine specific gravity. An additional advantage is that specific gravity can be determined using as little as one drop of clear urine. Most refractometers are temperature compensated between 60° and 100° F. One drop of urine is placed in the refractometer, and the specific gravity is read on a built-in scale. These meters utilize a hollow glass prism containing a hermetically sealed, stable liquid with an air bubble to allow for expansion or contraction of the liquid. Refractometers provide readings for specific gravity of urine with a degree of accuracy to 0.001 unit. Although these instruments are relatively expensive, they provide a rapid method for measuring specific gravity not only of urine but also of serum and plasma and may be utilized for determining total protein in these fluids.

The specific gravity of urine can also be estimated by use of a urinometer. Urine should be allowed to stand at room temperature for a few minutes prior to being read. This is particularly true if the urine has been refrigerated, as a decrease below room temperature will influence results. The technique for the use of the urinometer is as follows: (1) Fill the urinometer cylinder to within approximately 1 inch of the top. (2) Place the urinometer in the urine and spin it between the thumb and fingers so that the float will seek its proper level. (3) Read the specific gravity at the highest point at the bottom of the meniscus and record. Every attempt should be made to avoid bubbles on the top of the urine, as they interfere with an accurate reading of the meniscus. Urinometers for various quantities of urine can be purchased. For a small animal practice, a small sample urinometer is recommended. Using this small urinometer and a thin-walled centrifuge tube, specific gravity determination can be made on as little as 10 ml of urine.

The accuracy of the urinometer should be tested periodically by using distilled water. Distilled water at room temperature (approximately 20° C) should have a specific gravity of 1.000. If insufficient quantities of urine are present for use of even the small urinometer, the urine can be diluted with distilled water and the specific gravity recorded. To obtain the corrected reading, the last two figures of the specific gravity are multiplied by the dilution factor. If 5 ml of urine is diluted with an equal quantity of distilled water, the dilution factor is 2 (one part urine in a total of two parts); thus, if the specific gravity of the diluted urine is 1.015, the corrected value is 1.030.

Interpretation

Increased Specific Gravity

Transient increases in urine specific gravity occur physiologically as a consequence of decreased water intake, with hyperventilation, or in animals held in a high environmental temperature.

Increases in concentrations of urinary solids resulting in an increased specific gravity may occur in several disease conditions, including the following:

1. Dehydration resulting from diarrhea or prolonged vomiting.
2. Hypovolemic shock—if kidney function is normal.
3. Edema associated with circulatory failure.
4. Burns with considerable extracellular fluid loss.
5. High fever may produce a transient increase.

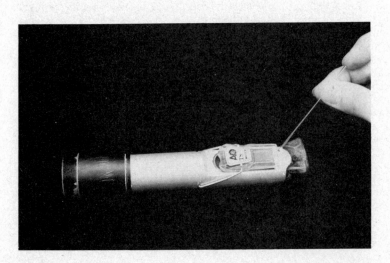

Figure 9–2. A hand-held refractometer is used for determining urine specific gravity and measuring total protein and fibrinogen. The easiest way to load the unit is with a capillary tube. The capillary tube is gently touched to the surface and fluid will flow into the chamber by capillary action.

6. Addition of excessively large quantities of solids.

Glucose and protein will affect urine specific gravity, but significant changes occur only when a large quantity is present. Each 0.27 gm of glucose/dl or 0.4 gm/dl of protein in urine will increase specific gravity approximately 0.001.

Only a careful correlation of the physical findings, history, and other laboratory examinations will reveal the actual cause of changes in specific gravity.

Decreased Specific Gravity

Decreased urine specific gravity (1.001 to 1.024) occurs physiologically as a result of increased fluid intake from excessive water consumption or iatrogenically following administration of corticosteroids, ACTH, diuretics, or parenteral administration of fluids.

A low urine specific gravity at a single reading on a randomly collected urine specimen suggests the presence of renal disease and warrants further study to evaluate renal function. A common cause of lowered urine specific gravity is renal failure. Urine specific gravity may also be lowered in the diuretic phase of toxic nephrosis or with chronic generalized pyelonephritis, advanced renal amyloidosis, or acute generalized nephritis. Other conditions in which lowered urine specific gravity is present include inherited generalized progressive renal diseases such as renal cortical hypoplasia, diabetes insipidus occurring as a result of lack of antidiuretic hormone (ADH), nephrogenic diabetes insipidus, hyperadrenocorticism, pyometra, diabetes mellitus, primary renal glucosuria, and some generalized diseases of the liver. Urine specific gravity may also be lowered when there is a rapid mobilization and excretion of edema fluid.[2]

As there are many conditions characterized by polyuria and a lowered urine specific gravity, care must be taken in evaluating the patient, and a systematic method for determining the underlying cause must be established. The first step is to confirm the presence of polyuria. This can be done by careful observation of the patient or preferably by measurement of 24-hour urine output. If the total output exceeds that anticipated for the animal species by $7\frac{1}{2}$ per cent, the presence of polyuria is confirmed. Because of the risk of producing dehydration in an animal with renal failure, free choice water should be provided during the 24-hour test. Once the presence of polyuria has been established, a urinalysis should be completed if it has not been done previously. If there is glucosuria, the blood glucose level should be evaluated to rule out the presence of an osmotic diuresis such as that occurring with diabetes mellitus or excess endogenous or exogenous glucocorticoids. In animals without glucosuria, the specific gravity should be measured (see Fig. 9–5).

In chronic renal disease, urine specific gravity may become fixed in a range of 1.008 to 1.012 (isosthenuria). As this is the range of specific gravity of glomerular filtrate, if a urine sample has a specific gravity within this range, further studies should be initiated. Normal animals have the ability to alter urine specific gravity in response to fluid consumption, and specific gravities in this range may occur normally. A urine specific gravity of 1.008 to 1.012 and a history of or hospital-confirmed polyuria in an animal with clinical signs of dehydration or laboratory findings such as increased packed cell volume and total protein indicates that the patient lacks the ability to conserve body water. When nonrenal causes of polyuria in a patient with a urine specific gravity less than 1.025 (1.030 in the cat and dog) are ruled out, further tests of renal function are indicated. In nonazotemic animals with a urine specific gravity that is constantly 1.012 or less, a water concentration or vasopressin (pitressin) test is indicated. A water deprivation test is contraindicated if serum urea nitrogen and creatinine concentrations are increased or the patient is already dehydrated.

WATER DEPRIVATION TEST. The water deprivation test (urine concentration test) is based on the fact that ADH is released from the posterior pituitary gland when a patient is deprived of fluids. This hormone enhances fluid reabsorption by the distal and collecting tubules of the kidney by increasing tubular cell permeability to water. If urinary function is normal, this hormonal control mechanism results in an increase in urine solutes. The procedure for conducting the concentration test is as follows:[2] (1) Deprive the patient of water and permit food with low moisture content. As urine concentration is dependent on the degree of hydration and rate of solute excretion, fasting is not recommended. (2) Weigh the patient as a baseline by which water loss can be estimated in evaluating dehydration. (3) Remove and discard all urine from the bladder approximately 12 hours after beginning water deprivation. (4) Permit sufficient time to lapse for urine to collect in the bladder, then determine urine specific gravity. If the specific gravity is above 1.030, the test can be discontinued, since this indicates ability to concentrate urine. If urine specific gravity is below 1.030, the test should be continued for 12 or more hours, and steps three and four should be repeated at the end of 24 hours. If at the end of 24 hours urine specific gravity is 1.030 or greater, the test can be discontinued. If urine specific gravity does not increase to at least 1.025, the clinician should determine the physical status of the patient, evaluate urea nitrogen or serum creatinine, and estimate the amount of dehydration by weighing the patient. If urea nitrogen (UN) and serum creatinine levels are abnormally elevated or body weight has decreased more than 5 per cent, the test should be discontinued. If UN and serum creatinine levels are normal and the patient has not lost more than 5 per cent of its body weight, the test can be continued for an additional six to 12 hours and urine specific gravity again determined.

Interpretation of a water deprivation test is relatively simple. If urine specific gravity is less than 1.030 after the patient has been deprived of water for a period of time adequate to stimulate ADH production, the following conclusions may be reached: (1) There is an impairment of ADH release as a consequence of diabetes insipidus. In animals with diabetes insipidus, urine specific gravity is usually below that of the glomerular filtrate and more likely to be in the range of 1.001 to 1.006, as renal tubular cells retain the ability to reabsorb solute in excess of water. (2) Ability of the kidney to concentrate urine has been decreased because of renal disease. (3) Antidiuretic hormone is released, but the nephron cannot respond to its stimulation (nephrogenic diabetes insipidus). (4) The lack of increase in urine specific gravity is a consequence of a mixture of dilute and concentrated urine because of a technical error in conducting the test. This may occur if the urinary bladder is not emptied at the end of the first 12 hours and the sample for specific gravity determination contains some urine that was present in the bladder prior to initiation of water deprivation.[2]

Prolonged polyuria can result in a loss of renal medullary hypertonicity (medullary washout). Such animals cannot concentrate urine during the usual water deprivation test. Normal hypertonicity can be re-established by an intravenous injection of a hyperosmolar (3 per cent) solution of sodium chloride or by gradually reducing water intake by 50 per cent for two or three days. Either method will correct the urine concentrating ability of the kidney that fails to respond to water deprivation because of medullary washout.

In animals with a urine specific gravity of less than 1.008 that do not respond to water deprivaton or ADH, a modified Hickey-Hare test can be used. The test is conducted as follows:

1. Give 20 ml/kg of water via stomach tube.
2. Administer a 2.5 per cent solution of sodium chloride intravenously at a rate of 0.25 ml/kg/minute over a 45-minute period.
3. Check urine specific gravity or serum and urine osmolality every 15 minutes during and after administration of the sodium chloride solution.
4. If the urine is concentrated (specific gravity above 1.025, or urine osmolality increases to 2 to 3 times that of serum) it supports a psychogenic polydipsia with medullary washout. If the urine is not concentrated the most probable cause is nephrogenic diabetes insipidus. Once the osmotic gradient in the kidney is re-established, an ADH test can be conducted and with pituitary diabetes the kidney will respond by concentrating urine.

VASOPRESSIN INJECTION TEST. If diabetes insipidus is suspected, the condition can be confirmed by use of the vasopressin test. The general principles of this test are similar to those of the water deprivation test except that the animal is given an injection of aqueous vasopressin. The test is conducted as follows: (1) Inject 0.25 unit of aqueous vasopressin per kilogram of body weight up to a maximum of five units. The injection should be given subcutaneously. (2) Withhold all fluids and food during the period of testing. (3) Thirty minutes after injecting the vasopressin, empty the bladder to remove any urine formed prior to the action of ADH. (4) Urine samples are collected at 30, 60, 90, and 120 minutes following administration of the vasopressin, and the specific gravity or osmolarity of each sample is determined.

An animal with normal ability to concentrate urine should excrete urine having a specific gravity higher than that of glomerular filtrate (1.008 to 1.012). Values of 1.020 to 1.035 or higher represent a normal response in the dog. Urine specific gravity remaining below 1.020 suggests (1) that generalized renal disease is present and is impairing the ability of the kidney to concentrate urine, (2) that renal diabetes insipidus is present and the nephrons are unable to respond to ADH (renal diabetes insipidus), (3) that a technical error has occurred as a consequence of a mixture of dilute and concentrated urine, or (4) that there is medullary washout.

This test can also be conducted using repositol vasopressin. In this technique, three to five units of vasopressin tannate in oil are injected intramuscularly; fluids and food are withheld during the test period; the bladder is emptied three hours after injection of repositol vasopressin; urine samples are collected at three, six, and nine hours following injection; and specific gravity is determined for each sample. Interpretation of results is similar to that suggested for the aqueous vasopressin test.

No attempt should be made to conduct a urine concentration test either with or without ADH in any uremic patient. To complete such a test on a uremic animal may precipitate a uremic crisis resulting in death. If animals are clinically dehydrated, there is no need to conduct a water deprivation test, as conditions that stimulate the kidneys to concentrate water already exist. Dehydration may become an acute problem in an animal with marked polyuria. If polyuria is present, special care should be taken to weigh the patient frequently during the period of water deprivation and to discontinue the test whenever the animal has lost 5 per cent of its body weight.

URINE OSMOLALITY

Osmolality measures the number of dissolved solute particles in a solution and is unrelated to the nature of those particles. Specific gravity, on the other hand, is the ratio of a mass of solution compared with the mass of an equal volume of water. Since specific gravity is a comparison of weights, it is not an exact measurement of the number of solute particles, because different atoms and molecules have different weights. Thus osmolality is a better measurement of total solute than is urine specific gravity. Osmolality is more difficult to measure than specific gravity as it requires instruments that determine changes in freezing point or vapor pressure. Although measurement of osmolality may provide a more accurate measurement of solute concentration in urine, the need for expensive equipment to make the measurements has limited its use.

The unit of osmotic concentration is the osmole. Because the osmole represents a large mass of solute, the milliosmole (mOsm) is used clinically. The osmotic pressure of intracellular and extracellular fluids is approximately 300 mOsm/kg of water. Slightly more than 90 per cent of serum osmolality is contributed by the electrolytes sodium, chloride, and bicarbonate, because they are present in the highest concentrations. Other extracellular fluid electrolytes such as serum proteins, glucose, and urea are responsible for the remaining percentage. A crude estimate for serum osmolality utilizes the formula:

Osmolality

$$= 2 \times Na + \frac{Glucose}{20} + \frac{Urea\ nitrogen}{3}$$

While serum osmolality remains fairly constant, urine osmolality is variable, since it depends on the state of hydration and renal function. With normal renal function in a dehydrated animal urine osmolality may approach 3000 and can be as low as 50 in individuals with polyuria and normal renal function. Calculation of the ratio of urine to serum osmolality (urine mOsm/serum mOsm) provides a method for determining the ability of the kidneys to concentrate or dilute glomerular filtrate. A ratio above 1.0 indicates that kidneys are concentrating urine above plasma and glomerular filtrate, while a ratio less than 1 indicates that renal tubules are capable of diluting the glomerular filtrate. Following water deprivation, the urine:serum osmolality ratio should increase dramatically. In dogs with normal renal function and response to ADH the ratio may be 7 or above.[3] If renal tubular function is decreased, there will be little or no change in the ratio. The same is true of animals with nephrogenic diabetes insipidus.

CHEMICAL EXAMINATION

Although urine contains a large number of organic substances, only a few are of clinical significance in urinalysis. Analysis of the chemical composition of urine routinely includes tests for acid-alkaline reaction (pH) and the presence of protein, glucose, ketone bodies, bile pigments, and blood.

Acid-Alkaline Reaction (pH)

The normal hydrogen ion concentration of urine is dependent upon the type of diet. Animals on a principally vegetable diet have a tendency to produce an alkaline urine, whereas acid urine is normal in animals that are consuming either a cereal diet with high protein content or a diet derived principally from an animal protein.

Determination of pH should be made on every urine specimen submitted for analysis, as it may reveal information relative to the metabolic status of that individual. Alterations from the normal pH are more commonly an indication of a systemic condition than they are of a localized disease of the urinary system.

Normal Values for pH. Normal values of the pH reaction of urine from any species of animal must be carefully considered, as the diet and state of metabolism play a marked role in determining the hydrogen ion concentration of any given specimen. In general, the reactions are as follows:

Bovine—alkaline (pH 7.4–8.4)
Ovine—alkaline
Caprine—alkaline
Porcine—acid or alkaline
Canine—acid (pH 6–7)
Feline—acid (pH 6–7)

As will be noted, the pig may have either an acid or alkaline urine. Since the pig is an omnivorous animal, the reaction will be alkaline if the diet is primarily vegetable and acid if the diet is high in animal protein. Any young animal that is nursing will have an acid urine, even if the adult of the same species characteristically has an alkaline urine.

Technique. The hydrogen ion concentration of urine can be readily determined by the use of litmus paper, hydrion pH paper strips, or other strips such as those produced by the Ames Co. (Elkhart, Indiana). Litmus paper can only determine whether urine is acidic or alkaline; it cannot detect the degree of acidity or alkalinity. With the use of hydrion paper or the pH test, an accurate estimation of pH can be determined.

Interpretation. Aciduria is normal in carnivorous animals, nursing calves and foals, and animals on diets containing excessive amounts of protein. Pathologically, increased acidity may result from starvation, fever, or acidosis (both metabolic and respiratory). Urine acidity is also increased following prolonged muscular activity. In addition, the administration of acid salts such as ammonium chloride, sodium chloride, calcium chloride, or sodium acid phosphate may result in an increased acidity in urine.

Alkaline urine is normal in herbivorous animals or carnivorous animals on a high vegetable diet. If urine is retained in the bladder as a result of an obstructive lesion or cystitis, the urine is usually alkaline. Alkaline urine frequently occurs in cystitis because many of the microorganisms that produce this lesion are capable of splitting urea to form ammonia. In addition, increased alkalinity may be associated with metabolic alkalosis and may also be a result of the ingestion of salts such as sodium lactate, sodium bicarbonate, sodium citrate, and nitrate. In the dog and cat, urine may become less acid after meals as a result of "alkaline tide" associated with gastric secretion of hydrochloric acid.[2]

Protein

Urine that is voided from the body does not contain detectable protein. Most protein that passes the glomerular filter is reabsorbed in the tubules. Consequently, normal urine when tested for protein is negative. The presence of protein in urine is always considered pathologic except at the time of parturition, during the first few days of life, following strenuous exercise, or during estrus. Since the presence of this substance is considered an abnormality, the detection of protein in the urine may be of clinical significance, and any persistent proteinuria should be investigated.

Techniques. A wide variety of methods for the detection of protein in the urine are available to the laboratory. One old and still reliable method is use of a strong acid such as that incorporated in Roberts' reagent. This reagent consists of one part of concentrated nitric acid in a saturated solution of magnesium sulfate prepared by the addition of 1970 gm. of magnesium sulfate to 1 liter of water. The technique is relatively simple, as the reagent is placed in a test tube and urine is gently layered onto the heavier fluid with a pipette or medicine dropper. Protein will react with the reagent to produce a white ring that varies in density with the amount present. If only a small amount of urine is available for the test, the reaction of urine and reagent can be observed with use of an eye dropper. A small quantity of urine is drawn into the eye dropper, and without releasing pressure on the bulb, a small quantity of Robert's reagent is sucked into the eye dropper. In the presence of protein a white ring will develop at the junction. One disadvantage of this test is the difficulty of reading the reaction in cloudy urine. If the specimen to be assayed by this method is cloudy, it should be centrifuged or filtered before being tested. If only small quantities of protein are present, development of the white ring may require two to three minutes.

Another commonly used chemical test for the detection of protein is the sulfosalicylic acid test. Commercial reagent tablets that contain all the required ingredients are available. Tablets are diluted in 1 ounce of water. Equal parts of reagent solution and urine are placed in a small test tube and the tube gently shaken. The amount of protein is estimated by the degree of turbidity produced. Cloudy urine cannot be used until it is centrifuged or filtered. This test is relatively accurate, but small amounts of protein may be overlooked, as it is often difficult to judge the degree of turbidity present.

The development of a reagent strip (Ames Company, Elkhart, Indiana), has simplified the detection of protein in urine. This strip contains tetrabromphenol blue, a citrate buffer, on a bibulous strip of cellulose. The basis of the reaction is the fact that at a fixed pH, certain indicators have one color in the presence of protein and another in the absence of protein. The citrate buffer present in these strips provides a hydrogen ion concentration of approximately pH 3. At this pH, the indicator tetrabromphenol blue has a yellow color if no protein is present and a green to blue color in the presence of an increasing amount of protein. To use this technique, dip the strip containing the reagent into the urine and compare the color with a chart furnished with the strips. The intensity of the color is proportional to the amount of protein present. If no color change occurs, the specimen is negative. In the presence of protein, the end of the test strip changes immediately to a yellow-green, green, or blue-green depending upon the quantity of protein. Many specimens will give a trace reaction. Therefore, weak reactions should be confirmed with sulfosalicylic acid or Roberts' test. A trace reaction is generally ignored, particularly in urine specimens from herbivorous animals. Use of the reagent strip is generally acceptable in testing urine with high concentration of protein; however, in highly alkaline urine, false-positive reactions may occur. For this reason we would not recommend the test for use in animals that normally have a highly alkaline urine. This method does not detect globulins with as great a sensitivity as it does albumin and therefore may be negative if myeloma proteins are present.

Interpretation. A transitory proteinuria may occur as a physiologic or functional reaction. It is believed that this appearance of protein may be due to a temporary increase in glomerular permeability resulting from a congestion of the capillaries. Physiologic transient albuminurias may follow (1) excessive muscular exertion, (2) emotional stress, (3) excessive ingestion of protein, and (4) convulsions.

An abnormal proteinuria may occur as the result of a wide variety of conditions. Renal proteinuria may occur in nephritis, in which it is a direct result of the increased permeability of the glomerular filter. Acute generalized nephritis results in a marked proteinuria and the presence of casts in voided urine. With chronic generalized nephritis, however, only a slight proteinuria may be observed. Pyelonephritis is accompanied by a marked proteinuria, depending somewhat upon the amount of tissue involved and acuteness of the process. Cattle with pyelonephritis usually have a strong urine protein reaction. Glomerular disease is accompanied by a marked and persistent proteinuria.

Certain drugs and chemicals may produce severe renal damage characterized by nephrosis. A marked proteinuria occurs in such intoxications. Agents included in this group are phenol, arsenic, phosphorus, lead, mercury, sulfonamides, turpentine, and ether. Amyloidosis is also accompanied by marked proteinuria, although in terminal stages proteinuria may decrease. Renal infarction, neoplasms, trauma, and acidosis may also result in a nephrosis and an accompanying proteinuria.

If passive congestion of the kidney occurs, a small amount of protein may appear. Passive congestion of the kidney often results from fever or toxemia in which cloudy swelling or tubular degeneration takes place and will cause a mild but transitory proteinuria. Congestion may also result from cardiac decompensation or pressure on abdominal veins resulting from tumors or ascites.

Postrenal proteinuria occurs when protein gains entrance to the urine after it leaves the kidney tubules. The most common causes of contamination by these exudates and blood include the following conditions: cystitis, vaginal or preputial discharges, prostatitis, pyelitis, urethritis, and urolithiasis. Hemorrhage in the urinary tract may be accompanied by high concentrations of protein in urine. Hemoglobin and myoglobin also give positive tests for protein. If protein is present in urine collected by catheterization or cystocentesis, it originated from the kidney, ureter, or urinary bladder.

Thus, a wide variety of conditions may culminate in proteinuria. The cause of proteinuria must be searched for with diligence, and a careful evaluation of the clinical signs must be made. In general, proteinuria points to a urogenital tract abnormality and may be a sensitive index of the presence of such abnormalities. However, the absence of protein in the urine does not rule out all urinary tract diseases.

If marked proteinuria persists, a 24-hour protein determination should be completed as described later in this chapter. On occasions one may wish to determine the type of protein being lost, particularly if myelomatosis is suspected. In such cases a urine specimen should be submitted for protein electrophoresis.

Glucose

No glucose is present in normal urine. Although glucose is readily passed through the glomerulus, complete reabsorption of this chemical occurs in the tubules. However, if the load in the blood exceeds the renal threshold, glucose may appear in the urine (glucosuria). Since glucosuria is an abnormality, a test for this condition should be included in each and every examination of urine.

Techniques. A number of methods are available for both qualitative and quantitative estimation of glucose in the urine. One of the simplest methods for semiquantitative estimation of sugar in the urine is the use of specially prepared reagent tablets (Clinitest Reagent Tablets, Ames Co., Elkhart, Indiana). The Clinitest Reagent Tablet contains copper sulfate, citric acid, sodium hydroxide, and sodium carbonate. Reducing sugars in urine react with copper sulfate to reduce the cupric ions to cuprous oxide, resulting in a color change that is dependent upon the amount of reducing substances present. This tablet is used as follows: (1) Place five drops of urine and 10 drops of water in a test tube. (2) Add one reagent tablet. (3) Wait 15 seconds after the boiling stops, shake the tube gently, and compare the color of its fluid contents with the color chart. If no sugar is present, the fluid in the tube will be blue. With the presence of reducing substances, the color will be green, tan, orange, or dark brown, depending upon the quantity of reducing substances present. This test does have limitations, as reducing substances other than glucose will result in a positive reaction.

The development of colorimetric strip tests has simplified the detection of glucosuria and provided an accurate method for estimation of glucose. These test strips contain glucose oxidase, peroxidase, and orthotoluidine. These paper strips produce a color reaction when moistened with urine containing glucose. The technique is simple, as it requires only the dipping of the test strip into urine or the brief passage of the strip through a urine stream. One minute after soaking in urine, the end of the strip containing the reagent is compared with a color guide. If no color change occurs, the urine specimen contains no glucose. However, if the end turns blue, glucose is present. It is advisable to use a more sensitive quantitative method if the glucose oxidase test strips are positive.

Canine urine may contain a high concentration of ascorbic acid, which interferes with development of the color reaction usually observed in the presence of glucose. In one study[4] the glucose oxidase–impregnated strip did not work efficiently in detecting low and high glucose concentrations in more than 85 per cent of all dog urine samples tested. In more than 50 per cent of the cases, the test failed to demonstrate the presence of a glucose concentration of 0.15 gm/dl. It is therefore recommended that these strips be used with caution and that the reducing sugar method be utilized in screening urine for glucose if the history and clinical signs suggest diabetes mellitus.

False-negative results have also been reported in urine containing formaldehyde or fluoride and in refrigerated samples that are not warmed before testing; also, large quantities of bilirubin or ketones may alter the color reaction.[5]

Interpretation. Glucosuria may result from conditions other than systemic disease. An emotional glucosuria may occur as a result of fear, excitement, and restraint. This appearance of glucose in urine is thought to be the result of the hyperglycemia that occurs subsequent to an increased secretion of epinephrine. Such epinephrine secretion leads to a rapid mobilization of glucose. A heavy meal of carbohydrates may elevate the blood glucose to such a level that glucosuria occurs. The administration of glucose solutions or a general anesthetic may be followed by glucosuria. In addition, glucose may occur in the urine with the following diseases: diabetes mellitus, acute or chronic pancreatitis accompanied by hyperglycemia, hyperthyroidism, overactivity of the adrenal cortex, chronic liver disease, hyperpituitarism with hyperglycemia, increased intracranial pressure, and enterotoxemia in sheep due to *Clostridium perfringens*, type D toxin. Glucose in the urine may also be a result of renal glucosuria due to the impairment of the tubular reabsorption or a lowering of the renal threshold for this substance.

False-positive reactions in the reducing test for glucose may be caused by a variety of drugs, including certain antibiotics (Streptomycin, chlortetracycline, tetracycline, penicillin, and chloramphenicol); reducing sugars such as lactose, pentose, maltose, or others; ascorbic acid; morphine; chloral hydrate; formalin; glucuronic acid; glucuronates; uric acid; and salicylates.

Ketone Bodies

Ketone bodies include acetoacetic acid, acetone, and beta hydroxybutyric acid. These are the results of lipid breakdown and the accumulation of acetyl coenzyme A that is not utilized for lipogenesis or in the citric acid cycle and that becomes converted to ketone bodies. If ketone bodies are present in the urine, there is a concomitant accumulation of these substances in the blood.

Techniques. The Ross test has been widely utilized for the detection of ketone bodies. The reagent consists of a powdered mixture of one part of sodium nitroprusside and 100 parts of ammonium sulfate. About one-half inch of the powdered reagent is placed in a dry test tube, 5 ml of urine is added, and the mixture is agitated. One to 2 ml of concentrated ammonium hydroxide is added to form a layer above the mixture. A flake of sodium hydroxide can be substituted for the ammonium hydroxide and should be added before the tube is agitated. If ketone bodies are present, a purple to black color will appear, the depth of color being dependent upon the amount of ketones present in the specimen. This test may also be applied to milk.

Correlation between blood ketone levels and the appearance of ketones in urine and milk is poor. In testing for urine ketones, the Ross test is very sensitive, false-positive results being common. It is recommended that bovine urine be diluted 1:10 with water to take advantage of the sensitivity of the Ross test and to increase diagnostic accuracy. The same test can be conducted on milk, with which it is not as sensitive and a 1+ reaction is of significance.

The dipstick routinely used in urinalysis measures the amount of ketones present as they react with nitroprusside. The strip is most sensitive to acetoacetic acid and reacts weakly with acetone and not at all with beta-hydroxybutyric acid. False-positive reactions are rare, but highly pigmented urine may sometimes give a false-positive result. False-negative reactions do not occur unless urine has been standing in an open container for several hours. Bacterial activity can also destroy ketones, resulting in low or negative test results.

Interpretation. In small domestic animals (dogs and cats) the principal cause of ketosis is diabetes mellitus. However, high fever and starvation may result in a ketonuria in puppies and kittens. Adult dogs and cats seldom show a ketosis except during very prolonged inanition.

In herbivorous animals, however, the situation is quite different. In the cow, ketosis may readily develop from a large variety of conditions in which carbohydrate metabolism does not keep up with the carbohydrate needs of the body. Ketosis may occur in high-producing milk cows that are improperly fed or that develop anorexia. Cattle may also develop ketosis in the absence of a primary disease.

In pregnant ewes, ketosis associated with hypoglycemia may occur, particularly in ewes carrying twin lambs.

If ketosis is detected, the clinician should conduct a careful examination before concluding that the condition is a primary disease and not a secondary reaction. Treatment of ketosis as a single clinical entity should not be initiated unless other causative factors have been detected and treatment of the primary disease has begun.

The method for the detection of bile pigments and their significance in urine have been discussed in Chapter 7.

Blood

Blood may be present in the urine (hematuria) or the pigment hemoglobin may occur independently of the presence of erythrocytes (hemoglobinuria). Differentiation between hematuria and hemoglobinuria is of considerable diagnostic significance. Hemoglobinuria is generally a sign of a systemic disease, whereas hematuria is more likely to occur in association with disease of the genitourinary system. It is possible, however, for erythrocytes that have ruptured in dilute or alkaline urine to rlease hemoglobin, leaving behind only their stroma as "ghost cells." Consequently, not all hemoglobinuria may be the result of this substance having passed through the glomerular filter.

Techniques. Test strips used for detection of blood in urine utilize the fact that oxygen is liberated from peroxide by the activity of heme from lysed erythrocytes or free hemoglobin. As heme catalyzes the oxidation of the reagent strip it produces a blue or green color depending upon the commercial brand of strip being used. The sensitivity of the strip will depend in part on the brand of reagent being used but is approximately 5000 to 10,000 intact erythrocytes per ml and 0.5 to 0.3 mg of hemoglobin/dl of urine.[6] This test will also give positive results with myoglobin. False-negative reactions occur if the ascorbic acid content of urine is high. The reagent strips lose their sensitivity if stored too long.

In urine that is relatively isotonic and not too alkaline, hematuria can be differentiated from hemoglobinuria by centrifugation of the specimen. Intact erythrocytes will sediment while hemoglobin and myoglobin remain in the supernatant. If urine is dilute or alkaline, the erythrocytes will rupture and the hemoglobin will be freed.

Interpretation. Hematuria with the presence of intact erythrocytes in the urine may occur as a resut of a wide variety of conditions primarily affecting the urogenital tract, although a few systemic diseases may be accompanied by hematuria. Among the conditions resulting in hematuria are: pyelonephritis; ureteritis; cystitis; urolithiasis; pyelitis; trauma to urinary bladder, kidney, or urethra (often from improper catheterization); prostatitis; neoplasms of the kidney, bladder, or prostate; passive congestion of the kidneys; renal infarction; acute nephritis; parasites such as *Dioctophyma renale, Capillaria plica,* and *Dirofilaria immitis* larvae; the administration or ingestion of toxic chemicals such as copper, mercury, arsenic, and thallium; thrombocytopenia; sweet clover poisoning; and capillary damage resulting from shock. Hematuria is also seen during estrus and postpartum, particularly in specimens collected as the animal urinates (midstream samples). In evaluation of hematuria, the bleeding can be inferred to be occurring in the bladder if only the last of the voided urine is contaminated with blood. If blood is present throughout the sample, it is probable that the hemorrhage is occurring in the kidney, bladder, or ureter. If blood appears at the onset of urination, it may be due to a lesion of the urethra, uterus, vagina, penis, or prostate.

Hemoglobinuria occurs as a result of an excessive hemolysis of erythrocytes and consequently is more commonly the result of systemic disease. Hemoglobinuria is found in association with the following: leptospirosis; piroplasmosis (babesiasis); photosensitization; chemical hemolytic agents such as copper and mercury; consumption of certain plants; severe burns; an incompatible blood transfusion; and hemolytic diseases of the newborn. *Clostridium haemolyticum* may cause bacillary hemoglobinuria, and hemoglobinuria may occur postparturiently. It has been reported that cattle may have an idiopathic hemoglobinuria after the ingestion of a large volume of cold water.

MICROSCOPIC EXAMINATION OF URINARY SEDIMENT

In healthy individuals, urine contains small numbers of cells and other formed elements from the length of the genitourinary tract; casts and epithelial cells from the nephron; mucous threads and spermatozoa from the prostate; and epithelial cells from the bladder, urethra, renal pelves, and ureters. In addition, a few leukocytes and erythrocytes reach the urine probably as a result of diapedesis in any part of the urinary tract. Urine from dogs, cats, and other carnivores will usually have some phosphate crystals. Horse urine characteristically has calcium carbonate crystals and mucous threads. Normal urine is bacteria free in the bladder but often contains small numbers of microorganisms accumulated as the urine is voided.

Extraneous materials resulting from fecal contamination may also appear in urine unless the specimen has been carefully collected. Typical contaminating substances include parasite eggs, plant spores, and other organic matter. If an excessive quantity of lubricant is utilized in collecting the specimen, this material may be observed microscopically.

Microscopic examination of the urine is of clinical importance and should never be omitted from a routine urinalysis. It will often reveal the presence of structures of diagnostic importance in urine that seems perfectly clear on physical examination. Conversely, microscopic examination of urine that is very cloudy and contains an abundant quantity of sediment may not disclose any structures of clinical significance.

The composition of urine sediment soon changes following its connection. Therefore, examination of sediment should be made using fresh specimens; if a delay must occur before examination can be made, the sample should be refrigerated or a preservative such as formalin should be added to preserve the structures present in the urinary sediment.

Technique

In most urine specimens it is necessary to concentrate the elements before conducting a microscopic examination. The successful interpretation of microscopic examination is dependent upon the technique of collection and examination. Examination of specimens contaminated with feces or other extraneous material is often inconclusive and can be misleading.

Urine to be examined microscopically should be gently agitated to suspend any sediment that may have settled to the bottom of the tube. Approximately 15 ml of urine is centrifuged at a low speed (not over 1000 revolutions per minute) for three to five minutes. All of the urine is poured out of the tube, and the fluid retained on the sides of the tube is used to resuspend the sediment. Sediment resulting from such centrifugation and resuspension should be examined. The color, type of aggregation, and amount of sediment should be recorded. If erythrocytes are present, the sediment will often have a red to brownish color. If bile pigments are present, the sediment is often yellow, whereas crystals are usually white. If fat is present, it will usually float to the top during centrifugation.

Supernatant urine can be used to dilute the sediment if the amount appears excessive. The dilution should be sufficient so that when microscopic examination is made, the elements are seen as a single layer without excessive overlapping. If it is necessary to dilute the urine in order to examine it microscopically, this fact should be recorded in the report.

After the sediment is resuspended, a drop is placed on a clean glass slide and a coverslip applied. The drop of sediment should be of the correct size—not so large as to float the coverslip and not so small that there is unoccupied space beneath the coverglass.

Microscopic examination of the urine must be conducted with care. The most common cause of failure to obtain accurate results is improper illumination. The light for microscopic examination of unstained urinary sediment should be central and subdued for oridinary work. Lowering the substage condenser is advised. The entire specimen should be examined under low power (100×), and high power (430×) should be utilized for detecting details of cell types and the presence of bacteria. Under low power, certain characteristics such as the presence or absence of casts, staining with bile pigments, the presence of crystals, and the amount of sediment can readily be recorded.

Satisfactory examination of a urine specimen that has dried on the slide is impossible. Organized structures are distorted beyond recognition and there may be a confusing deposition of urinary salts. A record of microscopic examination of the urine not only should state that a particular structure is present but should give an approximate idea of the number of such structures. The best plan is to record the average number of structures seen in a high-power field. This number is only an approximation, and interpretation should take this fact into consideration.

Addition of stain to urine sediment will facilitate identification of cells and structures. One drop of 0.5 per cent new methylene blue stain preserved by addition of a drop or two of formalin provides a most satisfactory stain and permits easy identification of cells and other organized elements. Commercial stains are available from a variety of sources. Although the light should be reduced for microscopic examination of stained specimens, the degree of illumination is not as important as it is in examination of unstained sediment.

Interpretation

Urinary sediment can generally be divided into organized and unorganized elements. The organized elements include leukocytes, erythrocytes, epithelial cells, microorganisms (protozoa, yeasts, fungi, bacteria), casts, parasites, and spermatozoa. Unorganized elements are fat droplets, crystals, and pigments. Both types of elements are illustrated in Figures 9–3 and 9–4.

In evaluating the number of cellular elements found in a urine specimen, the clinician must consider the specific gravity. A larger number of cells per unit of volume can be expected in highly concentrated urine, whereas the same number of cells present in urine of low concentration might be suggestive of renal disease. This consideration applies to all organized sediment in urine.

Leukocytes. Under normal conditions, only a few leukocytes are present in urine. Numerous leukocytes occur only as a result of a pathologic process. The presence of leukocytes in the urine constitutes pyuria. The diagnostician must consider the genital tract as a possible source for these cells, particularly in samples collected during micturition. If the specimen has been obtained by catheterization or cystocentesis, cells present must have been derived from the bladder, ureter, renal pelvis, or kidney. Diseases in which pyuria is observed include nephritis, pyelonephritis, pyelitis, urethritis, and cystitis.

Neutrophils may be difficult to distinguish in urinary sediment, as they are not as well preserved as they are in blood. Neutrophils in urine appear as granular, spherical cells somewhat larger than erythrocytes. Granularity may be due to the degeneration of the nucleus or to the presence of neutrophilic granules within these cells. The nucleus is often obscured by granules but may be brought clearly into view by running a little dilute acetic acid under the coverglass. Such a procedure will sometimes enable the technician to differentiate neutrophils from small, round epithelial cells. Additional differentiation can be made if a stain is used. Staining makes it possible to positively identify polymorphonuclear leukocytes. In some cells, the nuclei will have degenerated and will appear as several small, rounded bodies within the cell. If the urine is alkaline, the leukocytes are usually swollen, ragged in appearance, and very granular and have a tendency to

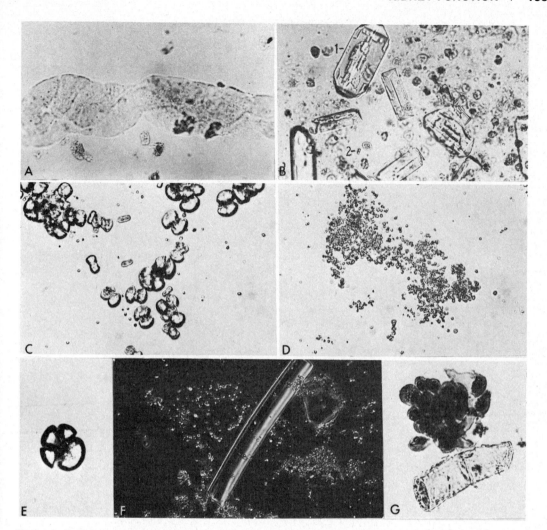

Figure 9-3. Urinary sediment (400×). *A*, Convoluted granular cast. *B*, (1) Triple phosphate crystal. (2) Small amorphous phosphate crystal. These crystals may be confused with bacteria but can be differentiated by their refractile appearance. *C*, Calcium carbonate crystals in equine urine. *D*, Amorphous phosphates in equine urine. *E*, Large calcium carbonate crystal in equine urine. *F*, Darkfield photograph of a large cylindrical phosphate crystal and amorphous phosphates. *G*, A cluster of epithelial cells just above an artefact that might be confused with a cast.

adhere in clumps. Cellular degeneration is frequent; it is often difficult to differentiate neutrophils from renal or transitional epithelial cells and lymphocytes.

The most severe pyuria occurs in patients with a bacterial infection of the urinary tract. If neutrophils are present in excess, the specimen should be carefully examined for microorganisms. If there is pyuria and no microorganisms are demonstrated, the urine should be submitted for bacterial culture. Occasionally, phagocytosed microorganisms can be found in the cytoplasm of neutrophils. Unless the neutrophils are incorporated within a urine cast, which would confirm a pyogenic infection of the kidney, it is impossible to identify the site of the infection.

Erythrocytes. Erythrocytes appear in urine in a variety of morphologic forms. In urine that is highly concentrated, they may be severely crenated and have a distorted appearance. In urine of low concentration and low specific gravity, erythrocytes are often ballooned into a spherical shape, in which case only faint, colorless rings are seen. These "shadow cells" are not always uniform in size and may be oval to pear shaped, although they are usually circular. In canine urine that has a specific gravity of approximately 1.020, the red blood cells present are typical biconcave discs, and this morphology can sometimes be detected as the cells move within the microscopic field. Erythroctes vary from colorless to yellow or orange and do not stain with new methylene blue.

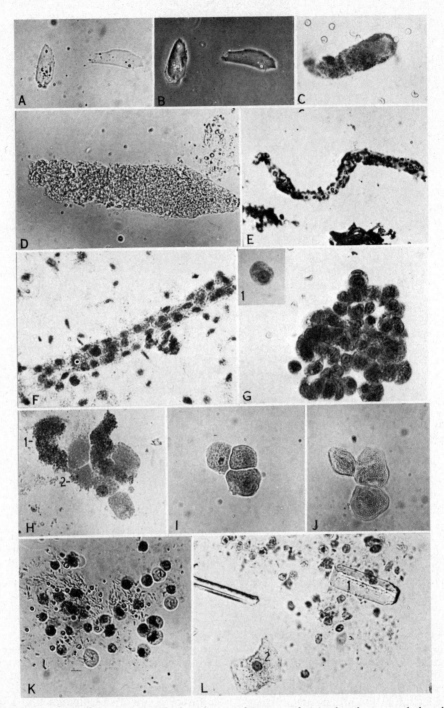

Figure 9–4. Urinary sediment photographed using 40 × objective and stained with new methylene blue stain. *A,* Hyaline casts. *B,* Hyaline casts visualized by phase-contrast condenser and objectives. *C,* Coarse granular cast and a few erythrocytes. *D,* Granular cast. *E,* Leukocyte cast. *F,* Sloughed renal tubule. *G,* Cluster of renal epithelial cells. Inset (1) shows a single cell. *H,* (1) Coarse granular cast. (2) Fine granular cast. *I,* Transitional epithelial cells. *J,* Squamous epithelial cells. *K,* Leukocytes and bacteria. (Not all leukocyte nuclei stain with new methylene blue.) *L,* (1) Triple phosphate crystal. (2) Squamous epithelial cell. There are several leukocytes in this field.

If the cell has been in the urine for a long period of time, hemoglobin may be completely dissolved away, leaving a colorless structure. Erythrocytes are smaller than leukocytes and can be confused with other objects such as fat globules, yeasts, and oxalate crystals. Red blood cells can usually be identified by examination with the high-power dry objective. If positive identification is still impossible even at this magnification, the addition of a small quantity of dilute acetic acid to the material on the slide will cause hemolysis of red blood cells. This will assist in identification, as other objects that can be confused with erythrocytes are not lysed by acetic acid.

The presence of erythrocytes in significant numbers in a urine specimen is an indication of hemorrhage somewhere in the genitourinary tract. Locating the exact source of hemorrhage can be difficult, although some information regarding its location can be inferred by noting at what point during the act of micturition voided urine is contaminated with blood.

Erythrocytes may also appear in the urine as a result of damage that occurred during catheterization. If the specimen was obtained by cystocentesis, the presence of red blood cells may be the result of rupturing a blood vessel during collection. Excessive manipulation of the bladder during physical examination may also be sufficient to produce hemorrhage.

Epithelial Cells. A wide variety of epithelial cells is normally observed in urine, but the number of such cells may be increased in animals with cystitis or other inflammation of the urogenital tract. Squamous epithelial cells are derived from the urethra, bladder, and vagina. These are the largest cells appearing in urinary sediment and have an irregular outline. They contain a small, round nucleus that is usually visible. Some of these cells may be rolled into a cigar shape and may be confused with casts. Squamous cells are usually seen in urine specimens not obtained by catheterization.

Cells derived from renal tubules are smaller and have a round to polyhedral shape. Although slightly larger than leukocytes, they may be confused with the latter. This is particularly true if the renal tubule cells are undergoing degeneration. These cells are most readily identified when they are incorporated in a cast.

No accurate data are available concerning the number of epithelial cells normally found in urine of domestic animals. Large numbers of cells characteristic of the bladder or kidney may be indicative of disease, as inflammatory changes may cause greater sloughing of the cells. Occasionally, degenerated cells containing fat may be observed. This is a frequent finding in renal epithelial cells in cat urine. The presence of large numbers of renal epithelial cells along with casts containing renal epithelial cells is suggestive of active tubular degeneration. Clumps of epithelial cells

may be seen in urine from an animal with acute tubular necrosis.

Microorganisms. Bacteria, yeasts, fungi, and protozoa may occasionally be seen in urine. Bacteria are most commonly observed as small objects that display active motility or brownian movement. The morphology of the organism may be detected by examination with the high-power objective; however, the use of new methylene blue or Gram's stain increases accuracy of identification. The significance of the presence of bacteria in urine is related to the method of collection and age of the specimen. In urine collected aseptically either by cystocentesis or by catheterization, the presence of bacteria is an indication of infection. Large numbers of bacteria may be seen in cystitis, pyelonephritis, or other bacterial infections of the urinary tract. Infections of the genital tract may cause the appearance of bacteria in urine sediment due to contamination of the specimen at the time of collection. No significance can be attributed to the presence of bacteria in urine specimens that have been standing at room temperature for any length of time.

Yeasts usually appear as colorless, round to ovoid bodies that are variable in size and have double refractile walls. Yeasts exist in urine usually as a contaminant, as yeast infection of the urinary tract of domestic animals is rare.

Fungi are characterized by the appearance of distinct hyphae that may be segmented, colored, or both. Fungi are common external contaminants and as such have little significance in the microscopic examination of urine.

Protozoan infections of the urinary tract are rare. The presence of protozoans usually results from contamination of the specimen with fecal material. Genital secretions containing trichomonads may contaminate the urine, but such contamination is rare.

Casts. These structures represent proteinaceous casts of the uriniferous tubules. Casts are principally formed in the lumen of the distal tubules, ascending loop of Henle, and collecting tubules of the kidneys, as it is in this portion of the tubules that urine reaches its maximum concentration and acidity. The presence of casts in the urine (cylindruria) usually indicates a pathologic change in the kidney, although this change may be only slight or transitory. The borderline between normal and abnormal findings is approximately two to four casts per low-power field (LPF).[3] In interpreting the significance of the presence of tubular casts, the number of casts per LPF must be related to urine specific gravity. The presence of two to four casts per LPF in urine of low specific gravity is more significant than the presence of a similar number in highly concentrated urine. If casts are present in large numbers, it is always an indication of renal disease, although temporary irritation and congestion of the kidneys may result in the appearance of a marked but transitory increase in casts. Casts do not in themselves imply organic disease of the kidney. They seldom occur in urine that does not contain or has not recently contained protein and have a significance similar to that associated with renal proteinuria.

The matrices of casts are Tamm-Horsfall mucoprotein that is secreted by collecting ducts, ascending loop of Henle, and distal tubules.

Casts represent molds of the tubules in which they are formed. These structures may be formed in the collecting ducts, distal convoluted tubules, and loops of Henle. If tubular lesions are present at the time a cast is formed, the products of degeneration are incorporated in the cast. Showers of tubular casts are frequently observed when urine production returns in a kidney that has been subjected to decreased perfusion. Finding numerous casts in the urine of a patient that has had oliguria or anuria is a favorable sign, as it indicates return of renal function.

The several types of casts that have been described in the urine of domestic animals may be categorized as follows: hyaline, granular, waxy, renal failure, epithelial, erythrocytic, fatty, and leukocytic.

HYALINE CASTS. Hyaline casts are composed of protein and mucoprotein. As visualized microscopically, they are hemogeneous, semitransparent, colorless, cylindric structures having rounded ends. These casts usually appear in acidic urine and are uncommon in the sediment of urine from larger domestic animals. They are difficult to demonstrate because of their refractive index and are seen in a relatively dark field or under conditions in which the light is arranged so that the beam is slightly oblique. They are more readily demonstrated in stained sediment. Hyaline casts indicate a mild form of renal irritation, and a few hyaline casts may be present in normal urine.

GRANULAR CASTS. Hyaline casts that contain granules, either fine or coarse, are called granular casts. The granules present in these casts are derived from the disintegration of tubular epithelium or are aggregates of serum protein.[6] The granular cast is the most common cast observed in the urine of domestic animals. Such casts may be observed in association with advanced irreversible renal disease such as amyloidosis and chronic nephritis. Generally, however, granular or hyaline casts are not a reliable index of severity of the kidney lesion.

WAXY CASTS. Waxy casts are similar in appearance to hyaline casts, being typically homogenous but frequently containing a few granules or an occasional cell. Under the microscope, the waxy cast appears more opaque than the hyaline cast, is grayish or colorless, and has a dull, waxy appearance. These structures are often found with a blunt, broken end, in contrast to the cigar shape of the hyaline cast. Waxy casts are an indication of chronic lesions of the tubules and accompanying degeneration. They may be seen occasionally in animals having amyloid degeneration of the kidney.

RENAL FAILURE CASTS. Renal failure (broad) casts are similar to but larger than granular casts. They are thought to originate in collecting ducts or dilated tubules of the nephron and indicate obstruction or loss of more than one nephron.[2]

EPITHELIAL CASTS. Epithelial casts are formed from the desquamated cells derived from the renal tubules. Cells within these casts vary in size and are often oval, elongated, or flat. Difficulty may be encountered in differentiating between epithelial and leukocyte casts if the cells have begun to degenerate. If differentiation is impossible, such casts should be reported as "cellular casts." Epithelial casts imply desquamation of the epithelium, which rarely occurs except in association with acute nephritis or tubular epithelial degeneration. Exceptionally good preservation of these cells may be an indication of acute nephritis.

ERYTHROCYTIC CASTS. Erythrocytic casts are homogeneous, cylindric masses having a deep yellow to orange color. Erythrocytes within these casts are often degenerate. Red cell casts are an indication of hemorrhage into the renal tubules originating from the glomerulus or the tubule. Although erythrocyte casts are infrequently observed, they have been associated with renal trauma.

FATTY CASTS. Fatty casts contain small droplets that appear as refractile bodies. The fat is usually colorless but can be stained with Sudan III. Fatty casts in the urine are an indication of degenerative tubular disease associated with deposition of lipoidal material in the renal tubules. Such casts are seen occasionally in dogs with diabetes mellitus and are the most frequent type in cats with renal disease.

LEUKOCYTIC CASTS. Leukocytic casts are characterized by the presence of many "pus cells" adherent to or within a hyaline matrix. These casts indicate the presence of a suppurative process such as pyelonephritis or kidney abscesses.

CAST-LIKE OBJECTS. There are some objects present in urine that may be readily confused with tubule casts. Mucous threads frequently appear in the urine and occur as long strands that are more ribbon-like and have less well-defined edges than do hyaline casts. Although mucous threads are present normally in horse urine, in other animals they may be an indication of irritation of the urethra. Most mucous threads, however, are usually the result of contamination by genital secretions.

Cylindroid is a term applied to certain structures that may appear in the urine that are more nearly allied to casts. They resemble hyaline casts in structure but differ from them in that one end tapers to a fine filament. This slender tail is often twisted or curled on itself. Cylindroids have a significance similar to that of hyaline casts.

PARASITES. Urinary sediment may contain ova of the following parasites: (1) *Capillaria plica*, the bladder worm of the cat, dog, and fox; (2) *Stephanurus dentatus*, the swine kidney worm; (3) *Dioctophyma renale*, the giant kidney worm of the dog and mink. Additional parasitic ova that may be observed in urinary sediment are the result of contamination by feces.

Spermatozoa. These cells are easily recognized by their characteristic structure and have little significance except to indicate that urine has been mixed with a quantity of semen. Spermatozoa are commonly encountered in urine collected from a male dog but are less commonly observed in urine from other species of domestic animals. Since the presence of spermatozoa indicates contamination of the specimen with semen, it is not unusual to find a small quantity of protein present in any specimen containing these cells.

Unorganized Elements. Included among the unorganized elements are fat droplets, crystals, and pigments.

Fat droplets appear in the urine as round, highly refractile bodies of various sizes. This variation in size may aid the technician in differentiating them from erythrocytes. Positive identification of fat droplets can be made by the addition of Sudan III to the urinary sediment. Fat droplets will stain orange to red. Fat that is present in the urine often originates from an extraneous source such as a lubricated catheter or a specimen container that has fat in it. Lipuria is a common finding in cat urine, occurring to some degree in most cats. Lipuria may occur pathologically as a result of fatty metamorphosis of the renal tubules. Rupture of a lymphatic may also lead to fat in the urine. In addition, lipuria has been reported to occur in association with obesity, diabetes mellitus, and hypothyroidism and in animals on a high-fat diet.

The type of crystal observed in urine depends upon the pH, solubility, and concentration of the crystalloid and colloids. Crystals in the sediment of animal urine seldom have any clinical significance. The appearance of struvite crystals ($NH_4MgPO_4 \cdot 6H_2O$) was associated with urethral obstruction in cats.[7] In a later report, no difference in the concentration of struvite crystals in cats with or without obstruction was demonstrated, and urine samples from many cats with obstruction contained few crystals.[8] Alkaline urine will contain triple and amorphous phosphates, calcium carbonate (especially in the horse), and, on rare occasions, ammonium urate crystals. Acidic urine most commonly contains amorphous urates and uric acid. Calcium oxalate and hippuric acid may be present but are less common. Large numbers of calcium oxalate crystals in the urine of animals with renal failure may suggest ethylene glycol toxicity. Uric acid and urate crystals are seen more abundantly in the urine of Dalmatians than in the urine of other breeds of dogs.

If calculi occur, a determination of the crystal type present in the sediment becomes important in order that therapy can be instituted to prevent recurrence. Leucine and tyrosine crystals have been reported in the urine in acute liver disease resulting from poisoning with carbon tetrachloride, chloroform, or phosphorus. Cystine crystals indicate the presence of a disturbance in protein metabolism and may result in formation of cystine calculi. Ammonium biurate crystals are associated with portal caval shunt and other liver diseases.

RENAL FUNCTION TESTS

As with the measurement of the function of any organ, the value of renal function testing is limited by the techniques available, accuracy of testing, frequency of testing, reserve capacity of the organ, biologic variability, lack of specificity of tests utilized, and interpretive ability of the clinician. In spite of these limitations, clinical laboratory examinations of organ function may be indicated and are of value in the diagnosis and prognosis of kidney disease. It must be recognized at the outset that a single determination or a single renal function test indicates only the functional capacity of the kidneys at the time the test was conducted. Renal function tests do not reveal the definitive cause of disease, whether the disease is in an acute or chronic stage, the eventual outcome of the normal repair mechanism and the likelihood that renal function will return, or the reversibility of the lesion. It is, therefore, obvious that in order to evaluate the status of a patient with renal disease, the functional status of the kidneys must be periodically re-evaluated. By periodic assessment of renal function, a more accurate prognosis can be achieved, and the regimen of treatment can be realistically evaluated.

Present knowledge concerning kidney physiology makes possible a rather precise determination of some individual phases of kidney function. Measurements can be made of the rate of renal blood flow, the glomerular filtration, and the maximum capacity of the renal tubules for excretion and reabsorption. Many of the most definitive test procedures are time consuming and require precise measurements. Thus, they do not lend themselves to a practice situation, although they are utilized in research studies of renal diseases. Because of the time-consuming nature of these determinations and the cost of conducting them, the veterinary clinician will usually utilize less specific tests in evaluating renal function. The methods of study that are employed most widely and are of the greatest value fall into several categories: (1) urine specific gravity and the effect of water deprivation, (2) estimations of nonprotein nitrogen levels in the blood, (3) studies of the ability of the kidney to excrete certain dyes, and (4) tests based on the clearance concept.

Urine Specific Gravity

Specific gravity as a measurement of renal function has been alluded to previously in this chapter, as has the water deprivation test. The measurement of specific gravity as a test of renal function is of value only if conducted in a serial fashion. However, there is little value in repeating this determination once the ability of the kidney to concentrate or dilute urine has been determined. Specific gravity determinations are of value in detecting functional changes that occur during the course of a renal disease.

If urine specific gravity is 1.030 or greater, it must be assumed that the kidneys are capable of performing their work and that this measurement is a reflection of functional collecting ducts and distal tubules that are responsive to ADH.

Fixation of specific gravity (isosthenuria) at or near that of glomerular filtrate (1.008 to 1.012) is a consistent finding in chronic and acute renal disease in which a great percentage of the functional tubules have been damaged. It has been estimated[2] that impairment of the ability of the kidneys to concentrate or dilute urine is usually not detectable by means of specific gravity determinations until at least two thirds of the total functional parenchyma has been incapacitated. In the uremic patient, a specific gravity greater than 1.030 may be a favorable prognostic sign. Such a specific gravity is usually an indication that there are enough functional nephrons present to concentrate urine and may suggest that the uremia is prerenal in origin.

Although a specific gravity of 1.001 to 1.006 is extremely low and may indicate a lack of ADH or a kidney that is incapable of responding to ADH, it is also a reflection of functional kidneys, since kidneys must be working in order for solute to be removed from the glomerular filtrate.

Urine Osmolality. As mentioned previously, another technique for measuring the ability to concentrate urine is the determination of osmolality. This is a measurement of the number of particles of solute per unit volume of solvent. The osmolality of a liquid is most readily determined by evaluating the freezing point. As the number of solute particles increases, the freezing point becomes progressively lower and can be measured utilizing an osmometer. Because of the cost of this equipment, the determination of osmolality is not a common practice in veterinary clinical laboratories.

One osmole is that quantity of an ideal solute in 1 kg of water that will have a freezing point of $-1.86°C$ as compared with the freezing point of pure water. The unit for recording the osmotic concentration of urine is the milliosmole (mOsm), which is equal to 0.001 osmole. Osmolality is expressed as mOsm per kilogram of solution. *Osmolarity* is frequently used in place of osmolality and is defined as the osmole content per liter of solution.

The normal osmotic concentration of the body fluids (transcellular, intracellular, and interstitial) is relatively constant at approximately 300 mOsm. Osmotic concentration of normal urine is variable and, as with specific gravity, is dependent upon the electrolyte and fluid balance of the body as well as the nitrogen content of the diet. Normal values for urine osmolality have been reported to be between 860 and 1920 mOsm/kg body weight in the cow,[9] 200 and 2000 mOsm/kg in the dog[10] and 500 and 1200 mOsm/kg in the cat.[2] These values assume normally hydrated animals, but in states of physiologic oliguria, values in excess of 2000 may occur. With extreme diuresis, urine osmolality may be as low as 50 mOsm/kg in the dog and cat.

The relationship between urine osmolality (total solute) and specific gravity is only approximate, as urine specific gravity is altered by abnormal solutes, such as protein and glucose. This change in specific gravity is dependent upon molecular size and weight of the solutes as well as the number of molecules of solute. As a consequence, equal numbers of molecules of albumin, globulin, fibrinogen, glucose, sodium, chloride, and urea each have different quantitative effects on specific gravity. In the measurement of osmolality, only the number of molecules present, not their mass, determines freezing point depression. It would thus appear that determination of osmolality would be a more sensitive technique than estimation of specific gravity. The significance of this sensitivity is, however, decreased when one considers the great biologic variability that occurs in serial determinations of urine osmolality. The same variations are reflected in specific gravity; thus the accuracy gained by determining osmolality tends to be minimized.

The ratio of urine osmolality (U_{osm}) to plasma osmolality (P_{osm}) may be a good index of renal function. The normal osmotic concentration of plasma is approximately 300 mOsm/kg of water. A ratio of U/P_{osm} greater than 1 indicates that the kidneys are capable of producing urine that is more concentrated than is plasma. After a 24-hour water deprivation test, the normal canine U/P_{osm} is 3 to 7.[3] A U/P_{osm} ratio of 1 indicates that water and solute are being eliminated in a state isosmotic with plasma. A U/P_{osm} ratio of less than 1 indicates that kidneys are capable of absorbing solute in excess of water.

Although use of the osmometer has some obvious advantages in terms of accuracy, determining specific gravity by the refractometer method remains the technique of choice in most veterinary clinical laboratories because of its simplicity and lower instrument cost.

Nonprotein Nitrogen Levels in Blood

The term *nonprotein nitrogen* (NPN) is used to identify nitrogen-containing components of serum or plasma that are not associated with protein. This group consists of a heterogeneous mixture of substances not precipitated by commonly used protein precipitants. Nonprotein nitrogens include urea, creatinine, creatine, uric acid, ammonia, amino acids, and a fraction designated "undetermined nitrogen." The NPN substances represent products of intermediary metabolism of both tissue and ingested protein.

Urea Nitrogen (UN)

Urea is formed in the liver and represents the principal end product of protein catabolism. This substance normally has no useful function in the body other than a possible mild diuretic action and is excreted almost entirely by the kidneys. The glomerulus filters urea in plasma, and under normal conditions approximately 25 to 40 per cent of filtered urea is reabsorbed as it passes through the tubules. Urine flow rates greater than normal diminish tubular reabsorption; conversely, low rates of urine flow increase urea reabsorption in the tubules.

INDICATIONS FOR TESTING. Urea nitrogen determinations should be completed (1) whenever decreased kidney function is suspected, (2) as a technique for measuring peripheral perfusion of tissues in animals subject to hypovolemic shock or decreased blood pressure, and (3) as a routine presurgical laboratory screening test. As with other tests of renal function, estimation of UN from a single randomly collected specimen is of less value than are serial UN determinations.

TECHNIQUE OF TESTS. As with all chemical determinations, specimen collection is of importance. Anticoagulants containing any nitrogen must be avoided. The anticoagulant of choice is ethylenediaminetetraacetic acid (EDTA), although heparin, sodium citrate, and sodium oxalate are acceptable. Urea nitrogen determinations are usually conducted on serum, and normal values are comparable to those in whole blood.

A variety of laboratory techniques have been developed for estimating urea nitrogen concentration in whole blood, plasma, or serum.

CHROMATOGRAPHIC TECHNIQUE. Chromatographic techniques for estimation of urea nitrogen have been marketed under the trade names Urograph (Warner/Chilcott Laboratories, Morris Plains, New Jersey) and BUN-O-Graph (Haver Lockhart Laboratories, Prairie Village, Kansas). The primary advantages of this method for determination of urea nitrogen are its simplicity, the fact that no special chemicals are necessary, and the small amount of serum or plasma required.

The chromatography paper is banded with different reagents. When the tip of the paper is placed in serum or plasma there is an upward migration so that the serum passes through a series of chemical reactions. This produces a color change the height of which is directly related to urea nitrogen concentration. The first band contacted by the serum or plasma is an excess of phosphate-buffered urease. In this band, urea is converted to an ammonia salt, which continues to migrate up the paper. The second band is potassium carbonate. Free ammonia is produced in this band and forced into the atmosphere of the test tube, first dropping toward the bottom, then building up in the tube. At this level a plastic barrier immediately above the potassium carbonate band prevents any further migration of serum or plasma. The top band is an indicator consisting of bromcresol green in tartaric acid. As ammonia accumulates in the test tube it comes in contact with the bottom of the band, neutralizes the acid, and produces a color change. The height of this color change bears a direct relationship to the amount of ammonia released. Details for conducting this analysis are presented in the Appendix, p. 443.

A word of caution concerning the use of this technique is warranted. Since the height of the reaction is dependent upon the accumulation of free ammonia in the test tube, any disturbing air currents may influence results. Therefore, the tubes should be placed in a position in which there will be minimal air movement. A distinct color change may also be produced in the indicator strip by smoke from a cigarette, cigar, or pipe. One should avoid placing the test tube containing the chromatographic strip in any area in which ammonia compounds are stored. Contamination and the influence of air currents may be minimized by covering the tube with a large glass beaker. This technique is of value in detecting UN levels up to 75 mg/dl and is useful in detecting increases in UN, but the limitations in accuracy and maximum levels detectable preclude its use in precise determinations.

MERCURY COMBINING POWER. In laboratories without access to a spectrophotometer this titration test can be used to estimate blood urea concentration. Mercury will combine with chemicals such as urea, creatinine, and uric acid when a mercuric salt solution is added to substances containing these products. A protein-free filtrate is prepared and mercuric chloride is added to it. When mercuric chloride has ceased combining with nonprotein nitrogen substances in the filtrate, it will combine with the test reagent sodium carbonate to produce a reddish brown precipitate. Details for this screening procedure are presented in the Appendix, pp. 442–443.

DIPSTICK METHOD. The Azostix testing system (Ames Co., Elkhart, Indiana) is a quick screening procedure that is useful in making an approximate estimation of the level of urea nitrogen. As with many other screening tests, it depends upon the ability of the individual to match colors and requires careful timing of all steps in order to achieve uniformity in results. Details for conducting the test are included with the reagent and should be strictly followed.

INTERPRETATION OF RESULTS. Urea nitrogen levels in the blood are affected not only by alterations in renal function but also by physiologic factors or diseases not primarily of renal origin.

Physiologically, urea nitrogen levels are increased with a dietary increase in protein. The UN concentration may be increased as much as 10 mg/dl if the animal is on a diet high in meat. Conversely, low dietary levels of protein may result in a decrease in UN. Experimental work in this laboratory revealed that a dog deprived of all food for 24 hours had a UN level approximately half that found in the same animal when it was fed free choice of protein. Changes in plasma urea and plasma creatinine concentrations following the feeding of three types of commercial diets were studied.[11] Plasma urea nitrogen concentration increased with all diets fed, with the peak concentration occurring about six hours after eating. Although the increases were statistically significant, 89 per cent of the values were less than 30 mg/dl. Plasma urea nitrogen levels in dogs on a dry food diet did not exceed 25 mg/dl, and the highest recorded was 43 mg/dl in one dog fed canned food. Plasma creatinine concentrations were not affected by the diet. If the serum urea nitrogen concentration is slightly increased and there is history of the dog having eaten within the last five or six hours, the test should be repeated.

The status of protein metabolism within the body regardless of diet may also influence urea nitrogen concentration. Catabolic breakdown of the tissues as a consequence of fever, trauma, infection, or toxemia may result in a moderate increase in UN concentration. A similar increase may be seen in association with hemorrhage into the gastrointestinal tract. UN may be increased iatrogenically by administration of drugs that increase protein catabolism (corticosteroids, thyroid compounds) or drugs that decrease protein anabolism (tetracyclines).

Anything that reduces the glomerular filtration rate (GFR) will cause an increase in blood or serum urea nitrogen. Alterations in fluid balance influence UN. Decreased plasma water may be associated with an increase in UN concentration. If dehydration becomes severe, a significant uremia may develop as glomerular filtration diminishes owing to decreased renal perfusion.

Decreases in the rate of excretion of urea nitrogen produce an increase in the concentration of UN. Azotemia resulting from a decreased excretory rate may be prerenal, renal, or postrenal.

Prerenal uremia is most commonly seen when renal function is reduced as a consequence of decreased blood flow through the kidneys. Examples of such conditions include shock, dehydration, cardiac disease, and hypoadrenocorticism. Glomerular filtration is dependent upon the maintenance of adequate blood pressure to provide the force required for filtration to take place in the glomerulus. Thus, a decrease in pressure below the critical level for filtration will result in anuria as glomerular filtration ceases. Prerenal uremia UN values are usually less than 100 mg/dl but oc-

casionally are higher if renal perfusion is drastically reduced. Anuria does not usually develop in animals until blood pressure approaches 60 mm. of mercury. Oliguria may, however, be seen in animals with a less severe reduction in blood pressure and glomerular filtration. Azotemia as a consequence of decreased renal perfusion occurs in animals having structurally normal kidneys that have no, or limited, blood flow. If the cause of decreased perfusion is rapidly corrected, the kidneys will return to a normal functional status. If the condition is permitted to persist, renal ischemia may develop and result in the destruction of organ structure. Prerenal uremia can sometimes be confirmed by demonstration of a significant increase in blood urea nitrogen with a urine specific gravity of 1.030 or greater.

Primary uremia occurs when the GFR is decreased. This happens in a variety of disease processes in which the common factor is destruction of at least three fourths of the total kidney parenchyma. Early stages of progressive kidney disease are accompanied by only minor changes in UN levels, although there may be destruction of a large quantity of renal parenchyma. As the disease advances, it usually reaches a stage at which destruction of a small number of nephrons may be accompanied by a large change in the UN concentration.

The following suggestions regarding the interpretation of the results of laboratory tests for blood urea nitrogen have been made.[2] (1) If UN concentration exceeds 35 to 45 mg/dl, GFR is diminished. (2) Abnormal UN concentration known to be caused by abnormal excretion may be due to prerenal, primary renal, or postrenal factors. Every effort should be made to determine the underlying cause of uremia in order to establish a meaningful prognosis and select an appropriate treatment. (3) Only a rough correlation can be made between the degree of elevation of UN and the severity of renal function impairment. This may be partly related to duration of renal disease, since progressive diseases that destroy renal parenchyma at a relatively slow rate permit remaining viable nephrons to undergo structural and functional compensation. Thus, in chronic renal diseases, more renal parenchyma may be destroyed before functional abnormalities are reflected in UN concentration than occurs with acute renal diseases. There is not an abnormal increase in UN during very early stages of acute renal shutdown, as time must elapse for a sufficient quantity of urea to accumulate to be considered abnormal. (4) A single determination of UN concentration, regardless of the value obtained, does not provide a reliable index of the reversibility or irreversibility of the disease process. Serial determinations of UN levels provide a more reliable index for prognosis. Progressive increases in the concentration of UN in spite of appropriate therapy are justification for a guarded to unfavorable prognosis.

Postrenal uremia occurs with obstruction or

rupture of the excretory pathway for urine. Thus, azotemia may be expected with obstruction of the urethra, bladder, or both ureters or a rupture of any of these structures. In postrenal uremia, the kidney structure initially remains normal, but if obstruction persists, varying degrees of renal disease may develop or the patient may, as is common in instances of ruptured excretory pathways, die of electrolyte and fluid abnormalities.

If a rupture of the lower urinary system is suspected, a urea nitrogen determination on fluid contained in the abdominal cavity is of value when compared with UN concentration in serum. The urea concentration in abdominal fluid is frequently greater than the UN concentration.

Creatinine. Creatinine is a nonprotein nitrogenous substance formed during muscle metabolism of creatin and phosphocreatin. It is excreted by glomerular filtration, and significant quantities are neither excreted nor reabsorbed by the tubules. If production remains constant, the measurement of serum creatinine may provide a crude index of glomerular filtration. Most factors influencing creatinine concentration are similar to those influencing blood urea nitrogen levels with the following exceptions: (1) Creatinine is not influenced by diet. (2) Daily production of creatinine from muscle metabolism is relatively constant. (3) Creatinine production is not as easily influenced by catabolic factors affecting urea formation. Therefore, conditions such as fever, toxemia, infection, and drug administration do not as readily influence creatinine levels.

As with urea, the rate of excretion is influenced by GFR, and any abnormality that decreases GFR will result in an increase in the concentration of serum creatinine. As there are fewer nonrenal factors that may influence creatinine concentration, it has had the reputation of being a more specific test for the diagnosis and prognosis of progressive renal disease than is the determination of serum UN level. Osborne et al.[2] make the following statement: "Although a marked elevation in serum creatinine concentration does indicate severe functional or organic impairment of nephron function, it is not of significantly greater value than BUN concentration in indicating the degree of reversibility or irreversibility of the underlying disease process, since it does not permit establishment of a specific diagnosis."

Techniques for determining serum creatinine level may not be as accurate as are those for urea nitrogen concentration. The alkaline picrate method measures some noncreatinine chromogens present in the plasma; thus it may give erroneously high creatinine values. The use of Lloyd's reagent reportedly permits measurement of true creatinine by removing these noncreatinine chromogens.

Normal serum creatinine concentrations are given as between 1 and 2 mg/dl, although normal values for any laboratory should be established on samples from normal animals within that practice area. Interpretation of creatinine concentration is similar to that for blood urea nitrogen level.

Other Blood Chemistry Determinations

As the kidneys play an important role in elimination and conservation of several chemical components of blood, renal disease may alter these blood chemical values. Although not usually of diagnostic significance, these alterations are of considerable importance in therapy and prognosis of renal disease.

Electrolytes

Detailed consideration of blood electrolytes will be found in Chapter 10; therefore, this discussion will be directed toward alterations observed in renal disease and some of the general mechanisms involved. It must be recognized that serum or plasma electrolyte values do not necessarily reflect total body concentration, and deviations from the normal level must be interpreted with this fact in mind. Electrolyte concentrations in plasma fluctuate rapidly with changes in the composition of extracellular and intracellular fluid. These fluctuations have as their net result a redistribution of water among the fluid compartments of the body in order to maintain osmolarity.

POTASSIUM. Potassium is removed from plasma by active reabsorption in the proximal tubules and is then actively excreted by cells of the distal tubules. The quantity of potassium handled by the kidneys is determined by the potassium intake. If a patient with renal disease becomes oliguric or anuric, potassium is retained and hyperkalemia may develop. If a patient with renal disease maintains adequate urine flow, the plasma potassium level remains normal unless acidosis develops.

SODIUM. Ability to retain sodium is frequently lost in the presence of generalized chronic renal diseases characterized by polyuria. This functional loss is accompanied by a deficiency in total body sodium that may or may not be reflected in plasma sodium concentration. Sodium loss through the diseased kidneys is accompanied by water loss as the body attempts to maintain body fluid isotonicity.

CHLORIDE. The chloride composition of the body tends to follow sodium concentration in patients with renal disease. Chloride insufficiencies may occur in patients with severe advanced renal disease.

BICARBONATE. The kidney functions to conserve bicarbonate. With advanced renal disease, deficiencies may occur, thus decreasing one of the most important buffers of hydrogen ions.

PHOSPHATE. Most of the phosphate excretion by the kidney is by glomerular filtration, with a variable amount of reabsorption by the tubules. Hyperphosphatemia occurs with regularity in dogs with chronic progressive and generalized acute renal diseases, as the GFR is reduced and the kidney loses its ability to eliminate phosphorus. Hyperphosphatemia is not a constant finding in cattle with azotemia. It has been suggested that the amount of serum phosphate increase may depend on prerenal factors as much as it does on renal excretory function in this species.[12] Horses with renal disease frequently have hypophosphatemia.

CALCIUM. No change in plasma calcium occurs in acute renal disease, but hypocalcemia may be observed with chronic generalized renal disease. Hypocalcemia is most commonly found in the terminal stages of the disease in dogs when values of 5 to 8 mg/dl may occur. If hypocalcemia develops, the parathyroid is stimulated, resulting in mobilization of bone calcium in an attempt to maintain plasma calcium concentration. Hypercalcemia has been observed in dogs with primary renal disease and no evidence of excess parathormone, parathormone-like substance, or vitamin D toxicosis,[13] but such a finding is not common. Hypercalcemia is frequent in horses with renal disease and is usually accompanied by a hypophosphatemia. Serum calcium levels range from 16 to 19 mg/dl, while phosphate is normal or decreased (less than 3.0 mg/dl). These changes are most frequently seen in horses with glomerulonephritis. Some horses with advanced renal disease do not have hypercalcemia. The relationship between hypercalcemia and primary or pseudohyperparathyroidism in such animals needs to be evaluated.

Nonelectrolytes

SERUM AMYLASE. Amylase is normally removed from plasma by renal excretion. In dogs and cats with uremia, serum amylase levels are usually increased. Results must, however, be interpreted with caution, and any other possible cause of the amylasemia must be ruled out. (See discussion in Chapter 8.)

BLOOD pH. Metabolic acidosis is a consistent finding in patients with renal failure. Lack of renal function reduces the ability of the kidney to remove H^+ from the blood as well as the capacity to remove accumulated acid breakdown products of metabolism. Such reduced ability is compounded by renal incapacity to conserve bicarbonate. Blood pH will be within the normal range if compensatory mechanisms are capable of handling the additional load, but if the capacity of the compensatory mechanisms is surpassed, blood pH will be lower than normal.

CHOLESTEROL. Although the mechanism remains unexplained, hypercholesterolemia frequently occurs in dogs with generalized glomerular disease or nephrosis.

SERUM PROTEINS. Total serum protein values reflect the state of hydration of the patient with renal disease. Hyperproteinemia will be present if the patient is dehydrated. Generalized renal disease in which there is a severe, persistent proteinuria may result in hypoalbuminemia. If protein (albumin) loss becomes marked, edema may result because of the decreased osmotic pressure associated with hypoalbuminemia. Hypoalbuminemia may be marked in animals with glomerulonephritis. If proteinuria is marked, a 24-hour urine collection should be made and the total protein loss calculated by measuring protein concentration as related to total 24-hour urine volume. Less than 300 mg/24 hours is considered normal. Losses of 3 to 13 gm/24 hours have been reported with severe glomerular disease.[14] If renal involvement is the result of an infectious disease or is immunologically mediated, plasma globulins may be increased. Evaluation of serum proteins in animals with renal disease should always include an estimation of albumin and globulin levels, as total protein determinations will not detect the alterations described.

Dye Excretion Tests

The most commonly used dye excretion test for renal function employs phenolsulfonphthalein (PSP). After being injected, this dye is bound to plasma proteins in a ratio that is dose dependent. The largest proportion of the dye is removed from blood plasma by tubular excretion. A comparatively minor fraction (5 per cent) is removed by glomerular filtration. The usual test dose of PSP is far below the maximum tubular clearance capability of the kidneys. Therefore, the 6-mg test dose is not a true evaluation of the excretory capacity of the tubules but is principally a test of renal plasma flow. The maximum tubular clearance capacity is approximately 50 times the test dose. Consequently, tubules would have to be extensively damaged before this test becomes a true measurement of tubular excretion.[2] This test appears to be most applicable for an assessment of kidney function in the canine species.

The PSP excretion test is conducted in the dog as follows:[2]

1. Empty the bladder by catheterization or permit the dog to micturate to remove the majority of accumulated urine.

2. Inject 6 mg of PSP dye intravenously, noting the exact time of injection.

3. If the animal has not been catheterized to remove accumulated urine, this procedure should be performed approximately 10 minutes following dye injection. The tip of the catheter should be positioned so that it is just beyond the junction of the neck of the bladder with the urethra.

4. Contents of the bladder are gently aspirated with a syringe, and all urine is collected in a flask. In order to minimize collection error, rinse the bladder with 10 to 15 ml of sterilized physiologic saline three or more times. Aspirate the saline rinse each time, adding it to the urine in the collection flask. Collection of

the fluid may be improved by injection and recovery of 10 to 15 ml of air following the final saline rinse.

5. The procedure should be completed exactly 20 minutes following dye injection.
6. Calculate the amount of dye that has been excreted according to the following technique:
   A. Place all urine and dye collected in a 1-liter graduated cylinder and dilute with water to 400 ml.
   B. Add 10 ml of 10 per cent sodium hydroxide and mix well. A pink color will develop following addition of the sodium hydroxide. If the color is deep pink, add enough water to bring the total volume to 1000 ml. If the alkalinized urine is light pink, add sufficient water to bring the total volume to 500 ml and divide the final result by 2. It may be necessary to filter the solution if it is turbid.
   C. The quantity of dye excreted can be found by measurement in a spectrophotometer set at a wave length of 560 mμ or by visually comparing the color of the unknown with color standards in a comparator block.

Sixty-seven per cent of normal dogs can be expected to excrete 33 to 55 per cent of the dye in 20 minutes; 95 per cent of normal dogs can be expected to excrete 21 to 66 per cent of the dye in 20 minutes.[2]

An abnormal decrease in urinary excretion of PSP may occur because of poor renal perfusion, which may be due to any one of several causes. Particularly significant causes are generalized renal disease, dehydration, congestive heart failure, and hypoadrenocorticism. PSP excretion is also decreased if there has been generalized destruction of proximal tubules of the kidney. The possibility that a technical error in collection of the dye from the bladder has resulted in an abnormally low value must always be considered.

It must be recognized that the necessity for careful timing of the sampling and complete removal of the urine constitute limitations for the application of this test.

Laboratory findings in diseases of the dog characterized by polyuria and polydipsia are summarized in Table 9–1 and Figure 9–5.

Renal Clearance Tests

As a part of its normal functioning, the kidney is said to clear blood of certain of its constituents. For example, urea clearance is defined as the volume of blood that one minute's production of urine clears of urea. Clearance also represents the minimum amount of blood required to furnish the amount of a specific substance excreted in the urine in one minute. The concept of renal clearance has contributed a great deal to the present understanding of renal function in disease and health.

In theory, a substance may be excreted by (1) glomerular filtration alone, (2) filtration plus tubular excretion, or (3) filtration plus tubular reabsorption. If a substance is completely filtered at the glomerulus and completely reabsorbed by the tubules, its clearance value is zero—e.g., glucose. As the degree of tubular reabsorption diminishes, the substance may appear in the urine. Its clearance then increases—e.g., urea—until if there is no reabsorption of a substance, its clearance will be equivalent to the rate of glomerular filtration—e.g., inulin and creatinine in the dog. If, in addition to being filtered through the glomerulus, the substance is also excreted by the tubular epithelium—e.g., phenol red—its clearance will exceed the rate of glomerular filtration by an amount equal to the extent of tubular excretion. Since the kidneys cannot excrete more of a substance in a given period of time than is brought to them in the blood, the maximum limit of renal clearance is determined by renal blood flow. These facts form the basis for quantitative determination of the various aspects of renal function.

ENDOGENOUS CREATINE CLEARANCE. Endogenous creatinine clearance is based on the same concept of renal clearance, but does not require administration of creatinine. The test is completed as follows:[15]

1. Remove residual urine by catheterization.
2. Rinse bladder several times with sterile physiologic saline. Discard urine and saline.
3. Begin timing urine formation upon completion of rinsing procedure.
4. Collect a serum sample approximately halfway through the test period.
5. At the end of timed urine collection (usually 20 minutes), collect all of the urine by catheterization and rinse the bladder with several milliliters of sterile saline. Urine and saline are mixed and the total volume is measured.
6. Analyze the serum sample and the final urine plus saline collection for the quantity of creatinine per dl.
7. Accurately determine the dog's weight.
8. Calculate creatinine clearance using the following formula:

$$C_{cr} = \frac{U_c V}{S_c \times T \times BW}$$

Where C_{cr} = ml/min/kg
U_c and S_c = mg/dl of creatinine in urine and serum respectively
V = urine volume in milliliters
T = time in minutes
BW = body weight in kilograms

The normal 20-minute C_{cr} for dogs is 2.8 ± 0.96 ml/min/kg.[16] The normal 24-hour C_{cr} for dogs has been reported to be 3.7 ± 0.77 ml/min/kg with a range of 1.7 to 4.5 ml/min/kg.[17] The C_{cr} for sheep

TABLE 9–1. Laboratory Findings in Diseases of the Dog Characterized by Polyuria and Polydipsia

Disease	Hemogram	Urinalysis					Blood Chemistry			Other Laboratory Tests
		Specific Gravity	Protein	Glucose	Others	Sediment	Creatinine and Bun	Electrolytes	Others	
Chronic generalized nephritis	Nonregenerative anemia; leukocytosis variable	1.008–1.012	N-trace to 2+	Neg.	pH ↓ if animal acidotic	Occasional hyaline or granular casts	↑	PO$_4$ ↑; Na, Cl, HCO$_3$ ↓ in advanced stages. Ca ↓ terminally	—	PSP excretion ↓ no increase in Sp. Gr. with water deprivation or vasopressin
Renal amyloidosis	Nonregenerative anemia if generalized and chronic	N to Low	++++	Neg.	pH ↓ if animal acidotic	Hyaline granular, and sometimes waxy casts	↑	As above if generalized advanced	Cholesterol ↑	PSP excretion ↓ Urine concentration test normal early but abnormal in advanced disease
Chronic pyelonephritis	Leukocytosis, nonregenerative anemia if generalized	N to fixed in generalized	+++	Neg.	Blood frequently +	Leukocytes, bacteria; erythrocytes, WBC and/or granular casts	↑ if generalized	If generalized as above	—	PSP excretion ↓ if generalized; urine culture frequently positive
Generalized acute nephritis	Leukocytosis may be present; if much stress ↓ lymphocytes and eosinophils	High or low depending on amount of renal damage	+++	Neg.	Blood may be +	↑ leukocytes, erythrocytes and casts—may be transient	No to ↑	Usually N	—	
Renal cortical hypoplasia	Nonregenerative anemia in later stages may be stress response if uremia marked	1.002–1.012	Trace to ++	May be present	—	No significant findings	↑	PO$_4$ ↑; Na, Cl HCO$_3$ and Ca ↓ if severe	—	PSP excretion ↓ Negative to urine concentration test

Disease									
Diabetes insipidus	No change	1.001–1.006	Neg.	Neg.	—	No significant findings	N	No change	—	Sp. Gr. increased in urine concentration test with vasopressin
Renal diabetes insipidus	No change	1.001–1.006	Neg.	Neg.	—	No significant findings	N	No change	—	No response to vasopressin
Diabetes mellitus	May be ↑ PCV and WBC may be normal	1.015–1.050	Neg.	+++	Ketones + pH low	Usually no significant findings; occasionally WBC, RBC, and bacteria	N to ↑	If acidotic HCO$_3$ ↓ and pH ↓	Hyperglycemia; hypercholesterolemia	PSP excretion usually N; glucose tolerance abnormal
Primary renal glucosuria	Normal	1.015–1.050	Neg. unless cystitis present ++ to +++	++++	—	No significant finding unless bacterial cystitis present	N	N	No increase in blood glucose	PSP excretion N
Pyometra	Marked leukocytosis with left shift; nonregenerative anemia may occur but not consistently	1.001–1.006	Neg.		—	Hematuria, possible pyuria	↑ if GFR <25–30%	Changes not consistent	↑ globulins; hyperproteinemia; cholesterol often ↑	
Hyperadrenocorticism	Eosinopenia, lymphopenia	1.008–1.018	Neg.	Neg. to +	↑ in ketogenic steroids	No significant findings	N	Usually N	Glucose slightly ↑; cholesterol ↑	PSP excretion N

N = Normal
↑ = Increase
↓ = Decrease

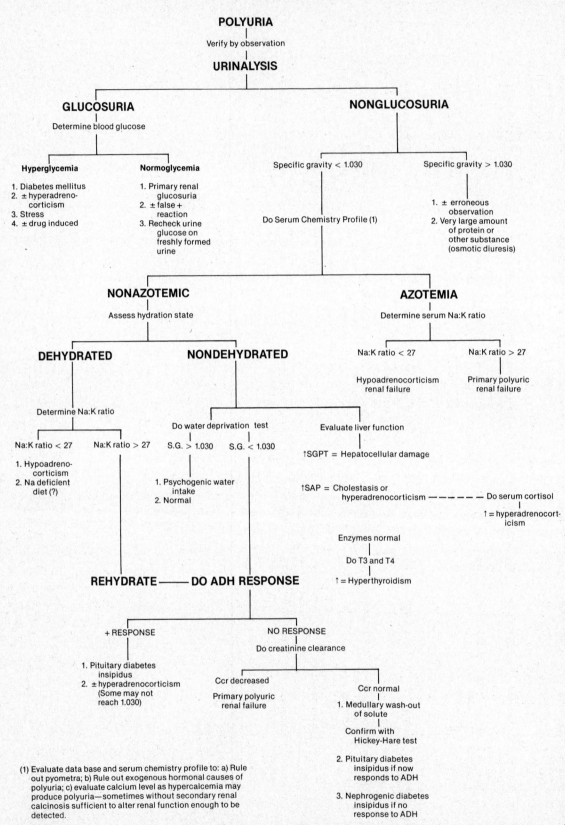

Figure 9–5. Investigation of polyuria in the dog. (Adapted from Polzin, D. J. and Osborne, C. A.: Conservation and management of canine chronic polyuric renal failure. *In:* Current Veterinary Therapy VIII. Small Animal Practice, edited by Kirk, R. W., W. B. Saunders Company, Philadelphia, 1985.

is 3.48 ± 0.12 ml/min/kg[18]; 1.95 ± 0.82 for the pony[19]; 1.47 ml/min/kg for the horse[20]; and 1.32 to 2.23 ml/min/kg in cattle.[20]

In interpreting the endogenous clearance one must remember that creatinine clearance is influenced by prerenal as well as renal factors. This necessitates a careful consideration of prerenal reduction in glomerular filtration such as that associated with dehydration, cardiac insufficiency, or other factors that would reduce renal blood flow.

The urine urea nitrogen/plasma urea nitrogen ratio (U_{un}/P_{un}), urine creatinine/plasma creatinine ratio (U_{cr}/P_{cr}), urine osmolality/plasma osmolality ratio (U_{osm}/P_{osm}), and fractional excretion of filtered sodium (FE_{Na}) were determined in horses with azotemia in an attempt to differentiate between prerenal and renal azotemia.[21] In horses with renal azotemia the U_{osm}/P_{osm}, U_{un}/P_{un}, and U_{cr}/P_{cr} were lower than in those with prerenal azotemia. The mean U_{osm}/P_{osm} in horses with renal azotemia, as confirmed by histopathology, was 1.11 ± 0.25 as compared to 2.71 ± 0.58 for those with prerenal azotemia. The mean U_{un}/P_{un} in renal disease was 6.93 ± 4.59 and 26.73 ± 11.43 in prerenal azotemia. The mean U_{cr}/P_{cr} was 17.09 ± 12.74 with renal azotemia and 109.43 ± 69.35 in prerenal azotemia. These means and standard deviations were calculated from data presented in this paper.[21] The means and ranges in six nonazotemic horses were: U_{osm}/P_{osm} = 4.1 (2.5–5.2); U_{un}/P_{un} = 67.2 (34.2–100.8); U_{cr}/P_{cr} = 151.5 (2.0–344.4); while the FE_{Na} was 0.17 (0.01–0.70). The mean FE_{Na} was calculated using the formula:

$$FE_{Na} = \frac{[Cr]_p}{[Cr]_u} \times \frac{[Na]_u}{[Na]_p} \times 100$$

Where $[Cr]_p$ = plasma creatinine (mg/dl)
$[Cr]_u$ = urine creatinine (mg/dl)
$[Na]_p$ = plasma sodium (mEq/L)
$[Na]_u$ = urine sodium (mEq/L)

The mean FE_{Na} was 0.24 ± 0.18 and 3.33 ± 3.14, respectively, for renal and prerenal azotemia.

These results suggest that these indices may be of value in an early identification of renal disease. However, the great variability reported, in part caused by the limited number of animals studied, resulted in overlapping values that make interpretation difficult. Additional data must be accumulated before these indices can be relied upon to differentiate between renal and prerenal azotemia in the horse.

The endogenous creatinine clearance method for determining GFR, if properly completed, provides a relatively precise measurement of renal function. It is more difficult to complete than determinations of urine specific gravity, serum UN, serum creatinine, urine osmolality, or PSP clearance but, because of its sensitivity, may be a more definitive measurement of early renal changes in generalized renal disease. Determination of GFR will not differentiate among prerenal, renal, or postrenal abnormalities but will detect alterations in renal function.

Sulfanilate Clearance

Sulfanilate is removed from the blood by glomerular filtration. Measurement of sulfanilate clearance should therefore be a method for evaluating glomerular filtration.

The sulfanilate clearance test is completed as follows:[22]

1. Inject sodium sulfanilate intravenously in a 10 per cent solution at a dosage of 20 mg/kg of body weight.

2. After injection, draw blood samples (2 to 3 ml.) at 30, 60, and 90 minutes.

3. Determine sulfanilate concentration of whole blood (details of analytical method in Appendix, p. 444).

4. Plot results on semilog coordinates and calculate $T_{1/2}$.

5. Sulfonamides are detected by the method used; thus this test should not be completed on dogs being treated with these drugs.

Sulfanilate $T_{1/2}$ for the dog was reported as 66.1 ± 10.8 minutes, but a range of 50 to 80 minutes was considered normal.[22,23] The same authors studied sulfanilate clearance in dogs with mild and severe renal disease and compared the results with those found in a group of normal dogs.[23] They concluded that sulfanilate clearance is most advantageous in evaluation of renal function loss in animals that are suspected of having renal disease but that have little or no increase in UN. Dogs with significantly increased UN values had sulfanilate $T_{1/2}$ values of 200 minutes or more. Dogs with borderline or normal UN values but with a reduction in renal function had sulfanilate $T_{1/2}$ times from 104 to 174 minutes. PSP excretion was within the normal range for this group of dogs.

In another evaluation of 13 clinically healthy dogs the mean sulfanilate $T_{1/2}$ was 58 ± 13 minutes, with a normal range (mean ± 2 standard deviations) of 32 to 84 minutes.[24] Sulfanilate clearance appeared to be more sensitive than serum creatinine or urea nitrogen as an indicator of early renal disease. In some cases the $T_{1/2}$ was increased in dogs with a urine specific gravity greater than 1.012. This suggests that renal disease may result in decreased sulfanilate clearance before complete loss of the ability to form urine with a specific gravity greater than that of the glomerular filtrate.[24]

This test is relatively simple to perform and appears to provide a degree of sensitivity not available with some of the other methods for evaluating renal function because (1) there is no need to collect urine specimens; (2) errors associated with removal of urine, flushing the bladder, and quantitative collection are avoided; (3) less time is required for test performance; and (4) accuracy in estimating renal functional capacity is improved.

This technique apparently is also applicable to the cat, although the $T_{1/2}$ of this animal is about half that of the dog (45.1 ± 7.0 minutes,[20] 44.2 ± 5.67 minutes[25]). Sulfanilate clearance was compared to glomerular filtration rate and renal blood flow in cats before and after reduction of renal mass.[25] Azotemia developed, but the cats retained considerable ability to concentrate urine. The sulfanilate clearance test was superior to PSP and urine concentration test for the clinical estimation of renal function.

Further clinical studies need to be completed in order to substantiate the use of the sodium sulfanilate clearance test as a measurement of renal function.

BACTERIAL CULTURE

If bacteria are observed in sediment from a freshly collected urine specimen or the clinician suspects bacterial infection, cultural examination is warranted.

Meaningful bacterial examinations can be made only if urine is properly collected. Normal urine is sterile until it reaches the neck of the bladder. Since the urethra, prepuce, vagina, and vulva have normal bacterial flora, urine collected as the animal micturates or by manual compression of the bladder will almost always contain bacteria. If urine collected in this fashion is used for culture, the first portion should be discarded and cultural examination completed on the last fraction excreted. The first part of urine flow flushes the urethra, reducing the number of contaminating bacteria. Specimens collected by catheterization or cystocentesis are preferred and should be used whenever possible. As with midstream collection, the first part of a sample collected by catheterization should be discarded and the latter portion cultured, as bacteria from the urethra may be forced into the bladder, contaminating the initial fraction. Urine collected by cystocentesis is the specimen of choice for cultural examination.

Urine must be cultured as soon as possible following collection, preferably within an hour. If urine is not immediately cultured, it should be refrigerated, but this should be avoided whenever possible.

Ideally, a urine culture should provide qualitative and quantitative information. A semiquantitative technique is acceptable, as precise enumeration is not required. Since a variety of gram-negative and gram-positive bacteria may be associated with disease of the urinary system, it is advisable to culture for both groups. This is read-ily accomplished by inoculating both a blood agar plate and a plate containing an agar medium selective for gram-negative bacteria (MacConkey, eosin-methylene blue, and so forth). If no quantitative estimation is to be completed, two or three loopfuls of well-mixed urine are streaked on each plate.

A semiquantitative urine culture can be completed by using a standard calibrated loop. Such loops are commercially available. A calibrated 4-mm loop holding 0.01 ml is acceptable. Plates for qualitative and semiquantitative urine culture are prepared as follows:

1. Place a small drop of sterile saline in the center of the agar plate.
2. Transfer one loopful (0.01 ml) of urine to the drop of saline.
3. Streak this inoculum over the surface of the plate using a bent needle.
4. Incubate at 35 to 37°C for 24 hours, then count the number of colonies, and multiply by 100 to estimate bacterial population.
5. After counting the colonies, select typical ones, identify organisms (at least to genus), and complete a sensitivity test.

Studies in human medicine suggest that less than 10,000 organisms per ml of urine are insignificant and that greater than 100,000 are indicative of urinary tract infections. Comparable studies in veterinary medicine are not available. The type of organism present must also be considered in interpretation of culture results. Finding 5000 *Staphylococcus aureus*/ml of urine is likely to be of more importance than five times that number of *Escherichia coli*.

If the patient has been receiving antibacterial therapy, urine cultures are often negative even if bacteria are observed in the urine sediment. Accurate cultural examination can be completed only when therapy has been discontinued for three to five days. If the clinician does not wish to discontinue therapy and a qualitative bacterial evaluation of urine is deemed necessary, the following technique may be helpful:

1. Centrifuge urine and discard the supernatant.
2. Replace urine volume with sterile physiological saline and completely resuspend the sediment.
3. Centrifuge the specimen, discarding supernatant.
4. Repeat steps 2 and 3 at least twice.
5. Prepare plates with washed sediment, using three or four loopfuls of material.

Washing urinary sediment in this fashion will sometimes reduce antibacterial concentration sufficiently to permit qualitative evaluation. If no bacteria are isolated with this technique, the possibility of a bacterial infection is not completely eliminated.

RENAL BIOPSY

Although not considered a routine laboratory examination, renal biopsy, if properly completed, will often be useful in evaluation of the patient with a renal problem. Since it is beyond the scope of this book to discuss renal biopsy techniques, the reader is referred to the text by Osborne et al.[2]

Biopsy should be considered when history, physical examination, laboratory data, and radiographic evaluation have been completed and additional information is needed as a basis for diagnosis, prognosis, and treatment. Other diagnostic aids may indicate renal dysfunction, but only a renal biopsy will reveal morphologic alterations. Evaluation of a renal biopsy may provide information needed to determine whether the condition is reversible or irreversible.

A renal biopsy is of more value in generalized renal disease, as there is less likelihood of missing the lesion when the specimen is obtained. Focal lesions may be missed during renal biopsy, but this is a minor consideration, as focal lesions do not produce signs of renal disease unless they are widely distributed throughout the kidney. As hemorrhage may be a problem following renal biopsy, it is advisable to evaluate the hemostatic status of the patient prior to surgery.

THE HEMOGRAM IN RENAL DISEASE

In advanced stages of renal disease, a slight to moderate normocytic normochromic nonregenerative anemia is common. This will become progressively more severe as the renal function deteriorates. Anemia results from reduction in erythropoietin and the subsequent hypoplasia of erythroid cells in the bone marrow. A progressive anemia in an animal with renal disease is an unfavorable sign, as it suggests chronic renal impairment. Evaluation of the degree of anemia must take into consideration the state of hydration of the individual. Polyuric animals that do not have free access to water become dehydrated, and the anemia will be masked in these patients. Correlation of the total plasma proteins with packed cell volume, hemoglobin, and total erythrocytes may assist in making such a differentiation.

In animals having a renal problem associated with blood loss, a typical regenerative anemia may be present if there is adequate renal production of the erythrocyte-stimulating factor.

Most renal diseases, even the acute inflammatory diseases, do not have an associated leukocytosis and neutrophilia. However, if pyelonephritis or renal abscesses are present, a classic leukocyte response can be expected. With a chronic renal disease and its accompanying stress, there may be a slight neutrophilia and lymphopenia.

REFERENCES

1. Altman, P. L., and Dittmer, D. S.: *Blood and Other Body Fluids*, Federation of American Societies for Experimental Biology, Washington, 1961.
2. Osborne, C. A., Low, D. G., and Finco, D. R.: *Canine and Feline Urology*, W. B. Saunders Company, Philadelphia, 1972.
3. Hardy, R. M., and Osborne, C. A.: Water deprivation test in the dog: Maximal normal values. J.A.V.M.A., *174*:479, 1979.
4. Watts, C.: Failure of an impregnated cellulose strip as a test for glucose in urine. Vet. Rec., *80*:48, 1968.
5. Chew, D. J.: Urinalysis. In: *Canine Nephrology*, edited by Bovee, K. C., Horwal Publishing Company, Philadelphia, 1984.
6. Meyer, D. J., and Senior, D. F.: Hematuria and dysuria. In: *Textbook of Veterinary Internal Medicine. Diseases of the Dog and Cat*, 2nd ed., edited by Ettinger, S. J., W. B. Saunders Company, Philadelphia, 1983.
7. Carbone, M. G.: Phosphocrystalluria and urethral obstruction in the cat. J.A.V.M.A., *147*:1195, 1965.
8. Rich, L. J., and Kirk, R. W.: The relationship of struvite crystals to urethral obstruction in cats. J.A.V.M.A., *154*:153, 1969.
9. Osbaldiston, G. W., and Moore, W. E.: Renal function tests in cattle. J.A.V.M.A., *159*:292, 1971.
10. Bovee, K. C.: Urine osmolarity as a definitive indicator of renal concentrating capacity. J.A.V.M.A., *155*:30, 1969.
11. Epstein, M. E., Barsanti, J. A., Finco, D. R., and Cowgill, L. M.: Postprandial changes in plasma urea nitrogen and plasma creatinine concentrations in dogs fed commercial diets. J.A.A.H.A., *20*:799, 1984.
12. Brobst, D. F., Parish, S. M., Torbeck, R. L., Frost, O. L., and Bracken, F. K.: Azotemia in cattle. J.A.V.M.A., *173*:481, 1978.
13. Finco, D. R., and Rowland, G. N.: Hypercalcemia secondary to chronic renal failure in the dog: A report of four cases. J.A.V.M.A., *173*:990, 1978.
14. DiBartola, S. P., Spaulding, C. L., Chew, D. J., et al.: Urinary protein excretion and immunopathologic findings in dogs with glomerular disease. J.A.V.M.A., *177*:73, 1980.
15. Polzin, D. J., and Osborne, C. A.: Conservative medical management of canine chronic polyuric renal failure. In: *Current Veterinary Therapy VIII. Small Animal Practice*, edited by Kirk, R. W., W. B. Saunders Company, Philadelphia, 1983.
16. Finco, D. R.: Simultaneous determination of phenolsulfonphthalein excretion and endogenous creatinine clearance in the normal dog. J.A.V.M.A., *159*:336, 1971.
17. Bovee, K. C. and Joyce, B. A.: Clinical evaluation of glomerular filtration: 24-hour creatinine clearance in the dog. J.A.V.M.A., *174*:488, 1979.
18. English, D. B., Hogan, A. E., and McDougall, H. L.: Changes in renal function with reduction in renal mass. Am. J. Vet. Res., *38*,1317, 1977.
19. Rawlings, C. A., and Bisgard, G. E.: Renal clearance and excretion of endogenous substances in the pony. Am. J. Vet. Res., *36*:46, 1975.
20. Osbaldiston, G. W.: Kidney function. In: *Clinical*

Biochemistry of Domestic Animals, 2nd ed., edited by Kaneko, J. J., and Cornelius, C. E., Academic Press, New York, 1971.

21. Grossman, B. S., Brobst, D. F., Kramer, J. W., Bayly, W. M., and Reed, S. M.: Urinary indices for differentiation of prerenal azotemia and renal azotemia in horses. J.A.V.M.A., *180*:284, 1982.

22. Carlson, G. P., and Kaneko, J. J.: Simultaneous estimation of renal function in dogs using sodium sulfanilate and sodium idohippurate 131. J.A.V.M.A., *158*:1229, 1971.

23. Carlson, G. P., and Kaneko, J. J.: Sulfanilate clearance in clinical renal disease in the dog. J.A.V.M.A., *158*:1235, 1971.

24. Maddison, J. E., Pascoe, P. J., and Jansen, B. E.: Clinical evaluation of sodium sulfanilate clearance for the diagnosis of renal disease in dogs. J.A.V.M.A., *185*:961, 1984.

25. Ross, L. A., and Finco, D. R.: Relationship of selected clinical renal function tests to glomerular filtration rate and renal blood flow in cats. Am. J. Vet. Res., *42*:1704, 1981.

WATER, ELECTROLYTES, AND ACID-BASE BALANCE

The role of electrolytes in the animal body is diverse, as there are almost no metabolic processes that are not affected by or dependent upon electrolytes. A number of instruments and techniques are available that permit accurate, reproducible analytical measurements of electrolytes and blood pH. With increasing knowledge about electrolyte balances in various animal diseases, the use of electrolyte replacement therapy has become routine practice in veterinary medicine. In order that therapy can be most efficacious, it is essential for the clinician to have an understanding of the basic mechanisms involved in electrolyte alterations and an ability to interpret results of laboratory estimations for electrolytes and acid-base balance.

The proportion of water in an animal body ranges from 45 to 70 per cent of total body weight, and the percentage is dependent upon the amount of fat in the body. As fat contains little water, a lean animal has a higher percentage of body water than a fat individual. Body fluid is divided into two compartments: (1) intracellular fluid (ICF), which constitutes from 65 to 75 per cent of the total body water and from 35 to 45 per cent of total body weight and (2) extracellular fluid (ECF). Approximately 25 per cent of the total body water and 15 per cent of body weight are found in ECF. The ECF compartment is composed of fluids found in three locations—intravascularly (plasma), interstitially (including lymph) and transcellularly. The so-called transcellular fluid is a small portion of the total ECF and includes the liquid found in cerebrospinal fluid and joint fluids as well as the liquid in the intestine.

Comprehension of the characteristics of the fluid compartments is essential before the various alterations that take place can be understood. The composition of ICF varies from tissue to tissue in a single animal as well as among the various species. ICF contains a higher concentration of potassium and phosphate and a lower concentration of sodium and chloride than does ECF. Unfortunately, it is impossible clinically to measure the electrolyte composition of intracellular fluid. Therefore, estimations of the status of ICF electrolytes are based on a knowledge of the fluid and electrolyte exchange between ICF and ECF. The electrolyte concentrations in ECF are measured, and findings are related to alterations that have taken place in the ICF.

Extracellular fluid is the liquid that bathes cells. The interstitial portion of ECF is essentially an ultrafiltrate of plasma. Water and major electrolytes move freely within this compartment and between it and intravascular fluids. The predominant ECF ions are sodium (Na^+), the cation, and chloride (Cl^-), the anion. These ions redistribute themselves in accordance with Donnan's equilibrium. Fluid in the intravascular portion of ECF has almost the same composition as does interstitial fluid except for its higher protein level.

Electrolytes and water move freely between the ICF and ECF compartments. Water is continually moving, and this movement is quite rapid. The movement of water is partially dependent upon the physical effects of hydrostatic pressure plus the osmotic effects of ECF proteins. These proteins counteract the tendency of fluids to move from areas of high intravascular pressure to areas of lower extravascular pressure. Shifts in water and electrolytes depend more on differences between the osmolarity of intracellular and interstitial fluids than on hydrostatic pressure. The homeostatic mechanisms of the body are designed to maintain the osmotic pressure of the extracellular fluid. If ECF osmotic pressure can be maintained, it will also serve to maintain cellular osmolarity. If the osmotic pressure of ECF is increased, water is removed from cells. When water moves from cells into extracellular fluid, it produces cellular dehydration, and a new state of equilibrium develops between ECF and ICF but at a new and different osmolarity. The net effect increases cellular osmolarity and decreases the hypertonicity of ECF.

A comparison of the concentrations of cations and anions in serum reveals that there is an exact equality of total anions and total cations. This electrical neutrality is maintained at all times. Any increase in one cation is accompanied by a decrease in some other cation or by an increase in one or more of the anions, or both, in order to maintain electrical neutrality. In a similar fashion, any decrease in cations is accompanied by an increase in some other cation or by a decrease in total anions, or both. Electrical neutrality should not be confused with acid-base neutrality (pH 7.0), as the former term is used to denote the equivalency of cations and anions. Plasma pH depends on the distribution of various compounds and their degree of dissociation.

The osmotic pressure of any fluid is directly related to the number of particles in a unit of solvent. Osmotic effect is measured in osmoles (Osm) or milliosmoles (mOsm). An osmole of an ionized substance is defined as being the gram molecular weight of the substance multiplied by the number of ions into which it dissociates. In the clinical laboratory, osmolality is measured in terms of milliosmoles per kilogram of water. The normal osmolality of plasma in domestic animals is about 300 mOsm/kg of plasma water. The main ECF cation is Na^+, and the primary anions are Cl^- and bicarbonate (HCO_3^-). In the ICF, the major cations are potassium (K^+) and magnesium (Mg^+), and the major anions are organic phosphates and protein. Sodium and potassium are mainly responsible for the osmotic pressures of ECF and ICF, respectively, as they are present in the greatest concentrations. Therefore, comprehension of the mechanisms for regulating the concentration of these electrolytes is essential to an understanding of electrolyte balance.

ELECTROLYTES

Sodium. Approximately half of the total body concentration of sodium is found in ECF where sodium has its primary function; most of the rest is present in bone in a form not readily available to ECF. The quantity of sodium is controlled by dietary intake and loss. Sodium is usually present in adequate concentrations in the diet of carnivores, but herbivores may occasionally experience a deficiency unless their diet is supplemented. Although sodium is constantly entering and being pumped out of cells, it is not used up in metabolism.

The most important route for sodium excretion is through the kidney. Most sodium presented to renal tubules is reabsorbed (approximately 90 per cent); this process is controlled by aldosterone. If there is a body excess of sodium, aldosterone secretion is reduced and sodium is excreted through the kidneys. If the total body concentration of sodium is decreased, aldosterone production is increased and sodium is almost completely reabsorbed. It must be remembered that sodium reabsorption requires an equivalent passage of hydrogen or potassium ions in the opposite direction. Sodium is also lost in sweat and in secretions of the digestive tract. In carnivores and most herbivores, sodium is reabsorbed in the lower intestinal tract. In herbivores with large quantities of fluid in the feces, such as the cow and the horse, there may be considerable fecal loss of sodium.

Potassium. Sodium concentration is higher in ECF than in ICF, and the reverse is true for potassium. Potassium concentration is low in ECF and high in most cells of the body. Sodium concentration within the cell is maintained at a lower level by active removal by means of the so-called "sodium pump." Dietary deficiencies of potassium are almost unknown, as the diets of carnivores and herbivores contain adequate potassium to meet body needs. In fact, most animals take in a great excess of potassium, and adequate excretion is essential in order to forestall potassium intoxication. Most potassium is excreted by the kidneys through glomerular filtration and tubular secretion. The ability of the kidney to conserve potassium is not as efficient as its ability to conserve sodium. It must be remembered that aldosterone facilitates excretion of potassium, since it causes increased sodium reabsorption by promoting the exchange of sodium in tubular fluid for potassium in the tubular cell. Potassium excretion by the kidneys is also controlled by competition between potassium and hydrogen ions for reabsorption. In addition to removal by the kidney, some potassium may be lost in feces, particularly in animals having a high fecal water content. Potassium may also be lost from the body in sweat and digestive fluids.

Chloride. Chloride is present in ICF in small quantities, but it is the anion in highest concentration in ECF. Chloride is adequate in the diet if major cations are present in the feedstuffs consumed, as it usually occurs in combination with these cations. Excretion, absorption, and distribution of chloride are passive, as chloride usually accompanies sodium, which is actively transported.

Bicarbonate. The maintenance of normal acid-base balance in the body is principally subject to the bicarbonate ion. Bicarbonate is mostly of endogenous origin, being produced by hydration of carbon dioxide to carbonic acid, which then dissociates to bicarbonate and hydrogen ions. Bicarbonate is lost through secretions to the digestive tract and in the urine. Regulation of the bicarbonate level by the lungs and kidneys will be discussed in the following section.

ACID-BASE BALANCE

Normal metabolic processes in an animal body result in the production of relatively large quantities of acids such as lactic acid, carbonic acid, sulfuric acid, beta-hydroxybutyric acid, and phosphoric acid. These acids are transported to the excretory organs, i.e., the lungs and the kidneys, without causing any marked alteration in body pH. Maintenance of pH is essential, as many metabolic processes that occur within cells are pH dependent and will cease to operate if the pH is altered. This sensitive control of blood pH in the normal range of 7.3 to 7.5 is accomplished by the combined effects of the blood buffer system, the respiratory system, and the renal system. In addition to their role in controlling blood pH, these systems are also of significance in maintaining the normal cation-anion composition of the body.

Blood Buffer Systems. A buffer is a mixture of a weakly dissociated acid and a salt of that acid. As such, buffers prevent a major shift in pH by binding or releasing hydrogen ions. For example, in the bicarbonate buffer system, if a strong acid is added to a solution containing bicarbonate (HCO_3^-) and carbonic acid (H_2CO_3), the hydrogen ion (H^+) reacts with HCO_3^- to form more H_2CO_3, which is a weak acid and causes only a slight increase in the H^+ concentration. On the other hand, if a base is added to the same buffer system, the hydroxide ion (OH^-) reacts with the H^+ to form HCO_3^- and water, and the pH change is again small.

The Henderson-Hasselbalch equation is of assistance in understanding and explaining pH control of body fluids. This formula is as follows:

$$pH = pK + \log \frac{salt}{acid}$$

In this formula pK = the negative logarithm of the dissociation constant K, salt equals the concentration of the ionized species, acid equals the concentration of the undissociated acid, and pH is the negative logarithm of the hydrogen ion.

The blood buffers that play a role in control of pH are: (1) the bicarbonate/carbonic acid system (HCO_3^-/H_2CO_3); (2) hemoglobin, which is available to accept H^+ from H_2CO_3; (3) the protein buffer system; and (4) the phosphate buffer system ($HPO_4^{--}/H_2PO_4^-$). When the hydrogen ion concentration is subject to change, all systems are affected, but the most important in control of blood pH is the HCO_3^-/H_2CO_3 system.

Bicarbonate/Carbonic Acid Buffer System. The Henderson-Hasselbalch equation as applied to this system is:

$$pH = 6.1 + \log \frac{HCO_3^-}{H_2CO_3}$$

Thus, the pH of plasma is dependent upon the *ratio* of HCO_3^- to H_2CO_3. The normal ratio is 20:1. As the log of 20 is 1.301, then 6.1 + 1.301 = 7.401 = normal pH of blood. As the bicarbonate buffer system is the most abundant in the body, the most easily controlled, and the easiest to measure, it is clinically the most important.

Carbonic acid is formed when hydrogen from cell metabolism combines with bicarbonate ($H^+ + HCO_3^- \rightarrow H_2CO_3$) or when carbon dioxide produced by cell metabolism is combined with water inside the erythrocyte to form carbonic acid under the influence of cellular carbonic anhydrase. Bicarbonate is formed when oxygen leaves oxyhemoglobin to form hemoglobin. Hemoglobin then takes up the extra hydrogen ion from the dissociation of carbonic acid, and bicarbonate is formed and diffuses out of the erythrocyte and into the plasma. Oxygen removed in this fashion passes from red blood cells through plasma and into the tissue cells. Carbon dioxide produced by the normal metabolic processes of the body is carried to the lungs by the blood. Because of the continuous production of carbon dioxide within tissue cells, there is a concentration differential for carbon dioxide from cells to plasma and erythrocytes. This causes a shift of physically dissolved carbon dioxide from tissue cells into the plasma and erythrocytes. A small portion of the carbon dioxide entering the plasma remains as dissolved carbonic acid, a second small portion reacts with water to form carbonic acid, and a third small portion combines with the amino groups of proteins to form carbamino compounds. Most of the carbon dioxide entering erythrocytes reacts with water to form carbonic acid. The dissolved carbon dioxide, carbamino compounds, and bicarbonate are transported by blood to the pulmonary capillaries and alveoli. Influenced by the comparatively low partial pressure of carbon dioxide (P_{CO_2}) in the alveoli, there is a shift of carbon dioxide from plasma and erythrocytes into the alveoli. Simultaneously, the high oxygen content in the alveoli results in a shift of oxygen into erythrocytes and plasma. This exchange results in a reversal of the reactions just described for the formation of carbonic acid, bicarbonate ion, and carbon dioxide.

Respiratory Control of Acid-Base Balance. The respiratory center found in the medulla oblongata is sensitive to blood levels of P_{CO_2}. If blood P_{CO_2} increases above the normal value, there will be an increase in the respiratory rate. This increase has a tendency to return P_{CO_2}, and consequently H_2CO_3, levels toward normal. This respiratory center will also respond to pH changes, and even if P_{CO_2} is normal and pH drops, the respiratory rate will increase and P_{CO_2} will be reduced. Conversely, if P_{CO_2} is low or blood pH is increased, the respiratory rate will decrease. Thus, regulation of the rate of pulmonary ventilation in response to changes in P_{CO_2} and pH serves as a basis for pulmonary compensation in alkalosis and acidosis.

Renal Control of Acid-Base Balance. The respiratory system of control deals only with changes in blood P_{CO_2} and, to a more limited extent, with other blood pH changes. Accumulation of nonvolatile acids and the subsequent depleting effect on bicarbonate ion content can be offset only by the renal ability to exchange sodium ions for hydrogen ions and the production of an acid urine. Most acids are not excreted in their free form by the kidneys, but only in the form of salts. Consequently, as nonvolatile acid anions are filtered through the glomerulus, they are accompanied by an equivalent number of cations (primarily sodium) in order to maintain electrical neutrality. Renal tubule cells, through the activity of carbonic anhydrase, combine carbon dioxide from their own metabolic activities with water to make carbonic acid, which dissociates to hydrogen and bicarbonate ions. The hydrogen ions pass into the tubule and an equivalent amount of sodium is returned to the blood accompanied by bicarbonate ions in an equivalent amount. Thus, bicarbonate ions are replaced, hydrogen ions and nonvolatile acid anions are excreted, and acid urine prevails.

Renal tubular cells have the ability to form ammonia from amides and some amino acids. This process is enhanced by acidosis and decreased by alkalosis. Ammonia (NH_3) produced by enzymatic action on the amide or amino acid diffuses into tubular urine where it combines with hydrogen to form ammonium (NH_4). This formation of ammonia in tubular cells permits an increased excretion of hydrogen ions and assists in sodium preservation.

It is well known that glomerular filtrates contain the same concentration of bicarbonate ions as does blood plasma. However, with increasing urine acidification, the bicarbonate ion content in urine decreases and the P_{CO_2} increases.

Along with the decrease of bicarbonate ions in tubular urine, there is an increase in chloride. These changes are accompanied by a simultaneous increase in bicarbonate ions and a decrease of chloride ions in the blood. Reabsorption of bicarbonate ions, no matter in what form, helps restore the bicarbonate ion:carbonic acid ratio, which is low in acidosis. Reabsorption of bicarbonate ions is decreased in alkalosis.

The control of pH occurs in steps, with buffer systems providing the immediate response to any alteration of pH, followed quickly by the respiratory response. Later, the kidney mechanism is initiated and sustains the corrective activity for a longer time span.

If control mechanisms are effective, blood pH is maintained. If, however, the compensatory mechanisms are overwhelmed, pH alterations occur. In compensated acidosis or alkalosis, absolute concentrations of bicarbonate ions and carbonic acid may be changed, but as long as the ratio remains in the range of approximately 20:1, the pH may be in the normal range. If an acid-base imbalance is uncompensated or if the compensatory capacity is overwhelmed, deviations in the bicarbonate ion:carbonic acid ratio as well as in the absolute quantities of bicarbonate ions or carbonic acid result in a pH change.

WATER BALANCE

With normal body function, water and electrolyte balance occur routinely and present no problem. The combination of water and other fluid consumption in the diet plus metabolic water produced during oxidation of foodstuffs meets the daily water requirements. This, in turn, is balanced by the steady loss of water through the skin and in expired air, feces, and obligatory urine loss. The volume of water discharged into the intestinal tract in the form of digestive juices is, for the most part, reabsorbed in animals with dry feces, but considerable water loss occurs in animals with more fluid feces. For example, it has been reported that the dairy cow may daily lose up to 19 liters of fluid in the feces. Water loss through the kidney is controlled by antidiuretic hormone (ADH) in response to plasma osmotic pressure and by aldosterone, which controls renal sodium excretion. A decrease in body water, plasma sodium, or both is compensated for by an equivalent decrease in water, sodium excretion, or both. There is also water loss through the skin and by evaporation from the lungs.

DISTURBANCES OF WATER AND ELECTROLYTE METABOLISM

WATER ABNORMALITIES

Dehydration. Dehydration occurs when loss of body water exceeds intake. This may result from excessive water loss without compensatory increased intake or from decreased intake with normal water loss. In spite of the compensatory mechanisms that assist in conservation of body water, dehydration is not uncommon in animals. The principal compensatory mechanism is consumption of water in amounts necessary to reduce the dehydrated state or to replace the water lost. In addition, the kidney is very sensitive, through the action of ADH, to any change in water balance and immediately acts to conserve water when plasma osmolarity is increased.

Excessive loss of body fluid may occur in any one of the following conditions: diarrhea, prolonged vomiting, sequestration of fluids in the digestive tract, prolonged fever, sweating, exudating burns or open wounds, excessive blood loss, and an uncontrolled polyuria if there is inadequate water intake to compensate for the loss. Although dehydration may occur in all of these conditions, if the loss is gradual and adequately compensated for by increased water intake and kidney conservation of water, dehydration may not be a major problem. If, however, loss is greater than can be compensated for, it may become a life-endangering problem. Many animals that have lost large quantities of body water may also have an alteration in sensorium that prevents compensatory water intake.[1]

The clinician must consider not only the possibility of water loss but the possibility that there has been a lack of water intake for one reason or another. Some conditions that may be associated with a lack of water intake include lack of access, inability to drink, nervous system disturbances, and failure of operation of normal thirst mechanism. In addition, an animal may be unable to retain water, as occurs in gastritis or other upper digestive tract irritation. This type of dehydration is usually of slow onset, as compensatory mechanisms come into operation. Water absorption from the digestive tract is one of the first compensatory mechanisms and is of considerable significance in animals that have a normally fluid feces. The supply of metabolic water from the oxidation of food may assist in preventing dehydration, as will restriction of urinary loss as ADH secretion increases.

Measurement of Dehydration. It is obvious that laboratory measurement of total body water is not a realistic procedure in a practice situation. One of the more commonly utilized methods for evaluating the status of body water is measurement of erythrocyte concentration. In the dehydrated animal, the packed cell volume, hemoglobin level, and total erythrocyte count are increased. Although this may seem a simple solution for detecting and evaluating dehydration, it does present problems in interpretation. Lack of knowledge concerning what these values were before the insult that altered ECF volume occurred presents a major problem. An anemic animal or one with a borderline anemia may have a considerable loss of plasma water without the erythrocyte parameters being increased above the normal range. The clinician must also take into consideration the possible effects that excitement and epinephrine release may have on increasing packed cell volume, erythrocyte count, and hemoglobin concentration. These parameters are of more value in following the response to treatment for dehydration than they are in making an original diagnosis.

Because of the interpretation problems associated with measurement of erythrocytes, it has been recommended that determination of plasma protein concentrations be used instead. Plasma protein concentration can easily be measured using a refractometer, so the technique does not present any problems. As with the erythrocyte count, the total plasma protein concentration is increased if there is water loss from the ECF. However, some of the same problems exist in interpreting plasma protein measurements as are present in interpreting erythrocyte counts. The only advantage that plasma protein estimations have over determination of the status of erythrocytes is that plasma protein levels are not influenced by excitement and epinephrine release. Again, the greatest value of plasma protein determinations is in following the course of dehydration. The changes in values for plasma proteins that occur over a relatively short time are usually reflective of the changing state of hydration. Blood urea nitrogen values frequently follow the same pattern as do plasma protein levels.

In the hands of an experienced clinician, physical examination may be a reliable method for evaluating a dehydrated patient. The status of a dehydrated animal can also be evaluated by following body weight changes on a daily or more frequent basis. This technique can be used to detect changes in the status of body fluid content as any sudden changes, either up or down, will usually reflect changes in body water content.

ELECTROLYTE ABNORMALITIES

Sodium. A decrease in plasma sodium concentration (hyponatremia) occurs most frequently because of excessive sodium loss. As with dietary lack of sodium, the renal compensatory mechanism will operate to conserve sodium. Sodium loss is most likely to occur from the gastrointestinal tract through diarrhea or vomiting or in renal disease in which the sodium conservation mechanism is operating deficiently because of tubular damage. Hyponatremia may occur with osmotic diuresis, such as seen in diabetes mellitus, or iatrogenically, following administration of diuretics. Excessive sweating without adequate dietary sodium intake may also produce a net loss. Adrenocortical insufficiency (Addison's disease) may result in sodium loss because of the lack of aldosterone. Sodium may be lost as a consequence of exudation from burns or open wounds when there is not a compensatory increase in dietary intake. In many of these conditions, water is also lost, therefore hyponatremia is not usually marked. Hyponatremia with concomitant dehydration or normal hydration is an indication of a total body deficiency of sodium. The principal problem occurs when fluid replacement, through either parenteral administration or water intake, does not contain sodium. Under such circumstances, body fluid is replenished but sodium is not, and the net result will be hyponatremia. Hyponatremia may occur with hyperglycemia in which ECF osmolarity is increased by glucose, and the response is sodium excretion to avoid creating hyperosmolarity. Lipemia in which lipid displaces a significant volume of the liquid phase of plasma may result in a low plasma sodium value simply because a smaller volume of the liquid phase is analyzed. If sodium is measured using an ion-specific electrode, the values are accurate in lipemic serum.

Hypernatremia is rare and occurs when there is loss of body fluids, containing less sodium than plasma and water intake is restricted. This condition can also occur if there is excessive sodium intake with limited liquid intake, in advanced chronic renal failure with a low glomerular filtration rate, and with primary hyperaldosteronism (not confirmed in animals).

Potassium. Serum levels of potassium may not reflect the true status of body potassium concentration. This occurs because most body potassium is in the ICF and there is no constancy of relationship between ECF potassium and ICF potassium. Serum potassium levels can be misleading if there has been massive cellular necrosis resulting in potassium release. In these circumstances, the serum potassium concentration may increase, but this is not an indication of an absolute alteration in intracellular potassium. The condition may be more confusing with acidosis, as cells tend to take in hydrogen and give up potassium. If this occurs, there may be an increase in serum potassium but a lack of cellular potassium. The

reverse is true in alkalosis in which a decrease in the serum potassium level is accompanied by an increase in the cellular potassium content as potassium replaces cellular hydrogen ions.

Plasma potassium increases about 0.6 mEq/liter for each 0.1 unit decrease in blood pH. The reverse is true for pH increases. Thus, if an acidotic animal has a normal plasma potassium level, it should be considered hypokalemic and corrective therapy should be initiated.

Hyperkalemia may occur with renal failure, particularly if the failure is acute; the intake of potassium remains high and the animal develops an anuria or oliguria. If urine flow remains normal, the serum potassium level may also be normal. Potassium is increased in animals with hypoadrenocorticism, in association with administration of potassium-sparing diuretics, and with increased intake when KCl is used as a salt substitute during salt restriction in congestive heart failure. The primary danger of hyperkalemia is the possibility of cardiac arrest. Death is likely to ensue when potassium exceeds 10 to 12 milliequivalents (mEq)/liter.

Hypokalemia may occur as the result of decreased potassium loss, or a shift of potassium from ECF to ICF. Potassium loss may develop as a consequence of vomition or diarrhea, particularly if fluid replacement is potassium free. Hypokalemia may occur iatrogenically with prolonged administration of mineralocorticoids or with true hyperadrenocorticism. Alkalosis may produce hypokalemia, as potassium is excreted in urine when hydrogen is retained.

Chloride. Chloride alterations generally follow those of sodium, as chloride is absorbed, excreted, and distributed passively, according to electrical gradients established by active transport of sodium. Thus, hypochloridemia may occur with (1) losses from the gastrointestinal tract, particularly

TABLE 10–1. Normal Values for Serum Sodium, Potassium, and Chloride

Species	Values (mEq/liter)		
	SODIUM	POTASSIUM	CHLORIDE
Bovine	132–152	3.9–5.8	97–111
			96–107
Calves (24 hr old)	126–146	4.5–6.9	94–112
Ovine	146.9 ± 4.9	4.85 ± 0.39	107.5 ± 4.0
Caprine	142–155	3.5–6.7	99–110
Porcine	110–154	3.5–5.5	88–115
	135–150	4.4–6.7	94–106
Equine	132–146	2.4–4.7	99–109
	141 ± 0.63	3.76 ± 0.075	102.5 ± 0.42
Canine	141.1–152.3	4.37–5.65	105.2–114.8
	141–153	4.2–5.2	102–118
	137–147	3.9–5.2	110–117
	146.2 ± 3.43	4.2 ± 0.39	111.9 ± 4.56
Feline	147–156	4.0–4.5	117–123

prolonged vomiting; (2) advanced renal failure; (3) adrenal insufficiency; or (4) exudation from burns or open wounds. Hyperchloridemia may occur with dehydration, and in humans has been reported in congestive heart failure in which there is decreased renal blood flow. Plasma chloride levels may be increased iatrogenically.

Techniques for Measuring Electrolyte Levels. The sample required for measuring ECF electrolyte levels is usually serum. Blood must be collected in containers that are chemically clean and free of contamination. Hemolysis should be avoided at all costs, as electrolyte concentrations within erythrocytes are different from those in serum. Serum should be separated as soon as possible to avoid any ion exchange between cells and serum.

A variety of techniques have been utilized for estimating the concentrations of serum sodium and potassium. Today flame photometry and ion-specific electrodes are used for estimating electrolyte levels in serum or plasma. Chloride levels are most frequently determined by a mercurimetric titrimetric technique, but ion-specific electrodes are available.

Normal Values. Normal values for serum sodium, potassium, and chloride levels are presented in Table 10–1. The concentration of these substances is usually expressed in milliequivalents per liter rather than as milligrams per deciliter. As with any other laboratory technique, normal values must be estimated for the specific laboratory and must be constantly subjected to a quality control program.

DISTURBANCES IN ACID-BASE BALANCE

Deviations that occur in acid-base balance are generally classified as respiratory or metabolic (nonrespiratory). More specifically, the classic disturbances in acid-base balance are respiratory acidosis, respiratory alkalosis, nonrespiratory (metabolic) acidosis, and nonrespiratory (metabolic) alkalosis. Mixtures of respiratory and nonrespiratory imbalances can occur.

Laboratory Tests Useful in Determining Acid-Base Balance. Tests of value in detecting disturbances in acid-base balance are basically those that can be substituted into the Henderson-Hasselbalch equation as applied to the bicarbonate/carbonic acid buffer system. These include determinations of blood pH, P_{CO_2}, and bicarbonate levels.

Blood pH is measured utilizing a pH meter with sufficient sensitivity to detect minor deviations (Fig. 10–1). The pH meter must be standardized with buffers that are accurate to 0.005 pH unit. The greatest limitation on the accuracy of blood pH determinations rests not with the instrument but with the manner in which the sample is collected and held prior to completing the examination.

Samples to be analyzed for pH and P_{CO_2} must be collected and handled under conditions in which exposure to air is avoided or kept at an absolute minimum. Venous blood is acceptable for such analyses, but must be carefully collected. A heparinized Luer-Lok Syringe is utilized, all air is removed, and a vein is entered. If a tourniquet is used, it should be removed after venous puncture, and blood should be permitted to flow freely for approximately one minute before the sample is withdrawn. A sample that is either removed from a vein that has been obstructed for some time or withdrawn immediately after release of the tourniquet will introduce substantial errors, since compounds accumulated during stasis will flush into the blood. A heparinized Vacutainer may be used if the tube is filled completely to avoid pH or P_{CO_2} changes that may result from diffusion of carbon dioxide into the vacuum. If a syringe is

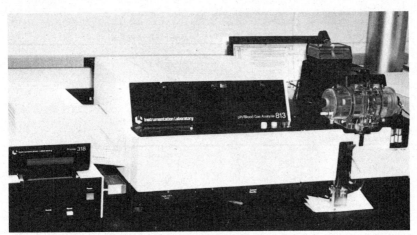

Figure 10–1. Automated units such as this have increased the accuracy and simplified the methodology for assaying blood pH and acid-base balance.

used, the tip should be sealed immediately. The simplest method is to insert the needle into a rubber or cork stopper. Analysis should be completed as soon as possible or else the sample must be chilled immediately. The pH of freshly drawn blood will decrease at a rate of 0.01 unit/10 minutes at 38° C and at about half that rate at 27° C. There is no measurable change in the pH of blood held for three hours at 4° C in an ice water bath. Measurements are made with the blood at a temperature of 38° C. Arterial blood may be utilized for pH, P_{CO_2} and carbonic acid measurements and is required for oxygen partial pressure (P_{O_2}) estimation. Arterial blood is usually collected from the femoral artery in small animals; from the saphenous artery in calves; from the brachial, carotid, iliac, radial, or coccygeal artery in mature cattle; and from the brachial artery of horses.

Carbon dioxide partial pressure is also determined utilizing a special electrode. P_{CO_2} is expressed in millimeters of mercury (Hg) and represents that part of the pressure of a mixed gas that is contributed by carbon dioxide. The level of bicarbonate may be determined directly by a titrimetric technique but is more frequently estimated from total carbon dioxide content or by use of a nomogram with which plasma bicarbonate levels can be estimated if blood pH and P_{CO_2} values are known. Carbonic acid is not measured directly but is calculated by multiplying the P_{CO_2} by 0.03. Total carbon dioxide determinations may be of value and can be accomplished by converting all of the bicarbonate to carbonic acid and then extracting the gaseous carbon dioxide from the liquid. Some automated biochemical profiling instruments include total carbon dioxide among the chemical determinations completed. It must be remembered that the total carbon dioxide value represents the dissolved carbon dioxide plus bicarbonate plus carbonic acid. Bicarbonate concentration can be estimated by subtracting 1.2 from the total carbon dioxide value.

Normal values for pH, P_{CO_2} and carbonic acid levels are presented in Table 10–2.

Respiratory Acidosis. Respiratory acidosis occurs when carbon dioxide elimination is decreased, and blood carbonic acid concentration and P_{CO_2} are increased. Such circumstances may be encountered with closed gas anesthesia when oxygen is adequate, but carbon dioxide removal is insufficient. Under these circumstances, there is no hypoxic stimulus for respiration, and carbon dioxide accumulates. This presents a particular problem to the surgeon because an animal may show no signs of cyanosis but may "die pink." Similarly, carbon dioxide may accumulate if the carbon dioxide absorbant in the closed anesthesia machine is not fresh. Other causes of respiratory acidosis include: drugs that depress the respiratory centers; interference with mechanical function of the respiratory cage; obstruction of the airways; intrathoracic lesions such as bronchitis, pneumonia, and asthma; circulatory disorders such as shock and congestive heart failure. The majority of these conditions, with the exception of closed anesthesia administration, are accompanied by cyanosis and are readily recognized.

Compensatory Mechanisms. Carbonic acid that accumulates in animals with respiratory acidosis is buffered by hemoglobin and protein buffer systems. The respiratory compensatory mechanism is an increased pulmonary rate if the primary cause is not respiratory center depression. This increase in respiratory rate increases carbon dioxide loss, which, in turn, decreases the carbonic acid level and the ratio of bicarbonate to carbonic

TABLE 10–2. Normal Values for Blood pH, P_{CO_2}, and Bicarbonate[1]

Species	Blood pH	P_{CO_2} mm Hg	HCO_3 mEq/liter
Bovine	7.378 ± 0.039	48.12 ± 12.4	—
	7.325–7.45	35–53	21–27
Calves (24 hr old)	7.38 ± 0.06	54.5 ± 5.8	30.9 ± 3.4
Ovine	7.401 ± 0.047	42.1 ± 4.9	—
	7.32–7.54	41.3 ± 4.7	20–25
Porcine	7.35	28.2	18–27
Equine	7.394 ± 0.0295(a)	37.9 ± 3.75(a)	22.5 ± 2.17(a)
	7.378 ± 0.0317	40.0 ± 4.05	22.7 ± 2.45
	7.489 ± 0.015	41.1 ± 1.24	29.4 ± 0.62
	7.38 ± 0.03	42.4 ± 2.0	20–28
	7.32–7.44	38–46	24–34
Canine	7.37–7.45	—	20–25
	7.30–7.45	29–42	16–24
	7.33–7.45	38–46	22–28
	7.31–7.42	38	18–24
Feline	7.24–7.40	36	17–21

[1] All values on venous blood unless otherwise noted.
(a) = arterial blood

TABLE 10–3. Laboratory Findings in Classic Uncompensated Acid-Base Imbalances (Acute)

	pH	P_{CO_2}	HCO_3^-	BE*
Respiratory acidosis	↓	↑	N	N
Metabolic acidosis	↓	N	↓	↓
Respiratory alkalosis	↑	↓	N	N
Metabolic alkalosis	↑	N	↑	↑

*BE = Base excess as estimated from the Siggaard-Andersen nomogram.
↑ = Increase
↓ = Decrease
N = Normal

acid approaches normal. Although slower to come into action, the renal mechanisms assist in compensating for respiratory acidosis. Sodium-hydrogen exchange is increased resulting in increased acid excretion and preservation of base. There is also increased formation of ammonia and reabsorption of bicarbonate.

Laboratory Findings. In uncompensated respiratory acidosis, the classic findings are: increased P_{CO_2} and therefore carbonic acid levels, a normal bicarbonate concentration, and a decreased blood pH (Table 10–3). If respiratory aci-

dosis is a clinical problem, by the time a clinician examines the animal, the acidosis is at least partially compensated. With partial compensation, the P_{CO_2} value (and therefore the carbonic acid value) is increased, the bicarbonate level is increased, blood pH is decreased, and the urine is acid (see Table 10–4).

Respiratory Alkalosis. Respiratory alkalosis occurs when there is a deficiency of carbonic acid as a consequence of P_{CO_2} loss. P_{CO_2} loss takes place with hyperventilation that develops accompanying pain or psychologic stress, with general anesthesia when there has been excessive artificial respiration, or in early heat prostration.

The compensatory mechanisms are principally renal. Renal control is manifested by a decrease in ammonia formation, a decrease in bicarbonate reabsorption, and an increase in excretion of bicarbonate instead of chloride. This results in an increase in plasma chloride and a decrease in bicarbonate that produces a decrease in the $HCO_3 : H_2CO_3$ ratio, and blood pH returns toward normal. The respiratory response is depression of the respiratory center, which causes carbon dioxide retention and a concomitant increase in carbonic acid. However, unless the cause of hyperventilation is removed, this compensatory mechanism cannot operate.

TABLE 10–4. Laboratory Findings in Clinical Acid-Base Imbalances— Partially Compensated

	pH	P_{CO_2}	HCO_3^-	BE	Causative Conditions
Respiratory acidosis	↓	↑	↑N	N to +	Anesthesia
Metabolic acidosis	↓	↓	↓	−	(1) Loss of HCO_3^- (2) Acid accumulation

Mixed—Acidosis
  Primary respiratory
    +
  Primary metabolic
	↓	↑	↓	−	(1) Prolonged surgical anesthesia
					(2) Circulatory and functional right-left shunt
					(3) Newborns

Respiratory alkalosis	↑	↓	↓	N (−)	(1) Hyperventilation (2) Pain (3) Early heat prostration
Metabolic alkalosis	↑	↑	↑	+	(1) Vomition (2) Renal alkalosis

Mixed—Alkalosis
  Primary respiratory
    +
  Primary metabolic
	↑	↓	↑	+	(1) Hyperventilation + vomition
					(2) Iatrogenic

Other Mixed
  Primary respiratory acidosis
    +
  Primary metabolic alkalosis
	N↑↓	↑	↑	+	Hypoventilation + vomiting

Primary respiratory alkalosis
    +
  Primary metabolic acidosis
	N↑↓	↓	↓	−	Hyperventilation + kidney, diarrhea

Primary respiratory alkalosis
    +
  Primary metabolic acidosis
	N↑↓	N↑↓	N↑↓	N + or −	Vomiting + kidney, or diarrhea

Laboratory Findings. In uncompensated respiratory alkalosis, the P_{CO_2} and carbonic acid are decreased and bicarbonate concentration is normal, and the blood pH is increased (Table 10–3). In partially compensated respiratory alkalosis, the P_{CO_2} is decreased, as are the carbonic acid and bicarbonate values; the pH is increased (Table 10–4); the chloride level is usually increased; and the urine pH is increased because of additional bicarbonate excretion and curtailed acid excretion.

Metabolic (Nonrespiratory) Acidosis. Metabolic acidosis occurs as a consequence of acid accumulation in excess of the rate of elimination. This may be seen in the diabetic animal in which there is an accumulation of keto acids. It may also be seen in situations in which lactic acid accumulation is associated with either excessive muscular activity or late heat stroke or in any condition, including anemia, in which there is cellular hypoxia.

In addition to being caused by acid accumulation, metabolic acidosis may develop as a consequence of bicarbonate loss associated with diarrhea, sequestration of intestinal contents (particularly in the horse), excessive loss of saliva, or renal inability to reabsorb bicarbonate. With renal failure, inability to reabsorb bicarbonate is compounded by the inability of the kidney to excrete hydrogen and by retention of phosphate, sulfate, and other acids.

Compensatory Mechanisms. The bicarbonate buffer system immediately enters into the attempts of the body to compensate for a metabolic acidosis, and the bicarbonate level decreases, which reduces the bicarbonate ion:carbonic acid ratio to less than 20:1. If the cause of the metabolic acidosis is not renal, renal compensation occurs as increased acid excretion, preservation of base by an increased rate of sodium-hydrogen exchange, increased formation of ammonia, and increased bicarbonate ion reabsorption. The respiratory response is an increase in the respiratory rate, which decreases P_{CO_2}, and thus the carbonic acid level, to bring the bicarbonate ion:carbonic acid ratio back toward normal.

Laboratory Findings. If metabolic acidosis is uncompensated, the classic findings are a normal P_{CO_2} with a decreased bicarbonate value and decreased pH (Table 10–3). As the majority of the metabolic acidoses are at least partially compensated, the more usual laboratory findings are decreased P_{CO_2}, decreased bicarbonate concentration, and decreased pH (Table 10–4). If there is a diabetic ketoacidosis, there will be an increase in organic keto acids in blood and urine and possibly a decrease in sodium and potassium levels because of the polyuria and resultant excretion of sodium and potassium as salts of acetoacetic and beta-hydroxybutyric acids. Most animals with acidosis have hyperkalemia as H^+ enters cells and K^+ moves into ECF.

Anion Gap. The presence of excess acids can be detected by calculating the anion gap. The formula is as follows:

$$Na - [Cl + HCO_3] = Anion\ gap$$

Some calculations of anion gap include potassium so that the formula is:

$$[Na + K] - [Cl + HCO_3] = Anion\ gap$$

The normal anion gap is 8 to 12 mEq/l when potassium is not included and 12 to 16 mEq/l when potassium is added to the sodium.

Organic acids and the inorganic acids, phosphates and sulfates, contribute to the anion gap. An estimation of the effect that phosphates and sulfates have on the anion gap can be made by multiplying the phosphate value by 1.2. Phosphate is normally reported in mg/dl and this is converted to mEq/l by multiplying that value by 0.6. Since sulfate and phosphate usually occur in approximately equal concentrations, multiplication of phosphate by 1.2 will account for most of the influence that these anions have. If the anion gap is calculated and the phosphate $\times$ 1.2 is subtracted, the result will give an approximation of the excess of organic anions.

An anion gap greater than 20 (if potassium is not included) or 25 (if potassium is included) suggests the presence of excess anions. Values over 22 (K^+ excluded) are significant and if over 27 represent a severe metabolic acidosis. In one study[2] the anion gap was calculated, without the inclusion of potassium, for 90 horses with signs of abdominal pain. Survival rates were calculated for horses whose anion gap concentrations were within a variety of ranges. The probability of survival decreased as the anion gap progressively increased above 20 mEq/l. Survival rates for increasing ranges of anion gaps were: <20 mEq/l, 81 per cent survival; 20–24.9 mEq/l, 47 per cent survival; and > 25 mEq/l, no survival). The presence of an anion gap was not of diagnostic significance as to the source of abdominal pain but did appear to be a good prognostic indicator.

Metabolic acidosis accompanied by an increased anion gap occurs when there is increased acid production as seen in ketotic animals, those with an increase in lactic acid production, and in individuals with an increase in an unknown organic acid such as occurs with ethylene glycol toxicity and paraldehyde poisoning. A decrease in acid secretion as seen in acute and chronic renal failure will increase the anion gap. With renal failure much of the increase may be due to retained phosphates and sulfates and this can be determined as just described. If phosphate and sulfate do not account for most of the excess anion gap one may assume that there is a concomitant increase in production of organic acids. Not all animals with metabolic acidosis have an increased anion gap. In some there may be a normal gap or a decrease in the gap.[3] Causes of metabolic acidosis that have a normal or decreased anion gap include loss of bicarbonate (either renal or gastrointestinal), hyperchloremic metabolic acidosis, and dilutional acidosis.

Metabolic Alkalosis. Metabolic alkalosis is accompanied by an accumulation of bicarbonate in extracellular fluid as a result of excessive acid loss due to: vomition, in monogastric animals; sequestration of abomasal juices in ruminants with high gastrointestinal (GI) tract obstructions; or potassium depletion as hydrogen ions move into cells to replace lost potassium. This condition may occur iatrogenically as a consequence of overtreatment with alkalinizing agents.

Compensatory Mechanisms. The renal compensatory mechanisms are as follows: sodium-hydrogen exchange is decreased, ammonia formation is decreased, and bicarbonate excretion is increased. The respiratory response is a decrease in respiration in order to increase P_{CO_2} and thus the carbonic acid level, which tends to reduce the ratio of bicarbonate ions to carbonic acid. In this instance both bicarbonate ions and carbonic acid are quantitatively increased, but the bicarbonate ion:carbonic acid ratio returns toward normal.

Laboratory Findings. In uncompensated metabolic alkalosis, the P_{CO_2} is normal and the bicarbonate ion concentration and pH are increased. With partially compensated metabolic alkalosis, P_{CO_2} and bicarbonate levels are increased, as is blood pH. If alkalosis accompanies prolonged vomiting, there will be a decrease in serum potassium and chloride values. If it has occurred as a result of sequestering of stomach contents, there will be a decerase in chloride and potassium levels. The urine in these animals may be more alkaline than normal, but paradoxical aciduria can occur.

Inappropriate (paradoxic) aciduria can occur in animals with a metabolic alkalosis. It is seen in individuals with hypochloremia and hypokalemia. With potassium depletion, sodium reabsorption is increased. If sodium reabsorption occurs while there is a chloride deficit, almost all chloride will be reabsorbed with the sodium. When chloride has been reabsorbed, additional sodium reabsorption proceeds by exchange with either potassium or hydrogen. In a hypokalemic animal potassium is not available in the usual concentration and is therefore being conserved by the kidney. As a consequence hydrogen ion secretion will occur and acidic urine is formed. Conditions under which paradoxic aciduria may occur include (1) avid sodium reabsorption, (2) potassium conservation, and (3) chloride depletion.[4]

Inappropriate aciduria occurs frequently in cattle that have metabolic alkalosis[4] but can be seen in any animal in which there is hypokelemia and hypochloremia.

Mixed Acid-Base Imbalances. Several combinations of the primary acid-base disturbances just mentioned may develop under specific circumstances in veterinary practice, and laboratory determinations may assist in identifying them. These findings are presented in Table 10–4.

Primary respiratory acidosis plus primary metabolic acidosis may occur during prolonged surgical anesthesia, in newborn animals, in pneumonia accompanied by anorexia with which there is a concomitant metabolic acidosis. Laboratory findings anticipated in this mixture of acid-base imbalances include increased P_{CO_2}, decreased bicarbonate ion level, and decreased blood pH.

Primary respiratory alkalosis plus primary metabolic alkalosis may be observed in an animal that is vomiting and hyperventilating. It may occur iatrogenically if the clinician, without benefit of laboratory results, initiates therapy to correct a nonexistent acidosis. Laboratory findings in this mixture of alkaloses are decreased P_{CO_2}, increased bicarbonate ion concentration, and increased blood pH.

Primary respiratory acidosis plus primary metabolic alkalosis may occur in a dog that is vomiting and hypoventilating, in cattle under anesthesia, or in cattle with nephritis-pneumonia complex. Laboratory findings include increased P_{CO_2} and increased bicarbonate ion values. Blood pH can be normal, increased, or decreased, depending upon the relative severity of the two imbalances.

Primary respiratory alkalosis plus primary metabolic acidosis could occur with hyperventilation compounded by either kidney disease or diarrhea. With this combination, laboratory findings would be represented by a decreased P_{CO_2}, a decreased bicarbonate ion level, and a blood pH that could be normal, increased, or decreased.

Primary metabolic alkalosis plus primary metabolic acidosis might occur in the nephritic uremic dog that is vomiting. Laboratory alterations are not definitive and would depend entirely upon the relative severity of the metabolic acidosis versus the metabolic alkalosis.

SOME COMMON CLINICAL CONDITIONS PRODUCING ABNORMALITIES IN WATER, ELECTROLYTES, AND ACID-BASE BALANCE

Bovine

Diarrhea of Young Calves. Diarrhea in young calves occurs in association with a number of different infections, and the calves are invariably dehydrated and have alterations in electrolyte levels and acid-base balance. There is typically a hyperkalemia with serum potassium values as high as 12.3 mEq/liter,[5] but there may be a total body deficiency of potassium. Plasma sodium values are normal to reduced, whereas chloride levels are in the normal range. Dehydration with its typical increases in packed cell volume, red blood cell counts, and plasma protein levels is a universal finding. There is a metabolic acidosis as indicated by the decreased pH and bicarbonate ion concentration. Acidosis is complicated by an increase in organic acid production and a decrease in hydrogen ion excretion by the kidneys. Other laboratory findings include increased urea nitrogen (UN), phosphate, and magnesium levels.[5] These undoubtedly are related to renal insufficiency occurring because of a decrease in renal perfusion that is associated with the hypovolemia and dehydration. Thus, the UN level increase is classified as prerenal azotemia. In severe acute diarrhea, hypoglycemia may develop.

Abomasal Displacement and Torsion. Alterations in electrolyte values and acid-base balance seen in any obstruction of the upper intestinal tract in the bovine are consequences of the sequestration of large volumes of abomasal juices. When sequestration occurs, there is a significant loss of chloride from plasma and interstitial fluid. There is almost invariably a hypokalemia and hypochoridemia with an increase in plasma bicarbonate concentration and metabolic alkalosis.[6] Cows with metabolic alkalosis associated with abomasal displacement and other abomasal disorders often have acidic urine.[4] Dehydration is usually present and may produce other alterations in normal function that are associated with decreased levels of body fluids. The acid-base alterations in cattle with other digestive disturbances are not as characteristic. Alkalosis with hypokalemia and hypochloremia may occur in vagus indigestion, early in abomasal impaction, and occasionally in intussception and cecal torsion. This occurs only if the intestinal blockage is complete and prevents escape of abomasal fluids into the intestine. If the blockage is not complete, metabolic acidosis usually ensues.[7]

Carbohydrate Intoxication. Carbohydrate intoxication is also accompanied by metabolic acidosis, as large quantities of low-weight organic acids are absorbed across the ruminal epithelium.

Equine

Acute Diarrhea (Salmonellosis). The disturbances of anion-cation balance in the horse with acute diarrhea are characteristic. There are hyponatremia, hypokalemia, hypochloridemia, and metabolic acidosis.[1] Serum potassium values may be in the normal range until the acidosis is corrected; then the decrease becomes obvious.[1] If the serum potassium concentration in a severely acidotic animal is low or subnormal, the presence of severe potassium depletion is suggested.

Anesthesia in a Closed System. With the development of closed systems for the administration of gas anesthesia to the horse, the potential development of a respiratory acidosis must become a consideration, particularly in prolonged procedures. No significant electrolyte changes were found with either halothane or chloroform anesthesia, but a moderate respiratory acidosis developed and was of the same degree with both anesthetic agents.[8] There was a slight increase in the serum potassium level, but it was not considered significant. Tasker[1] remarks that in his experience clinically ill patients have often had more severe abnormalities than those reported in the experimental study.

Intestinal Obstruction. Metabolic acidosis and dehydration may develop in a horse with intestinal obstruction.[1] The electrolyte changes are not predictable, but most alterations seen are undoubtedly the result of the accumulation of large volumes of intestinal secretions in the digestive tract plus the shock that accompanies the condition.

Fasting and Water Deprivation. Horses were deprived of food and water for eight days; plasma bicarbonate and potassium values decreased as did the pH, whereas the P_{CO_2} and plasma protein levels increased.[9] One of the outstanding physiologic responses was the rapid reduction in urine volume from approximately 5 liters per day to less than 2 liters. The decreases in blood pH and plasma bicarbonate concentration were interpreted as being an indication of a tendency toward metabolic acidosis that was consistent with the starvation. The author had no explanation for the increased P_{CO_2} levels observed.

Strenuous Exercise. The pH of arterial blood decreases immediately following exercise and returns to normal by 60 minutes after exercise. The arterial carbon dioxide tension decreases immediately following exercise but returns to normal in 30 minutes. Lactic acid concentrations follow a similar pattern.[10]

Canine

Renal Failure. Classically, the electrolyte and acid-base balance disturbances observed with renal failure in the dog include dehydration and, if the animal is uremic, metabolic acidosis with a lack of hydrogen excretion and a decreased blood pH and plasma bicarbonate level. Sodium values are usually normal to decreased, whereas serum potassium levels are variable and in some dogs may be increased. If there is anuria or oliguria in acute renal failure, hyperkalemia may develop. With an oliguric renal failure, if urine specific gravity is 1.030 or greater and the UN value of serum is increased, prerenal uremia should be considered until other laboratory tests prove otherwise.[11] Depending upon the degree of oliguria, the animal can be normally hydrated, overhydrated, or dehydrated. Hyperkalemia will ultimately develop unless urine volume is adequate, in which case there is no increase in potassium.[11] Hypernatremia may develop, and this perpetuates fluid retention. Metabolic acidosis supervenes with its decrease in plasma bicarbonate concentration.

With polyuric renal failure, there is an excess loss of fluids and electrolyes including bicarbonate, chloride, and calcium. Serum potassium levels are usually normal, although hypokalemia may develop. Excesses of phosphate, sulfate, nonprotein nitrogenous substances, and acids may be present, causing metabolic acidosis.

Diarrhea. Alterations in fluid, electrolyte, and acid-base balances may be problems associated with diarrhea in young dogs or in older dogs if this condition is severe and prolonged and dietary intake of food and water is low. Depending upon the length of time the diarrhea has persisted, dehydration may develop. If the animal has not continued to eat or drink, metabolic acidosis develops because of bicarbonate loss from the intestinal tract. Blood pH and plasma bicarbonate levels are decreased, whereas serum sodium and chloride values are often normal. Serum potassium concentration may increase as cellular potassium moves into ECF because of acidosis. On the other hand, if there has been a great lost of potassium in the diarrheal fluid and potassium intake has been inadequate, the serum level may be decreased or normal. It must be remembered that these alterations develop only in the dog that has not continued to eat and drink. If water intake is increased by fluid treatment or excessive drinking, electrolyte concentrations may be subnormal.

Vomiting. If vomiting persists and there is a great loss of gastric juice, dehydration may develop. Dehydration is frequently compounded by an inability of the patient to retain fluids taken by mouth. If vomiting is severe and prolonged, metabolic alkalosis develops because of the loss of gastric juice. In this circumstance, there is an increase in blood pH and plasma bicarbonate with a decrease in serum potassium and chloride values. These conditions do occur, but urine often remains acid. Although this is the classic finding in the vomiting dog, it must be remembered that if vomition persists, reverse peristalsis of the duodenum may result in regurgitation of intestinal contents. If this occurs, there will be a loss of bicarbonate that may mask the alkalosis or make it less severe. This trend toward reversal of alkalosis is unlikely if vomiting is due to pyloric obstruction.

Variations in the severity of vomiting, its duration, and composition make an absolute prediction of the effect on electrolytes difficult.

Diabetes Mellitus. Diabetes mellitus in the dog is frequently accompanied by ketoacidosis with the accumulation of organic acids. Under these circumstances, blood pH and plasma bicarbonate levels are decreased, whereas serum sodium and potassium values may be normal to decreased. If there is osmotic diuresis, serum sodium and potassium levels decrease. If severe ketoacidosis is present, potassium may leave cells as hydrogen enters. The hyperkalemia occurs even though there is a total body potassium deficit. What appears to be a life-threatening hyperkalemia may be followed by a life-threatening hypokalemia after correction of the ketoacidosis.[12]

Adrenal Malfunction. Hypoadrenocorticism is accompanied by an increase in serum potassium values and a decrease in serum sodium levels. There is usually no abnormality in acid-base balance. Hyperadrenocorticism in the dog is not usually accompanied by any major deviation in serum electrolytes. It would be anticipated that aldosterone secreted by the hyperactive gland would tend to cause sodium retention and potassium excretion, but these electrolyte changes are rarely observed in the dog. Hyperkalemia may occasionally occur, but it is not a constant finding.

Hypovolemic Shock. Shock occurring because of decreased blood flow is usually accompanied by metabolic acidosis resulting from cellular hypoxia. Blood pH may decrease from 7.4 to 7.0 if blood flow is reduced to 25 per cent of normal and doubling the ventilation rapidly increases the pH to 7.4 to 7.6.[13] If shock becomes sufficiently severe, renal failure may develop, and oliguria and anuria complicate changes in electrolyte balance.

Congestive Heart Failure. With congestive heart failure, there is an increase in extracellular fluids.[14] Sodium is conserved, with the level of extracellular sodium being increased and the level of serum sodium being normal. Dehydration may occur in some nonedematous portions of the body. There is also reduction in the concentration of serum proteins. Frequently there are no detectable alterations in serum electrolyte levels or acid-base balance unless there are other complicating factors.

Leptospirosis. Alterations in water, electrolyte, and acid-base balance in experimental leptospirosis were studied.[15] Forty-eight hours following infection there was a decrease in serum sodium, chloride, and potassium levels. Serum sodium and chloride values continued to decrease, but potassium concentration increased as the disease progressed. A moderate to severe metabolic acidosis developed in the later stages accompanied by a decrease in the amount of plasma bicarbonate. Serum calcium content decreased slightly in the later stages of the experiment, whereas phosphorus and UN levels increased.

Diabetes Insipidus. Diabetes insipidus is characterized by an uncontrollable loss of water.

There are usually no electrolyte or acid-base disturbances as long as drinking water is freely available. Assessment of plasma and urine osmolality along with a water deprivation test will assist in the diagnosis of diabetes insipidus (see Chapter 11).

Adrenal Insufficiency. Hypoadrenocorticism is characterized by a decrease in mineralocorticoid activity. This leads to hyperkalemia and hyponatremia. This is followed by a negative water balance due to the sodium diuresis that results in hypovolemia and dehydration. The ratio of Na to K in the serum is a more obvious indication of mineralocorticoid deficit than are absolute values of either ion. For a more complete discussion on mineralocorticoid deficit see Chapter 11.

In the normal animal the Na:K ratio is approximately 30:1 (range 27 to 40:1) and will be decreased in animals with hypoadrenocorticism to as low as 13 to 16:1. Any ratio below 27:1 should be viewed with suspicion in a patient presented with clinical signs and history suggestive of hypoadrenocorticism.

Care must be taken in interpreting the results of sodium and potassium analyses, because other factors may influence the ratio. Other causes of hyperkalemia include acute renal failure, some severe gastrointestinal diseases, and rapid release of potassium in response to severe acidosis or as the result of increased tissue breakdown. It may also occur in cats with feline urologic syndrome. Artefactual elevations can be associated with use of excessively hemolyzed blood for the analyses or in animals that have a thrombocytosis if the sample is hemolyzed or refrigerated. Most of these causes of hyperkalemia are not associated with the characteristic hyponatremia of Addison's disease.

Hyponatremia from any cause will also alter the Na:K ratio. Conditions in which hyponatremia may occur include inadequate sodium intake, vomiting, diarrhea, renal tubular disease, and diuretic loss of sodium. It can occur in diabetics with sodium loss accompanying osmotic diuresis. A significant lipemia may cause a false depression of sodium because fat displaces a significant amount of the aqueous phase of plasma. When a lipemic sample is measured by flame photometry, less aqueous phase is obtained, causing an erroneously low sodium estimation. If sodium is measured by use of an ion-specific electrode, it is expressed as sodium concentration in plasma water rather than whole plasma and the measurement will be accurate in lipemic blood. Before evaluating the significance of a low serum sodium estimation, the presence or absence of lipemia should be noted and the clinician should consider the analytic method used.

Anorexia. Dehydration due to decreased water intake may occur and result in some increase in serum electrolyte values if the water loss is proportionally great. There is a tendency toward metabolic acidosis caused by a breakdown of tissue.

References

1. Tasker, J. B.: Fluids, electrolytes and acid-base balance. In: *Clinical Biochemistry of Domestic Animals*, Vol. 2, edited by Kaneko, J. J. and Cornelius, C. E., 2nd ed., Academic Press, New York, 1971.
2. Bristol, D. G.: The anion gap as a prognostic indicator in horses with abdominal pain. J.A.V.M.A., *181*:63, 1982.
3. Feldman, B. F., and Rosenberg, D. P.: Clinical use of anion and osmolar gaps in veterinary medicine. J.A.V.M.A., *178*:396, 1981.
4. Gingerich, D. A., and Murdick, P.W.: Paradoxic aciduria in bovine metabolic alkalosis. J.A.V.M.A., *166*:227, 1975.
5. Tennant, B., Harrold, D., and Reina-Guerra, M.: Physiologic and metabolic factors in the pathogenesis of neonatal enteric infections in calves. J.A.V.M.A., *161*:993, 1972.
6. Schotman, A. J. H.: The acid-base balance in clinically healthy and diseased cattle. Neth. J. Vet. Sci., *4*:5, 1971.
7. Hoffsis, G. F., and McGuirk, S. M.: Diseases of the abomasum and intestinal tract. In: *Current Veterinary Therapy: Food Animal Practice*, edited by Howard, J. L., W. B. Saunders Company, Philadelphia, 1981.
8. Tevik, A., Nelson, A. W., and Lumb, W. V.: Chloroform and halothane anesthesia in horses: Effect on blood electrolytes and acid-base balance. Am. J. Vet. Res., *29*:1791, 1968.
9. Tasker, J. B.: Fluid and electrolyte studies in the horse: V. The effects of fasting and thirsting. Cornell Vet., *57*:658, 1967.
10. Krzywanek, H., Milne, D. W., Gabel, A. A., and Smith, L. G.: Acid-base values of standard bred horses recovering from strenuous exercise. Am J. Vet. Res., *37*:291, 1976.
11. Osborne, C. A., Low, D. G., and Finco, D. R.: *Canine and Feline Urology*, W. B. Saunders Company, Philadelphia, 1972.
12. Tasker, J. B.: Fluids electrolytes and acid-base balance. In: *Clinical Biochemistry of Domestic Animals*, 3rd ed., edited by Kaneko, J. J., Academic Press, New York, 1980.
13. Whittick, W. G.: Shock, J.A.A.H.A., *8*:456, 1972.
14. Hamlin, R. L.: Fluid and electrolyte balance in congestive heart failure. J.A.A.H.A., *8*:224, 1972.
15. Finco, D. R., and Low, D. G.: Water, electrolytes and acid-base alterations in experimental leptospirosis. Am. J. Vet. Res., *29*:1799, 1968.

ADRENAL AND PITUITARY FUNCTION

Although diseases of the adrenal and pituitary glands are not common, they occur with sufficient frequency to present diagnostic problems. Adrenal and pituitary diseases in the dog and cat are fairly well delineated, but similar conditions in the other species have not been as completely studied.

Diseases of the adrenal and pituitary are manifestations of endocrine insufficiency or endocrine excess. Theoretically, the causes of endocrine insufficiencies fall into one or more of the following categories:

1. Hyposecretion of hormone as a consequence of atrophy, neoplasia, destruction of the endocrine gland, or lack of availability of hormonal precursors.

2. Increased degradation or excretion of hormone.

3. Excessive binding of the hormone.

4. Failure of the target organ to respond, creating an apparent endocrine insufficiency.

5. Secretion of an inactive hormone that is either an abnormal hormone or a normal hormone in an unusual form.

Endocrine excesses, on the other hand, may occur in association with the following:

1. Increased hormone secretion as a result of functional neoplasms of hormonal tissue, failure of feedback mechanisms to function, or production of hormones by ectopic nonendocrine tissue.

2. Decreased excretion or destruction of hormone.

3. Decreased binding of the hormone.

4. Functional overresponse of the target organ.

5. Iatrogenic causes.

Hormonal assays are procedures requiring specialized equipment. Thus, many of the endocrine function tests are performed by commercial laboratories. Delays occurring as a result of utilizing commercial laboratories are usually insignificant, as an animal with an endocrine abnormality usually has had the problem for some time, and a few days more is seldom important in the final outcome of the case. If the animal's condition is critical, as with adrenocortical insufficiency, there is seldom time to complete definitive laboratory tests, and therapy must commence immediately. In these circumstances it is wise to collect specimens prior to treatment and preserve them for later examinations as required.

ANTERIOR PITUITARY (ADENOHYPOPHYSIS)

The adenohypophysis produces a number of important hormones including adrenocorticotropic hormone (ACTH) and melanocyte-stimulating hormone (MSH) by the chromophobe cells, somatotropic hormone (GH, growth hormone) and luteotropic hormone (LTH) by the acidophils, follicle-stimulating hormone (FSH), luteinizing hormone (LH) and thyroid-stimulating hormone (TSH) by the basophils.

In considering adenohypophyseal deficiencies or excesses, one must take into consideration the functional aspects of the hormones produced and the target organ upon which they act.

One of the most significant hormones in terms of its activity and manifestations of disease is ACTH, which has as its target organ the adrenal cortex. Functionally, ACTH is responsible for cortisol secretion by the zona fasciculata of the adrenal. In addition, it has some stimulating effect on the melanocytes but not to the same extent as does MSH.

Growth hormone (GH) affects all tissues in young animals and does not have a specific end organ. It is known that growth hormone is diabetogenic in dogs when given with dexamethasone.[1]

Luteotropic hormone (LTH) affects the ovaries and mammary glands to maintain the corpus luteum and to initiate and sustain lactation.

Follicle-stimulating hormone (FSH) acts upon the ovaries to initiate follicular development and on the testes to stimulate spermatogenesis.

Luteinizing hormone (LH) affects the graafian follicle, causing its rupture, and initiates luteinization. The male homolog of LH is interstitial cell-stimulating hormone (ICSH), which serves to maintain androgen production in the testicle.

Thyroid-stimulating hormone (TSH) acts on the thyroid gland and is essential for the normal functioning of that organ.

Melanocyte-stimulating hormone (MSH) is responsible for cutaneous pigmentation by its action upon melanocytes.

DISEASES OF THE ADENOHYPOPHYSIS

Hypofunction. Decreased function of the adenohypophysis occurs as a consequence of pressure changes due to tumors, degenerative changes with hemorrhage and necrosis, panhypopituitarism, and, less commonly, a congenital lesion involving lack of development. Most biochemical effects associated with decreased anterior pituitary function are caused by hypofunction of the target organs, particularly the adrenal and thyroid.

Panhypopituitarism. What appears to be a hereditary panhypopituitarism has been reported in German shepherd dogs.[2] Affected animals are dwarfs, and while their littermates progress normally, they have a very slow growth rate and retain their puppy hair coat. Permanent dentition is greatly delayed or absent. The epiphyses have delayed closure and external genitalia remain infantile. These dogs have a short life span, resulting mostly from the secondary endocrine dysfunction that accompanies panhypopituitarism. Affected animals have a low serum plasma level of growth hormone, low somatomedin activity, and do not respond to ACTH or TSH because of atrophy of the thyroid and adrenal glands. A similar condition has been reported in other breeds of dogs.

Growth hormone (GH) deficiency in the adult dog has been reported.[3] Nine dogs were identified. The dogs had moderate to severe skin changes that included hair loss and hyperpigmentation that

was most pronounced on the trunk. The hair loss and skin changes apparently began two to three years prior to presentation. Routine endocrine studies were normal, including baseline plasma cortisol, plasma cortisol response to ACTH and dexamethasone, as well as basal plasma T_4 and response to TSH. Growth hormone secretory capacity, as determined by measurement of plasma GH during clonidine stimulation, was subnormal in all dogs. Growth hormone could not be detected at any time in four dogs. In three dogs there was a slight increase in GH levels following administration of clonidine, and in two dogs there was a distinct but subnormal increase in GH. As other endocrine functions were normal, it was concluded that these dogs had isolated GH deficiency. However, it could not be determined whether GH deficiency was of primary pituitary or primary hypothalamic origin.[3]

Hyperfunction. Adenohypophyseal hyperfunction is infrequently encountered, except with neoplasia. If there is a functional eosinophilic adenoma, growth hormone will be produced in excess resulting in the appearance of gigantism or acromegaly. In the young animal, there is excessive growth of long bone, which produces gigantism, whereas in the older animal, hyperfunction is more likely to produce acromegaly. Diabetes mellitus has been reported in association with acromegaly in the dog. Similarly, reports show that eosinophilic tumors of the adenohypophysis that are associated with diabetes but without acromegaly have been found in the horse and dog. Iatrogenic acromegaly has been recorded in dogs that have been frequently administered large doses of a progestational drug.[5] In one experiment female dogs were given medroxyprogesterone acetate at a dosage level of 75 mg/kg every three months for 17 months. Some animals developed typical clinical evidence for acromegaly that included thickening of the skin of the face, trunk, and forelegs as well as an increased incidence of mammary nodules. During this time growth hormone levels were elevated in all of the bitches with acromegaly. Serum cortisol levels were significantly reduced in these dogs.[4]

Excessively high GH levels were reported in a cat with diabetes mellitus.[6] The cat received high doses of insulin but the diabetes could not be controlled. The cat had an enlarged abdomen, a large head, enlarged paws, and a protruding mandible. Hyperglycemia was constant even though serum insulin levels were extremely elevated. Serum GH levels were approximately 100 times greater than normal. Other measurements of endocrine function (cortisol, ACTH response, T_4, and TSH response) were normal. A mass in the pituitary was detected by a computed tomographic brain scan and gamma camera imaging. This finding led the authors to postulate that the cat had a pituitary tumor that was producing excess GH.[6] The high

GH levels created a peripheral insulin resistance that caused hyperglycemia and diabetes mellitus. This case raised a question regarding the possible association of nonresponsive diabetes mellitus in the cat with the presence of pituitary neoplasia. Further studies are needed to clarify this possibility.

Clinical manifestations observed in animals with chromophobic and basophilic adenomas are mostly associated with excessive production of ACTH and the associated hyperadrenocorticism. Clinical laboratory alterations associated with hyperadrenal function will be discussed later.

POSTERIOR PITUITARY (NEUROHYPOPHYSIS)

The neurohypophyseal hormone most frequently altered by disease is antidiuretic hormone (ADH), which has as its target organ the distal renal tubular collecting ducts. Its action increases the permeability of these structures to water. In addition, ADH may reduce the glomerular filtration rate, increasing water retention. Oxytocin, which is also from the neurohypophysis, increases the contractibility of the uterus, stimulates prolactin production, and is of significance in the mammary gland, where it causes "letdown" of milk.

Hypofunction (Diabetes Insipidus). A lack of ADH produces diabetes insipidus. This condition, characterized by polyuria and polydipsia, usually occurs when (1) the hypothalamus fails to synthesize ADH, (2) hypothalamic osmoreceptors do not detect increases in extracellular osmotic pressures, or (3) ADH does not reach the neurohypophysis or is not released from the neurohypophysis. It must be remembered that ADH is produced in the hypothalamus and released into the bloodstream by the neurohypophysis. Thus, lesions of either the hypothalamus or posterior pituitary may be responsible for production of diabetes insipidus. Other than the obvious changes in urine specific gravity previously described, there are no additional biochemical alterations of significance if the condition is not secondary to panhypopituitarism. In panhypopituitarism, clinical signs of diabetes insipidus may not be detected because the absence of glucocorticoids reduces the glomerular filtration rate to a point at which urine specific gravity is normal although ADH secretion is markedly reduced. Replacement of glucocorticoids will often disclose the existence of diabetes insipidus.

Hyperfunction. Although excess production of ADH has been reported in humans, there are no confirmed reports of such a condition in domestic animals.

ADRENAL CORTEX

The adrenal cortex is the most active organ in the body in production of steroids, and more than 40 different compounds have been isolated. Included among these are the corticosteroids, which are produced only by the adrenals, as well as androgens, progesterone, and estrogens, which are also secreted by the gonads.

As mentioned previously, adrenal activity is governed by the anterior pituitary hormone ACTH. From a physiologic as well as a quantitative basis, corticosteroids are the most important group of adrenal steroids. The major corticosteroids secreted by the adrenal cortex include cortisol, corticosterone, and aldosterone. These have been subdivided into glucocorticoids and mineralocorticoids. Both cortisol and corticosterone are classified as glucocorticoids, whereas aldosterone is a mineralocorticoid. This classification is not meant to imply that these hormones act strictly on either carbohydrates or minerals, as cortisol may have an effect on salt and water metabolism and aldosterone may affect carbohydrate metabolism.

Although the term glucocorticosteroid suggests that action of these substances is on carbohydrate metabolism, these hormones have dramatic effects on other metabolic activities not associated with carbohydrates. Biologically the glucocorticoids influence carbohydrate metabolism because they are insulin antagonists. They impair peripheral utilization of carbohydrates and increase hepatic gluconeogenesis, both of which have a tendency to produce hyperglycemia.

The glucocorticoids are involved in protein metabolism as they reduce synthesis and increase protein catabolism. Such catabolic actions of glucocorticoids on muscle may result in myopathies and muscle wasting.

Glucocorticoids also function to increase lipolysis; this results in a release of free fatty acids and glycerol.

In addition to their effects to increase glycogen stores and increase gluconeogenesis in the liver, glucocorticoids also increase or induce the production of liver enzymes and in particular cause production of a unique alkaline phosphatase isoenzyme by the canine liver. Once hepatocytes have been induced to produce this isoenzyme, they will continue to do so for several months. As a consequence, serum alkaline phosphatase activity may remain increased long after glucocorticoid levels have returned to normal. The amount of excess glucocorticoid needed to induce the formation of this isoenzyme by the dog liver may be very small. Most but not all dogs produce this isoenzyme and the minimum dosage required varies among individuals. A careful history to detect any previous treatment with steroids should always be taken in a dog with increased serum alkaline phosphatase activity, and the increase should be interpreted in light of the information obtained.

One outstanding effect of glucosteroids is suppression of inflammatory and immune responses. Glucocorticoids participate in anti-inflammatory activity by reducing capillary permeability, preventing vasodilation by reducing the histamine level, increasing the constricting effect of norepinephrine, retarding liberation of kinins that are active vasodilators, reducing leukocyte diapedesis, reducing collagen formation, decreasing antibody production by impairing antigen processing by cells of the reticuloendothelial system, and decreasing immunoglobulin production. Although phagocytosis is increased by small doses of glucocorticoids, they suppress phagocytosis when present in excess.

There is a marked reduction in calcium uptake from the intestine because glucocorticoids inhibit vitamin D activity.

Glucocorticoids have a remarkable effect on circulating leukocytes. There is an increase in circulating neutrophils and thrombocytes with a concomitant decrease in lymphocytes and eosinophils. In some species monocytes increase. Neutrophilia is probably due to a decrease in the escape of neutrophils from blood into tissues as well as increased influx of cells from the bone marrow. Circulating lymphocytes decrease because of cytolysis of the short-lived lymphocyte population and suppression of lymphocyte mitosis. Polycythemia has been noted in animals receiving glucocorticoid therapy. The origin of such an increase is not well understood.

Glucosteroids affect water metabolism by increasing free water clearance, producing the polyuria associated with endogenous or exogenous increases in glucocorticoids. Finally, glucocorticoids participate in a weak effect, causing sodium retention and potassium excretion by the kidney.

Aldosterone is the mineralocorticoid. The principal functions of aldosterone are related to electrolyte regulation and include sodium retention, potassium excretion, retention of water, and expansion of extracellular fluid volume. Aldosterone also plays an important role in raising blood pressure.

DISEASES OF THE ADRENAL CORTEX

Hyperfunction

Hyperfunction of the adrenal cortex may involve increased secretion of the glucocorticoids (Cushing's syndrome), mineralocorticoids, androgens, or estrogens.

Most clinical signs observed with Cushing's syndrome result from excessive production of glucocorticoids. The first clinical signs include polydipsia and polyuria. As the disease progresses, symmetrical alopecia develops, and in severely affected dogs, hair loss extends over most of the body, with the exception of the head and the lower portion of the legs. Alopecia occurs one year following development of polydipsia and polyuria. Pendulousness of the abdomen appears later in the disease and is usually observed when the condition has existed for one year or longer. If androgens are also secreted, an enlarged clitoris may be observed in females. Testicular atrophy occurs in some intact males. Osteoporosis of spinal vertebrae can sometimes be detected radiologically.

Other clinical signs in hyperadrenocorticism include hyperpigmentation of the skin; cutaneous mineralization; centripetal redistribution of adipose tissue, with prominent fat pads on the dorsal midline of the neck; atrophy of the temporal muscles; hepatomegaly; and an increased susceptibility to infections of the skin, urinary tract, eye, and lung.

Hyperadrenocorticism may have several different causes. Theoretically, canine Cushing's syndrome can result from (1) adrenocortical hyperplasia caused by excess pituitary ACTH (pituitary-dependent hyperadrenocorticism), (2) adrenal tumor, (3) ectopic production of ACTH, and (4) iatrogenically from excessive administration of ACTH or glucocorticoids.

Pituitary-dependent hyperadrenocorticism (PDH) is a consequence of ACTH-producing neoplasms of the pituitary that results in bilateral hyperplasia and hypertrophy of the adrenal cortex. The existence of pituitary neoplasms may be undetected unless the pituitary gland is carefully and systematically examined at necropsy. The majority of the cases of hyperadrenocorticism in dogs are a consequence of such neoplasia.

Adenoma and carcinoma of the adrenal gland occur and produce a typical hyperadrenocorticism. When present unilaterally, such neoplasia usually results in atrophy of the opposite adrenal gland.

Clinical signs closely resembling natural cases of hyperadrenocorticism may also be induced by long-term administration of large doses of ACTH or corticosteroids in the treatment of other diseases.

In humans, Cushing's syndrome may occur as a consequence of ectopic ACTH production by a variety of tumors. Although this condition has not been documented in domestic animals, we must keep this mechanism in mind, as it could occur.

Laboratory Findings

Laboratory findings associated with endogenous or exogenous excesses of glucocorticoids include the following:

1. Lymphopenia.
2. Eosinopenia, which should be confirmed by a direct eosinophil count. A total direct count

less than 100 eosinophils/μl is suggestive of increased glucocorticoids.

3. Neutrophilia and leukocytosis with some neutrophil hypersegmentation.

4. Fasting blood glucose is sometimes, but not always, increased. In dogs serum glucose is frequently in the 120 to 130 mg/dl range.

5. Hypercholesterolemia and lipemia.

6. A marked increase in serum alkaline phosphatase activity in most dogs.

7. An increased serum ALT activity. This is not a constant change.

8. A low urine specific gravity, often 1.003 to 1.005, which must be differentiated from other causes of low urine specific gravity.

9. Serum sodium and potassium are usually in the normal range. A slight elevation in sodium and a depression in potassium may be present in some cases. These changes may become important in the patient that develops anorexia, diarrhea, or vomiting.

10. An increased plasma cortisol; in animals with adrenals that remain under pituitary control there is an exaggerated response to ACTH and a normal response to dexamethasone.

11. Thyroid tests are abnormal because the T_4 is usually low.

A definitive diagnosis can be made by the demonstration of an increased plasma cortisol concentration or an exaggerated ACTH response.

The development of acceptable laboratory techniques for cortisol assay has facilitated confirmation of the presence of a hyperfunctioning adrenal cortex. As with other laboratory assays, normal values should be established for each laboratory according to the technique utilized.

With hyperadrenocorticism, serum cortisol values are usually increased. However there may be an overlapping of the normal and hyperadrenocorticism levels of plasma or serum cortisol.

Because of the overlapping of cortisol levels in normal animals, and in some animals with hyperadrenocorticism, an elevated serum level of cortisol does not enable the veterinarian to identify and differentiate between pituitary-dependent hyperadrenocorticism (PDH) and adrenal neoplasia. Therefore, additional tests are necessary.

ACTH Stimulation Test

The ACTH stimulation test is reliable in the study of canine hyperadrenocorticism. The secretory ability of the adrenal is evaluated by determining its response to the administration of a high dose of exogenous ACTH. Although this test is of value in evaluating PDH, it has limited use in the diagnosis of functional adrenal neoplasia. The adrenals of dogs with PDH have been continually stimulated by high levels of ACTH and are capable of rapid response to any additional increase in ACTH.

The test is conducted as follows: (1) Obtain a baseline plasma sample for cortisol estimation. (2) Administer ACTH intramuscularly or intravenously. The dose and route of administration is dependent on the preference of the clinician and the laboratory to which the samples are to be submitted for assay. If in doubt, check with the laboratory you are using before conducting the test. The dosages recommended range from 0.25 IU of aqueous ACTH administered intravenously to a high of 40 IU of ACTH gel given intramuscularly. Some authors suggest the use of a synthetic ACTH at a dosage of 0.25 mg given IV or IM.[7] (3) Obtain a poststimulation plasma sample for cortisol determination. If an aqueous solution of ACTH is used, this should be done one hour following administration, whereas with a gel a two-hour poststimulation cortisol is recommended.

In animals with PDH, baseline cortisol values are usually elevated although some may be in the high normal range. Following ACTH stimulation there is a remarkable increase in plasma cortisol (four- to eightfold increase). Plasma cortisol will increase two- to fourfold in dogs with a normal adrenal gland. The ACTH stimulation test is not reliable in the diagnosis of hyperadrenocorticism caused by a functional adrenal cortical neoplasm. ACTH stimulation of dogs with functional adrenal tumors provides variable results, and interpretation is difficult if not impossible. Some dogs with an adrenal neoplasm, particularly those with adrenal carcinoma, tend to over-respond to ACTH. Therefore, an absolute differentiation between a PDH and adrenal neoplasia is difficult.

Dexamethasone Suppression

Dexamethasone suppression tests have been used for determining the primary cause of hyperadrenocorticism. Dexamethasone suppresses pituitary ACTH secretion by the negative-feedback principle and may also depress the release of CRF from the hypothalamus. Dexamethasone is used because it depresses ACTH release but does not interfere with the usual plasma cortisol assays.

Dexamethasone can be used as a low-dose, high-dose, or megadose suppression test. The low-dose suppression test can be used to confirm the presence of hyperadrenocorticism but cannot be used to differentiate between PDH and a functional adrenal neoplasm.

A low-dose dexamethasone suppression test is done by obtaining a baseline plasma sample for cortisol assay. Dexamethasone is administered at the rate of 0.015 mg/kg intramuscularly, and additional plasma samples are collected two, four, six, and eight hours after injection. Alternately, dexamethasone can be administered at the rate of 0.01 mg/kg body weight intravenously. In order to avoid excessive costs for multiple samples, the two-, four-, and six-hour samples can be eliminated and only the eight-hour collection assayed for cortisol. In a normal dog this dosage of dexamethasone will reduce the serum cortisol of the eight-hour sample to less than 1.4 µg/dl. Many dogs will have values less than 1.0 µg/dl. Dogs with PDH and those with an adrenal neoplasm do not respond to this extent. One report[8] suggested that a cortisol concentration less than half the baseline at three hours but greater than 1.5 µg/dl at eight hours most probably indicates PDH while a concentration greater than half the baseline at three hours and greater than 1.5 µg/dl at eight hours could indicate either PDH or adrenal neoplasia. In another report,[9] the results of a low-dose dexamethasone suppression test in dogs with PDH and those with adrenal tumors were compared with normal dogs. In many dogs with PDH the cortisol was suppressed to near-normal concentration two and four hours after injection but rose to presuppression levels by the eighth hour while in normal dogs suppression continued throughout the test. In dogs with adrenal neoplasia there was a slight depression of plasma cortisol two hours after injection, but the level did not decrease after the two-hour reading.

The high-dose dexamethasone suppression test appears to be more useful in determining the cause of canine hyperadrenocorticism. As with the low-dose test, samples for plasma cortisol assay are collected before and two, four, six and eight hours after administration of dexamethasone at the rate of 1.0 mg/kg of body weight. In normal dogs there is a rapid reduction in plasma cortisol at two hours and it remains low for the remainder of the test period. Dogs with PDH respond to high-dose dexamethasone with the suppression becoming greatest at six and eight hours after injection. Dogs with a functional adrenal tumor do not respond to the high-dose dexamethasone test, and the eight-hour cortisol level is near or only slightly less than the preinjection value.

Occasionally dogs with PDH will fail to respond to the high-dose dexamethasone suppression test. Most of these, however, will respond if treated with a megadose of dexamethasone, but in some dogs suppression does not occur even with a dose as high as 2.0 mg/kg.[9]

A combined dexamethasone/ACTH stimulation test can be conducted as follows:

1. A baseline blood sample is drawn and an intramuscular injection of dexamethasone (usually a high or megadose) is given immediately after the blood sample is taken.
2. Two hours later a blood sample is drawn and this is immediately followed by intravenous administration of ACTH at the dose recommended by the laboratory that will complete the cortisol assay.
3. One hour after ACTH administration a blood sample is drawn.

4. Plasma cortisol is measured on all samples using a radioimmunoassay procedure.

In a dog with hyperadrenocorticism under pituitary control, dexamethasone will reduce plasma cortisol and the ACTH stimulation will increase it. As with any test of adrenal response, the veterinarian should check with the reference laboratory for recommendations regarding the dosages to be used. Such laboratories, if staffed by a qualified veterinary clinical pathologist, have experience with a particular method and can assist the clinician in interpretation of test results.

Aldosteronism is not a usual finding in hyperplasia of the adrenal cortex in domestic animals. In humans, both primary and secondary aldosteronism are observed. The primary condition is characterized by hypertension, hypokalemia, and polyuria. Hypernatremia may also develop. Secondary hyperaldosteronism is reported in humans with nephrosis, hepatic cirrhosis, and congestive heart failure.

Hypofunction

Decreased adrenocortical function may occur as a primary condition or secondary to pituitary ACTH deficiency.

Primary Hypoadrenocorticism

Primary adrenal insufficiency (Addison's disease) is usually a progressive disease of varying etiology. Adrenocortical atrophy is the most common pathologic change observed, but its pathogenesis remains undetermined except for some evidence that it may be the consequence of an autoimmune reaction. Adrenocortical insufficiencies may also occur as a result of any destructive lesion of the adrenals, such as those seen with metastatic tumors, adrenal infarction, or amyloidosis or those caused by infectious agents that colonize both glands. These lesions occur rarely in animals.

Clinical findings associated with the chronic phase of adrenocortical hypofunction include, in descending order of frequency, depression, weakness, weak pulse, dehydration, slow mucus refill time, bradycardia, and abdominal pain.[10] Dehydration is compounded by vomiting and diarrhea as well as by loss of sodium and water through the kidney. Hemoconcentration, hypotension, and circulatory collapse may also be observed. The history often includes reports of an episodic course of illness in which the patient had been well for some time followed by a period of unexplained illness, then recovery followed by another unexplained illness.

HEMATOLOGY. Leukocyte counts in dogs with Addison's disease are variable. Some animals have an elevated total leukocyte count reflecting a response to a simultaneously occurring inflammation or infection. Some animals exhibit an absolute eosinophilia, a few have no eosinophils, while others have a normal eosinophil count. Finding a normal eosinophil count in a sick dog is unusual. Most sick dogs are stressed and have eosinopenia. A normal eosinophil count in a stressed dog may suggest hypoadrenocorticism.

Lymphocytosis may occur in canine adrenocortical insufficiency but is an inconstant parameter. As with eosinophils, normal lymphocyte counts in a sick dog are unusual, as one would expect a normal stressed dog to have lymphopenia. Therefore, hypoadrenocorticism might be suspected when normal or elevated lymphocyte counts are present in sick dogs.

Some dogs with classical clinical signs of Addison's disease and with laboratory findings that support that diagnosis have a characteristic "stress leukogram" complete with neutrophilia, monocytosis, lymphopenia, and eosinopenia.

Although hypoadrenocorticism is accompanied by normocytic, normochromic, nonregenerative anemia, this finding is frequently masked by the presence of hemoconcentration secondary to dehydration. When rehydrated, the dogs have a characteristic mild anemia.

UREA NITROGEN AND CREATININE. Azotemia occurs secondarily in many dogs with hypoadrenocorticism. This prerenal azotemia occurs as a consequence of decreased blood flow to the kidneys that accompanies hypovolemia associated with fluid loss through diarrhea, vomiting, a reduction in cardiac output, and a drop in blood pressure. Urea nitrogen values vary from a mild to a marked increase with values in excess of 100 mg/dl not uncommon. Creatinine follows the same pattern with levels ranging from 2 to 10 mg/dl. When the animal is rehydrated the urea nitrogen and creatinine usually return to normal. If this does not occur it may suggest inadequate rehydration or the possibility of renal disease. Unless the clinician is careful in his assessment of the patient, this azotemia, along with a vague clinical history that resembles that of renal disease, may lead to a mistaken diagnosis of primary renal failure. This is particularly true when the urea nitrogen and creatinine fail to decrease following replacement of body water. In such cases the clinician should rely on a urinalysis to assist in evaluating renal function. If the azotemia is prerenal in origin the urine specific gravity should be 1.025 to 1.030 or greater. With renal disease the urine is frequently isosthenuric (specific gravity 1.008 to 1.012) or is less than 1.030.

SERUM ELECTROLYTES. Electrolyte changes in an Addisonian dog include hyponatremia, hyperkalemia, and hypochloremia. Such electrolyte alterations occur as sodium and chloride are lost into the urine and the kidney does not excrete potassium. These electrolyte alterations occur because of an inadequacy of mineralocorticoids.

The sodium:potassium ratio is frequently used as a diagnostic tool in detecting Addison's disease. In the normal animal the sodium:potassium ratio is approximately 30:1 (range 27 to 40:1) and will be decreased in animals with hypoadrenocorticism to as low as 13 to 16:1. Any ratio below 27:1 should be viewed with suspicion in a patient presented with clinical signs and history suggestive of hypoadrenocorticism.

Care must be taken in interpreting the results of sodium and potassium analyses as there are other factors that will influence the ratio. Other causes of hyperkalemia include acute renal failure, some severe gastrointestinal diseases, and rapid release of cellular potassium in response to severe acidosis or as the result of increased tissue breakdown. It is seen in cats with feline urologic syndrome. Artefactual elevations can be associated with use of excessively hemolyzed blood for the analyses or in animals that have thrombocytosis if the sample is hemolyzed or refrigerated. Fortunately, most of these causes of hyperkalemia are not associated with the hyponatremia characteristic of Addison's disease.

In addition to other causes of hyperkalemia, hyponatremia from any cause will alter the serum Na:K ratio. Conditions in which hyponatremia may occur include inadequate sodium intake, vomiting, diarrhea, renal tubular disease, a diuretic loss of sodium, and in diabetics with sodium loss that accompanies osmotic diuresis.

If there is significant lipemia, it may cause a false depression of sodium and potassium as fat displaces a significant amount of the aqueous phase of plasma. When a lipemic sample is measured, less aqueous phase is obtained, causing an erroneously low estimation of sodium and potassium concentration. If these electrolytes are measured by use of an ion-specific electrode, they are expressed as the concentration in plasma water rather than whole plasma and will be normal in lipemic blood. Before evaluating the significance of a low serum sodium or potassium, the presence or absence of lipemia should be noted and the clinician should consider the methodology used. If sodium and potassium in lipemic serum have been measured by flame photometry the reported values will be falsely low. The values are reliable if measured by an ion-specific electrode.

One cannot rely solely on the presence of a decreased Na:K ratio for the diagnosis of Addison's disease. All factors must be taken into consideration before arriving at a final diagnosis. The Na:K ratio is most useful in animals that are presented when ill. Animals between the recurrent bouts of illness often have a normal Na:K ratio.

Hypercalcemia has been reported in dogs with hypoadrenocorticism.[11] Sixteen (28 per cent) of dogs diagnosed as having Addison's disease had an increased serum calcium level (mean 13 ± 0.3 mg/dl). Some of this increase might be explained by an elevated total serum protein, but there was no statistical correlation between total protein, total albumin, and calcium levels. Protein/albumin levels were not exceedingly high (7.4 ± 0.3 gm/dl and 3.6 ± 0.2 gm/dl, respectively). The hypercalcemia abated when the dogs were treated with adequate amounts of corticosteroids.

PLASMA CORTISOL. Dogs with Addison's disease, whether primary or secondary, have plasma cortisol concentrations below normal or within the normal range. Following ACTH stimulation plasma cortisol will be below normal. One report indicates that some dogs had a 60-minute cortisol concentration that was less than the baseline. The lack of response to ACTH confirms the inability of the adrenal gland to respond. If the lack of adrenal function has occurred as a result of prolonged corticosteroid therapy, the ACTH stimulation test may be abnormal, since the gland has become atrophied because of disuse. In such individuals the ACTH stimulation may need to be repeated several times before the adrenal will respond to ACTH. The same thing will occur in animals with secondary hypoadrenocorticism caused by pituitary failure.

PLASMA ENDOGENOUS ACTH. Tests for endogenous ACTH are relatively expensive and are not available in all laboratories. When such a test does become available, it will provide conclusive evidence concerning the presence of hypoadrenocorticism. As ACTH release is regulated by the amount of cortisol in the plasma, animals with primary hypoadrenocorticism provide little or no negative feedback to the pituitary and ACTH levels are high. In contrast, an animal with secondary hypoadrenocorticism should have a low ACTH reading, as there is no release by the diseased pituitary gland. The same finding would prevail in patients with a history of long-term corticosteroid therapy.

The endogenous ACTH assay may also aid in detecting dogs with adrenal neoplasia. In such animals the ACTH would be low. There is a great overlap of ACTH levels between normal animals and those with a pituitary neoplasm. This overlap may be even greater in patients under severe stress that have an increase in ACTH production.

The measurement of endogenous ACTH will probably remain a research tool in major hospitals until the test becomes available in a larger number of laboratories and the cost is reduced.

Special care must be taken in handling specimens for analysis. ACTH disappears rapidly from whole blood, and in order to avoid erroneously low values the specimen must not be allowed to stand at room temperature even for short periods of time. As ACTH adheres readily to glass, contact with glass must be avoided during collection, separation, and storage. Plastic syringes and test tubes must be used. The sample must be kept cold by collecting it in a cold syringe, placing it immediately into a cold tube, and submersing it in icewater. Centrifugation for separation should be done in a refrigerated centrifuge and the sample frozen immediately and kept frozen until presented for analysis.

THORN TEST. The status of adrenal function may be assayed by use of the Thorn test if cortisol assays are not available. This test is based upon the observation that circulating eosinophils rapidly disappear following administration of ACTH in the presence of a functional adrenal cortex. The test procedure includes administration of a test dose of ACTH and determination of the decrease in circulating eosinophils at various intervals following ACTH injection.

Eosinophils may be enumerated directly by utilizing a special diluting fluid and hemocytometer (see Appendix, p. 436). Indirect estimations of the

TABLE 11–1. Laboratory Findings in Diseases of the Adrenal Cortex

Condition	Plasma Cortisol Level			Plasma Glucose	Serum Na	Serum K	Eosinophils	Lymphocyt
	BASE	ACTH RESPONSE	DEXAMETHASONE RESPONSE					
Normal	N	↑	↓	N	N	N	N	N
Adrenocortical neoplasia	↑	No change	No change	N-↑	N	N	↓	↓
Functional pituitary neoplasm	N-↑	↑↑	No change to slight ↓ [1]	N-↑	N	N	↓	↓
Primary hypoadrenocorticism	↓	No change	Not indicated	N-↓	↓	↑	N-↑	N-↑
Secondary hypoadrenocorticism-hypopituitarism	↓	↑	Not indicated	N-↓	↓	↑	N-↑	N-↑

N = Normal
↑ = Increased
↑↑ = Greatly increased
↓ = Decreased
[1] Decreased with high- or megadose dexamethasone test.

total eosinophil count can be made by multiplying the total leukocyte count by the per cent eosinophils observed in a differential leukocyte count. The latter technique is not as accurate as the direct method but may suffice if in the differential count a minimum of 500 to 1000 white blood cells are examined and classified. If the clinician suspects an adrenocortical insufficiency and the Thorn test results are positive (i.e., a decrease in circulating eosinophils does occur), these findings may suggest that there is a lack of ACTH production by the pituitary gland.

If hypopituitarism is the cause of adrenal insufficiency, it may be necessary to repeat the injection of ACTH two or three times before a typical response is obtained. Adrenal glands that have reduced function because of ACTH deficiency may require a "priming" before regaining the capability to respond to ACTH. This test is rarely used today, as more definitive laboratory tests are available.

Secondary Hypoadrenocorticism

Adrenal hypofunction occurs secondary to an insufficiency of pituitary ACTH. In such diseases, other clinical signs of panhypopituitarism are also observed. The plasma cortisol decreased in a fashion similar to that seen in primary adrenal insufficiency; however, increased secretion will occur following parenteral administration of ACTH. If the condition has been present for some time, two or three injections of ACTH may be required before the adrenal gland can be stimulated to produce these corticosteroids. Clinical and laboratory signs are less severe than those seen in primary adrenal insufficiency, as aldosterone secretion is not controlled by ACTH, and, therefore, electrolyte disturbances are not observed.

The classic laboratory findings associated with adrenocortical malfunction are presented in Table 11–1.

ADRENAL MEDULLA

The medulla of the adrenal gland produces the catecholamines, epinephrine, and norepinephrine. Secretion of catecholamines appears to be under neural control with no involvement of any tropic hormones. The principal actions of the catecholamines are mobilization of glucose and fatty acids and increase of metabolic rate.

Hypofunction of the adrenal medulla does not occur as a clinical entity because there is no base-line production of catecholamines, as their release is under neural control.

Hyperfunction of the adrenal medulla may occur in association with functional neoplasia. Pheochromocytomas have been detected postmortem in cattle, sheep, dogs, and horses. Although there are no accurate records of clinical laboratory findings in this condition, it could be assumed that it would be accompanied by hyperglycemia, glucosuria, and an increased packed cell volume (PCV). In humans it is characterized by hypertension associated with severe headaches, palpitations, sweating, anxiety, pallor, hyperventilation, and occasionally nausea and vomiting.

REFERENCES

1. Greve, T., Dayton, A. D., and Anderson, N. V.: Acute pancreatitis with coexistent diabetes mellitus: An experimental study in the dog. Am. J. Vet. Res., 34:179, 1978.
2. Scott, D. W., Kirk, R. W., Hampshire, J., and Altszuler, N.: Clinicopathological findings in a German shepherd with pituitary dwarfism. J.A.A.H.A., 14:183, 1978.
3. Eigenmann, J. E., and Patterson, D. F.: Growth hormone deficiency in the mature dog. J.A.A.H.A., 20:741, 1984.
4. Concannon, P., Altszuler, N., Hampshire, J., Butler, W. R., and Hansel, W.: Growth hormone, prolactin, and cortisol in dogs developing mammary nodules and an acromegaly-like appearance during treatment with medroxyprogesterone acetate. Endocrinology, 106:1173, 1980.
5. Rjinberk, A., Eigenmann, J. E., Belshaw, B. E., Hampshire, J., and Altszuler, N.: Acromegaly associated with transient overproduction of growth hormone in a dog. J.A.V.M.A., 177:534, 1980.
6. Eigenmann, J. E., Wortman, J. A., and Haskins, M. E.: Elevated growth hormone levels and diabetes mellitus in a cat with acromegalic features. J.A.A.H.A., 20:747, 1984.
7. Feldman, E. C.: The adrenal cortex. In: *Textbook of Veterinary Internal Medicine. Diseases of Dogs and Cats*, edited by Ettinger, S. J., W. B. Saunders Company, Philadelphia, 1983.
8. Meijer, J. C.: Canine hyperadrenocorticism. In *Current Veterinary Therapy VII. Small Animal Practice*, edited by Kirk, R. W., W. B. Saunders Company, Philadelphia, 1980.
9. Peterson, M. E.: Hyperadrenocorticism. In: *Current Veterinary Therapy VIII. Small Animal Practice*, edited by Kirk, W. J., W. B. Saunders Company, Philadelphia, 1983.
10. Mulnix, J. A.: Hypoadrenocorticism in the dog. J.A.A.H.A., 7:220, 1971.
11. Peterson, M. E., and Feinman, J. M.: Hypercalcemia associated with hypoadrenocorticism in sixteen dogs. J.A.V.M.A., 181:1982.

CHAPTER

12

THYROID FUNCTION

The thyroid gland is unique among endocrine organs in that its secretions include a specific chemical element, iodine. The thyroid is the principal gland in the body that accumulates iodide and converts it to an organic form, although the gastric and intestinal mucosa, kidney tubules, mammary glands, and salivary glands also have some iodide activity. Because of this unique capacity, measurements of physiologic activities related to iodine metabolism serve as a basis for laboratory tests of thyroid function.

Morphologically, the thyroid gland consists of a number of small follicles lined by a simple epithelium, the cells of which vary in size depending upon the state of activity of the follicle. Contained within the follicle is thyroglobulin, which on hematoxylin-eosin–stained sections appears as a homogeneous acidophilic mass sometimes containing vacuoles. There is no excretory duct system; therefore, material must leave through the follicular epithelium.

In order to better understand the laboratory tests utilized for determining thyroid function, it is essential to review briefly iodine metabolism. Iodine is absorbed mostly from the gut as an inorganic iodide. From 20 to 40 per cent of absorbed inorganic iodide is trapped by the thyroid gland. Iodine that is not trapped is mostly excreted by the kidneys. The follicular cells of the thyroid trap iodine by means of an active transport mechanism. Thyrotropin (thyroid-stimulating hormone; TSH), which is produced by basophil cells of the anterior pituitary, is the principal stimulator for iodide transport into the thyroid, although an iodine deficiency will also accelerate transport. A chronic excess of iodide will depress the thyroid's iodine-trapping mechanism.

Iodide trapped by the thyroid is oxidized and reacts with tyrosine groups on thyroglobulin to form monoiodotyrosine (MIT) and diiodotyrosine (DIT). Following this reaction, two molecules of DIT on thyroglobulin couple to form tetraiodothyronine (T_4), while one molecule of DIT and one molecule of MIT couple to form triiodothyronine (T_3).

Thyroglobulin is a large glycoprotein with a molecular weight (MW) of 650,000, each molecule of which has many tyrosine residues (110–120). Thyroglobulin is formed by the rough endoplasmic reticulum of the follicular cells and is secreted into the follicular lumen. It is here that thyroglobulin is iodinated and the final structure of thyroid hormone is determined.

The release of thyroid hormone is controlled by TSH. Iodinated thyroglobulin near the cell-colloid interface is hydrolyzed by proteases and peptidases, releasing MIT, DIT, T_3, and T_4 into the cell. The MIT and DIT are rapidly deiodinated, and the released iodine is salvaged for reutilization. T_3 and T_4 are released into the blood.

In the plasma, T_4 and T_3 are bound to proteins. The binding affinity for T_4 is lower in the dog than in humans. As a consequence, the total T_4 concentration is lower, the hormone turnover rate is more rapid, and the unbound, free fraction of circulating T_4 is higher. When T_4 is released from the thyroid, approximately 40 per cent remains in the plasma. Most of the remaining T_4 is taken up by the liver and equilibrates rapidly with the plasma. T_3 is less firmly bound to the plasma proteins and enters peripheral cells more readily than does T_4. Because of their characteristic activities, the ratio of T_4 to T_3 in canine plasma is approximately 25:1. The turnover rate for both T_3 and T_4 in the dog is extremely high, and it has been estimated that the equivalent of 115 per cent of total extrathyroidal T_4 and 205 per cent of extrathyroidal T_3 is metabolized and must be replaced daily.

The feedback control mechanism that governs the production of thyroxine is related to the concentration of this hormone in the plasma. Any reduction in the level of thyroid hormone stimulates the pituitary gland to release TSH, which stimulates increased secretion of thyroxine to restore the plasma concentration. An excess level of thyroid hormone will reduce the secretion of TSH.

The biologically active form of thyroxine is thought to be T_3. It has been established that in the dog, T_4 is converted to T_3 at the site of the target cell.

Although its precise mechanisms remain to be determined, thyroxine has a number of physiologic effects. In addition to increasing oxygen consumption, it affects glycogenolysis, pulse rate, cardiac output, sensitivity to epinephrine, glucose absorption, lipid metabolism, bone resorption, and body temperature. Moreover, thyroxine is required for growth and maturation and is related to various phases of reproduction including fertility, pregnancy, and ovulation. Thyroxine also decreases formation of phosphocreatine.

The thyroid gland is also the site of formation of thyrocalcitonin in some animal species. This substance, which acts upon calcium metabolism, will be discussed in Chapter 13.

DISEASES OF THE THYROID

Hyperthyroidism in Dogs. Hyperthyroidism in the dog is almost always associated with neoplasia. Most (approximately two thirds) of neoplasms are classified as adenocarcinomas. By the time animals are presented, approximately 40 per cent of the adenocarcinomas have already metastasized.[1] Extension of the malignancy frequently involves the retropharyngeal nodes, and metastasis to the lungs is frequently an early observation.

The first clinical sign of hyperthyroidism is usually polydipsia that can occur gradually or have an abrupt onset. The dog will have a history of weight loss in spite of a ravenous appetite. Other signs depend on the extent of the hyperthyroidism and its duration. Other clinical signs noted include a preference for a cool environment even though the rectal temperature is normal, fatigue, a forceful apex beat and arterial pulse, and restlessness.

The thyroid gland function should be carefully evaluated in any dog with a history of polyuria.

Hyperthyroidism in Cats. Recently the presence of hyperthyroidism in cats has received considerable attention.[2,3] The condition develops in elderly cats (9 to 22 years) of both sexes. The hyperthyroidism results from presence of adenocarcinomas, adenomas, or simple adenomatous hyperplasia. Clinical signs develop gradually and include weight loss in spite of polyphagia and stools that are abundant and soft; some cats have diarrhea. There is thirst and polyuria that accompanies restlessness, a tendency to pace, and evidence of extreme nervousness. Affected cats are so tense that they will not relax even when fondled and reassured.[3] Palpation in the areas of the thyroid just below the larynx will reveal enlargement of one or rarely both thyroid lobes. As with the dog, T_3 and T_4 levels are increased.

In a study of 131 cats with hyperthyroidism,[4] laboratory findings included mild to moderate erythrocytosis and high serum alkaline phosphatase, alanine transferase, aspartate transferase, and lactic dehydrogenase activity. All cats had increased T_4 values, while T_3 concentrations were normal in four (3 per cent) of the cats. Little or no increase in resting serum T_4 concentration was seen following TSH administration. Such results may have occurred either because the hyperfunctioning adenomatous thyroid glands secreted thyroid hormones independent of TSH control or because the gland was already producing at the maximum rate. There was an increase in thyroidal uptake of radioiodine in cats with hyperthyroidism.

Hypothyroidism. Decreased thyroid function is not uncommon in the dog. The clinical features of hypothyroidism are present in the following order of approximate relative frequency in the adult dog[5]:

1. Lethargy and easy fatigability.
2. Cold intolerance.
3. Changes in skin and hair coat (dry, scaly skin; brittle, easily epilated hair; and hyperpigmentation).
4. Abnormal estrous cycles, infertility, and decreased libido.
5. Either constipation or a mild diarrhea.
6. Bradycardia.
7. Weight gain.

PRIMARY HYPOTHYROIDISM. The etiology of primary hypothyroidism has not been definitely determined in all animal species; however, decreased thyroid function in the adult dog is presented as two distinct entities.[1] Thyroid atrophy occurs when there is progessive destruction of the follicles in animals with chronic lymphocytic thyroiditis. Studies in beagles have shown that it has a familial occurrence.[6] The presence of antibodies to thyroglobulin[7,8] supports the possibility that the inflammatory process is immune mediated.

Another common form of thyroid atrophy in the dog is noninflammatory; the pathogenesis of this condition remains unknown.

Goiter, a condition characterized by an enlargement of the thyroid gland other than that produced by malignancy or inflammation, is not frequently diagnosed in domestic animals.

SECONDARY HYPOTHYROIDISM. Secondary hypothyroidism occurs when there is a lack of TSH due to a pituitary lesion. Animals with this type of hypothyroidism have other clinical signs of pituitary malfunction if the problem is panhypopituitarism.

Congenital secondary hypothyroidism occurs in animals with pituitary dwarfism such as the condition described in German shepherd dogs. An acquired secondary hypothyroidism can occur when there is a compression atrophy or replacement of the pituitary pars distalis by a tumor.

Tertiary hypothyroidism is the result of a deficiency in release or production of thyroid releasing hormone (TRH). This has been reported[1] in a dog as a congenital defect of apparently an isolated TRH deficiency and as an acquired disorder in adult dogs when it occurred alone or in combination with a moderate adrenocortical insufficiency.

The clinical signs of secondary and tertiary hypothyroidism are similar to those with primary hypothyroidism, except that they are not as extensive or as progressive.

Failure of the thyroid to produce normal quantities of hormone because of an inborn defect in synthesis (dyshormonogenesis) has been recorded in sheep, cattle, and dogs. In merino sheep, the condition occurs as a result of formation of abnormal iodoproteins, whereas in cattle an abnormal thyroglobulin is produced.[9]

Equine goiter due to excessive dietary iodide was reported. The condition occurred in thoroughbred foals on three farms, although some yearling and adult horses on these same farms were also affected. The dietary intake of inorganic iodide by mares bearing goitrous foals ranged from 48 to 432 mg/day compared with values of 7 mg/day or less for horses on a farm where goiter did not occur. Dried seaweed (kelp) was found to be the principal source of iodide in these goitrogenic diets. These authors believed that the consumption of as little as 50 mg of iodide per day by pregnant mares caused congenital goiter in some foals.

THYROID FUNCTION TESTS

Because of thyroxine's great diversity of activities, excesses or deficiencies of thyroid function produce a plethora of clinical signs, so that without the use of laboratory tests, a definitive diagnosis is almost an impossibility. The picture is complicated by the fact that routine laboratory determinations that are useful in the diagnosis of malfunction of other organs are not applicable to the detection of thyroid abnormalities. However, in the past several years more specific determinations that are of value in detecting thyroid diseases have become available. Many of these tests require highly specialized equipment; therefore, it is unlikely that many, if any, veterinary practitioners will be conducting these tests in their own laboratories.

Because of the sensitivity of the determinations and the necessity for careful controls, selection of a laboratory to complete the tests is an important factor. Before a reliable interpretation of data can be made, the veterinarian must establish normal values for the particular practice situation and reference laboratory. This should be done when the laboratory is first selected, and normal specimens should periodically be submitted to the laboratory in order to detect any deviation that may have developed in procedures. The following discussion of interpretation assumes that the laboratory is performing tests in an acceptable manner and that the results are reliable.

Hematology. Hematologic alterations in diseases of the thyroid are not definitive.

A normocytic, normochromic anemia of moderate intensity may occur if the animal has hypothyroidism. This is the nonregenerative type with no observable signs of erythropoiesis such as polychromasia, anisocytosis, reticulocytosis, or the presence of nucleated erythrocytes in the peripheral circulation. The anemia may develop because the animal requires less oxygen, since less is needed in the reduced metabolic state that exists in hypothyroidism. Hypochromasia and the appearance of variable numbers of leptocytes may occur.

In primary hypothyroidism, the total leukocyte count is variable, with values usually in the low normal range, although counts may exceed 20,000 cells/μl. The distribution of cell types is usually within the normal range. A differential leukocyte count may assist the clinician in distinguishing between primary and secondary hypothyroidism.

In secondary hypothyroidism, lymphocytosis and eosinophilia may be present if there is panhypopituitarism and a concomitant lack of adrenocorticotropic hormone (ACTH) production. If secondary hypothyroidism occurs only because of a lack of TSH, and ACTH production is normal, there will be no alteration in numbers of lymphocytes or eosinophils.

Serum Cholesterol Determination. For years, veterinarians relied on the estimation of serum cholesterol levels to assist them in diagnosing hypothyroidism in the dog. It is a well-known fact that the level of serum cholesterol is affected by thyroid activity and that it varies inversely with the degree of activity. Hypothyroidism is frequently associated with an increase in serum cholesterol values. However, it is extremely difficult to interpret these changes, as serum cholesterol concentration has a wide normal range and may be elevated in a variety of conditions not associated with thyroid function. Hypercholesterolemia is frequently seen in animals on a high-fat diet, and in those with biliary obstruction, glomerular disease, nephrosis, general hepatic dysfunction, adrenocortical hyperfunction, or diabetes mellitus.

Normal serum cholesterol levels are presented in Table 12–1. It will be noted that normal cholesterol values for the dog are variable. This is undoubtedly a reflection of the techniques utilized as well as the diet of the animals being tested. It is this variability in normal values that makes serum cholesterol levels difficult to utilize diagnostically.

The diagnostic accuracy of serum cholesterol determinations for hypothyroidism in the dog is about 60 per cent.[10] However, when serum cholesterol levels are greater than 500 mg/dl and diabetes mellitus can be eliminated as a possibility, the diagnostic accuracy of the test is greatly increased, and it can be of value in determining hypothyroidism. The greatest diagnostic significance of serum cholesterol level occurs when the test is employed in combination with other measurements of thyroid function.

Serum cholesterol determination may be of some assistance in evaluating therapy instituted in the treatment of hypothyroidism. If diet can be controlled and specimens are collected from a fasted animal, total serum cholesterol levels may indicate the success or lack of success of treatment.

T₃ and T₄ Assay. The development of radioimmunoassay and competitive protein assay techniques for the quantitation of serum T_4 and T_3 has greatly enhanced detection of hypothyroidism in the dog. As normal levels for T_3 and T_4 are much lower in domestic animals than in humans, commercial laboratories conducting such determinations must alter their techniques in order to provide reliable results. Normal values for T_4 and T_3 should be established for each laboratory conducting the determination. Several commercial kits are available for assaying T_4 and T_3 levels. As commercial laboratories often change the method they are using, it may be necessary to resubmit specimens from normal animals to validate the results.

Normal T_4 values range from 1.5 to 4 μg/dl, whereas T_3 values range from 50 to 200 ng/dl. These values are decreased in the hypothyroid dog. If the reference laboratory provides consistently reproducible results, the T_3 or T_4 assay may be relied upon to detect hypothyroidism. One endocrinologist[11] suggests that the T_3 assay is preferred. He points out that T_3 is the active hormone at the cellular level, and when T_3 is administered there is complete suppression of T_4. When T_4 is administered to a hypothyroid dog, reversal of the clinical signs does not occur unless T_4 is converted to T_3. Another author[12] commented that measurement of T_3 was of little additional value in the evaluation of thyroid function in the dog.

The plasma concentration of T_4 in dogs can be depressed by glucocorticoid excesses, either endogenous or exogenous. One report[1] suggests that half of the dogs with excess glucocorticoids will have a moderate to severely depressed plasma T_4 concentration. Other drugs that will depress T_4 concentration include phenytoin, phenobarbital, phenylbutazone, and o,p'DDD ([Lysodren] Calbio Pharmaceuticals, La Jolla, California). There are no studies that reveal the exact mechanism by which each of these drugs affects the plasma T_4 concentration in the dog. In man, however, it has been found that glucocorticoids decrease TRH release, TRH-induced release of TSH, and T_4 binding capacity of thyroxine-binding globulin. Phenytoin interferes with T_4 binding to plasma proteins and increases the rate of conversion of T_4 to T_3.

TSH Response Test. Because of the low values for T_4 and T_3 and the irregularity in obtaining consistent results, it has been suggested[13] that a thyroid-stimulating hormone response test would have advantages over single assay techniques. The test is conducted by drawing a preinjection blood sample, then administering 10 IU of TSH subcutaneously in dogs, 2.5 IU intramuscularly in cats, and 5 IU in horses. A blood sample is taken 16 hours postinjection, and the preinjection and postinjection samples are assayed for T_4. In the normal dog, a twofold or greater increase in the T_4 level should be expected in the postinjection sample. The dog with primary hypothyroidism would have little or no response to the injection

TABLE 12–1. Serum Cholesterol Levels in a Variety of Animal Species

Species	Serum Cholesterol (mg/dl)		
	TOTAL	FREE	ESTER
Bovine	110 ± 32	37 ± 15	73 ± 15
Ovine	64 ± 12		
Caprine	80–130		
Porcine	64–104		
Equine	92.8 ± 2.8	15.7	81.1
Canine	110 ± 28	51 ± 20	59 ± 19
	125–250		
Canine	211 ± 32		
Low fat diet	140		
High fat diet	280		
Male	107–325		
Female	116–380		
Feline	93 ± 24	30 ± 10	63 ± 23
	95–130		

of TSH. In dogs with a drug-induced low plasma T_4, the TSH response is normal. In cats the T_4 level is double baseline by 8 or 12 hours after TSH administration, while in the horse T_4 values double by three hours.

Response to TSH is our choice of a test for evaluating the functional status of the thyroid in a clinical situation in which thyroxine analyses are completed in a commercial laboratory that has not revised its techniques to adapt for the T_4 levels in dog serum. If primary hypothyroidism is suspected, a serum T_4 test on day one followed immediately by a single injection of TSH and a second T_4 test the following day may serve to identify the condition. If secondary hypothyroidism is suspected, a T_4 determination should be completed on day one, and a series of three or four injections of TSH should be followed by a second T_4 determination on the day following the final injection. Confirmation of secondary hypothyroidism is obtained by demonstrating an increase in T_4 concentration. For all practical purposes, failure to respond to even a single injection of TSH should be sufficient justification to commence replacement therapy.

TRH Stimulation. TRH stimulation is useful in differentiating between secondary and tertiary hypothyroidism. Such a test is run only in cases of hypothyroidism in which the thyroid responds to TSH stimulation. The test is conducted by administering 0.2 mg of TRH intravenously. Plasma samples are collected immediately before and four hours after TRH administration. In normal dogs the increase in plasma T_4 has been reported to range from as little as 0.5 to as much as 2.0 µg/dl above basal concentration.[1] In hypothyroid dogs that respond to TSH, an additional finding of an increase in plasma T_4 of at least 1.0 µg/dl after TRH suggests that the underlying cause of the hypothyroidism is a defect in transport, production, or release of TRH.

Thyroid Radioiodine Uptake Test. Radioactively labeled iodine is metabolized in the same fashion as is nonradioactive iodine. Therefore, administered or ingested radioactive iodine will follow the same metabolic pathways as nonradioactive iodine and will eventually become trapped in the thyroid gland. Although the radioactive iodine uptake technique is limited to facilities capable of handling radioactive substances and monitoring the amount of iodine taken up by the thyroid gland, it remains one of the most definitive tests available for detecting thyroid abnormalities.

The standard technique is to monitor the amount of radio-labeled I taken up by the gland using an external scintillation detector placed over the thyroid gland. Uptake is expressed as a percentage of the injected dose. In the dog, a single 72-hour measurement is usually satisfactory for detection of hypothyroidism, but a timed uptake curve constructed over a three- to four-day period is required for the differential diagnosis of hyperthyroidism.[14]

Because the requirements of time, personnel, and facilities and equipment are great, this test is used only in research or teaching institutions.

REFERENCES

1. Belshaw, B. E.: Thyroid diseases. In: *Textbook of Veterinary Internal Medicine. Diseases of the Dog and Cat*, edited by Ettinger, S. J., W. B. Saunders Company, Philadelphia, 1983.
2. Holzworth, J., Theran, P., Carpenter, J. L., Harpster, N. K., and Todoroff, R. J.: Hypothyroidism in the cat: Ten cases. J.A.V.M.A., 176:345, 1980.
3. Theran, P., and Holzworth, J.: Feline hyperthyroidism. In: *Current Veterinary Therapy VII. Small Animal Practice*, edited by Kirk, R. W., W. B. Saunders Company, Philadelphia, 1980.
4. Peterson, M. E., Kintzer, P. P., Cavanaugh, P. G., Fox, P. R., Ferguson, D. C., Johnson, G. F., and Becker, D. V.: Feline hyperthyroidism: Pretreatment clinical and laboratory evaluation of 131 cases. J.A.V.M.A., 183:103, 1983.
5. Siegel, E. T.: Endocrinology. In: *Scientific Presentations and Seminar Synopses*, 39th Annual Meeting, A.A.H.A., South Bend, Ind., 1972.
6. Musser, E., and Graham, W. A.: Familial occurrence of thyroiditis in purebred beagles. Lab. Anim. Care, 18:58, 1968.
7. Mizejerski, G. J., Barron, J., and Poissant, G.: Immunologic investigations of naturally occurring canine thyroiditis. J. Immunol., 107:1152, 1971.
8. Gosselin, S. J., Capen, C. C., Martin, S. L., and Targowski, S. P.: Biochemical and immunological investigations on hypothyroidism in dogs. Can. J. Comp. Med., 44:158, 1980.
9. Rac, R., Hill, G. N., Pain, R. W., and Mulhearn, C. J.: Congenital goiter in merino sheep due to an inherited defect in the biosynthesis of thyroid hormone. Res. Vet. Sci., 9:209, 1968.
10. Kaneko, J. J.: Thyroid function. In: *Clinical Biochemistry of Domestic Animals*, 3rd ed., edited by Kaneko, J. J., Academic Press, New York, 1980.
11. Nachreiner, R. F.: Using the commercial endocrine diagnostic laboratory. Bull., Am. Soc. Vet. Clin. Pathol., 5(3):14, 1976.
12. Peterson, M. E., Ferguson, D. C., Kintzer, P. P., and Drucker, W. D.: Effects of spontaneous hyperadrenocorticism on serum thyroid hormone concentrations in the dog. Am. J. Vet. Res., 45:2034, 1984.
13. Kaneko, J. J., Comer, K. M., and Ling, G. V.: Thyroxine levels by radioimmunoassay (T4-RIA) and the thyroid stimulating hormone response test in normal dogs. Calif. Vet., 32(1):9, 1978.
14. Kaneko, J. J.: Thyroid function. In: *Clinical Biochemistry of Domestic Animals*, 2nd ed., edited by Kaneko, J. J. and Cornelius, C. E., Academic Press, New York, 1970.

MINERAL BALANCE AND PARATHYROID FUNCTION

In the animal body, the mineral substances calcium, phosphorus, and magnesium are of importance in a number of physiologic activities and may be found in either increased or decreased quantities in association with certain diseases.

CALCIUM AND PHOSPHORUS METABOLISM

The control of calcium metabolism, and in particular the extracellular level of calcium ions, is mediated primarily through the effects of the hormones parathormone, calcitonin (thyrocalcitonin), and vitamin D. Although these are the primary hormones involved in calcium control mechanisms, other hormones—such as estrogens, corticosteroids, somatotropin, glucagon, and thyroxine—may contribute to calcium homeostasis.

Approximately 99 per cent of body calcium and 80 to 85 per cent of body phosphorus are found in the skeleton and teeth. Only a small percentage of the total body concentration of these elements is found in the blood, but their presence in extracellular fluids is essential. Calcium ions are required for: (1) preservation of skeletal structure, (2) muscle contraction, (3) blood coagulation, (4) activation of several enzymes, (5) transmission of nerve impulses, and (6) decreasing cell membrane and capillary permeability. Phosphorus ions have an important role in major metabolic intermediates and in high-energy phosphate bonds associated with carbohydrate metabolism. This element is an important constituent of bone and of nucleic acids, phospholipids, nucleotides, and other chemical moieties. Phosphorus is located in all cells and is concerned in many metabolic processes including body fluid buffers.

Dietary calcium and phosphorus are absorbed primarily in the upper small intestine, with the amount absorbed dependent upon (1) dietary levels of calcium, phosphorus, vitamin D, iron, aluminum, manganese, and fat; (2) the source of the minerals; (3) intestinal pH; and (4) lactose intake. The efficiency of absorption increases as body needs for calcium and phosphorus become greater. Intestinal absorption of calcium and phosphorus requires an acid pH for formation of readily absorbable soluble salts. Insoluble nonabsorbable salts are formed in an alkaline pH. Lactose enhances calcium absorption by a mechanism that is not yet understood but that may be related to intestinal pH. The principal role of vitamin D is in relation to intestinal and cellular absorption of calcium. As the dietary calcium:phosphorus ratio increases, body requirements for vitamin D are increased.

Calcium and phosphorus absorption will be reduced when there is (1) a decrease in vitamin D or vitamin D activity (as in presence of excess glucocorticoids); (2) an alkaline gut; (3) an excess of dietary fat or poor fat digestion, which enhances formation of insoluble nonabsorbable calcium soaps; and (4) an accumulation of dietary oxalate, which combines with calcium to form insoluble salts that are lost in feces. The high concentration of phytates in cereal grains and oil seeds is significant in comparisons of calcium and phosphorus metabolism in monogastric and ruminant animals. Sixty to 80 per cent of the total phosphorus present in these feedstuffs exists organically bound as phytic acid. This organically bound phosphorus is generally unavailable to monogastric animals because they lack the enzyme phytase, which is normally present in the rumen. This enzyme hydrolyzes organically bound phosphorus, making it available for absorption.

Calcium and phosphorus absorbed from the gut are readily transported by blood and are removed from it according to body needs. During periods of bone and tooth growth, the removal rate may be great; in the adult animal, total body requirements for calcium are somewhat reduced, although some of this element is incorporated into bone. In the adult, bone serves as a reservoir of calcium and phosphorus that can be drawn upon to maintain normal plasma concentrations.

Calcium and phosphorus are lost through the feces and urine. Fecal calcium is mostly of dietary origin, but some may be endogenous as a result of calcium excretion into the intestinal lumen. This may be of considerable significance in cattle in which endogenous calcium loss has been estimated to be as much as 4 to 7 gm daily. Phosphorus is also lost through feces. Calcium and phosphorus loss through urine is regulated, since kidney tubules have the capacity to reabsorb these elements. The renal threshold of calcium has been estimated to be between 6.5 and 8 mg/dl, and little urine loss will occur at blood levels less than this. In most ruminant animals, renal excretion of phosphorus is low and may be related to the alkaline pH of urine. Considerable calcium and phosphorus loss occurs through the milk of these animals.

CALCIUM AND PHOSPHORUS IN BLOOD

Almost all calcium in blood is found in the plasma, as erythrocytes contain very little calcium. Calcium is present in two forms in the plasma: (1) a nondiffusible protein-bound form that constitutes 40 to 50 per cent of total plasma calcium and (2) a diffusible nonprotein-bound form. Diffusible nonprotein-bound calcium exists in two forms: (1) as a complex with citrate and phosphate and (2) as physiologically active ionized calcium. Approximately 5 per cent of nonprotein-bound diffusible calcium is in the complex form, with the remainder being the ionized physiologically active form. Ionized calcium is the most important physiologically. A decrease in ionized calcium produces tetany. The hydrogen ion concentration is a major chemical factor influencing the concentration of ionized calcium. An increase in pH (alkalosis) decreases ionized calcium but does not change the total serum calcium concentration.

Total serum calcium concentration is affected by total plasma protein concentration. An increase in plasma proteins increases the amount of protein-bound calcium and thus the total serum calcium concentration. Serum calcium concentration is decreased with hypoproteinemia because of the reduced amount of protein-bound calcium. Under these circumstances, the amount of ionized diffusible calcium will not usually be altered. In interpretation of a serum calcium level, the concentration of serum protein and the acid-base status of the animal must be considered. Normal values for serum calcium are presented in Table 13–1.

Phosphorus is present in blood as an organic ester within erythrocytes or as phospholipid and inorganic phosphate in plasma. The inorganic fraction is usually measured to determine serum phosphorus levels. As there is considerable phosphorus in erythrocytes, samples to be analyzed for phosphate must be handled carefully to avoid hemolysis. Phosphoric esters released from erythrocytes may undergo hydrolysis and liberate phosphate, thus increasing serum levels. Abnormally high serum phosphate levels may be seen in nonhemolyzed samples exposed to high ambient temperatures. Normal values for phosphate are presented in Table 13–2.

TABLE 13–1. Concentration of Calcium in Serum of Normal Animals

Species	Calcium (mg/dl)	
	Mean	Standard Deviation
Bovine	11.08	±0.67
Bovine	7.4*	±0.8
Bovine at parturition	8.07	
Ovine	12.16	±0.28
	9.8	±0.1
Caprine	10.7	
	10.3	
Porcine	11.0 (10.2–11.9)	
Porcine (6 months)	9.65	±0.99
Porcine (pregnant sow)	10.11	±1.08
Equine	12.8	±0.58
Canine		
Large dogs	10.15	±0.4
Beagle dogs 13 mo ± 1 mo	10.8	±0.39
Giant breeds		
up to 3 mo	11.1	±0.4
3–6 mo	10.8	±0.6
6–9 mo	10.5	±0.5
9–12 mo	10.3	±0.5
Adult	9.9	±0.8
Feline	8.22	±0.97

*Whole blood.

TABLE 13–2. Normal Serum Phosphorus Levels in Domestic Animals

Species	Phosphorus (mg/dl)	
	MEAN	STANDARD DEVIATION
Bovine	5.56	±1.56
Calves	8.9	±0.6
Heifers	6.2	±0.6
Cattle	5.5	±0.8
Ovine	5.21	±0.11
	6.4	±0.2
Porcine	7.8	
After 115 hr fast	5.8	
6 mo	10.94	±0.98
Pregnant sow	7.87	±1.42
Equine	3.6	±1.0
<1 yr	5.1	
1–5 yr	4.2	
>5 yr	2.85	
Canine		
Beagles 13 mo ± 1 mo	4.5	±0.62
Large dogs	3.7	±0.5
	5.6	
Giant breeds		
Up to 3 mo	8.7	±0.7
3–6 mo	8.7	±0.7
6–9 mo	7.5	±0.8
9–12 mo	8.0	±2.0
Adult	4.2	±0.9
Feline	6.4	
	2.6–4.7	
Caprine	3.1	±0.71

FACTORS INFLUENCING SERUM CALCIUM AND PHOSPHORUS LEVELS

Parathormone. This hormone from the parathyroid has three target organs: bone, kidney, and intestinal mucosa. The major function of parathormone is the maintenance of a normal serum calcium level by action upon target cells. This is accomplished by mobilization of calcium from bone.

Parathormone is produced by the secretory cells of the parathyroid and stored in small quantities in these cells, providing an immediate source of parathormone that is released according to the ionic calcium concentration. Secretion of this preformed hormone can be rapid, whereas increased hormone synthesis occurs more slowly.

Parathormone acts on the kidney to assist in maintenance of a normal plasma calcium concentration. This hormone enhances renal tubular reabsorption of calcium and decreases tubular reabsorption of phosphate, thus increasing urinary loss of phosphate. This decrease in tubular reabsorption of phosphate tends to decrease serum phosphorus levels and assists in maintenance of the calcium:phosphorus ratio. Parathormone action on intestinal mucosa promotes ab-

sorption of dietary calcium. Intestinal mucosa is, however, the least sensitive target organ.

The fact that the serum calcium concentration decreases following parathyroidectomy, although the calcium level never reaches zero, indicates that there is another calcium control mechanism. This control, which is independent of parathyroid, is physicochemical and depends on the solubility equilibrium between skeletal calcium and the extracellular fluids that bathe bone crystals. These bone crystals are described as having both a "labile" and a "stable" fraction. The labile crystals readily exchange calcium, phosphorus, and other ions with plasma; rapidly sequester foreign ions; and make a net contribution of calcium and other ions by means of strictly physicochemical processes. The stable fraction apparently is not in direct contact with body fluids, and it is this portion that is acted upon by parathormone.

Although the kidney is a target organ for parathormone, it must be remembered that the stimulus for parathormone release is strictly dependent upon calcium ion concentration in blood and is not affected by serum phosphate concentration.

Calcitonin (Thyrocalcitonin). Calcitonin's activity is the opposite of that of parathormone. If blood calcium levels are high, calcitonin acts to store calcium in bone by inhibiting bone resorption. This hormone is produced by the parafollicular cells, which are found immediately outside the cells bordering the thyroid follicles in most mammals. These cells represent ultimobranchial tissue and in most animals are found within the thyroid and parathyroid. There is continual secretion of calcitonin that is increased by an elevation of plasma calcium. Preformed calcitonin is stored in secretory granules of the parafollicular cells and is released in response to hypercalcemia. Calcitonin does not affect calcium absorption and, although it has been hypothesized that it may have a direct effect on the kidney, this has not been unequivocally confirmed. This hormone acts by its inhibitory effects on parathormone-stimulated bone resorption. In humans, thyrocalcitonin promotes phosphaturia but decreases urinary excretion of calcium, magnesium, and hydroxyproline.

Fine control of plasma levels of calcium is dependent on the action of both parathormone and calcitonin. Parathormone secretion and production are stimulated by calcium ion decrease, whereas calcitonin release is dependent on increased calcium ion levels in plasma.

Vitamin D. The activity of vitamin D in the control of serum calcium and phosphate levels is similar to that of parathormone, although its major target organ is intestinal mucosa. Vitamin D stimulates bone resorption by dissolution of mineral salts and destruction of collagen fibers. It may promote phosphaturia, but to a lesser extent than does parathormone.

Vitamin D must be metabolically activated before it can participate in mineral metabolism. Vitamin D_3 (cholecalciferol) is converted by the enzymes of the liver into 25-hydroxycholecalciferol. This metabolite is then converted to 1,25-dihydroxycholecalciferol by enzymes in kidney cells. This conversion is enhanced by parathormone and consequently by conditions that stimulate parathormone release and production. Calcitonin has the opposite effect.

This activated form of vitamin D acts on target cells in the bone and intestine to increase the rate of calcium absorption and to increase bone resorption. Because of its mode of action and chemical composition, vitamin D is now considered a hormone.

Age and Breed. As can be seen by the data presented in Tables 13–1 and 13–2, serum calcium and phosphorus concentrations vary in a manner that appears to be age related. This is especially true of phosphorus levels. Normal serum phosphorus levels in the equine have been reported to be 3.6 ± 1.0 mg/dl,[1] but in the same study, animals of less than one year of age had a mean serum phosphorus level of 5.1 mg/dl. Of particular significance is the high serum phosphorus level in the giant breeds of dogs.[2] Values of 8 to 8.7 mg/dl were observed in dogs of giant breeds that were less than one year of age as compared with a value of 4.2 mg/dl for adult animals of the same breed. These facts must be taken into consideration in evaluating serum phosphorus levels in the various breeds of dogs.

DETERMINATION OF SERUM CALCIUM AND PHOSPHORUS LEVELS

Serum calcium and phosphorus levels should be determined whenever there is clinical evidence suggesting a disturbance in mineral metabolism. Many disturbances in mineral metabolism are accompanied by clinical or radiologic evidence of bone disease. Therefore, if there are any signs of bone disease, determination of total serum calcium and phosphorus levels should be considered. Total serum protein and alkaline phosphatase activities should be determined at the same time that serum calcium and phosphorus levels are measured. As previously discussed, serum protein values are necessary to interpret accurately the results of a total serum calcium determination, whereas alkaline phosphatase activity reflects bone activity. Total serum calcium and phosphate estimations are also indicated if paralytic conditions exist or if an animal has convulsions.

In addition to estimation of the levels of calcium and phosphorus in the serum, determination of the concentration of these two elements in the urine may be of significance and will be discussed later in this chapter.

Techniques for Determination. Calcium and phosphorus determinations are made using serum, although plasma may also be used if it is in an anticoagulant that does not depend upon the binding of calcium for its activity. Such anticoagulants include sodium citrate, sodium oxalate, and heparin. A wide variety of chemical techniques are available for completing calcium determinations. The most accurate is atomic absorption spectrometry, although the flame photometer will also provide accurate results. Relatively simple colorimetric techniques have been developed and are useful in estimating total serum calcium levels. Most automated biochemical profiling equipment has channels for calcium and inorganic phosphate estimations.

Techniques are now available for determining the concentration of ionized calcium by use of a calcium ion-specific electrode. Because of the physiologic significance of the ionized calcium fraction, this technique may prove to be valuable.

ABNORMALITIES IN SERUM CALCIUM AND PHOSPHORUS CONCENTRATIONS

Increases in total serum calcium levels (hypercalcemia) may be seen in the following conditions: (1) hypervitaminosis D, (2) primary hyperparathyroidism, (3) pseudohyperparathyroidism, (4) osteolytic bone lesions, (5) primary renal disease (particularly in the horse), (6) hypoadrenocorticism, (7) hyperproteinemia, and (8) laboratory error.

Decreases in total serum calcium concentrations (hypocalcemia) may occur in the following conditions: (1) vitamin D deficiency, (2) hypoparathyroidism, (3) parturient paresis, (4) eclampsia, (5) transport tetany in cattle and horses, (6) secondary hyperparathyroidism (not constant), (7) bovine ketosis, (8) acute necrotizing pancreatitis, (9) hypoproteinemia, (10) hypomagnesemic tetany in ruminants, and (11) hyperadrenocorticism.

A positive linear relationship between total calcium and albumin and between total calcium and total protein in serum of 209 dogs has been reported.[3] The authors suggest that use of a correction formula is essential for correct interpretation of calcium values and detection of abnormalities in calcium metabolism. The formulas are[3]:

1. Calcium corrected for albumin concentration:

$$\text{Adjusted Ca (mg/dl)} = \text{Ca (mg/dl)} - \text{Albumin (gm/dl)} + 3.5$$

2. Calcium corrected for total protein:

$$\text{Adjusted Ca (mg/dl)} = \text{Ca(mg/dl)} - (0.4 \times \text{total serum protein [mg/dl]}) + 3.3$$

Elevations in total serum inorganic phosphate values (hyperphosphatemia) may be found in: (1) reduced glomerular filtration rate in dogs and cats, (2) secondary hyperparathyroidism associated with renal failure, (3) nutritional secondary hyperparathyroidism, (4) young growing animals, and (5) hypoparathyroidism. The serum inorganic phosphate level may increase slightly with healing fractures and be falsely elevated in hemolyzed serums or in blood held at a high ambient temperature.

Decreases in total serum inorganic phosphate levels (hypophosphatemia) may occur in: (1) primary hyperparathyroidism, (2) pseudohyperparathyroidism, (3) postparturient hemoglobinemia in the bovine, (4) parturient paresis, and (5) hypercalcitoninism. Sometimes the concentration of total serum phosphate decreases with secondary nutritional hyperparathyroidism resulting from vitamin D or calcium deficiency. An inadequate intake of dietary phosphorus will also cause a decline in total serum phosphate levels.

DISEASES OF THE PARATHYROID

Hyperparathyroidism in domestic animals occurs as a primary condition with functional parathyroid adenoma. As a secondary condition, hyperparathyroidism may develop from renal failure or it may have a nutritional origin. Pseudohyperparathyroidism has been reported in the dog and cat.

Primary Hyperparathyroidism. A functional adenoma of the parathyroid, which produces excessive quantities of parathormone, is rare in domestic animals. The neoplastic parathyroid gland fails to respond to the normal control mechanism—serum calcium concentration—and continues to produce parathormone, although it is not required. The consequence of excess hormone production may be observed in the increased amount of phosphate and calcium excretion by the kidneys plus the continual removal of minerals from the skeleton and replacement by fibrous connective tissue.

Clinical signs associated with primary hyperparathyroidism are often related to skeletal changes. Fractures of long bones following a slight traumatic injury are not uncommon, and compression fractures of the vertebrae may occur. Facial hyperostosis may develop and result in the loss or loosening of teeth and, occasionally, in varying degrees of nasal cavity obliteration. Classic signs of "rubber jaw" may be encountered in advanced cases. If hypercalcemia is significant, an affected dog may have a history that includes periods of vomiting, generalized muscular weakness, constipation, and anorexia.

Clinical laboratory findings include hypercalcemia; hypophosphatemia, unless the animal is uremic (in which case serum phosphorus levels may be normal to increased); normal or increased serum alkaline phosphatase activity, with the amount of increase dependent upon severity of bone involvement (the greater the bone involvement, the higher the serum alkaline phosphate); increased urinary excretion of phosphate; and increased excretion of calcium if kidney function is normal. Laboratory findings in diseases of the parathyroid are summarized in Table 13–3.

Primary hyperparathyroidism in the dog usually results in a serum calcium level of from 12 to 20 mg/dl or greater. In one case the serum calcium level was 27.5 mg/dl. Calcium values consistently exceeding 11.5 mg/dl in the mature dog should be considered in the hypercalcemic range. It would be anticipated that both ionized and total serum calcium would be increased. If this disease

TABLE 13–3. Summary of Clinical Laboratory Findings in Diseases of Parathyroid

Condition	Serum		Urine		Serum Alkaline Phosphatase[1]	Other Tests
	Ca^{++}	HPO_4^{--}	Ca^{++}	HPO_4^{--}		
Primary hyperparathyroidism	↑	↓	↑	↑	N to ↑	UN–N to ↑ Creatinine N to ↑
Renal secondary hyperparathyroidism	N to ↓	↑	N to ↑	↓	N to ↑	UN ↑ Creatinine ↑
Nutritional secondary hyperparathyroidism	N to ↓	N ↑	↓	↑	N to ↑	UN–N Creatinine N
Pseudohyperparathyroidism	↑	↑ to N or ↑ [2]	↑	↑	N to ↑	UN–N to ↑ Creatinine–N to ↑
Hypoparathyroidism	↓	↑	↓	↓	N	Renal function tests—N

[1] Alterations in serum alkaline phosphatase activity is related to the degree of bone involvement.
[2] Increased or normal if uremia develops.
↑ = Increase
↓ = Decrease
N = Normal
UN = Urea nitrogen

is permitted to continue, it may culminate in renal failure, which may obscure the classic hypercalcemia and hypophosphatemia. Such renal disease would have a tendency to cause phosphate retention and a decrease in the serum calcium value.

Secondary Hyperparathyroidism with Renal Failure. Hyperparathyroidism in the dog may develop secondary to progressive renal disease. If the glomerular filtration rate is significantly reduced, the net effect is phosphate retention. Although phosphate retention itself has no direct effect on parathyroid function, there may be a concomitant decrease in the blood calcium level. The decrease in blood calcium concentration occurs as the body attempts to balance total mineral content by increasing urinary excretion of calcium. As the calcium ion concentration in the plasma decreases, parathyroid activity increases. Another effect of the severe renal damage may be impaired intestinal absorption of calcium because of an acquired defect in vitamin D metabolism, particularly the decrease in conversion of 25-hydroxycholecalciferol to its active form (1,25-dihydroxycholecalciferol).

Laboratory findings associated with hyperparathyroidism secondary to renal failure include normal to decreased serum calcium concentration; increased serum phosphorus level; normal to increased serum alkaline phosphatase value, depending upon the amount of bone resorption; and an increase in blood urea nitrogen level and other laboratory evidence of renal failure. Urinary calcium may be either normal or increased, and urine phosphate excretion is decreased (see Table 13–3).

Clinical signs of secondary hyperparathyroidism resulting from chronic renal failure are a combination of the clinical manifestations of renal disease and those associated with hyperparathyroidism. Predominant clinical signs include polyuria, polydipsia, dehydration, and, if uremia occurs, vomiting and typical uremic depression. Skeletal lesions may vary from extremely minor alterations to marked changes resembling those present in the later stages of primary hyperparathyroidism. Varying degrees of demineralization may be detected radiographically in most animals with advanced renal disease. In all cases, every attempt should be made to evaluate renal function using the tests previously described.

Secondary Hyperparathyroidism of Nutritional Origin. Parathyroid activity increases as the body compensates for alterations in mineral homeostasis occurring as a result of improper nutrition. This condition occurs in dogs, cats, horses, goats, and pigs. It has also been reported in nonhuman primates and in a variety of zoo animals.

Dietary imbalances involved in the production of nutritional hyperparathyroidism include a low content of calcium, an excessive phosphorus level with either normal or low calcium content, and inadequate amounts of vitamin D_3. No matter what the dietary deficiency, the physiologic alteration is a decrease in the serum calcium level, which stimulates the parathyroid glands.

If the calcium content of the diet is low and fails to satisfy the minimum daily requirements of the animal, hypocalcemia may develop. If excessive phosphorus is ingested, a hyperphosphatemia may be produced, which indirectly causes a decrease in blood calcium. According to the mass-law equation, when serum becomes saturated with calcium plus phosphorus, hypocalcemia may develop because of an excess of phosphorus. If the diet contains inadequate quantities of vitamin D_3, calcium absorption by the intestine is decreased, and hypocalcemia may develop.

In response to these nutritionally induced hypocalcemias, the parathyroid glands undergo hyperplasia. In most affected animals, kidney function is normal and parathormone will act upon the kidneys to decrease renal tubular reabsorption of phosphate and increase reabsorption of calcium, which has a tendency to return serum levels to normal. Bone resorption is also activated, and the release of calcium may elevate serum levels of this element to normal or only slightly below normal. If dietary imbalances are temporary, parathyroid activity will decrease when the dietary imbalance is corrected. If, however, the diet remains deficient, compensatory parathyroid hyperplasia continues and may lead to the development of the bone lesions characteristic of hyperparathyroidism.

In cats, the disease is most frequently seen in the young animal being fed a predominantly meat diet, especially one high in beef heart and liver. This condition in cats has been referred to by a number of names including juvenile osteoporosis and osteogenesis imperfecta. Dogs are also subject to nutritional hyperparathyroidism if fed exclusively meat diets that are low in calcium and high in phosphorus. The condition in horses is characterized by pyramidal enlargement of the facial bones, thickening of the rami of the mandible, and temporary lameness. It has been produced experimentally in horses by feeding the animal a diet with optimal calcium content but with excessive amounts of phosphorus.[4]

Clinical laboratory results derived from tests of single specimens are not definitive. If the diet contains an excessive amount of phosphorus and a normal amount of calcium, the blood phosphorus concentration may be elevated or within normal limits and the serum calcium level normal or slightly decreased. If obvious bone changes are present, serum alkaline phosphatase activity may be increased. If nutritional hyperparathyroidism has occurred because of a deficiency of calcium or vitamin D_3 but with adequate phosphorus intake, the patient will have a mild hypocalcemia or a normocalcemia with a slightly reduced to normal serum phosphorus value. In a study of nutritional secondary hyperparathyroidism in horses,[5] low urine calcium and high urine phosphorus levels were considered of greater diagnostic value than measurements of serum calcium, inorganic phosphorus, and alkaline phosphatase activities (see Table 13–3).

Pseudohyperparathyroidism in the Dog (Hypercalcemia of neoplasia). The production of hormone-like substances by neoplastic tissue of nonendocrine origin has been known in humans for some time. It was only recently, however, that such a condition was confirmed in domestic animals. A number of different malignant neoplasms secrete parathyroid hormone–like polypeptides. Pseudohyperparathyroidism has been reported in dogs with lymphosarcoma, apocrine adenocarcinomas in the perirectal area, adenocarcinoma and squamous carcinoma of the mammary gland, thyroid carcinoma, testicular interstitial cell tumors, and gastric squamous carcinomas. By far the most common cause is lymphosarcoma. Cats with lymphosarcoma may also develop pseudohyperparathyroidism. Clinical laboratory findings in these cases include hypercalcemia with a decreased serum phosphorus level unless the animal is uremic. Alkaline phosphatase activity is normal to increased. As renal damage becomes more severe, blood urea nitrogen and creatinine concentrations may be increased. Diminution in kidney function has a tendency to increase serum phosphorus concentration while decreasing urine calcium concentration. The degree of hyperphosphatemia is usually greater in dogs with secondary renal hyperparathyroidism than in dogs with renal failure caused by pseudohyperparathyroidism or primary hyperparathyroidism (see Table 13–3).

Hypoparathyroidism. Hypoparathyroidism is a metabolic condition resulting from a lack of parathormone activity. It is seen following complete thyroidectomy in which the parathyroid glands are removed or damaged. It also occurs idiopathically. Idiopathic hypoparathyroidism is most frequent in small breeds of dogs but has been reported in larger breeds.[6] A transient hypoparathyroidism can be seen following surgical removal of a neoplastic parathyroid gland. Because of the excess production of parathormone by the neoplastic gland, the other parathyroids have become atrophic from disuse. Upon proper stimulation these atrophied glands will resume function.[6]

Clinical signs associated with hypoparathyroidism are characteristic for patients with hypocalcemia. Neuromuscular irritability, seizures, and tetany are the predominant findings. Muscle spasms, particularly in muscles of the face and forelimbs, sometimes occur spontaneously but at other times are revealed only following stimulation.

The most common clinical laboratory abnormality is hypocalcemia. Serum inorganic phosphate is increased. Renal function tests are normal. Hypomagnesemia frequently accompanies hypocalcemia, and the serum magnesium level should be monitored in patients with hypocalcemia.

Parathormone assays, although expensive, are now commercially available. The test can be used to differentiate between primary and pseudohyperparathyroidism. Parathormone activity is increased in the serum of patients with primary hyperparathyroidism and is within normal range in those with pseudohyperparathyroidism. Serum activity of this hormone is low in patients with hypoparathyroidism. This test will probably not be widely used until the cost is reduced.

OTHER CAUSES OF MINERAL IMBALANCE

Rickets and Osteomalacia. Dietary insufficiencies of calcium, phosphorus, or vitamin D may result in the development of rickets or osteomalacia. Rickets is a disease of the young growing animal and is manifested by a failure to form calcium deposits in the bone matrix. Osteomalacia is a disease of the adult animal occurring in association with parathyroid hyperactivity or as the result of a continued demand for calcium and phosphorus not supplied by the diet. The result is resorption of formed bone.

The signs observed in a rachitic animal occur because of a lack of calcium salt deposits in the ground substance of bone. Typical lesions are most likely to develop in the long bones, more specifically, in areas of provisional calcification. Whether the cause is vitamin D deficiency or lack of dietary calcium or phosphorus, the signs are similar and characterized by enlargement of the ends of long bones and costochondral articulations. The most frequent cause of rickets in young animals, particularly those raised in close confinement, is vitamin D deficiency. In vitamin D–deficient animals there is a progressive decrease in total serum calcium level, with a slight decrease in the amount of serum inorganic phosphate. There is usually, but not always, an increase in serum alkaline phosphatase activity. If rickets is produced by a diet low in phosphorus, serum inorganic phosphate levels are low, whereas serum calcium levels may be normal. Calcium-deficient diets may occasionally produce rickets and a concomitant hypocalcemia. Serum calcium levels may be within normal limits in young calves. The effects of a diet with excess phosphorus in relation to calcium has been discussed in the section on secondary nutritional hyperparathyroidism.

Osteomalacia, sometimes termed adult rickets, is pathophysiologically similar to rickets in the young. There may be irregular thickening and softening of the diaphyses. Flat bones in the head and pelvis may become thickened and distorted, particularly in the horse. Although the evidence of osteomalacia is similar in all domestic animals, its etiology varies according to the type of diet used for the different animal species. In cows and sheep, it occurs generally as aphosphorosis; in pigs as acalcicosis; in dogs as avitaminosis; and in horses as hyperphosphorosis.

Aphosphorosis is characterized by a decrease in inorganic serum phosphate values with a normal serum calcium and magnesium level. Acalcicosis is accompanied by a decrease in serum calcium concentration, with serum phosphate activity usually in the normal range. With vitamin D deficiency, there is a decrease in both serum calcium and inorganic phosphate levels. With a dietary imbalance resulting in hyperphosphorosis, serum phosphate concentration is increased, whereas serum calcium values may be normal to decreased.

With both rickets and osteomalacia, clinical laboratory findings must be interpreted with care, since hormonal control of calcium may compensate for anticipated alterations in serum mineral levels.

Estimation of Parathormone Excess. In the conditions just discussed, an excess of parathormone is characteristic. It has been suggested[7] that such an excess can be detected by determining the clearance of phosphorus:clearance of creatinine ratio (Cp:Ccr). Calculation of this ratio requires phosphorus (p) and creatinine (cr) determinations for a random urine sample and a serum sample collected at the same time. The ratio is calculated as follows:

$$\frac{Cp}{Ccr} = \frac{\text{urine p}}{\text{serum p}} \times \frac{\text{serum cr}}{\text{urine cr}}$$

Normal clearance ratios are 0.15 to 0.30, suspect ratios 0.30 to 0.75, and with a parathormone excess exceeding 0.75. In addition to having diagnostic value, this test may be useful in assessing the response to dietary change initiated following diagnosis of secondary nutritional hyperparathyroidism. This ratio does not change immediately following diet correction and may require one or two weeks to return to normal.

Parturient Paresis. Milk fever is a classic disease associated with hypocalcemia and hypophosphatemia. There is a reduction in both bound and ionized calcium, with serum levels as low as 3 mg/dl having been reported. Studies of the serum calcium level of cattle at parturition indicate that there is a decrease in the amount of total calcium, but the ionized calcium concentration remains the same if parturition is not followed by development of parturient paresis. Several theories to explain the mechanisms responsible for development of parturient paresis have been advanced, but the precise mechanism responsible for the hypocalcemia has not been elucidated.[8]

Several methods for preventing milk fever have been proposed, including administration of vitamin D_2 in the feed, injection of vitamin D_3, dietary adjustment of the calcium:phosphorus ratio, and drenching of cattle with a calcium chloride solution. Experimental evidence suggests that any one or all of these may be somewhat effective in prevention of milk fever.

A condition similar to parturient paresis in cattle has been reported in other animal species. A subnormal serum calcium level may be observed in lambing sickness in ewes and in lactation tetany or transit tetany in mares.[8] Hypocalcemic tetany or paresis has been reported in the sow, the goat, the bitch, and the rabbit. As with parturient paresis, the basic mechanisms responsible for these conditions remain unknown, and the only known factors are the decrease in serum calcium and the usual rapid response of the individual to injection of substances containing calcium.

MAGNESIUM BALANCE

Metabolism. Another major cation in the body is magnesium. This cation is present in all tissues with approximately three fourths of the total body magnesium being found in the skeleton, where it is available for mobilization to other body tissues if dietary intake is insufficient. The magnesium not found in bone occurs principally intracellularly. The intracellular magnesium concentration is approximately 36 mg/dl, as compared with a plasma concentration of approximately 2.4 mg/dl.[8]

Intracellularly, magnesium functions as an enzyme activator. It is of particular significance in activation of enzymes responsible for reactions involving adenosine triphosphate (ATP). Extracellular magnesium plays an important role in production and destruction of acetylcholine, a compound required for impulse transmission at neuromuscular junctions.[8] Thus, if fluid surrounding the neuromuscular junction is deficient in magnesium, tetany may result.

Absorption of magnesium occurs primarily in the small intestine, although it has been reported that in young calves, absorption may also occur in the large intestine. Ruminants have a low efficiency of magnesium absorption and a great loss of dietary magnesium occurs through the feces. It has been suggested that magnesium moves passively across the wall of the small intestine. Magnesium absorption is not influenced by vitamin D level.

Magnesium is excreted through the intestinal tract, the kidneys, and, during lactation, the mammary glands. The gastrointestinal tract is the main excretory route both for magnesium that has been ingested and not absorbed and for magnesium of endogenous origin. If magnesium is absorbed in excess of body needs, it is excreted by the kidneys. In lactating cattle, a considerable amount of magnesium may be lost in the milk. Such loss modifies the dietary needs for magnesium and should be taken into consideration.

Serum Magnesium Levels. Normal values for serum magnesium are presented in Table 13–4. The mean normal values for serum magnesium vary from 2 to 5 mg/dl. Magnesium occurs at a higher concentration in erythrocytes than in plasma in all animal species except the bovine.

Although there is no specific hormonal control of magnesium levels, the adrenal, thyroid, and parathyroid glands may be involved in regulating serum magnesium. Although no definitive action has been detected, it has been shown in humans that hyperaldosteronism is accompanied by hypomagnesemia. With adrenal insufficiency, however, serum magnesium concentration is increased. Similar findings may occur in domestic animals. Likewise, the thyroid gland has been indirectly involved; hypomagnesemia has been observed with thyrotoxicosis, and there may be a depression of the serum magnesium level following the feeding of thyroprotein to lactating cows.

Hyperparathyroidism in humans is also associated with hypomagnesemia. There is evidence to suggest that hypomagnesemia stimulates parathormone release. In spite of these proposed mechanisms for control of serum magnesium levels, dietary intake remains the primary factor involved in diseases associated with alterations in magnesium metabolism.

TABLE 13–4. Normal Values of Magnesium in Blood of Various Animals

| Species | Blood Fraction | Magnesium (mg/dl) | |
		MEAN	STANDARD DEVIATION
Bovine	WB	2.4	± 0.32
	S	2.05	± 0.32
	P	2.8	± 0.25
	S	2.3	± 0.17
Ovine	WB	3.3	± 0.13
	S	2.5	± 0.30
	P	2.9	± 0.13
Caprine	WB	3.7	± 0.65
	P	3.2	± 0.35
Porcine	WB	6.4	± 0.78
	P	3.2	± 0.49
	S	2.07	
Equine	WB	4.0	± 0.62
	P	2.4	± 0.32
	S	2.5	± 0.31
	S	1.86	± 0.15
Shetland ponies	S	1.54	± 0.16
Canine	S	2.1	± 0.30
Feline	S	2.2	

WB = whole blood, P = plasma, S = serum.

Hypomagnesemia. Hypomagnesemia as a clinical entity produces tetanic conditions in cattle and sheep. In calves and beef cattle, the disease generally has a slow onset, whereas in the majority of the cases in lactating cattle and sheep, onset is rapid. This syndrome often occurs coincidentally with the first appearance of green grass in the spring. Depletion of magnesium ions in the extracellular fluid bathing neuromuscular junctions is apparently responsible for the tetanic syndrome. Therefore, the clinician should be alert to the primary signs of this condition, which include twitching of muscles, excitement, staggering, restlessness, increased sensitivity to noise, and, terminally, convulsions and death.

In calves, hypomagnesemia is associated with feeding of whole milk for an abnormal length of time. The disease mainfests itself because of a simple dietary deficiency of magnesium. A growing calf requires considerably more of this mineral than is supplied by the magnesium content of cow's milk. Sudden death losses of rapidly growing four-month-old beef calves were attributed to hypomagnesemia.[9] Clinical signs included weakness, stiffness, unsteady movement, bulging eyes, and tetanic spasms. Serum magnesium levels were less than 2.0 mg/dl, and affected calves responded to magnesium salts administered intravenously. There was a deficiency of magnesium in silage and hay being consumed by the cattle.

Slowly Developing Hypomagnesemia. In the slow form of hypomagnesemia, cattle may have a low serum magnesium level for some time, even for months. When the level approaches a critically low value, it is accompanied by mild clinical signs including nervousness and increased excitability. Fasting and reduced feed intake may also precipitate tetany and paresis. The Norwegian tetany-paresis syndrome resulted[10] from special conditions existing during World War II. At that time, Norwegian farmers were forced to feed rations containing herring meal and fodder cellulose, both of which were low in magnesium. Subnormal values for both serum magnesium and calcium were found in paretic cows as well as in cows suffering from tetany. Some cows had pronounced hypomagnesemia without clinical signs, whereas in others, hypomagnesemia was accompanied by tremors, muscular irritability, and twitching.

Rapidly Developing Hypomagnesemia. The rapid type of hypomagnesemia, more commonly referred to as grass tetany, is a metabolic disturbance that affects cattle and has been referred to by a variety of other names including wheat pasture poisoning, grass staggers, Hereford disease, and lactation tetany. The disease is most commonly seen in spring soon after cattle are turned onto lush spring grass, but in some areas of the United States, it may occur with some frequency in the fall when animals are on wheat pasture.

Both magnesium and serum calcium concentrations are decreased in the majority of cases of hypomagnesemic tetany. Serum phosphate levels are normal or slightly decreased.

The incidence of grass tetany varies from year to year and from pasture to pasture and is undoubtedly related to chemical constituents and their concentration in the grass. The content of phosphorus and crude protein decreases during the growing season, whereas magnesium and crude fiber content slowly increases. Thus, the minimum level of magnesium in pastures occurs in the early spring and late autumn when clinical cases of grass tetany are most frequently observed.

The mineral content of pastures is also altered by treatment with fertilizer. Herbage from "tetany pastures" has a higher phosphorus and potassium content and a lower sodium, calcium, and magnesium content than herbage from pastures in which grazing produces no tetany. The frequency of hypomagnesemia is also increased when a high grass nitrogen content occurs in conjunction with a high potassium content. There is also evidence to suggest that plant magnesium may decrease as a consequence of potassium applications.

Simesen[8] discussed the trigger effects that might induce or precipitate clinical signs of hypomagnesemic tetany. Precipitating factors may include: (1) suddenly reduced feed intake; (2) adverse weather; (3) estrus; (4) oral application of relatively high doses of sodium phosphate, or sodium sulfate, or both; and (5) sudden reductions in dietary supplies of magnesium. He cautioned that even the mere handling of a susceptible cow, pricking of the animal with a needle, unexpected noise, or anything similar might provoke an acute state of tetany.

Hypomagnesemia in Sheep and Dogs. Hypomagnesemia in sheep has also been reported and the factors involved are undoubtedly similar to those of grass tetany in cattle.

Hypomagnesemia has also been reported in dogs following removal of the parathyroid glands as a treatment for hyperparathyroidism. If dietary magnesium intake is low and parathyroid function is depressed, hypomagnesemic convulsions may occur.

REFERENCES

1. Simesen, M. G.: Some clinical-chemical values in normal thoroughbreds and trotters. Nord. Vet. Med., 24:85, 1972.
2. Fletch, S. M., and Smart, M. E.: Blood chemistry of the giant breeds—bone profile. Bull. Am. Soc. Vet. Clin. Pathol., 2:30, 1973.
3. Meuten, D. J., Chew, D. J., Capen, C. C., and Kociba, G. J.: Relationship of serum total calcium to albumin and total protein in dogs. J.A.V.M.A., 180:63, 1982.
4. Krook, L., and Lowe, J. E.: Nutritional hyperparathyroidism in the horse. Pathol. Vet. I, Suppl. 1, 1964.
5. Joyce, J. R., Pierce, K. R., Romane, W. M., and Baker, S. M.: Clinical study of nutritional secondary hyperparathyroidism in horses. J.A.V.M.A., 158:2033, 1971.
6. Lees, G. E.: Hypoparathyroidism. In Current Veterinary Therapy VIII. Small Animal Practice, edited by Kirk, R. W., W. B. Saunders Company, Philadelphia, 1983.
7. Moore, W. E.: Screening profiles: How to read and what next. Sci. Proc. 44th Ann. Meet. A.A.H.A., A.A.H.A., South Bend, IN, 1977.
8. Simesen, M. G.: Calcium, inorganic phosphorus and magnesium metabolism in health and disease. In: Clinical Biochemistry of Domestic Animals, edited by Kaneko, J. J., and Cornelius, C. E., Academic Press, New York, 1970.
9. Haggard, D. L., Whitehair, C. K., and Langham, R. F.: Tetany associated with magnesium deficiency in suckling beef calves. J.A.V.M.A., 172:495, 1978.
10. Ender, F., Halse, K., and Slagsvold, P.: Undersodelser Uedrorende Krampe og lammeleser hos kur. Hypomagnesemia hos melkekyr frambrakt under kontrollerte foringsbetingelser, E.T. Tifelle av hypomagnesemia med dodelig utank. Nord. Vet. Tidsskr., 60:14541, 1948.

DIAGNOSTIC CYTOLOGY, SYNOVIAL FLUID, AND MISCELLANEOUS FLUIDS

DIAGNOSTIC CYTOLOGY

Microscopic examination of blood, bone marrow, urine, and cerebrospinal fluid has been accepted for years as a valuable adjunct to laboratory diagnosis. Today, microscopic examination of preparations made from tissues and fluids is an integral part of the services provided by the veterinary clinical laboratory.

Cytologic examination of body fluids is utilized to reveal the cellular characteristics of the fluid so that the presence or absence of inflammation or neoplasia can be detected. Such examinations are of value in detecting infectious agents such as bacteria, mycoplasmas, fungi, parasites, and viral inclusions. In addition to its application in the examination of body fluids, cytologic analysis is of value in identifying tissue cell types and distribution by use of impressions and scrapings. This type of study also finds a place in the preliminary examination of tissue biopsy specimens, scrapings from the body surface, and material obtained from body orifices.

The principal advantage of cytologic examination is the rapidity with which such an examination can be completed, enabling the clinician to begin treatment as soon as possible. Cytologic examinations often provide a definitive diagnosis and preclude the necessity for other more refined and time-consuming techniques.

SPECIMEN COLLECTION AND SLIDE PREPARATION

Collection of Fluid Specimens. **Abdominal Paracentesis.** Removal of fluid from the abdominal cavity is indicated when there is excessive fluid accumulation or if the clinician suspects the presence of a lesion characterized by cellular exfoliation. The equipment required for obtaining a specimen for cytologic examination is minimal. An assortment of hypodermic needles and syringes is needed. Such an assortment should include an aspirating needle of sufficient length to enter the abdominal cavity without forcing the needle hub against the skin. It should be long enough to permit ready access to the abdominal cavity without penetrating or damaging any of the abdominal organs and of sufficient gauge to allow for easy aspiration. Most fluid transudates can be collected through a 16- to 18-gauge needle, whereas a 14- to 16-gauge needle may be required for exudates. Since abnormal abdominal fluids frequently clot, a test tube or small flask containing ethylenediaminetetraacetic acid (EDTA) as an anticoagulant should be available. The puncture site is selected to avoid major abdominal organs including the urinary bladder, liver, and spleen. Except for avoiding these organs, the puncture site is not critical. If the clinician wishes to remove large quantities of fluid, however, the most dependent portion of the abdominal cavity should be chosen.

We have found that a midline approach, 1 to 2 inches caudal to the xiphoid cartilage, is an acceptable site in most animal species. The skin over the area to be punctured is surgically prepared and, depending upon the temperament of the patient, sedation and local anesthesia may be used. The skin should be slightly displaced cranially or caudally and the needle with syringe attached carefully introduced through the abdominal wall.

As the needle is advanced, a gentle vacuum is created in the syringe by gentle pressure on the plunger. If this technique is followed, fluid will appear in the syringe as soon as the abdominal cavity is entered. If fluid is not readily obtained, it may be necessary to choose another puncture site. The quantity of fluid removed depends upon the amount of effusion in the abdominal cavity. Only a small quantity is needed for cytologic examination.

In the horse, the preferred site for abdominal paracentesis is at the lowest point of the abdomen between the xiphisternum and umbilicus. A 19-gauge, 2-inch needle is quickly introduced through the skin, then slowly advanced through the linea alba and into the abdominal cavity. When the cavity is entered, the needle will move with each respiration. Fluid will usually begin to flow, but if it does not, the needle should be gently rotated. A syringe may be used, but the end of the needle frequently becomes occluded by tissue. The procedure should be conducted using a sterile technique.

Thoracentesis. Fluid accumulations in the thoracic cavity may present diagnostic problems, since physical and radiographic examinations do not permit differentiation among the various types of fluids that may accumulate. Microscopic and chemical examinations of these fluids assist in differentiation among hemothorax, hydrothorax, chylothorax, and pyothorax.

As with abdominal paracentesis, the equipment required is minimal. Select a needle that is of sufficient length to enter the pleural cavity without the hub touching the skin but not long enough to damage thoracic viscera. Under most circumstances a 1- to 1½-inch needle will suffice, except in some large domestic animals in which a 2- to 2½-inch needle may be required, particularly if the animal is fat. A 16-gauge needle is usually adequate, although a 14-gauge needle may be required if the fluid is excessively viscid.

Before attempting thoracentesis, the clinician should carefully evaluate the patient to determine the fluid level in the pleural cavity. This is most readily accomplished in smaller animals by use of a radiograph. In larger animals, auscultation will assist in determining the extent of fluid accumulation.

The site selected for thoracentesis varies, but the seventh or eighth intercostal space is chosen in most animals. The puncture should be made in the middle of the intercostal space to avoid entering or causing damage to intercostal vessels found just caudal to the ribs. As with abdominal paracentesis, the skin over the puncture site is surgically prepared, and local anesthesia may be required. Stress must be avoided in patients with marked pleural effusion to prevent suffocation. Thoracentesis is preferably performed with the animal in a standing position, which permits fluid to accumulate in the lower portion of the cavity.

Fluid is removed in a fashion identical to that used for abdominal paracentesis.

If the needle enters the lung, blood will appear and the fluid will be frothy. Placement of the needle too far caudally may lead to penetration of the liver. Occasionally, damage to an intercostal vessel will produce a bloody fluid. In cases of accidental blood contamination, blood will be apparent either during the first or very last portion of the aspiration. If a sudden movement of the patient is accompanied by an almost immediate appearance of blood, it may be an indication of contamination from one of the above sources. Blood will be present throughout the aspiration if the effusion is hemorrhagic. If aspirate is accidentally contaminated with blood, the needle should be withdrawn and another site selected for thoracentesis.

Pericardicentesis. Fluid is less frequently removed from the pericardium, but if there is an abnormal accumulation of pericardial fluid, pericardicentesis may be of diagnostic and therapeutic value. An 18- to 20-gauge needle of sufficient length to reach the pericardium is required. This will vary according to animal species, with a 3-inch needle being adequate for most pet animals.

Before attempting pericardicentesis, the clinician determines the cardiac position by palpation of the cardiac apex beat. Sedation and local anesthesia are usually required for this procedure. A dog or cat is placed in lateral recumbency and the skin over the selected puncture site is surgically prepared. After the cardiac apex beat is located by palpation, the needle is carefully advanced toward the heart. A constant negative pressure should be kept in the syringe. When the needle enters the pericardial sac, fluid will appear in the syringe. If the needle is advanced sufficiently to touch or penetrate the cardiac wall, pulsation occurs and the needle will move, coinciding with the heart beat. Should this occur, the needle location should be slightly altered in order to prevent damage to the heart or its blood vessels.

A small quantity (0.5 to 1.0 ml) of pericardial fluid is adequate for cytologic evaluation. If the fluid collected is bloody and clotted, this usually indicates that a blood vessel has been damaged or that a chamber of the heart has been entered during collection. If a bloody fluid does not clot, this is an indication that defibrinated blood is present in the pericardial sac.

Slide Preparation of Fluid Specimens. Slides should be prepared as quickly as possible following collection, in order to minimize cellular degeneration. Cytologic examination may be conducted on smears prepared from unconcentrated fluids or on sediment, following centrifugation of the fluid specimen. Centrifuged sediment has the advantage of providing a greater number of cells for examination, but interpretation of such slides is more difficult, since it is impossible to estimate cell concentration. Also, because of the time required and the physical damage to cells, centrifugation may produce cellular distortion. Many reference laboratories use a special centrifuge in which cells are centrifuged directly on a glass slide. This method is particularly useful for fluids that have a low cell count.

In the preparation of slides for microscopic examination, care should be taken to ensure that a thin film of material is present. If smears are too thick, cells will not stain adequately and will not flatten. As a consequence, they will be difficult to identify. A smear of a fluid specimen is prepared in a fashion similar to that used for preparation of peripheral blood smears, the technician taking care to ensure the presence of a "feathered edge" on the slide. Many larger cells accumulate in this area, and if a smear covers the entire slide, such cells may be lost.

If the fluid is viscid, the usual rapid smearing technique will not suffice. Slow spreading of the material with a "pusher" slide may be adequate if the fluid is not too thick. With extremely viscid material it may be necessary to make a "squash" preparation. For a squash preparation, material to be examined is placed on a slide, a second slide is placed on the specimen, and the two slides are gently drawn apart. If too much pressure is utilized, a majority of cells may be damaged or distorted, but adequate areas can usually be located if the slide is carefully prepared. Fluids containing fibrinogen present a problem in slide preparation, and it is with such specimens that the squash preparation is most frequently used. The use of an adequate anticoagulant will usually reduce or eliminate fibrin unless it is already present in the fluid at the time of collection. EDTA is the anticoagulant of choice, since it does not severely affect cell morphology.

Depending upon the type of stain to be utilized, the slide is either air dried or fixed while wet.

Staining. The choice of stain for slides prepared from body fluids will depend to a great extent upon experience and personal preferences. For most practical clinical uses, the technique selected should be simple and rapid, and the stain should provide sufficient cellular detail to permit identification.

Wright's stain is suitable for cytologic studies and has the advantage of being the stain most frequently used for blood films. Quick dipstains can be used and generally permit good cell differentiation. This stain is particularly useful in making permanent preparations.

The new methylene blue stain is excellent for routine use. Staining can be completed quickly and staining properties are consistent. Results are similar enough to those obtained with Wright's stain that an individual who is experienced in examining Wright's-stained blood films will find little difficulty in interpreting the results of a new methylene blue preparation.

The method for utilizing new methylene blue stain is as follows: (1) Permit slide to air dry completely, (2) place a small drop of stain on the preparation and (3) add a coverslip. This procedure requires only a few seconds before the slide is ready for examination. A preliminary report is immediately submitted to the clinician. More definitive studies should be completed later using slides stained in a more permanent fashion.

In addition to Wright's and new methylene blue stains, other staining techniques such as Papanicolaou's or Shorr's stain may be utilized. These techniques are presenated in the Appendix. If these stains are to be used, it is imperative that fixation be completed as quickly as possible. The preferred fixative consists of equal parts of diethyl ether and 95 per cent ethyl alcohol. An alternative fixation technique for fluids is the addition of fresh material to an equal amount of 50 per cent ethyl alcohol at the time of collection with smears prepared later. Fixation should proceed for a minimum of 30 minutes, although slides may be left in the fixative for several days.

Examination. After the slide has been stained, it is rapidly scanned with the low power of a good microscope to determine specimen cellularity. This also is a quick method for detecting giant cells and polymorphonuclear neutrophil leukocytes (PMN's), which can be identified at this power. The presence or absence of sheets and cell clusters should be noted. During examination under low power, areas for a more detailed examination are selected and the × 40 objective is utilized to identify specific cellular characteristics. For a definitive examination, the oil immersion objective is utilized to identify infectious agents such as bacteria, parasites, and fungi and to determine nuclear and cytoplasmic detail.

Collection and Slide Preparation of Tissue Specimens. Biopsy techniques and their diagnostic value in small animal practice have been discussed in detail in a series of papers.[1-4] The reader is referred to this excellent series for more precise descriptions.

Biopsy is indicated when clinical examination, radiographic evaluation, and laboratory data suggest a diagnosis that cannot be confirmed by these methods. Results of a biopsy frequently will confirm or eliminate a clinical diagnosis. Although a long list of contraindications to biopsy has been proposed, the clinician should not hesitate to perform this procedure to assist establishment of a final diagnosis or evaluation of therapy. The only absolute contraindications are hemorrhagic tendencies in the patient or an inexperienced clinician.[2] There may be some risk that a needle biopsy may induce malignant metastases and, although this possibility seems somewhat remote, it must be considered before a biopsy is completed.

Several different biopsy techniques may be used to prepare material for cytologic examination. These include aspiration by needle; excisional or incisional biopsy; and exfoliative cytology, including irrigation of hollow organs and serous cavities, direct smears, scrapings, curettage, and pressure massage.

Needle Aspiration Biopsy. This technique may be employed for any lesion in which examination or identification of cells may be of value in establishing or eliminating a clinical diagnosis. It is particularly desirable in differentiating between inflammation and neoplasia. The advantages of needle biopsy over an excisional or incisional biopsy are that it (1) is less time consuming, (2) permits sampling of multiple sites during a single procedure, (3) provides an opportunity for consecutive sampling at intervals, and (4) can establish a diagnosis that may eliminate the need for major surgery. In addition to the advantages of this technique for cytologic evaluation, specimens obtained by needle biopsy can be used for microbiologic examination. It must be recognized that a needle biopsy does not always permit a positive diagnosis, but a study of cellular morphology may reveal information that supports or contradicts a tentative clinical diagnosis. Structural changes in tissues are not identified in a specimen collected by needle biopsy.

COLLECTION. A needle of adequate size and a tight-fitting syringe are required for a needle biopsy of most soft tissue. Needle gauge and length depend upon location of the lesion to be aspirated. Both syringe and needle should be absolutely dry, since even a small quantity of fluid may cause cellular distortion and artifacts.

Before the needle biopsy is performed, the skin over the tissue or organ is surgically prepared, and the area is anesthetized. If skin is to be traversed, a small incision is made to prevent plugging of the needle lumen with skin debris. The lesion, if palpable, is localized and immobilized with one hand, and the needle is guided through the tissues to the mass with the opposite hand. The needle should not yet be advanced into the mass. If the needle contains a stylet, it should be removed and a syringe attached. Negative pressure is created within the syringe, but care should be taken not to create excessive pressure.

With moderate negative pressure in the syringe, the needle is advanced into the lesion. If the lesion is firm, it may be necessary to pass the needle through the lesion in two or three different directions in order to obtain a satisfactory sample. Care must be taken to avoid extensive tissue trauma if this is deemed necessary. By maintaining negative pressure within the syringe while the needle is in the lesion, tissue is aspirated. Tissue may or may not appear in the syringe barrel. If it does not, it is usually present in the needle lumen.

Upon completion of the biopsy, the negative pressure should be slowly released before the needle is removed from the lesion. If this is not done, the specimen will be contaminated with extraneous material. Failure to release the negative pressure when the needle is removed will also cause biopsy material to be sucked or sprayed into the syringe barrel, making removal for slide preparation difficult.

SLIDE PREPARATION. Following collection, the methods of handling the sample will depend upon its characteristics. If fluid is obtained, a slide is immediately prepared as described earlier. If small fragments of tissue are removed slides may be prepared by gently squashing the fragments between two slides and pulling the slides apart. If larger tissue fragments are collected and are too large or too firm to prepare by squashing, imprints are made on clean, dry glass slides. For specimens that are to be utilized for later histologic sectioning, fixation fluid may be drawn into the syringe. In cases in which culture examination is deemed necessary, the needle is placed into the appropriate culture medium and gently swirled before fixation of the specimen or slide preparation.

Punch Biopsy. Punch biopsies are accomplished by use of a biopsy needle designed specifically for that purpose. A variety of such needles are commercially available. A punch biopsy is indicated when structural relationships within the lesion are considered essential for evaluation.

Specific techniques for punch biopsy will depend upon the instrument selected, and reference should be made to these techniques before attempting a punch biopsy.

It must be recognized that punch biopsy techniques may have a greater risk of postbiopsy complications than do needle biopsies.

Upon completion of a punch biopsy, the specimen is carefully removed from the needle and immediately placed in an appropriate fixative or used to prepare impression smears.

Excisional Biopsy. Excision of a lesion has advantages over the needle or punch biopsy techniques. This is a preferred method for biopsy, since both treatment and diagnosis are frequently incorporated in the same procedure. Removal of a relatively large specimen of tissue permits examination by conventional histologic and cytologic methods. The primary disadvantage is that excisional biopsy is more time consuming and may be more costly to the client than is needle biopsy.

Acceptable surgical procedures must be utilized, and excision should include adjacent normal tissue along with the lesion. Upon completion of surgery, the specimen should be carefully incised and imprints prepared on clean, dry glass slides. The most acceptable method for preparation of an imprint for cytologic examination is as follows: (1) Carefully blot the surface of the tissue with absorbent material, such as a paper towel, to remove any blood or other fluid that might be present. (2) The cut surface of the lesion is gently touched to the surface of a clean, dry slide. If too much pressure is utilized, excessive numbers of cells will be present, making cytologic examination difficult. (3) Several imprints can be placed on the same slide, which is then either permitted to air dry or immediately fixed. (4) The slide is stained with new methylene blue or a permanent stain. (5) The remaining portion of excised material is incised in several places or, if large, sliced into thin sections and placed in a fixative for histologic sectioning.

Touch imprints from solid tissues may be relatively acellular. Carefully scraping the cut surface of the excised tissue with a scalpel blade will provide a more acceptable slide. The first scraping obtained in this fashion is frequently contaminated with blood and should be discarded. The tissue is again carefully and gently scraped, and the material is applied to a slide and spread in a thin layer. Slides prepared in this fashion can be air dried and stained or wet fixed and a permanent preparation completed.

Incisional Biopsy. Incisional biopsy, in which only a small portion of a lesion is surgically removed, may also be utilized. Incisional biopsy has the same advantages and disadvantages and requires the same equipment and technique as excisional biopsy. Slides for examination are prepared in a similar manner.

Other Collection Techniques. Cytologic examination of material collected by use of a swab, scraping of a surface lesion, preparation of an impression smear by placing a glass slide on a lesion, irrigation of a lesion or hollow body organ, and curettement may all be of value.

NASAL SECRETIONS. Cotton swabs or pledgets moistened with saline are frequently used for obtaining material from the nasal passages in an animal with a continuing nasal discharge or other evidence of upper respiratory tract involvement. If the secretion is tenacious, moistening a cotton swab with saline will often prove advantageous. Material collected in this fashion is transferred to a clean glass microscope slide by gently, but firmly, rolling the cotton swab over the slide surface. If material is especially thick and tenacious, a drop of saline placed on the slide may assist in preparation of the specimen. Nasal secretions may be collected utilizing a tongue depressor to remove fluid from the anterior nares of the larger domestic animals. Nasal secretions or exudates are collected and smeared immediately on a microscope slide. Some nasal exudates are of a consistency that will permit pressing a slide against the nostril in order to obtain material for cytologic examination. Additional techniques suitable for examination of the nasal cavity include aspiration of fluids utilizing a plastic or glass pipette or a blunt needle and syringe. Occasionally, irrigation of the nasal cavities may be indicated. A small quantity of sterile saline is introduced into the nasal cavity, the fluid is collected, centrifuged at slow speed, and a slide is prepared from the sediment.

ORAL CAVITY LESIONS. Cytologic examination of lesions of the oral cavity may also be of diagnostic value. Ulcers, tumors, inflammatory tissue proliferation, and undiagnosed swellings may all indicate the need for collecting material for cytologic examination. Impression smears can be readily prepared from open lesions. Such lesions are carefully cleaned, and a clean glass microscope slide is gently pressed to the surface. Several slides are prepared, air dried or wet fixed, and immediately forwarded to the laboratory for staining and examination. Scraping or curettement of nonulcerated lesions is the method of choice for cytologic evaluation of tumors or other undiagnosed swellings. Slides are prepared from such curettements by suspending the material in a small quantity of saline and preparing a thin slide for further examination.

MAMMARY GLAND MATERIAL. Material collected from the mammary glands may also be examined cytologically. Inflammation or masses in the mammary glands are indications for microscopic examination of material collected from the glands. In small domestic animals, breasts to be examined are gently massaged, and an effort is made to remove the accumulated material from the nipple. The small quantity of material collected is thinly smeared on a microscope slide for staining and evaluation. Milk can be examined in a similar fashion, and if an infection is present, the causative agent can frequently be identified by direct microscopic examination or by cultural techniques.

RECTAL AND COLONIC TISSUE. It has been suggested that a detailed examination of the rectum and colon is indicated when there is colitis, the persistent presence of fresh blood in the feces, recurrent bleeding from the anus, a mass or masses detected in the colon or rectum by either rectal or abdominal palpation, or persistent diarrhea of undetermined cause.[3] These authors recommend that the animal be prepared by undergoing a 24-hour fast followed by a warm-water enema about two hours before the examination is begun.

The colon is irrigated until the water is clean, and a proctoscopic examination is performed with the patient under general anesthesia. If lesions are observed, a basket type biopsy forceps is utilized and a small portion of tissue is removed. A plastic pipette attached to a syringe or rubber bulb can also be used to aspirate material from lesions. If it is necessary to irrigate the area, the fluid is centrifuged and the sediment is examined. Cells can be collected by curettement and the collected material smeared on a slide for staining. The principal disadvantage of aspiration and curettage is that only surface cells are collected. With disease of the colon, however, it is desirable to collect deeper tissue as well.

VAGINAL DISCHARGES. Vaginal discharges are also amenable to collection and cytologic examinations. If there is abundant discharge present in the vagina, the material can be collected by pipette, by cotton swab, or by everting the lips of the vulva, so that the vaginal mucosa is exposed and direct impression smears can be prepared. Occasionally curettement of the vaginal mucous membrane may be indicated, and this can be readily accomplished. If only small quantities of exudate are present, it may be necessary to irrigate the vagina with a small quantity of sterile saline (1 to 3 ml), so that the material may be aspirated and a smear prepared.[3]

PROSTATE GLAND MATERIAL. Prostatic enlargement, persistent urethral discharge thought to be of prostatic origin, and undiagnosed hematuria are all indications for collection of material from the prostate gland. If there is a continuous and persistent urethral discharge of prostatic origin, a single drop of the exudate may be placed on a glass slide for examination. If the quantity of exudate is small or there is a prostatic enlargement without an exudate, prostatic fluid may be obtained by massaging the prostate gland vigorously by means of a gloved finger inserted into the rectum. Such massage will frequently result in gravitation of fluid out of the urethra. Alternatively, a urethral catheter can be passed into the urethra, stopping short of entering the bladder, and sterile saline can be introduced into the proximal urethra. This solution is collected at the urethral orifice and centrifuged, and the sediment is examined microscopically.

TRACHEAL WASH. In animals with chronic respiratory infection transtracheal washes can be used to assist in arriving at a diagnosis. Such a procedure is indicated in animals with a chronic cough or in those with evidence of a parenchymal disease of the respiratory tract. Material collected in this fashion can be used for both cytologic and bacteriologic examination. Equipment required includes a local anesthetic, sterile saline, a syringe of appropriate size (10 to 25 ml), a skin disinfectant, a needle-catheter device (usually 18 or 20 gauge) of appropriate length for the species.

An area on the ventral aspect of the neck is clipped and prepared with an appropriate skin germicide. The site is infiltrated with a local anesthetic, the neck is extended, and a needle-catheter device is introduced into the lumen of the trachea. The needle is introduced between two cervical tracheal rings or through the cricothyroid ligament of the larynx. The cricothyroid ligament can be located by palpation of the trachea. A finger is placed on the trachea and moved upward until the ridge of the cricoid cartilage is felt. Just cranial to this ridge is a small depression where the cricothyroid ligament is located. Once the needle has entered the tracheal lumen, the catheter is advanced through the needle and down the trachea. The catheter is passed down the trachea until it reaches the mainstream bronchi. At this point the needle is withdrawn from the tissues so that only the catheter remains in the trachea. The catheter stylet is removed and a syringe is attached. Negative pressure is applied to the syringe and if there is a considerable quantity of secretion it can be aspirated. If no material is aspirated, 2 to 5 ml of sterile saline is introduced and suction is applied immediately after injection. It may be necessary to repeat the procedure until an adequate sample is obtained. Unaspirated saline is quickly absorbed by the respiratory mucosa and presents no major problems. Complications include air leakage from the puncture site into the subcutaneous tissues. This can usually be avoided by maintaining digital pressure over the puncture site for several minutes following removal of the catheter.

The aspirated material can be cultured directly and prepared for cytologic evaluation. If there are strands of mucus they can be placed onto a glass slide, smeared, and stained. If the cell concentration is relatively low the sample should be gently centrifuged and smears made from the sediment. In low cell count samples, use of a cytofuge is advantageous. Prepared slides can be stained with any of the usual stains.

Samples for cytologic examination can also be obtained by tracheobronchoscopy. A variety of bronchoscopes are available and the directions for the particular instrument should be followed in obtaining specimens. Samples are obtained by mucosal brushings. Samples obtained in this manner are frequently better than those obtained by a transtracheal wash.

TRANSUDATES AND EXUDATES

Fluid is always present in the serous body cavities. Serous fluid is thought to originate as a dialysate of plasma, although it has been suggested that fluid flow may be regulated by the mesothelial cells lining serous cavities. The chemical characteristics of normal serous fluid are dependent upon the blood concentration, membrane permeability, charge of the ion, and concentration of nondiffusable ions. Serous fluids are generally of low protein content (less than 3.0 gm/dl) and contain a small quantity of fibrinogen, but they do not usually clot. The specific gravity is less than 1.015, and the chemical composition in terms of electrolytes is probably similar to that of interstitial fluids. Electrolyte concentrations are governed by Gibbs-Donnan equilibrium between plasma and serous fluids.

The cellular composition of serous fluids is rather constant and characteristic. The cell population is usually low in normal fluids, although as fluid quantity increases, the types of cells and their numbers may be altered. Mesothelial cells occur in low numbers in normal serous fluid and are of two types. Reactive mesothelial cells are large (15 to 25 microns) and have a brush border, a basophilic cytoplasm, and a dark-staining hyperchromic nucleus that contains single or multiple large nucleoli. Because of these characteristics, reactive mesothelial cells can be confused with neoplastic cells, particularly if mitotic figures are present. If serous fluid accumulation is excessive, this fluid, which contains all the essentials for cell growth, will support mesothelial cell multiplication, and mitotic figures may become frequent. Occasionally, clusters of these basophilic mesothelial cells are present.

In addition to the reactive mesothelial cell, a lighter-staining, large, transformed mesothelial cell may be seen in serous fluids and transudates. These cells are frequently phagocytic, having a considerably less hyperchromic nucleus, and a pale blue, vacuolated cytoplasm. Such cells are difficult to differentiate from macrophages.

In addition to the two types of mesothelial cells, small numbers of leukocytes and erythrocytes may be found in serous fluids. These may be increased in number in transudates, and, more dramatically, in exudates. For a comparison of a transudate and an exudate, see Table 14–1.

Transudates. The increased formation of serous effusions, more frequently referred to as transudation, results from increased capillary pressure, increased interstitial fluid pressure, decreased plasma osmotic pressure, and increased interstitial osmotic pressure. Although the classic transudate has the physical, chemical, and cellular characteristics of normal serous fluid, typical transudates are seldom encountered in veterinary medicine. The more usual finding is a modified transudate that has all or some of the characteristics of an exudate. Since there are several factors involved in the increased production of serous fluids, it is obvious that the composition may vary considerably.

Hypoproteinemia associated with excessive protein loss, lack of protein production, or decreased nutritional intake of protein produces a pure transudate of a rather specific character. This transudate is transparent and has a low specific gravity.

Transudates associated with an interference in circulation may have a different consistency. Liver cirrhosis will obstruct hepatic flow and may be a cause of ascites. Such an obstruction also produces excessive hepatic lymph flow, which escapes through the capsule into the peritoneal cavity. A transudate formed in this fashion is high in protein, since hepatic lymph contains almost as much protein as does plasma.

Lymphatic obstruction may also result in transudation and accumulation of serous fluids. This may occur in association with a neoplasm arising from the mesothelium or with any other neoplastic mass that obstructs normal lymph flow. Such effusions vary considerably in their characteristics from a blood-tinged fluid, occurring because of the escape of blood from the vessels, to a rather typical noninflammatory transudative effusion.

Chylothorax occurs when there is rupture of the thoracic duct, and the fluid has the chemical characteristics of a transudate except for its high protein content. Such fluid contains large numbers of chylomicrons, is extremely high in the number of total mature lymphocytes, and is a white or light pink, opaque fluid. The presence of chylomicra can be confirmed by use of a fat-specific strain (oil red O, Sudan III or IV) or by the addition of ether to the fluid. The fluid is centrifuged and equal portions placed in each of two tubes. One or two drops of 1N sodium hydroxide are added and an equal volume of ether is added to one sample and water to the second. If the effusion is chyle, the portion receiving ether will clear after mixing while that mixed with water remains cloudy.[5]

Pseudochylous effusions also occur and grossly cannot be distinguished from a chylous effusion. These fluids contain cholesterol and lecithin resulting from cellular degeneration or chronic inflammation. Such effusions do not clear when mixed with ether.

Chemical analysis of a chylous or pseudochylous effusion may assist in differentiating between

---

TABLE 14–1. Comparison of a Transudate and an Exudate

Transudate	Exudate
1. Thin and watery, resembles lymph, no tissue fragments present	1. Thick, often creamy, contains tissue fragments
2. Clear and odorless	2. Cloudy and may have an odor
3. Colorless or pale yellow (color may depend on the species and breed of animal)	3. White, red, or yellow
4. Specific gravity 1.015 or below	4. Specific gravity 1.018 or above
5. Less than 3 per cent protein	5. More than 4 per cent protein
6. Alkaline	6. Acid
7. Does not coagulate (may contain few fibrin strands)	7. Coagulates (both *in vitro* and *in vivo*)
8. No bacteria present	8. Bacteria often present
9. Only a few or no leukocytes or erythrocytes	9. Many leukocytes and erythrocytes
10. Low enzyme content	10. High enzyme content
11. Not associated with inflammation	11. Associated with inflammation

them. Chyle has a lower cholesterol level than serum while pseudochylous effusions have a greater concentration. Triglyceride levels are lower than serum levels in pseudochylous effusions and higher in the typical chylous effusion.

Chemical Properties of Transudates. As mentioned earlier, the chemical composition of transudates is dependent upon the cause of transudation and may vary from having the chemical and physical properties of normal serous fluid to having those that are more characteristic of an exudate. Specific gravity is usually less than 1.018, the protein content is under 3 gm, and the principal protein is albumin. Fibrinogen is present in a low concentration. The typical transudate does not clot, but strands of fibrin may be observed in sediment.

Cellular Composition of Transudates. As mentioned earlier, a number of cells may be present in transudates, including mesothelial cells, blood leukocytes, erythrocytes, and macrophages. Mesothelial lining cells are found in purely transudative effusions, and if the fluid accumulation is transitory, mesothelial cells are normal. Basophilic reactive mesothelial cells tend to decrease as the fluid becomes modified and cellular debris accumulates. Mesothelial cells are capable of phagocytosis and transformation into tissue macrophages. As they are transformed they assume the characteristics of a macrophage by losing their cytoplasmic basophilia and hyperchromic nucleus.

A few mononuclear phagocytes may be found in a transudate. They probably have their origin from the emigration of monocytes from the blood.

Erythrocytes may be found in transudates, and they probably enter the fluid through damaged blood vessels when transudation is produced by a decrease in colloid osmotic pressure. If a transudate has been produced by an alteration in hydrostatic pressure, erythrocytes may passively escape into the serous fluids. In terminal cases of congestive heart failure, ascitic fluid becomes greatly modified and large numbers of erythrocytes may appear. Erythrocytes in these body fluids are morphologically altered and usually appear crenated. If erythrocytes have been present in the effusion for some time, erythrophagia may be noticed in macrophages and phagocytic mesothelial cells. (See Fig. 14–1.)

Although neutrophils may be demonstrated in transudates, they are usually present in low numbers, the concentration of neutrophils increasing as the transudate becomes modified. The morphology of neutrophils found in serous effusions is of considerable interpretive significance. In noninflammatory transudates, neutrophils are usually identical to those found in peripheral

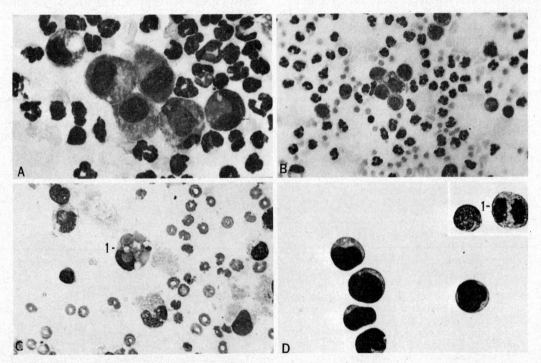

Figure 14–1. Effusion into body cavities. *A*, Peritoneal fluid from a dog. Note the many neutrophils and the large epithelioid cells characteristic of a chronic granuloma (1000 ×). *B*, Thoracic effusion. An exudate with many neutrophils and a cluster of macrophages near the center (400 ×). *C*, Peritoneal fluid from an anemic dog. The cell at (1) has engulfed several erythrocytes (erythrophagocytosis). Several such cells were observed as a part of a posthemorrhagic reaction (1000 ×). *D*, Ascitic fluid from a dog with malignant lymphoma. Mitotic figures (1) may be present (1000 ×).

blood. They have a typical shape, clear nuclear detail, and minimal degenerative changes. Occasional degenerate forms may be found in small numbers. As a transudate approaches the characteristics of an exudate, a greater number of degenerate cells may be present (Plate 14–1).

Eosinophils are not frequently found in the typical transudate, although eosinophils are common in modified transudates associated with the ascites resulting from congestive failure due to dirofilariasis.

Lymphocytes are present in all transudates. They are usually present in low concentration, although with lymphatic rupture or chronic granulomatous inflammation, they may be increased. The presence of lymphocytes as the principal cells may be indicative of a ruptured lymphatic or other lymphoid tissue injury. In lymphosarcoma, particularly in the cat, pleural effusions are not uncommon and are characterized by the presence of neoplastic cells. Neoplastic lymphocytes have a variable morphology. Classically, blast cells are present and have an increased nucleus to cytoplasm ratio, nucleoli, a highly basophilic cytoplasm, and nuclear chromatin that is usually finer than that in the mature lymphocyte. Large lymphocytes may be observed that have a finer nuclear chromatin than do the mature small cells, but nucleoli are absent and the cytoplasm is less basophilic. If there has been escape of lymph into the body cavity, the majority of the cells are characteristic of the mature lymphocyte seen in peripheral blood.

Neoplastic cells may occasionally be observed in transudative serous effusions. Care must be taken in making a diagnosis of neoplasia not to mistake reactive mesothelial cells for malignant forms of cells originating from other tissue. The characteristics of neoplastic cells will be discussed later in this chapter.

Exudates. An exudate is the fluid of an inflammatory reaction. Classically, it has a chemical composition in which the protein concentration is less than that of plasma, but is usually greater than 3 gm/dl. The specific gravity of an exudate is usually greater than 1.015 to 1.018. It may vary in appearance from a watery fluid to a thick, creamy pus, with or without the presence of blood. If such a fluid is discovered, it can be positively classified as an exudate. However, since the line of division between transudate and exudate is tenuous, exudative fluids may have some of the properties of transudates, just as a transudate may become modified and have some of the characteristics normally attributed to an exudate.

Inflammatory exudation into a body cavity is not a rare occurrence, but its frequency varies among animal species. The character of an inflammatory effusion is dependent upon the type of disease present in the animal species in question.

In the bovine, for example, a frequent cause of exudative fluid in a body cavity is traumatic reticulitis and the resultant perforation of the pericardial sac, pleura, diaphragm, or various abdominal organs. In the normal animal, peritoneal fluid contains approximately equal numbers of lymphocytes and neutrophils, with a tendency toward more lymphocytes. Mesothelial cells are commonly observed. With inflammatory processes, the percentage of segmented and band neutrophils increases. Fluid volume also increases and assumes the physical characteristics of serum. As the condition becomes more chronic and recovery imminent, the proportion of neutrophils decreases, and monocytes and lymphocytes predominate. With neoplasia, characteristic cell types may be observed.

The cat is frequently affected with pyothorax arising as a complication of a variety of infectious and parasitic diseases of the respiratory tract. Feline leukemia frequently results in pleural and peritoneal effusions that are sometimes classified as transudative and at other times as exudative. Infectious peritonitis of the feline is associated with relatively acellular fluids of high protein content.

Accumulation of exudative fluids in the serous body cavities of the dog is not uncommon. A variety of bacterial and fungal infectious agents may be responsible for the appearance of an exudate in either the pleural or peritoneal cavity. Nocardiosis and actinomycosis occur in both dogs and cats and produce exudation. Trauma resulting in hemoperitoneum may be observed in any animal, but is more commonly seen in the dog and cat. Autotransfusion of red blood cells frequently occurs, and, in spite of the accompanying hemorrhage, the fluid may have all the characteristics of an exudate with only a small number of erythrocytes.

Inflammatory exudation into a serous cavity may result from a variety of causes, and it behooves the clinician to attempt to ascertain the primary cause when exudative fluid is encountered.

Cellular Composition of Exudates. Exudative effusions have a high leukocyte content, but precise enumeration of the cells is of little diagnostic value. Owing to the nature of the agents causing some inflammatory exudates, neutrophils degenerate rapidly, and total counts may be misleading. Probably of more significance is an evaluation of leukocyte morphology. In most transudates, leukocytes have a morphology similar to that of blood cells, whereas with exudative lesions, neutrophils are frequently degenerate, particularly if the causative agent produces toxins. Pyknosis, karyolysis, and karyorrhexis of leukocytes suggest the presence of microorganisms. Phagocytic macrophages are present and often contain phagocytized material, including bacteria or other infectious agents. Remnants of neutrophils and erythrocytes may also be seen in the cytoplasm of

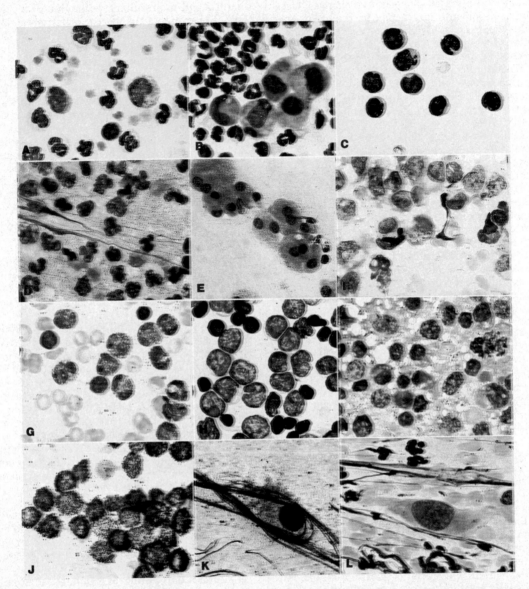

Plate 14–1. Wright-stained preparations from body fluids, lymph node impressions and biopsies. *A,* Fluid from the thoracic cavity. Note the numerous well-preserved neutrophils. The larger cells are phagocytes (1000×). *B,* Fluid from the abdominal cavity. The large cells are epithelioid type, characteristic of a chronic granulomatous condition (1000×). *C,* From the abdominal cavity of a cat with lymphoma (1000×). *D,* An exudate from the thorax. Some of the neutrophils are degenerate. The stippled background is characteristic of effusions containing large quantities of protein. Unless care is taken in examining this area one might mistake this for bacteria (1000×). *E,* These are hepatocytes aspirated when the liver was accidentally penetrated in an attempt to remove fluid from the thoracic cavity. They could easily be confused with neoplastic cells (400×). *F,* Impression smear from the spleen of a dog with histoplasmosis. The organisms are found in a phagocyte just left of center (1000×). *G,* Impression smear from a lymph node. The cells with cytoplasmic granules are eosinophils (1000×). *H,* Impression smear of a lymph node from a dog with lymphoma (1000×). *I,* Impression smear from a reactive lymph node. Note the plasma cells and plasmoid lymphocytes (1000×). *J,* Biopsy of a cutaneous tumor on a dog. The cells with basophilic granules are mast cells. Diagnosis was mastocytoma (1000×). *K,* A single cell typical of many demonstrated in a biopsy from a cutaneous tumor. Diagnosis was melanoma (1000×). *L,* Impression smear from a cutaneous granuloma. The large cell is a young, active fibroblast (1000×).

phagocytic cells. Lymphoreticular cells, including plasma cells, may be present in relatively large numbers in chronic infections. With some granulomatous diseases, mononuclear cell aggregates and giant cells may be found.

Exfoliated organ cells may be present in addition to leukocytes, erythrocytes, macrophages and lymphoreticular cells. Although these organ cells are observed infrequently, exfoliation may take place if the inflammatory reaction has invaded an organ of the serous cavity. Organ cells are encountered when an organ has been inadvertently entered during collection because of organ displacement or improper specimen collection. (See Plate 14–1E.)

The occurrence of neoplastic cells in the fluids of body cavities has been alluded to previously. Mesotheliomas and adenocarcinomas of the ovary are frequently associated with massive fluid accumulation. In both circumstances, difficulty may be encountered in distinguishing between neoplastic cells and reactive mesothelial cells present in an effusion. The fluid associated with neoplasia may have characteristics of both exudates and transudates. If there is an increase in the amount of fluid in a body cavity, care should be taken to detect the presence of any neoplastic cells.

CYTOLOGIC FINDINGS IN FLUID ACCUMULATIONS

Acute Suppurative Inflammation. With acute suppurative inflammation, the first cell to appear is the segmented neutrophil. If the accumulation has been induced by bacteria, the cells may become degenerate. The degree of cellular degeneration is dependent upon the type of bacteria and the potency of their toxic products. In general, gram-negative organisms produce potent toxins, whereas *Actinomyces* and *Corynebacterium* organisms produce fewer toxic products. Typical signs of cell death are karyorrhexis and pyknosis. Karyorrhexis of neutrophils is not frequent, but when it occurs it is a manifestation of rapid cell death, whereas pyknosis is generally indicative of a slow cell death.[4] If neutrophils tend to be hypersegmented and actively phagocytic, possess normal nuclear detail, and are found as the major component of an inflammatory exudate, the interpretation is of a nonseptic etiology. If there is considerable cellular degeneration, a search for the causative agent should immediately be instituted. Under some circumstances, microorganisms may be infrequent (infection with organisms of the genera *Nocardia*, *Actinomyces*, and *Staphylococcus*), whereas in other conditions, many bacteria are present and can be found in almost every field as well as in the cytoplasm of phagocytic cells. The feathered edge of the slide should be carefully examined for microorganisms, since they tend to be carried to this area

during preparation of a smear. If microorganisms are discovered in a body fluid, the finding must be interpreted with care, since slides or tissues may become contaminated after collection. Such extraneous contamination can be confused with a true infection unless care is exercised in sample collection and preparation.

As an inflammation becomes chronic, lymphocytes and plasma cells may appear. The presence of plasma cells in considerable number is an indication of a chronic process of long duration.

Chronic Suppurative Inflammation. The cellular pattern observed in chronic suppurative inflammatory exudates is similar to that observed in an acute reaction, including the presence of neutrophils, lymphocytes, and macrophages, with an increased number of plasma cells. Eosinophils, basophils, and tissue mast cells may be present in low numbers.

With chronic inflammation caused by the development of granulomas, the neutrophil number is usually low. Macrophages, monocytes, and lymphocytes usually predominate. Epithelioid cells that have an appearance similar to that of macrophages may accumulate in sheets and clusters. (See Plate 14–1B.) Multinucleate giant cells are frequently encountered in chronic granulomatous inflammations.

Allergic Reactions. Fluids associated with an allergic reaction are characterized by the presence of a large number of eosinophils in a fluid with a high protein matrix. Neutrophils, lymphocytes, and plasma cells may be present in variable numbers.

Trauma. The characteristics of fluids accumulating as a consequence of trauma depend upon the end result of the injury. Hemothorax and hemoperitoneum may occur if a major organ or blood vessel has been ruptured. Whenever a clinician is faced with a patient having a history of trauma and there is indication that fluid is present in a body cavity, thoracentesis or peritoneocentesis should be performed. Although hemopericardium is a possibility following trauma, it does not occur with great frequency. If trauma is of recent origin, the fluid resembles peripheral blood. With hemoperitoneum, erythrocytes may soon be reabsorbed into the circulation. If this occurs, there will be little gross evidence of whole blood, although microscopic examination almost invariably reveals the presence of erythrocytes in the cytoplasm of macrophages or neutrophils (Fig. 14–1C). In addition, hemoglobin pigments may be found in the phagocytic cells. Thus, even if blood is not grossly evident, microscopic examination may reveal that hemorrhage has occurred.

Rupture of the thoracic duct results in chylothorax. Thoracentesis reveals a milky fluid containing variable quantities of blood. Microscopically, the fluid is high in mature lymphocytes and chylomicrons. Chylomicrons are identified as refractile lipid droplets ringing the cells (particularly the RBC's). If such fluid is centrifuged, chyle appears as a whitish opaque ring on the top of the fluid, whereas erythrocytes and other cells are found in the sediment.

Reticuloperitonitis of cattle resulting from penetrating hardware is characterized by a predominance of neutrophils with an increase in the total cell count. As with any other inflammatory reaction, if the condition is prolonged, lymphocytes and macrophages predominate.

CYTOLOGIC FINDINGS IN SPECIFIC INFECTIOUS PROCESSES

Feline Infectious Peritonitis. Thoracic and peritoneal fluid collected from a cat with effusive infectious peritonitis is usually relatively low in cells (1500 to 5000/μl) but on occasion may be high (25,000/μl)[6] and high in protein. The fluid is usually viscid, clear to slightly cloudy, and yellow. The high protein content (5 to 10 gm/dl) may be recognized by the presence of a stained background on which other cells rest. When Wright's stain is used, the protein assumes a granular appearance and may sometimes be confused with bacteria. The fluid usually clots, but bacteria are rarely seen. In the acute form of FIP, well-preserved, intact neutrophils predominate with a few mononuclear cells. In more chronic cases, macrophages, lymphocytes, and mesothelial cells are more numerous then neutrophils.

Nocardiosis. Nocardiosis may produce a pyothorax in cats and dogs that is characteristically a typical purulent exudate. Fibrinous material with flakes or small granules is frequently collected. Microscopic examination reveals clumps of branching, often beaded, filaments that are gram positive and slightly acid fast (see Plate 18–1). Fragments resembling rods or cocci may also be present. Neutrophils are, for the most part, well preserved, and there is little sign of toxin production.

Actinomycosis. The purulent exudate associated with actinomycosis has many of the characteristics of the exudate seen with nocardiosis. "Sulfur granules" may be observed grossly. Microscopically, they appear to be tangled masses of gram-positive filaments with coccoids and rods. Occasionally, filaments may have a beaded appearance. It is difficult to differentiate between nocardiosis and actinomycosis.

Blastomycosis. The chronic purulent exudate associated with blastomycosis contains spherical, single, budding yeast cells with a thick wall and a broad base. Cellular changes are typical of a chronic inflammatory process.

Cryptococcosis. Cryptococci appear as spherical budding yeast cells with a very thick capsule. The organism can be readily observed with a new

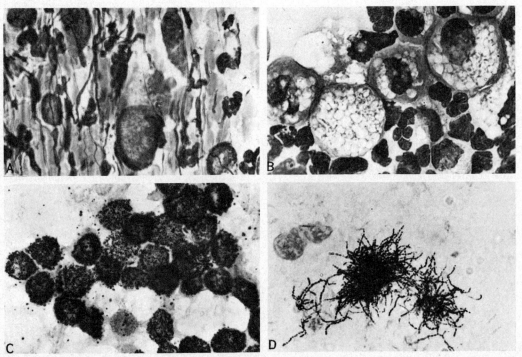

Figure 14–2. *A,* Impression from an active granulomatous lesion on the carpus of a dog. The large cells are young, active fibroblasts (1000×). *B,* Aspirate from a cystic enlarged abdominal mass diagnosed as cystic prostate. Note the many lipid-filled cells (1000×). *C,* Biopsy of a cutaneous tumor diagnosed as a mastocytoma (1000×). *D,* Colonies of *Nocardia* sp. from an exudate. Note the beading of the branched filaments (1000×).

methylene blue stain, although classically an India ink preparation is utilized.

Histoplasmosis. Confirmation of histoplasmosis can be made by demonstrating typical *Histoplasma capsulatum* yeast forms in cells of the reticuloendothelial system. In animals with a disseminated form of histoplasmosis the yeast forms can occasionally be demonstrated in peripheral blood monocytes. Examination of blood for histoplasma is best made by preparation of a slide from the buffy coat of a centrifuged microhematocrit tube. With the intestinal form of histoplasmosis, occasionally the organism can be demonstrated in macrophages present in feces or from rectal scrapings. If the lungs are involved, a transtracheal wash can be utilized. Occasionally lung biopsies will reveal presence of the organism. If lymphadenopathy is present, a needle biopsy of enlarged nodes will sometimes be positive. Failure to demonstrate the organism in any of these samples does not rule out a diagnosis of histoplasmosis. However, if the organism is present it will permit a rapid confirmatory diagnosis. (See Plate 14–1F.)

CYTOLOGIC FINDINGS IN NEOPLASIA

As previously suggested, there may be a fluid increase associated with certain types of neoplasia. In order to identify neoplastic cells, it is necessary to be familiar with the morphology of malignant cells. The cytologic characteristics of malignant cells were summarized[7] as follows: (1) They vary in size, being larger or smaller than normal cells of the same origin. (2) Unusual shapes are not uncommon, and shape varies as growth of the cells results in crowding and distortion. (3) Malignant cells are frequently shed in clusters or sheets as well as singly. (4) The cytoplasm is variable but frequently is intensely basophilic when treated with Romanowsky type stains. (5) Cytoplasmic inclusions (melanin, mast cell granules, and the like) can be demonstrated if present. (6) Highly undifferentiated cells have a low cytoplasm to nucleus ratio. (7) Variations in nuclear size and shape are frequently observed, as is nuclear hyperchromasia. (8) Young, undifferentiated malignant cells have a finer chromatin pattern than do normal cells of the same origin. (9) Nucleoli are frequently observed in malignant cells and in immature nonmalignant cells but are seldom seen in mature cells. (10) Irregular mitotic figures are sometimes observed in malignant cells.

No single criterion is sufficient to identify a cell positively as being malignant. However, if many of these characteristics are present, the existence of malignancy should be suspected. The characteristics just enumerated apply to malignant cells found in fluids as well as to cells found in imprints or scrapings made from neoplastic tissue. Although cytologic evidence of malignancy may provide a presumptive diagnosis, a more definitive classification can be made by histologic examination of tumorous growths. The ease and rapidity with which the cytology of a lesion can be determined does, however, make such laboratory procedures useful.

Cytologic Examination of Solid Tissue. Cytologic studies of solid tissues are particularly useful in differentiating between neoplasia and inflammatory reactions. Solid tissue specimens are usually obtained by imprints of excised or incised masses, by needle biopsy, or by needle aspiration biopsy. Tissue masses especially amenable to routine cytologic study are tumors located in the cutaneous and subcutaneous tissues.

Tumors most readily diagnosed by cytologic techniques include mast cell sarcoma, malignant melanoma, malignant lymphoma, lipoma, anal gland adenoma, and histiocytoma.[7] Although sarcomas are difficult to differentiate, the malignant nature of the lesion can be identified.

In a similar study[8] on cytologic examination of 250 canine specimens, the Papanicolaou or Sano staining method was used. Specimens were placed in classes one though five, with five being definite cellular evidence conclusive for malignancy. Most specimens were sectioned histologically, and the results were compared. Cytologic evidence was considered conclusive for the presence of malignant lesions in 47 specimens from which tissue for histologic sectioning was also available. Histologic diagnosis confirmed the cytologic diagnosis of malignancy in 46 of 47 specimens. Eight cytologic specimens collected from areas in which malignancy was diagnosed by histologic studies failed to contain recognizable malignant or suspicious cells.

Exfoliative cytologic diagnosis of cancer provides a fast and simple method that requires a minimum of skill, provides little discomfort to the patient, permits the lesion to remain virtually undisturbed, and, most importantly, permits cellular examination of closed body cavities without major surgery. Careful specimen collection is essential, since detection of cancer is possible only if malignant cells have fallen free and appear on prepared slides. The number of smears failing to contain malignant cells when cancer is present can be reduced by careful specimen collection and proper handling following collection.[8]

Mast Cell Sarcoma. Mast cell sarcomas can be quickly and readily identified by means of cytologic examination using new methylene blue stain. Characteristically, there are dark-staining basophilic cytoplasmic granules present in varying numbers. Some granules may be found outside cells. With a Romanowsky stain, the granules appear to be basophilic, but do not usually stain as darkly or distinctly as they do with new methylene blue. Cells are usually present in packets or singly. Cytoplasmic granules in rapidly growing metastatic mast cell sarcomas are often undifferentiated and are not highly basophilic. Some inflammatory cells and eosinophils may be numerous. (See Plate 14–1J.)

Malignant Melanoma. The typical cell in a malignant melanoma is round to oval, although considerable pleomorphism may be observed. Melanin granules remain unstained with new methylene blue, appearing as greenish black, small cytoplasmic granules. The number of granules within a cell varies, and occasionally only very minute melanin granules can be demonstrated. This lack of staining quality readily enables the cytologist to differentiate between melanin granules and mast cell granules. (See Plate 14–1K.)

Lipoma. Lipomas occur with relative frequency in the dog and do not usually present diagnostic problems. Cytologic examination reveals a relatively acellular preparation with numerous small oil droplets of varying size. The tissue specimen is usually oily and at times may contain large quantities of liquid fat. Use of a fat-specific stain (Oil Red O, Sudan III or IV) will confirm the presence of fat.

Anal Gland Adenoma. Anal gland adenomas do not usually present diagnostic problems when present in the usual location.[7] However, similar adenomas may be found in other locations on the body, and clinical diagnosis under these circumstances is difficult. Cytologic preparations from anal gland adenomas contain cells that are characteristically well defined and have the appearance of hepatocytes. Secretion droplets may be found in the cytoplasm.

Lymphadenopathy. A clinician is often faced with a patient having localized or generalized lymph node enlargement. Clinical differentiation of such lymphadenopathies can be difficult, but cytologic examination will often separate the malignant from the benign lesion. It may also be possible to identify the presence of a metastatic neoplasm (Fig. 14–3).

Specimens may be obtained by needle biopsy, excision, or incision. Cytologically, specimens taken from normal nodes are characterized by the appearance of predominantly small- to intermediate-sized lymphocytes. These cells have the same characteristics as circulating lymphocytes with a mature nucleus containing coarse chromatin and a slightly basophilic cytoplasm. Mature lymphocytes have a relatively small nucleus, whereas an intermediate cell has a somewhat larger nucleus and a greater quantity of cytoplasm. If germinal centers are aspirated or an impression smear contains material from a germinal center, lymphoblasts will be present. A few mitotic figures may be encountered in these areas.

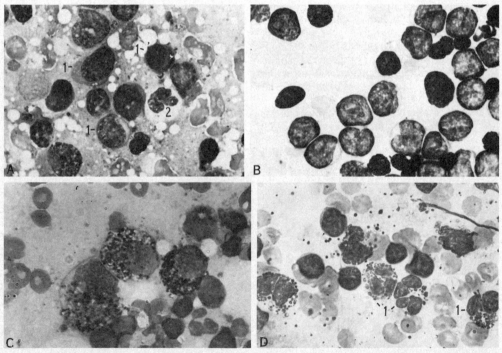

Figure 14–3. Lymph node impressions and aspirates. *A*, Impression from a reactive lymph node. Several plasma cells or plasmoid lymphocytes are present (1) as well as a neutrophil (2) (1000×). *B*, Impression of a lymph node from a dog with malignant lymphoma (1000×). *C*, Lymph node aspirate from a dog. The cells with dark cytoplasmic granules are mast cells (1000×). *D*, Impression of a mesenteric lymph node of a dog with chronic diarrhea. The cells with cytoplasmic granules (1) are eosinophils (1000×).

In addition to the lymphocytes, macrophages having an abundant, slightly basophilic cytoplasm may be identified. The nucleus of these macrophages is round to slightly oval, and the chromatin pattern is finer than that of the mature lymphocyte.

Plasma cells are also present in a normal lymph node and are characterized by a basophilic cytoplasm and an eccentrically placed nucleus with the chromatin frequently arranged in a spoke-wheel fashion. There is usually a light area in the cytoplasm immediately adjacent to the nucleus. These characteristics make the plasma cell easy to differentiate from the lymphocyte. (See Plate 14–1I.)

Very small numbers of mast cells and eosinophils may be present.

The clinical pathologist should become familiar with these cell types and their relative distribution in preparations from normal nodes, since this provides a basis for interpretation.

LYMPHOID HYPERPLASIA. An impression smear prepared from a hyperplastic lymph node is similar to a smear from a normal lymph node but has greater numbers of macrophages and plasma cells. Mitotic figures may be increased, but in the usual aspiration or impression smear they are not found with great frequency.

LYMPHOSARCOMA. The cytologic features of enlarged lymph nodes occurring as a result of lymphosarcoma are variable from animal to animal, although in an individual case there may be a rather homogeneous cell population. (See Plate 14–1H.) The majority of the cells are immature lymphoblasts or prolymphocytes having a basophilic cytoplasm, nucleoli, and a fine nuclear chromatin pattern. Mitotic figures are frequent and may be as numerous as three to four or more per high-power field. Normal cellular constituents are lacking and only a few mature lymphocytes, macrophages, and plasma cells are observed. There is frequently a monotony of cells, with a high percentage having an identical morphology. Abnormal, large prolymphocytes may be observed in some individuals, with an irregular, sometimes folded nucleus and an occasional bi-

nucleate form. Vacuoles may be present in the cytoplasm.

INFLAMMATORY LESIONS OF THE LYMPH NODES. As with all other inflammatory lesions, inflammation of the lymph nodes results in the appearance of large numbers of both acute (neutrophils) and chronic (macrophages and plasma cells) cells. Frequently, the infectious agent can be demonstrated by cytologic examination of an inflamed lymph gland.

ALLERGIC REACTIONS. If lymphadenopathy has resulted from an immune mediated (IgE) response, many eosinophils will be present (Fig. 14–3, Plate 14–1G).

CYTOLOGIC FINDINGS IN SPECIFIC BODY SECRETIONS

Equine Peritoneal Fluid. Specific diagnosis of abdominal disease in the horse may present diagnostic problems. The results of hematologic examinations are not specific and frequently fail to provide the clinician with the information needed to make judgments related to diagnosis, treatment, and prognosis. Cytologic and physicochemical determinations using peritoneal fluid may be of assistance.

Normal values for the cytologic and physicochemical characteristics of equine peritoneal fluid have been reported.[9–12] Although there are differences in the normal values reported, it is generally agreed that normal peritoneal fluid is colorless to straw or pale pink, is clear to slightly turbid, and does not coagulate following collection. Other normal values are summarized in Table 14–2.

Ten major criteria for classification of equine peritoneal fluids as transudates have been suggested.[10] These are failure to clot; low cellularity; essentially normal neutrophil morphology; a preponderance of neutrophils on smears of sediment; few mononuclear cells, lymphocytes, or eosinophils; occasional reactive mesothelial cells; virtual absence of fibrin strands; a specific gravity of less than 1.020; a protein content of less than 1.6

TABLE 14–2. Normal Values for Equine Peritoneal Fluid

Characteristic	Value			
	MEAN	RANGE	MEAN ± SE	RANGE
Protein (gm/dl)	1.1	0.1–3.4	1.05 ± 0.97	0.1–2.5
Specific gravity	1.001	1.000–1.093	1.013 ± 0.006	1.006–1.030
Fibrinogen (mg/dl)	—		<50	
Nucleated cells ($10^3/\mu$l)	3.244	200–9000	2.097 ± 1.715	0.05–4.6
Neutrophils (%)	59.5	36–78	90.1 ± 9.7	80–98
Lymphocytes (%)	10	0–29	4.4 ± 3.06	1–11
Mononuclear cells (%)	30.4	3–50	7.4 ± 5.33	1–17
Eosinophils (%)	0–2	0–3	2.1 ± 1.77	0–7

gm/dl; and a fibrinogen concentration of less than 50 mg/dl.

A slightly modified transudate differs from a transudate primarily in cellular composition. Smears from a slightly modified transudate contain moderate numbers of fibrin strands and a relative increase in mononuclear cells, eosinophils, lymphocytes, or reactive mesothelial cells.

A modified transudate is characterized by a protein content of greater than 1.6 gm/dl; a fibrinogen content of greater than 50 mg/dl; a specific gravity of more than 1.020; the presence of significant numbers of neutrophils, sometimes showing evidence of autolysis; and an increase in reactive mesothelial cells.

It is not possible to supply definitive criteria for distinguishing between modified transudates and nonpurulent exudates.[12] A classic purulent exudate is characterized by remarkable increase in cellularity, with degenerative neutrophils, evidence of phagocytosis, a fibrinogen level of 100 to 400 mg/dl, a specific gravity of 1.029 to 1.035, a total protein content of 4.3 to 5.1 gm/dl, and coagulation following collection. Total nucleated cell counts range from 60,600 to 278,000 cells/μl.

Peritoneal fluid from horses with impaction of the large colon is abnormal, with a total protein content of 2 to 2.5 gm/dl, specific gravity of 1.018 to 1.020, fibrinogen level of 50 to 300 mg/dl, a total nucleated cell count of 7000 to 18,400 cells/μl with well preserved neutrophils, prominent mononuclear cells, and an occasional lymphocyte, eosinophil, or mast cell.[12] Fibrin strands are numerous, but the fluid does not clot.

Internal abdominal abscesses caused by *Streptococcus equi, S. zooepidemicus* or *Corynebacterium pseudotuberculosis* produced characteristic alterations in abdominal fluids.[13] Abdominal fluids from such animals have the characteristics of an exudate. Grossly, the material is yellow and cloudy to opaque. Specific gravity is greater than 1.017, the total protein content is more than 2.5 gm/dl, total nucleated cell counts are more than 10,000 cells/μl, and neutrophils predominate. Most samples have great quantities of fibrinogen and tend to clot following collection. Although cultural results using peritoneal fluid are often negative, samples may contain readily identifiable intracellular bacteria. In addition to having alterations in peritoneal fluid, horses with internal abdominal abscesses also have a depression anemia and increased plasma fibrinogen and plasma protein levels with a hypergammaglobulinemia and hypoalbuminemia.

Conjunctival Cytology. Conjunctival sampling for cytologic evaluation is most easily accomplished by pulling down the lower eyelid and carefully scraping the inflamed conjunctiva until a small drop of fluid is collected on the end of a small spatula. Care should be taken to avoid scraping the margin of the eyelid. A droplet is transferred to a clean glass slide, carefully spread, and allowed to air dry. The slide is stained in the usual manner for a cytologic determination. Gram's stain may be helpful in identification of an infectious agent and in selection of a therapeutic drug. The scraping should be made from the most severely involved area of the conjunctiva.

Scrapings from normal animals usually contain sheets of epithelial cells with a small number of bacteria and an occasional leukocyte. Melanin granules may be observed in some epithelial cells.[14]

In inflamed conjunctivas of dogs and cats, acute and chronic bacterial conjunctivitis is characterized by the presence of a great number of neutrophils.[14] Mononuclear cells are present, particularly with chronic infections. Mononuclear cells predominate early in viral infections and are followed by an increase in the number of neutrophils.

Mycoplasmal conjunctivitis in the cat is accompanied by a marked increase in the number of neutrophils with concurrent demonstration of basophilic, coccoid, or pleomorphic organisms on the cell membrane. Chlamydial conjunctivitis can be identified by the presence of basophilic cytoplasmic inclusions early in the disease. With this infection, epithelial cells tend to occur singly or in groups of two or three cells, in contrast with the sheets of cells observed in a normal conjunctival scraping.

Conjunctivitis resulting from an allergic reaction can be identified by the presence of eosinophils and occasionally basophils in the conjunctival scraping. Neutrophils are also increased in number.

With keratoconjunctivitis sicca, the epithelial cells are keratinized, there is a marked neutrophil response if infection accompanies the condition, and goblet cells are sometimes present. Goblet cells are identified by a large quantity of mucus in the cytoplasm and a nucleus displaced to the cell periphery. Goblet cells may also be seen in smears made from the conjunctivas of animals with chronic bacterial conjunctivitis.

SYNOVIAL FLUID

Examination and analysis of synovial fluid in joint diseases has proved to be of value as a diagnostic test.

Synovial fluid is a protein-containing dialysate of plasma. It also contains mucin secreted by the synovial cells as plasma diffuses through the synovial membrane into the joint cavity. The nonelectrolytes of joint fluid pass readily in either direction between the blood and synovial fluid, whereas electrolytes are present in accord with the Gibbs-Donnan theory of membrane equilibrium.

Thus, synovial fluid is a tissue fluid that changes with disease and is characterized by alterations in synovial tissues and the metabolism in the intra-articular space. The normal exchange of substances between the vascular and lymphatic systems and synovial fluid may be disturbed or there may be altered formation, destruction, or utilization of various components in the fluid within the joint. Theoretically, it is therefore possible that synovial fluid analysis could yield information concerning the degree and type of change occurring within joints.

EXAMINATION OF SYNOVIAL FLUID

The routine laboratory examination of synovial fluid should include the following: (1) Determination of the total number of cells, both leukocytes and erythrocytes, and an estimation of the percentage distribution between polymorphonuclear and mononuclear cells. (2) Examination of the characteristics of the mucin following precipitation with acetic acid. (3) Observation of physical characteristics, including quantity, color, specific gravity, clot formation, viscosity, and turbidity. (4) Comparison of glucose content with serum glucose level. Other analyses to be performed when indicated include a bacteriologic and microscopic examination of a Gram-stained slide prepared from sediment; an assay of enzyme activity (aspartate amino transaminase [GOT], lactic dehydrogenase, alkaline phosphatase); and determinations of the total protein content and the albumin-globulin ratio.

Cytologic Examination. **Specimen Collection.** Arthrocentesis should be performed aseptically, and the fluid should be aspirated with a sterile needle of the proper length and gauge. A needle of at least 18 gauge having a short bevel and equipped with a stylet is preferred. Five to 10 ml of the synovial fluid may be collected from certain joints of large animals, and smaller quantities are removed from the joints of smaller domestic animals. The aspirated specimen should be transferred to a tube containing EDTA. EDTA salts inhibit alkaline phosphatase activity and will affect mucin clot formation.

Characteristics of Synovial Fluid. Normal synovial fluid is transparent, pale yellow, and free of flocculent material, although an occasional sample may be slightly opaque and contain a few small flecks of debris. With degenerative diseases, cartilaginous material may give the fluid a definite flocculent appearance. In such diseases, the samples vary from pale yellow and transparent to pale yellow and opaque.

Occasionally, blood is observed in the sample, and it becomes important to determine whether hemorrhage occurred prior to or during the aspiration. With an acute traumatic arthritis, the sample is markedly hemorrhagic, whereas samples that are streaked with whole blood usually indicate hemorrhage at the time of aspiration. Dark yellow to amber samples are seen in chronic traumatic arthritis and usually indicate a prolonged low-grade hemorrhage or massive hemorrhage that occurred prior to collection.

Normal synovial fluids and fluid collected from horses with degenerative joint diseases do not clot. Fluids collected from joints with acute to subacute arthritis and acute to chronic septic or infectious arthritis tend to clot rapidly.

Total Cell Count. Attempts should be made to count the cells in undiluted synovial fluid, using a white cell pipette. If dilutions are necessary, they should be made in normal saline solution, as acetic acid will produce a clot. Crystal violet in a concentration of 1 per cent may be added to the saline to make the leukocytes more readily visible. The total cell count is calculated based on the dilution factor required and the area that was counted in the hemocytometer. If the fluid is frankly hemorrhagic, a hypotonic (0.3 per cent) sodium chloride solution is used to lake the erythrocytes.

A normal count must be interpreted based on the reported counts for the individual joint, as total cell count may vary from joint to joint. Total leukocyte counts per microliter in the fluid from normal carpal, elbow, shoulder, hip, stifle, and hock joints of dogs have been reported to be from 0 to 2900 cells/μl, with a mean of 430.[15] The following range of total leukocyte counts in the joints of horses have been reported: radiocarpal, 25 to 3000 cells/μl; intercarpal, 9 to 555; metacarpophalangeal, 44 to 1350; tibiotarsal, 25 to 466; and metatarsophalangeal, 66 to 411.[16] Average total cell counts reported by others for the horse were found to vary greatly from joint to joint[17]; atlantooccipital, 358 to 1162 cells/μl; elbow, 107 to 366; knee, 390 to 1638; radiocarpal, 40 to 453; and temporomandibular, 412 to 2350.

Differential Cell Counts. In differential cell counts, the synovial fluid smear may be prepared by the use of coverglasses. Alternatively, one or two drops of synovial fluid may be placed between two microscope slides and the slides pressed together by a circular sliding movement and separated by sliding one off the other with a quick motion. The cytology centrifuge is most useful in preparation of slides from joint fluids. Smears for microscopic examination should be treated with Wright's or other polychrome stain. Schalm's new methylene blue is also recommended. The stained smear should be examined under the oil immersion objective.

Normal synovial fluid should have less than 10 per cent polymorphonuclear leukocytes (PMN's). Lymphocytes predominate in normal equine fluids. Mean values for lymphocytes range from a low of 33.86 per cent for the metacarpophalangeal joints to a high of 56.50 per cent for the intercarpal joints.[16] In this study, the lymphocytes had a dense, homogeneous, dark blue nucleus with a minimal amount of pale blue cytoplasm. These cells were well rounded to oval in shape and varied in size from somewhat larger than an erythrocyte to slightly smaller than the small synovial fluid monocyte. The relative number of PMN's ranged from none in the metatarsophalangeal joints to a high mean value of 7.55 per cent for the radiocarpal joint. The PMN's had a nucleus with a dense homogeneous chromatin material surrounded by a pale cytoplasm with indistinct granules. Occasionally, a few degenerate PMN's that had a single hyperchromatic pyknotic nucleus were present. Other cells appeared to be undergoing a ballooning type of degeneration.

Monocytes almost approximated the mean values obtained for lymphocytes, ranging from a mean low of 31.44 per cent for the intercarpal joints to a high of 56.86 per cent for the metacarpophalangeal joints. These cells were spherical or oval with an eccentrically placed nucleus folded upon itself. The nuclear material was not homogeneous and tended to be irregular and clumped.

Large mononuclear cells are relatively rare. On stained smears these are the largest synovial fluid cells. Characteristically, they contain a round to oval nucleus that is relatively small when compared with total cell size and usually eccentrically located. The mean values range from a low of 4.06 per cent for the intercarpal joints to a high of 9.27 per cent for the radiocarpal joints. Eosinophils were rare, varying from none for the metatarsophalangeal joints to a high mean value of 1.0 per cent for the intercarpal joints. Morphologically, eosinophils closely resembled those seen in blood.

In the dog, the following mean values for cells: monocytes, 39.72 per cent; lymphocytes, 44.16; large mononuclear cells, 4.20; and PMN's, 1.38 have been reported.[15]

In the cow, the differential count in the tarsal joint is monocytes, 36.4 per cent; PMN's, 2.2; large mononuclear cells, 15; and lymphocytes, 40.1, with a mean total nucleated cell count of 181.8/μl. In the carpometacarpal joint, the percentages were: monocytes, 63; PMN's, 1.2; large mononuclear cells, 7.2; and lymphocytes, 23.[18] In another report[19] synovial fluid from the normal bovine tarsus had a mean leukocyte count of 103.5 ± 14.23/μl with a range of 0 to 725/μl. Differential leukocyte counts were made from smears stained with Wright's stain. The mean differential counts were: neutrophils, 6.0 ± 1.24 per cent; lymphocytes, 49.0 ± 2.77; monocytes, 38.22 ± 2.47; macrophages, 5.93 ± 1.38; and eosinophils, 0.77 ± 0.22.

Monocytes were characterized by a nucleus that was usually kidney shaped and at times appeared to be convoluted. The nuclear material stained less intensely than that in the lymphocytes as the chromatin material tended to be scattered and formed coarse strands that sometimes clumped.

Occasionally, the pale gray to blue-gray cytoplasm contained minute vacuoles, phagocytosed particulate matter, erythrocytes, nuclei of other cells, and cellular fragments.

Cell Changes in Disease. Information concerning the cytologic alterations occurring in joint diseases in domestic animals is increasing. The most striking cell increase in synovial fluid from hip joints of dogs with dysplasia[15] was in the number of large mononuclear cells. A similar change was found to occur in other cases of traumatic arthritides, including ruptured anterior cruciate ligaments, osteochondritis dissecans of the shoulder, ununited anconeal osteoarthritis, and traumatic arthritides of unknown cause. Synovial fluid in 20 cases of possible septic arthritis was examined.[15] In these cases, total leukocyte and total erythrocyte counts were considerably increased. The absolute number of PMN's was increased, as was the number of large mononuclear cells.

Nonseptic polyarthritis in dogs is characterized by an extremely high leukocyte count in a synovial fluid that coagulates immediately upon removal.[20] LE cells are sometimes present in the synovial fluid of dogs with rheumatoid arthritis associated with canine systemic lupus erythematosus.[20] Synovial fluid analysis in six dogs with rheumatoid arthritis revealed a pronounced increase in total leukocytes with a preponderance of neutrophils in four dogs and mononuclear cells in two dogs.[21]

In the horse, the synovial fluid in traumatic equine joint effusions is clear and viscid, the total cell count is usually 100 cells or less per microliter, and mononuclear cells predominate. In bacterial joint infections, the aspirated fluid is cloudy, less viscid than normal, and the total cell counts range from 5000 to 10,000/μl. These cells are predominantly PMN's.[22]

The data available on the properties of synovial fluid in joint diseases of horses have been summarized.[22a] With degenerative joint disease, the total leukocyte count varies from 110 to 8250 cells/μl, with mean leukocyte percentages as follows: neutrophils, 14.9 ± 5.8; lymphocytes, 52.4 ± 7.6; monocytes, 30.4 ± 6, macrophages, 2.2 ± 0.8, and eosinophils, 0.1 ± 0.1. In horses with tarsal hydrarthrosis, the mean leukocyte count is 79 ± 13 cells/μl, with the following distribution: neutrophils, 3.0 ± 0.9 per cent; lymphocytes, 66.9 ± 5.0; monocytes, 27.5 ± 4.2; macrophages, 2.4 ± 0.8; and eosinophils, 0.2 ± 0.2. With idiopathic septic arthritis, the total mean leukocyte count is 20,862 ± 7.703/cells μl, with the following percentage distributions: neutrophils, 68.9 ± 12.3; lymphocytes, 18.5 ± 8.5; monocytes, 10.4 ± 5.1; macrophages, 0.4 ± 0.2; and eosinophils, 1.8 ± 1.8. With infectious arthritis, the mean total leukocyte count is 105,775 ± 25,525 cells/μl, with a distribution as follows: neutrophils, 90.5 ± 4.7 per cent; lymphocytes, 7.3 ± 5.4; and monocytes, 2.3 ± 1.9, with no macrophages or eosinophils.

Traumatic arthritis in cattle is characterized by the presence of a transudative synovial effusion.[24] Although total cell counts range from 700 to 12,000/μl, the predominant cell is the lymphocyte. In contrast, total leukocyte counts obtained from synovial fluids of cattle with infectious arthritis are considerably higher. In 18 animals with septic arthritis, total counts range from 2000 to over 3,000,000/μl, with a mean of 226,000/μl. The predominant cell was the neutrophil. Similar observations were reported in the synovial fluids of calves with idiopathic septic arthritis.[24]

Chemical Examination. The most commonly studied chemical components of synovial fluid are mucin and proteins.

Mucin. Synovial mucin is an acidoglycoprotein that is demonstrated by the addition of acetic acid to synovial fluid. Mucin clot formation in equine synovial fluid is determined by adding 0.1 ml of 7N-glacial acetic acid to 4 ml of distilled water in a test tube and thoroughly mixing the solution. To this solution 1.0 ml of synovial fluid is added slowly, taking care that the sample does not come in contact with the glass. The resulting dilution is gently swirled to mix the synovial fluid thoroughly, then allowed to stand for one hour at room temperature and graded as follows: normal (N), a tight ropy clump in a clear solution; fair (F), a soft mass in a very slightly turbid solution; poor (P), a small friable mass in a turbid solution; and very poor (VP), a few flecks present in a turbid solution. Mucin clot quality ranged from 88.5 to 100 per cent normal in studies conducted on clinically normal radiocarpal, intercarpal, metacarpophalangeal, and metatarsophalangeal joints.[16]

Mucin clot quality, as determined by the precipitation of synovial fluid in an aqueous solution of acetic acid, is a representative indication of the viscous property and quality of hyaluronic acid present in synovial fluid. In articular disease processes, reduced polymerization of the hyaluronic acid molecules will result in clots of poor quality and variable degrees of flocculation appearing in a cloudy solution.[19]

In the synovial fluid from animals with traumatic or degenerative joint lesions, the mucin concentration is usually normal, the viscosity is within normal limits, and the acetic acid test results are normal. With infectious arthritides the mucin concentration and viscosity are lowered owing to bacterial degeneration of mucin. An abnormal result in the acetic acid test usually occurs under such circumstances.

Proteins. Normal bovine synovial fluid has been reported to have an albumin:globulin ratio of 1.21 ± 0.02 and to contain albumin, alpha 1, beta, and gamma 2 globulins.

In an analysis of the protein constituents of synovial fluid in 10 normal horses, the following average percentages as determined by electrophoresis were reported: albumin, 39.6 ± 4.47; alpha globulins, 10.5 ± 2.3; beta globulins, 21.3 ± 4.2; and gamma globulins, 28.7 ± 4.0.[25] In acute non-infectious inflammations, the percentage of albumin decreased and that of gamma globulins increased. An increased gamma globulin percentage and decreased albumin concentration were consistently observed in acute purulent joint infections. Chronic noninfectious joint involvement resulted in a synovial fluid with an increase in the percentage of beta globulins.[25]

The increase in nonmucin protein that occurs in pathologic joint conditions is a result of a change in the permeability or a degeneration of the blood vessels immediately adjacent to the joint cavity. Nonmucin protein levels may double in concentration in association with traumatic and degenerative joint conditions, whereas mucin levels are only slightly lowered. Therefore, it has been suggested that total protein levels will be established from a summation of the changes of the various proteins involved including the mucoproteins and fibrinogen.

Glucose. Variations in the concentration of glucose in the synovial fluid may be of diagnostic value in the interpretation of various arthritides. The relationship between the sugar in synovial fluid and that appearing in the blood and plasma of 83 healthy cattle was examined.[26] The ratio of plasma sugar level to synovial fluid sugar level was 1.3:1.0 in a group of cattle that had not been fed for approximately 18 hours. In cattle maintained on full feed prior to being tested, the plasma sugar level:synovial fluid sugar level ratio was 1:1.

The synovial fluid sugar level was compared with serum sugar concentration.[16] The mean serum value for 29 samples was 97.50 ± 3.99 mg/dl. The mean synovial fluid sugar concentration proved to be higher than the serum sugar concentrations for the radiocarpal, metacarpophalangeal, and metatarsophalangeal joints, respectively. Synovial glucose levels rose significantly in horses and cattle following intrarticular injection of 6α-methylprednisolone acetate.[27]

Synovial fluid glucose levels may be of diagnostic value. Cell-free synovial fluid has little or no glycolytic activity, in contrast with effusions containing high numbers of leukocytes. Glycolytic enzymes are probably entirely confined to the polymorphonuclear neutrophils. It would be anticipated that glucose levels would be decreased as a result of the glycolytic activity of these cellular constituents.

The synovial fluid sugar level was compared with the serum sugar level in horses with a variety of joint diseases. In nondiseased adult horses, the sugar content of synovial fluid closely paralleled that of the serum. With increasing inflammation, synovial fluid sugar values fell below those of the simultaneously measured serum sugar and sometimes even approached a value of zero. With degenerative joint disease, the sugar level of synovial fluid was an average of 28 mg/dl less than that of the serum. In animals with tarsal hydrarthrosis there was less than 1 mg/dl difference between the two sugar levels, whereas in horses with idiopathic septic arthritis, the mean sugar concentration was 25 mg/dl less in synovial fluid than in plasma. With infectious arthritis, the mean decrease was 35 mg/dl.

Alkaline Phosphatase. Alkaline phosphatase values of synovial fluid of horses were much lower than those of serum from the same animal.[16] The mean alkaline phosphatase activity of serum for a series of 21 animals was 4.81 ± 0.46 Sigma units/ml. The mean values for synovial fluid were significantly lower than those for serum having a range of 0.10 to 1.95 Sigma units/ml and a mean that ranged from 0.53 to 0.93 Sigma units/ml. In a later study[27] a mean synovial fluid alkaline phosphatase value of 2.11 Sigma units/ml was reported in seven horses having traumatic effusions. Horses with idiopathic septic arthritis had a mean alkaline phosphatase activity of 2.72 ± 0.41 Sigma units/ml and those with infectious arthritis had a mean of 23.20 ± 8.4 Sigma units/ml. Similar changes were noted for lactic dehydrogenase (LDH) and aspartate amino transferase (GOT) activity in synovial fluids from diseased joints. The injection of 6α-methylprednisolone acetate resulted in a marked decrease in synovial fluid alkaline phosphatase activity. In the same animals, serum alkaline phosphatase activity remained constant preinjection and postinjection. In cattle, there was likewise a significant drop in synovial fluid alkaline phosphatase activity following injection of 6α-methylprednisolone acetate.[26]

GENITAL FLUIDS

VAGINAL AND CERVICAL FLUIDS

The study of vaginal and cervical fluids in domestic animals has been directed principally toward methods for determining the proper timing for breeding, recognizing reproductive disorders, and for detecting early pregnancies.

Bovine. The chemical and physical properties of cervical and vaginal secretions of the bovine have been studied in some detail, and considerable information is available, although little is utilizable in the diagnosis of disease.

Considerable work has been done on the flow-elasticity of cervical mucus, and it was found that during diestrus the cervical mucus had low elasticity. A fern-like pattern formed by cervical mucus on drying is characteristic of estrus or high estrogenic activity. This fern pattern occurs in cervical mucus obtained from about three days proestrus to nine days postestrus. One author[28] reported that the fern-like pattern was formed in cervical mucus from 13 cows with cystic corpora lutea. This finding suggested either an abnormal output of progesterone or the production of estrogens by these abnormal corpora lutea.

Studies of the pH of vaginal mucus have shown that vaginal secretions have a lower pH in vivo (6.57) than they do in vitro (7.45). The lowest pH occurs in early estrus, with the mucus becoming more alkaline as estrus progresses. There is apparently little, if any, relation between the pH of vaginal secretions and fertility.

The appearance of antibodies in vaginal and cervical fluid has been of interest as an aid to diagnosis. Vaginal mucus has been shown to contain agglutinins against *Brucella* and *Campylobacter* organisms. In the case of bovine vibriosis, such specimens may be used for diagnostic purposes to confirm the infection serologically and to attempt to isolate the causative agent.

Many studies have been conducted on the cytologic alterations in this fluid. Inflammatory cells are normal constituents of all vaginal fluids during certain phases of the reproductive cycle, particularly metestrus. In inflammatory and infectious processes, these cells become more predominant, occurring at all stages of the estrous cycle. Neutrophils are most commonly observed in acute processes, whereas mononuclear cells are more likely to occur in chronic diseases. A wide variety of bacteria may be present in the exudates resulting from pyometra, metritis, cervicitis, and vaginitis and following abortion. In order to evaluate the importance of the presence of bacteria, cultural examination and identification of the organism should be completed. Organisms of the enteric group are commonly encountered, and occasionally organisms of the genera *Streptococcus, Pasteurella, Listeria, Corynebacterium, Pseudomonas,* and *Mycoplasma* may be isolated. The isolation of any organism from the reproductive tract is not positive proof that it is the cause of the disease under question. It is difficult to determine whether the abnormality is due to the presence of the bacteria or whether the bacteria are present as a result of the abnormality.

Canine. Characteristic elements may occur in vaginal smears that coincide with external signs of estrus and morphologic changes occurring in the genital tract throughout the cycle. The elements present in a vaginal smear may vary among individuals as well as during the same phase of the estrous cycle. The techniques for examination of vaginal smears include staining by one or more of the Romanowsky stains or by supravital stain.

Supravital staining provides more exact preservation of the details of the cells present. The dog should be placed on her back in a semi-upright position. The vulva is wiped clean with a pledget of cotton, and a sampling spatula or a small, blunt-pointed cannula is inserted into the upper boundary of the vestibule. A small quantity of warm saline solution (1 to 2 ml) is placed in the cannula with the attached rubber bulb to gently flush the vagina as fluid is withdrawn for examination. A drop of 0.1 to 0.25 per cent toluidine blue O in saline solution is placed on the slide, and the spatula sample is added. The preparation is sealed by a coverslip, which is rimmed with paraffin, and examined. New methylene blue or Wright's stain may also be used.

In the dog there are characteristic cellular changes in the various stages of the estrous cycle. These are as follows (Fig. 14–4):

1. Proestrus. The outstanding finding is the presence of large numbers of erythrocytes. This is accompanied by some neutrophils as well as parabasal, intermediate, and a few superficial vaginal epithelial cells. The parabasal cells are small round epithelial cells with a large nucleus. The intermediate epithelial cells are about twice the size of the parabasal cells and have a round nucleus with a readily identifiable chromatin-parachromatin pattern. Superficial epithelial cells are the largest cell present; the nuclei are small, dark (somewhat pyknotic), and centrally located. By the middle of proestrus neutrophils decrease in number and by late proestrus may have disappeared. As the neutrophils disappear the number of superficial epithelial cells increases.

2. Estrus. Vaginal smears taken during estrus have no neutrophils and the erythrocytes have decreased. Erythrocytes may be absent in some dogs but may be present in low numbers throughout estrus in others. Superficial epithelial cells with a pyknotic or no nucleus predominate, because intermediate and parabasal cells are no longer present.

3. Metestrus. As the bitch enters the number of superficial epithelial cells decreases, the number of parabasal and intermediate cells increases, and neutrophils begin to appear in variable numbers. "Metestral cells," which are parabasal cells containing a neutrophil in the cytoplasm, are often present, as are parabasal cells containing cytoplasm vacuoles ("foam cells").

4. Anestrus. Intermediate and parabasal epithelial cells predominate in vaginal smears taken during anestrus. Neutrophils are variable in number. In some bitches there are none while in others a small number may be present.

Bacteria may be abundant in smears prepared throughout the estrous cycle but unless accompanied by a marked increase in neutrophils are probably of little significance.

Although not used as frequently, cytologic examination of the vaginal epithelium will reflect

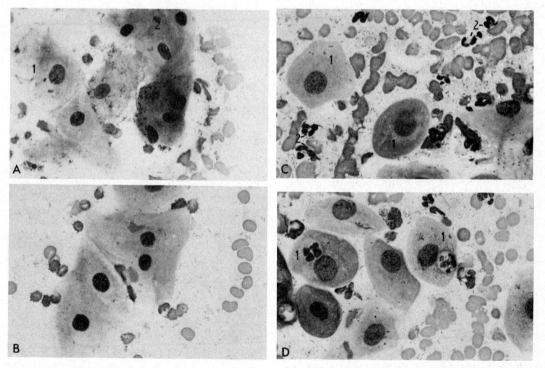

Figure 14–4. Cells from canine vaginal smears stained with Wright's stain. A, Smear made during late proestrus showing noncornified (1) and partially cornified (2) epithelial cells and numerous erythrocytes. B, Smear made during estrus showing typical cornified epithelial cells. C, Metestrous-stage smear showing noncornified epithelial cells (1), segmented neutrophils (2), and erythrocytes. Most dogs in metestrus have no erythrocytes in a vaginal smear. Occasionally, erythrocytes may persist in metestrus. D, Smear made during metestrus showing two noncornified epithelial cells containing segmented neutrophils (1). This has been reported to be characteristic of this stage of the cycle.

ovarian activity and stages of the estrous cycle in cats.[29] There are no erythrocytes in vaginal smears from the queen as there are in the bitch. Vaginal cytology during estrus in the queen is as follows[29]:

1. Anestrus. There are many small round epithelial cells with a high nuclear to cytoplasmic ratio.

2. Proestrus. Nucleated epithelial cells decrease in number but are larger and now have a low nuclear to cytoplasmic ratio.

3. Estrus. There are many large cornified cells with no or pyknotic nuclei and curled edges.

4. Early metestrus. Cornified epithelial cells remain but their margin becomes ragged and the cells are hazy. Leukocytes may appear in some but not all queens.

5. Late metestrus. The number of smaller cells increases while leukocytes are still present.

Equine. The vaginal smear from the mare is not distinctive during estrus, as no cell type is characteristic for any stage of the cycle. Slight variations in pH have been found to occur throughout the cycle, but, in general, the pH of the vaginal secretion in the mare is unimportant, as semen deposition during copulation takes place in the uterus through the open cervix. In general, the vaginal mucus is more alkaline prior to ovulation and less so following ovulation.

Ovine. In the ewe at estrus, there is a copious flow of thin mucus with relatively few cells. On the following day (metestrus), the volume of mucus decreases and the viscosity increases. Smears prepared from this fluid contain large quantities of desquamated cells, many of which are cornified. Cornified cells may appear in small numbers on the day of estrus, and some may be present in proestrus. The maximum number of these cells occurs two days after estrus. These changes are not as typical as those observed in the dog and probably play little part in determining the stage of estrus for breeding purposes.

SEMEN

The laboratory examination of semen has assumed ever-increasing importance, as the veterinarian is being called on for examination of males to determine their ability to produce viable spermatozoa in a high quality semen. The assessment of semen quality can be grouped into four distinct categories: (1) microscopic methods, including spermatozoal density and motility estimations, differentiation of live and dead spermatozoa, and enumeration of abnormal forms; (2) biochemical methods for measuring metabolic changes produced by or within semen; (3) determination of spermatozoal resistance to changes of temperature or to the effects of dilution; and (4) physical and other methods for objectively measuring the rate of spermatozoal movement and the associated

electrical changes in the semen and other changes. In the clinical laboratory, the first two methods may be used to advantage and will be discussed here. The last two methods of semen evaluation are seldom, if ever, used in the clinical laboratory. Such determinations should be made in a central laboratory that routinely deals with determination of semen quality.

Microscopic Examination. The microscopic appearance of bovine spermatozoa is shown in Figure 14–5.

Spermatozoal Density. Originally, spermatozoal density was measured by use of a hemocytometer, and this remains an excellent procedure. This method provides the veterinarian with a relatively accurate method for measuring the number of spermatozoa. The technique is simple, resembling that for a blood cell count. The dilution fluid for enumeration of spermatozoa is prepared as follows:

Sodium bicarbonate	5 gm
Formalin	1.0 ml
Distilled water	1000.0 ml

The sample is mixed by inverting the tube, and the red cell pipette is filled to either the 0.5 or the 1.0 mark with semen. The semen is diluted with special fluid to the 101 mark, and the counting chamber is filled after adequate mixing. The sperm on the four large corner squares and the entire central square are counted, enumerating only the heads and disregarding the tails. In calculating the total number of spermatozoa per microliter of semen, the total of the five squares is multiplied by 2. This figure is then multiplied by 100 if the pipette was filled to the 1.0 mark, by 200 if it was filled to the 0.5 mark, or by 20 if a white cell pipette was used.

Other methods for estimating spermatozoal density include the use of a calibrated absorbtiometer for comparing spermatozoal suspensions of known density with the unknown density and standard opacity tubes for comparing the opacity of diluted semen with the opacity of a standardized spermatozoal suspension. These techniques are most applicable in the large artificial insemination unit in which the dilution of samples is dependent upon spermatozoal density. In addition, spermatozoal density may be estimated by measuring the packed cell volume of semen samples centrifuged at 10,000 rpm for 10 minutes in capillary hematocrit tubes. This method may be sufficiently accurate for clinical work.[30] For every 1 per cent increase in packed cell volume, the number of spermatozoa was estimated to increase by 206.1 million. It has been suggested that each per cent represented 220 million spermatozoa. The electronic cell counter may also be utilized to advantage.

Motility of Spermatozoa. This is a subjective measurement, and results obtained by different observers cannot be reliably compared. An initial

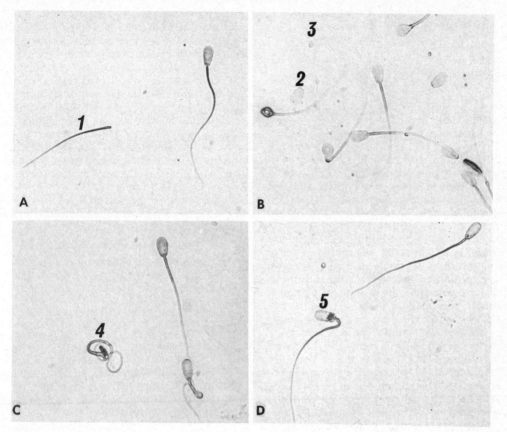

Figure 14–5. Bovine spermatozoa. *A*, The sperm at the right is normal. At (1) is shown a headless tail. The head may have been lost as a result of an accident; large numbers of such tails may be of significance. *B*, There are two heads without tails (2). A leukocyte is located at (3). Leukocytes are not present in any number in normal semen. *C*, The sperm at (4) has a coiled tail and a very small, dark-staining head. *D*, The head of the sperm at (5) is beginning to undergo degeneration.

motility estimation in comparison with the motility of stored semen can be used to detect gross differences in semen quality, but such comparison has limited value in detecting small fertility differences. The usual practice is to rate the sample by the character of the wave observed in a fresh smear of uniform thickness and the movement of the individual spermatozoa in the semen. The character of the wave is dependent upon the activity of individual spermatozoa and their concentration. The following conditions are usually estimated: the degree of motility, the percentage of motile spermatozoa, the type of motility, and, occasionally, the duration of motility. Since spermatozoa are sensitive to changes in temperature and their motility will be affected by a low temperature, every attempt should be made to maintain the slide temperature as near 37° C as possible throughout the examination. The types of motility will vary and are classified as:

1. Rapid, progressive movement.
2. Undulating movement with slow progression.

3. Oscillatory or stationary bunting in which spermatozoa do not move from place to place.

The following classification has been proposed for bovine semen[31]:

0 = No motility discernible.
1 = Less than 50 per cent in motion, most weak and oscillatory.
2 = More than 50 per cent motile, vigorous, rapid, with waves and eddies.
3 = 75 to 85 per cent motile, vigorous waves and eddies moving slowly.
4 = 90 per cent motile, rapid waves and eddies.
5 = 100 per cent motile, waves and eddies extremely rapid.

Although this categorization is adequate for bull semen, other techniques are used to assess spermatozoal number and motility in the ram. Evaluation of ram semen involves the visual examination of physical properties and a scale developed that may be used to approximate the sperm count[32]:

Type of Semen	Approximate Sperm Count in 10^8/ml
Very thick creamy	30
Thick creamy	25
Creamy	20
Thin creamy	15
Thick milky	10
Milky	5
Cloudy	1
Less than cloudy	1

This classification is combined with an assessment of motility that is based on a 1 to 5 scale in which 1 represents 20 per cent motility and each successive higher number represents a 20 per cent increase, ending with 5, which represents 100 per cent motility.

The ejaculate of the boar is voluminous and has an average density of about 100 million spermatozoa per milliliter, although there may be a great variation in density among boars. In contrast to findings in semen from the bull, wave motion is not seen in the boar's ejaculate. These factors should be taken into consideration in interpreting a microscopic examination of boar semen.

In the horse, it has been estimated that to establish a normal conception rate, the stallion must produce no less than 10,000 spermatozoa per microliter of ejaculate and that 65 per cent of these should be normal. Assessment methods generally depend upon the examination of samples for spermatozoal density, motility, and extent of maintenance of motility.

In the dog, an examination for motility should be made immediately following collection. Normal semen will present a picture of tremendous activity, the whole mass appearing to have a rippling movement unlike the wave motion of bovine semen. Individual movements of spermatozoa in fresh semen are intense. Although visual examination of the density of an ejaculate will give fairly reliable information regarding the quality of the semen, an exact expression of density can be made only be defining the spermatozoal concentration per unit volume. This is carried out in the usual manner using a hemocytometer and diluting the samples 1:20 in formol-saline. It must be remembered that density will vary according to the method of collection adopted and is dependent upon whether the whole or only part of the ejaculate is collected.

Differentiation of Live and Dead Spermatozoa. A stain used to differentiate living and dead spermatozoa is prepared as follows[33]:

(a) 1. Water-soluble eosin, 2 gm
　　2. M/8 phosphate buffer, pH 7.4, 100.0 ml
(b) 1. Opal blue, 1 part
　　2. Phosphate buffer as just described, 1 part

Mix equal parts of (a) and (b) just prior to use. The staining is completed as follows:

1. Place one drop of stain on a slide.
2. Add one drop of semen and mix.
3. Drop a second slide on the preparation, causing it to spread between the slides.
4. Carefully draw the slides apart, preparing a thin film on each side.
5. Dry on a warm plate at approximately 40° C.
6. Examine with oil immersion objective.
7. Count 500 spermatozoa, classifying the stained and unstained organisms to determine the percentage of living sperm (Fig. 14–6).

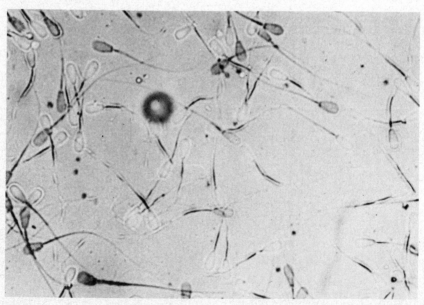

Figure 14–6. A live/dead sperm stain of bovine semen. The living spermatozoa remain unstained, whereas those that are dead take up the stain and appear darker.

The unstained sperm were alive when staining was instituted, whereas stained sperm were dead. The significance of the relationship between living and dead spermatozoa varies with individual workers, but, in general, a semen sample should contain 75 per cent or more viable sperm.

Morphology of Stained Sperm. The presence of abnormal spermatozoa in an ejaculate is important, as samples having a high percentage of abnormal forms tend to be of low fertility. Although published reports indicate that morphologic examination is of limited value in the assessment of fertility, it should be completed, as there are definite spermatozoal abnormalities associated with complete infertility.

It is important that in the collection, handling, smearing, and staining of semen care be taken to avoid damaging the spermatozoa and thereby increasing the number of abnormal cells. Perhaps the simplest method for delineating spermatozoa is the use of India ink.

Spermatozoal abnormalities that are often observed include: (1) coiled tail, in which the tail is coiled in a sharp hook; (2) piriform head—the posterior part of the head is contracted; (3) swollen head—the middle part of the head is swollen; (4) double head, two heads to one tail; (5) double tail, two tails to one head; (6) tailless, head without a tail; and (7) beaded middle piece, an expansion or enlargement at the center of the middle piece. In addition, semen may be abnormal owing to the presence of bacteria and cellular debris or other cells, such as leukocytes and erythrocytes.

In preparing a smear for staining, extreme care should be taken to avoid any physical damage to spermatozoa. Slides are best prepared by placing a small drop of semen on one end of a slide and tilting it to a 75-degree angle and allowing the semen to flow down the slide. The slide is allowed to dry and is stained by any one of a variety of techniques.

REFERENCES

1. Osborne, C. A., Perman, V., and Low, D. G.: Biopsy techniques and their diagnostic value. Part I. General principles of biopsy. *Scientific Presentations and Synopses of the 40th Annual Meeting A.A.H.A.*, p 548, American Animal Hospital Association, South Bend, IN, 1973.
2. Osborne, C. A., Low, D. G., and Perman, V.: Biopsy techniques and their diagnostic value. Part I. Biopsy techniques of specific organs and tissues. *Scientific Presentations and Seminar Synopses of the 40th Annual Meeting A.A.H.A.*, p 564, American Animal Hospital Association, South Bend, IN, 1973.
3. Low, D. G., Perman, V., and Osborne, C. A.: Biopsy techniques and their diagnostic value. Part III. Collection of material from natural body orifices. *Scientific Presentations and Seminar Synopses of the 40th Annual Meeting A.A.H.A.*, p 593, American Animal Hospital Association, South Bend, IN, 1973.
4. Perman, V.: Biopsy and cytology as an aid to clinical diagnosis. *Scientific Presentations and Seminar Synopses of the 39th Annual Meeting A.A.H.A.*, American Animal Hospital Association, South Bend, IN, 1972.
5. Kagan, K. G., and Stiff, M. E.: Pleural diseases. In *Current Veterinary Therapy VIII. Small Animal Practice*, edited by Kirk, R. W., W. B. Saunders Company, Philadelphia, 1983.
6. Barlough, J. E., and Weiss, R. C.: Feline infectious peritonitis. In: *Current Veterinary Therapy VIII. Small Animal Practice*, edited by Kirk, R. W., W. B. Saunders Company, Philadelphia, 1983.
7. Perman, V.: Diagnostic cytology in canine medicine. *Proceedings 16th Gaines Symposium*, 1966, p 6.
8. Roszel, J. E.: Exfoliative cytology in diagnosis of malignant neoplasms. Vet. Scope, *12*:14, 1961.
9. Coffman, J. R.: Technic and interpretation of abdominal paracentesis. Mod. Vet. Pract., *54*:79, 1973.
10. Bach, L. G.: Exfoliative cytology of peritoneal fluid in the horse. In: *The Veterinary Annual*, edited by Grunsell, C. S. G., and Hill, F. W. G., John Wright, Bristol, 1973.
11. Bach, L. G., and Ricketts, S. W.: Paracentesis as an aid to diagnosis of abdominal disease in the horse. Equine Vet. J., *6*:116, 1974.
12. McGrath, J. P.: Exfoliative cytology of equine peritoneal fluid—an adjunct to hematologic examination. *First International Symposium on Equine Hematology*, p 116, East Lansing, MI, 1975.
13. Rumbaugh, G. E., Smith, B. P., and Carlson, G. P.: Internal abdominal abscesses in the horse. J.A.V.M.A., *172*:304, 1978.
14. Lavach, J. D., Trhall, M. A., Benjamin, M. M., and Severin, G. A.: Cytology of normal and inflamed conjunctivas in dogs and cats. J.A.V.M.A., *170*:722, 1977.
15. Sawyer, D. C.: Synovial fluid analysis of canine joints. J.A.V.M.A., *143*:609, 1963.
16. Van Pelt, R. W.: Properties of equine synovial fluid. J.A.V.M.A., *141*:1051, 1962.
17. Davies, D. V.: The cell content of synovial fluid. J. Anat., *79*:66, 1945.
18. Warren, C. F., Bennet, G. A., and Bauer, W.: The significance of the cellular variations occurring in normal synovial fluid. Am. J. Pathol., *11*:953, 1935.
19. Van Pelt, R. W., and Conner, G. H.: Synovial fluid from the normal bovine tarsus. II. Relative viscosity and quality of mucopolysaccharide. Am. J. Vet. Res., *24*:537, 1963.
20. Perman, V., and Cornelius, C. E.: Synovial Fluid, In: *Clinical Biochemistry of Domestic Animals*, edited by Kaneko, J. J. and Cornelius, C. E., 2nd ed. Academic Press, New York, 1971.
21. Pederson, N. C., Pool, R. C., Castles, J. J., and Weisner, K.: Noninfectious canine arthritis: Rheumatoid arthritis. J.A.V.M.A., *169*:295, 1976.
22. Wheat, J. D.: The use of hydrocortisone in the treatment of joint and tendon disorders in large animals. J.A.V.M.A., *127*:64, 1955.
22a. Van Pelt, R. W.: Interpretation of synovial findings in the horse. J.A.V.M.A., 165:91, 1974.
23. Van Pelt, R. W.: Traumatic arthritis in cattle. Am J. Vet. Res., *29*:1883, 1968.
24. Van Pelt, R. W., and Langham, R. F.: Synovial fluid

changes produced by infectious arthritis in cattle. Am J. Vet. Res., 29:507, 1968.

25. Eggers, H.: [Clinical cytology of synovial fluid]. Wien. Tierartzl. Monatsschr., 46:24, 1959.

26. Van Pelt, R. W., and Conner, G. H.: Synovial fluid from the normal bovine tarsus III. Blood plasma and synovial fluid sugars. Am. J. Vet. Res., 24:537, 1963.

27. Van Pelt, R. W.: Clinical and synovial fluid response to intrasynovial injection of 6 alpha-methylprednisolone acetate into horses and cattle. J.A.V.M.A., 143:738, 1963.

28. Bone, F. F.: Crystalline patterns in vaginal and cervical mucus smears as related to bovine ovarian activity and pregnancy. Am J. Vet. Res., 15:542, 1954.

29. Lein, D. H., and Concannon, D. W.: Infertility and fertility treatments and management in the queen and tom cat. In: *Current Veterinary Therapy VIII. Small Animal Practice*, W. B. Saunders Company, Philadelphia, 1983.

30. Foote, R. H.: Estimation of bull sperm concentration by packed cell volume. J. Dairy Sci., 41:1109, 1958.

31. Herman, H. A., and Swanson, E. W.: Variations in dairy bull semen with respect to its use in artificial insemination. Univ. Mo. Agr. Esp. Sta. Bull., 326, 1941.

32. Gunn, R. M. C., Sanders, R. N., and Granger, W.: Studies in fertility in sheep. 2. Seminal changes affecting fertility in rams. Bull. Counc. Sci. Industr. Res. Aust., 148:140, 1942.

33. Lasley, J. F., Easley, G. T., and McKenzie, F. F.: *A Staining Method for Differentiation of Live and Dead Spermatozoa*, Univ. Mo. Agr. Exp. Sta. Cir., p 242, 1944.

CEREBROSPINAL FLUID

In human medicine, examination of cerebrospinal fluid (CSF) is considered an essential aid to the diagnosis of diseases of the central nervous system. With modern techniques, it is possible for a veterinary practitioner to obtain cerebrospinal fluid and utilize the results of laboratory examination as an aid to differential diagnosis of diseases of the central nervous system (CNS).

Cerebrospinal fluid is formed within the ventricles of the brain by a mechanism that is not fully understood. The choroid plexus undoubtedly plays an important role, as do the ependymal cells and the blood vessels of the pia-arachnoid membranes. The choroid plexus is a vascular fold of the pia mater located on the floor of the lateral ventricles and in the lateral recesses of the fourth ventricle. Cerebrospinal fluid is formed by both filtration and secretory processes. Filtration undoubtedly takes place through the selective permeable membrane of the choroid plexus. Some of the constituents of the spinal fluid are quantitatively dependent upon the concentration of these substances in the blood plasma. Thus, cerebrospinal fluid might be considered a dialysate that is in osmotic and hydrostatic equilibrium with blood. However, the composition of spinal fluid differs materially from that of blood plasma. The process of formation of cerebrospinal fluid is more complicated than simple filtration, and it appears that the choroid plexus contributes to this process by means of active transport mechanisms that utilize energy.

In addition to the ventricular formation of CSF, there is evidence to support the fact that there is considerable CSF production in the subarachnoid space. The subarachnoid system has a large space directly below the posterior portion of the cerebellum and over the medulla. This enlarged space is referred to as the cisterna magna and is the site of puncture for withdrawal of CSF from most domestic animals.

Cerebrospinal fluid circulates from the ventricles into the subarachnoid space where it bathes the surface of the brain and spinal cord. As the cranial cavity is a closed space consisting of blood, CSF, and brain parenchyma, any change in the volume of one component will result in a change in the volume of the others. This can be readily demonstrated by compression of the jugular veins, which will result in an increase in venous blood volume in the cranial cavity and a subsequent increase in CSF pressure.

Absorption of CSF occurs primarily at the arachnoid villi located in a cerebral vein or a venous sinus. Removal may also occur in the veins and lymphatics located around the spinal nerve routes as well as in the spinal nerves and the first and second cranial nerves at the point where they leave the skull. In addition, there is evidence to suggest that some CSF enters directly into the subarachnoid blood vessels and some CSF enters the brain parenchyma through the ependyma and is absorbed by the blood vessels there. Such absorption occurs more frequently when intraventricular CSF pressure is elevated.

Functionally, CSF protects and nourishes the parenchyma and maintains homeostasis. The CSF is important in the regulation of intracranial pressure and serves as a chemical buffer to the central nervous system by assisting in the maintenance of the proper ionic concentrations.

INDICATIONS FOR CEREBROSPINAL FLUID EXAMINATION

Removal and laboratory examination of CSF are indicated whenever there is clinical evidence suggesting CNS disease. Occasionally, CSF examination may be of value as a prognostic method for evaluation of disease and of response to treatment. It is also necessary to puncture the cerebrospinal fluid space for an x-ray procedure to assist in visualization of the CNS or for the treatment of disease.

Punctures of the lumbar region and cisterna are relatively simple and safe procedures but should not be performed indiscriminately—there should be definite indications for such procedures. Before performing a puncture of the CSF space, the clinician should be familiar with the anatomic structures that will be invaded and the exact procedure that should be utilized. Care must be taken to avoid contamination from the skin. An examination of CSF would be contraindicated if a localized skin infection existed over the area where the puncture is to be made.

TECHNIQUES FOR OBTAINING CEREBROSPINAL FLUID

Bovine. Cerebrospinal fluid may be removed from the cow by either suboccipital or lumbar puncture. Both techniques have proved satisfactory. A lumbar puncture may be used in calves or cows. A right-handed individual stands on the left side of the cow and by palpation locates the soft depression between the dorsal process of the last lumbar vertebra and the anterior end of the median sacral crest (Figs. 15–1 and 15–2). This point is at the level of a line joining the anterior borders of the tubera coxae. Before puncture is attempted, the area should be carefully clipped, shaved, and disinfected. The puncture is made using a sterile 5-inch, 14- to 16-gauge needle with stylet. The principal problem encountered in entering the subarachnoid space at this point is the thickness of the skin and struggling of the animal. Struggling by the patient is accentuated when the subarachnoid space is entered. In order to complete the procedure as safely as possible, it is of importance that the operator make the puncture directly on the midline. If the fluid does not flow readily after the subarachnoid space is entered, 5 ml may be withdrawn by means of a sterile syringe. If the animal is in lateral recumbency, difficulty may be encountered in entering the subarachnoid space at the lumbosacral junction.

Although the lumbar puncture is widely recommended, CSF can be readily obtained by use of the suboccipital approach (Fig. 15–3B). Utilizing a 3- to 4-inch 16-gauge needle complete with stylet, cerebrospinal fluid can be removed from an animal in the standing position or, preferably, from one that has been placed in lateral recumbency. If the animal is in lateral recumbency, the head should be fully flexed and firmly held in this position by one or two assistants. The space can be readily approached if the needle and stylet are forced through surgically prepared skin on the midline at the level of a line that joins the anterior borders of the wings of the atlas. In most animals, CSF will readily flow from the needle following removal of the stylet. If the flow does not occur spontaneously, 5 ml of fluid may be removed by a sterile syringe. In animals having an excessively high CSF pressure, as much as 100 ml of fluid has been collected.

Ovine. Suboccipital puncture is the most sat-

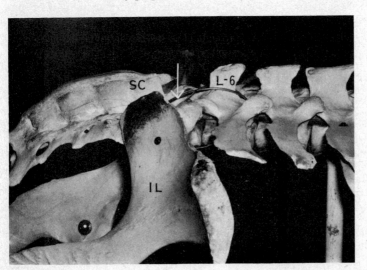

Figure 15–1. Lateral view of the skeleton of the cow. The arrow identifies the site for collection of cerebrospinal fluid from the lumbosacral junction. SC = sacrum. L-6 = sixth lumbar vertebra, IL = ilium.

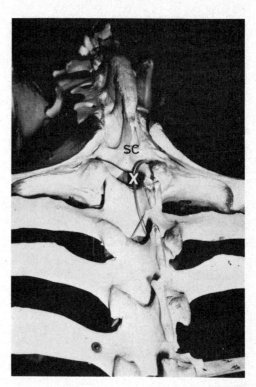

Figure 15–2. Dorsal view of the skeleton of the cow. SC = sacrum, X = the site for collection of cerebrospinal fluid from the lumbosacral junction.

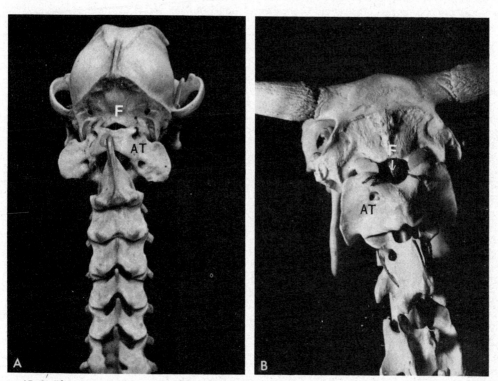

Figure 15–3. The anatomical location of the point of entry for collection of cerebrospinal fluid from the cisterna magna (F) of the dog (A) and the cow (B). AT = Atlas.

isfactory technique for collection of CSF from sheep. A needle of appropriate size should be inserted vertically at a midpoint in line with the anterior edge of the atlas. As with cattle, the area should be clipped, shaved, and disinfected before any attempt is made to remove fluid. Because of the thickness of overlying muscles and the steep edge of the occipital bone, the method is sometimes difficult and may result in hemorrhage.

The lumbar puncture technique is similar to that for the cow; however, inadequate quantities of fluid are obtained unless the animal is held in a sitting position. In this position, restraint may be a problem and undue struggling by the animal after the subarachnoid space has been entered may result in trauma. For lumbar punctures a 3½-inch 16- to 18-gauge needle is recommended.

Porcine. The suboccipital cerebrospinal puncture is difficult in swine. In order to obtain adequate restraint for fluid removal by this method, a general anesthetic is essential. Lumbosacral puncture is the method of choice in hogs weighing more than 300 lb. As with sheep, the puncture and aspiration of fluid are most easily performed with the hog in a sitting position. The lumbosacral space is rather easily palpated in a thin animal but may be difficult to locate in one that is fat. Care should be taken never to make the puncture anterior to the lumbosacral junction since in this area the spinal cord completely fills the dural sac and cord damage can occur easily.

Equine. In the horse, the suboccipital puncture is the method of choice; punctures made between the atlas and the axis have been described but are less satisfactory. Unless the animal is comatose, sedation is usually necessary.

For completion of a suboccipital puncture, the horse should be placed in lateral recumbency; the puncture site should be clipped, shaved, and disinfected; and the head should be flexed ventrally. This flexion should be continued until the tangents of the nasal line and neck produce a 90 degree angle. The puncture site is draped and sterile gloves are used. The needle is inserted at the intersection of lines created by drawing (1) an imaginary line between the anterior edges of the wings of the atlas and (2) a line representing the median of the neck. The needle is slowly inserted and penetration of the subarachnoid space may be detected by a sudden decrease in resistance to the needle. At this point, the animal will often show reflex movements, and care should be taken to avoid any damage to the nerve structures in the area. The stylet should be removed, and clear CSF will appear if the needle is properly located. The depth of penetration necessary for entering the space will, of course, depend upon the breed of animal and its nutritional status. A needle and stylet that are approximately 3½ inches long and 18- to 20-gauge are recommended.

Cerebrospinal fluid can also be collected from the lumbrosacral region.[2] The horse should be lightly restrained in a standing position and a tranquilizer used if the animal is excitable. This site may be used for a horse in lateral recumbency but the procedure is more difficult than it is for a standing animal. As with any CSF collection, the area should be surgically prepared and draped, and surgical gloves should be used.

The preferred site for penetration of the skin is within the depression that is bordered laterally by the medial rim of the tuber sacrale, caudally by the cranial edge of the second sacral spine, and cranially by the caudal edge of the sixth lumbar spine. This site can be tentatively located by finding the intersection of a line joining the caudal border of each tuber coxa with the dorsal midline. Palpate the lumbar spines, and by moving caudally locate the caudal edge of the spines of the fifth and sixth lumbar vertebrae. The spine of the sixth lumbar vertebra is usually shorter than the fifth, and there is often a depression at the caudal edge of the fifth lumbar vertebra. This site can be mistakenly identified as the point for completion of the puncture.

When the site is located, it should be anesthetized and a small stab incision made through the skin using a sterile surgical blade. In ponies and foals, a 3½-inch, 18- or 20-gauge spinal needle is used, whereas a longer, 6-inch, 18-gauge, thin-walled needle with stylet is used on horses up to 17 hands tall. On very large horses, an 8- or 9-inch needle may be required.

A right-handed person should stand on the horse's right side and rest the wrist of the right hand on the dorsal midline of the horse, cranial to the site of the skin incision. While the stylet is held in place, the needle is advanced along the median plane toward the lumbosacral space. The needle usually moves toward the space without much resistance, and penetration of the lumbosacral interarcuate ligament is felt as a sudden loss of a slightly increased resistance. The dura mater and arachnoid may be entered at the same time. Occasionally, there is some distance separating the ligament from the dura mater and arachnoid, and it may be necessary to advance the needle a few millimeters. When the dura is penetrated, the animal will frequently respond by tail movement and a slight flexion of the pelvic limbs. Some horses will react with sudden violent movements. If it is impossible to prevent such movement, the animal should be appropriately anesthetized or sedated. At this time the stylet should be removed. If CSF is not obtained, the stylet should be replaced and the needle advanced to the floor of the vertebral canal, then slowly withdrawn while being slowly rotated. As the position of the needle is changed, the stylet should be removed frequently until CSF is obtained. Occlusion of both jugular veins may increase intracranial and intraspinal pressures and enable the operator to obtain CSF. At times, it may be necessary to use a 5-ml syringe to obtain the CSF. Rotation of the needle within the subarachnoid space will often free the lumen of any meninges or nerve roots that might occlude it. Care must be taken to avoid creating hemorrhage during the collection procedure.

Canine. Cerebrospinal fluid can be removed from the dog at the cisterna magna (Fig. 15–3A) at the atlanto-occipital articulation. Lumbar puncture is extremely difficult in the dog owing to the lumbar vertebral arches and the small subarachnoid area. Light anesthesia or sedation is recommended, since the cisterna magna is in a vital area. Any struggling by the patient might result in irreparable damage. The area from the posterior portion of the sagittal crest to the wings of the atlas is clipped and surgically prepared. In order to prevent contamination, it is wise to drape the field with sterile towels. Following preparation, the subject is placed on its right side on a table with its back toward the operator and its head to the operator's right. The head is flexed by an assistant and maintained at a right angle to the long axis of the neck. The nose should be elevated so that the head is parallel to the table top. This position will separate the occipital condyles from the atlas and increase the area for puncture. An imaginary line is drawn across the neck between the anterior borders of the wings of the atlas. A second line is drawn from the occipital crest to the dorsal border of the axis. Puncture is then made in the exact middle of the dog's neck at the point of intersection of these lines. A 20-gauge, 1½- to 3-inch spinal needle with stylet is passed through the skin and fascia at right angles to the dorsal line of the neck. As the needle passes into the cisterna magna, a slight "give" can be felt. At this point, the stylet is withdrawn and cerebrospinal fluid will normally drip slowly from the needle. Compression of the jugular veins may increase the rate of flow. If the CSF pressure is excessive, the fluid will flow rapidly. If it is necessary to utilize a syringe, not more than 1 ml of fluid per 30 seconds should be removed until a sufficient quantity has been obtained for the laboratory. It may be dangerous to remove more than 4 to 5 ml of fluid.

Feline. In the cat, suboccipital puncture is recommended for removal of CSF. The technique is similar to that described for use in the dog. It must be emphasized at this point that no more than 0.5 to 1 ml of fluid should be removed from the cat, as this animal is susceptible to meningeal hemorrhage if too much fluid is withdrawn. In kittens, no more than 10 to 20 drops of cerebrospinal fluid should be removed.

LABORATORY EXAMINATION OF CEREBROSPINAL FLUID

The following tests should be included in all laboratory examinations of CSF: (1) physical examination, (2) total and differential cell counts, (3) qualitative and quantitative protein determinations, and (4) total glucose.

If these tests reveal the presence of abnormalities, additional tests might be performed. These additional procedures include bacteriologic culture, Gram's stain for detection of bacteria, determinations of chloride level and other chemical examinations as indicated by the clinical signs.

PHYSICAL EXAMINATION

Color. Normal cerebrospinal fluid is clear and colorless, resembling distilled water. The most common change in color is the appearance of a bright red fluid, resulting from the addition of fresh blood to the specimen because of a blood vessel rupture occurring at the time of collection. When centrifuged, such specimens have a clear supernatant in contrast to the yellow supernatant that may appear if an old hemorrhage exists.

A dull red to brown color is usually due to hemorrhage, which may be the result of either a chronic hemorrhagic pachymeningitis (intracranial hemorrhage) or a previous trauma.

Yellow (xanthochromic) CSF is usually attributed to bilirubin, which appears as a result of the disintegration of red blood cells within the subarachnoid space. Erythrocytes enter this space because of hemorrhage or a change in the permeability of the lining, which allows pigments in the blood plasma to enter the CSF. Some of the more common causes of xanthochromia of CSF include subarachnoid hemorrhage, spinal block, neoplasms, acute inflammations, abscesses, and severe systemic jaundice.

It has been suggested that a gray to greenish discoloration of the fluid may be the result of a suppurative condition.

Turbidity. Normal cerebrospinal fluid has no turbidity but is completely transparent. Turbidity usually occurs when cells are present. Turbidity does not become grossly evident until there are 500 or more cells per microliter. In acute infections of the meninges, the fluid may be slightly cloudy or purulent in appearance. Hemorrhage resulting from puncture of a blood vessel during collection produces a turbid red fluid.

Coagulation. Normal CSF does not coagulate. Coagulation occurs if there is an increase in fibrinogen, although a fibrin net containing blood cells may occasionally be observed in association with a meningeal reaction. In acute suppurative meningitis, a heavy coagulation may occur. The CSF will coagulate if contaminated with large quantities of blood, as a result of internal hemorrhage or contamination at the time of collection.

TOTAL AND DIFFERENTIAL CELL COUNTS

Total Cell Count. Cells in CSF degenerate rapidly. Consequently, the total cell count must be performed as soon after collection as possible. Most cells encountered in normal fluid are small lymphocytes. Only on rare occasions are larger mononuclear cells present.

A special diluting fluid consisting of 10 ml of glacial acetic acid, 90 ml of distilled water, and 0.1 gm of crystal violet is used. This diluting fluid should be filtered prior to use. For completion of a total cell count, diluting fluid is drawn to the 1 mark on a white cell-diluting pipette, and the pipette is filled to the 11 mark with cerebrospinal fluid. This mixture is shaken, and two or three drops are discarded. Each side of a standard hemocytometer is filled and allowed to stand for two minutes in order for the cells to settle. All cells within the entire ruled area on both sides of the counting chamber are enumerated and multiplied by 0.6 to obtain the number of cells per microliter.

If the sample is grossly contaminated with whole blood, a total red and white cell count may be indicated. Since the approximate ratio of erythrocytes to leukocytes is 500:1 in normal blood, any relative increase in leukocytes can be roughly estimated. This method should be used only when it is impossible to obtain uncontaminated specimens, as the results are not reliable. In one study, blood contamination had little effect on leukocyte counts even when several thousand erythrocytes were present.[3]

Normal cerebrospinal fluid contains less than five leukocytes/μl.

An increase in the number of nucleated cells (pleocytosis) in CSF may be the result of an inflammatory lesion or an irritation of the meninges, brain, or spinal cord. Extremely high counts are observed in acute pyogenic meningitis, and increases may also be observed in association with neoplasms; with chronic, focal, or degenerative lesions; in brain or spinal cord abscesses; and in association with encephalitis. Pleocytosis may also occur with chronic inflammation and toxic conditions.

Differential Cell Count. If the total cell count is increased, a differential count should be made. If the total cell count is less than 500/μl, the sample should be centrifuged at a low speed (600 revolutions per minute or less) and a smear made of the sediment. The sediment can be stained with any polychrome stain, such as those used for blood films.

A simple method for sedimentation of cells in CSF is performed as follows:

1. Cut a glass test tube with a glass cutter to create an open-ended cylinder.
2. Dip the smooth end of the cylinder in melted paraffin wax.
3. Warm a glass slide and place the waxed end of the cylinder on the slide.
4. Allow the paraffin wax to cool; this will seal the cylinder to the slide.
5. Place 0.25 to 1.0 ml of freshly collected CSF into the cylinder and let it stand undisturbed for 20 to 25 minutes.

6. Carefully aspirate the CSF and remove the cylinder. Excess fluid remaining on the slide is removed by gently absorbing it with filter paper.
7. Allow the small drop of CSF on the slide to dry.
8. Fix the material to the slide using a spray fixative.
9. Remove the excess paraffin wax with a scalpel blade and stain the slide.

Slides prepared in this fashion are coverslipped and are then ready for microscopic examination.

Excellent preparations for cytologic examination can be made using a special centrifuge in which cells are centrifuged directly onto a glass microscope slide.

If the total cell count is high (greater than 500/μl), a direct smear of the fluid can be made or a wet mount preparation can be utilized. For a wet mount, a drop or two of 0.5 per cent new methylene blue is added to 1 ml of CSF or CSF sediment. A medium size drop of this mixture is placed on a slide, a coverslip added and the slide examined under a microscope.

Cytologic examination of CSF should be made as soon as possible (within 30 minutes) after collection. Cells have a tendency to degenerate rapidly because CSF is relatively protein deficient. If a delay in cytologic examination is necessitated, CSF should be centrifuged, the supernatant removed, and a drop of homologous serum added to the sediment. The CSF-serum combination can be held for two or three hours before examination. Alternatively, equal volumes of 95 per cent ethanol may be added to a part of the collected CSF to preserve cells. If chemical examinations are needed, CSF without alcohol should be retained and submitted to the laboratory.

In a smear from normal CSF, only small lymphocytes and an occasional monocuclear cell are present. The observation of neutrophils is usually a sign of a pyogenic or bacterial infection—such as an abscess, bacterial encephalitis, or bacterial meningitis—or evidence of hemorrhage. An increase in total cells that is primarily lymphocytic may be a sign of viral infection, chronic infection, toxic condition, or fungal infection. Such an increase may also be found in an animal with uremia. The presence of neoplastic cells indicates that there is a neoplasm within the central nervous system.

If a patient undergoes a series of CSF examinations, a continuing increase in neutrophils may be a sign of a progressing lesion and is considered an unfavorable prognostic indication. If the cell pattern changes and a rising lymphocyte count is observed, it may be a favorable prognostic sign.

Membrane Filtration Technique. A membrane filtration method for cytologic examinations of canine and feline CSF has been described.[4–6]

In this technique, CSF is passed through a millipore filter. CSF (10 drops to 1 ml) is mixed with

2 ml of 40 per cent ethanol. This will prevent cellular degeneration. A Swinny-type hypodermic adapter (Gelman Instrument Co., Ann Arbor, Michigan) is attached to a syringe. The CSF-ethanol mixture is added to the syringe and gently passed through the millipore filter by placing pressure on the plunger of the syringe. Because the pores of the millipore filter are smaller than cells, all CSF cells are collected. The membrane filter is lifted from the adapter with forceps and placed in 95 per cent ethanol for two minutes. The filter is now ready for staining, which is completed as follows: (1) Place into distilled water for 30 seconds. (2) Place into the Harris hematoxylin for 10 to 15 seconds. (3) Place into distilled water for 30 seconds. (4) Place back into 95 per cent ethanol for 30 seconds. (5) Put into absolute alcohol for one minute and finally in xylene for another minute. The treated membrane is now transparent and can be placed on a standard glass slide. A few drops of mounting media and a glass coverslip are applied and the specimen is ready for microscopic examination.

The principal advantages of the technique are (1) a small quantity of spinal fluid can be readily examined, (2) samples collected into a fixative permit a semiquantitative evaluation of cell population, and (3) the morphologic features of the cells are clear in specimens that remain in 40 per cent ethanol for as long as 120 hours prior to membrane filtration and staining. This technique undoubtedly has value in detecting the presence of infectious agents that may be present in small numbers and also for detecting neoplastic cells that might otherwise be overlooked because of their small numbers.

Protein Determinations. In normal CSF, protein is present at a very low level (12 to 40 mg/dl) and consists almost entirely of albumin. The total protein concentration in CSF is increased in both inflammatory and noninflammatory diseases of the CNS. Globulins are the fraction of chief interest, since they are increased in pathologic conditions. If a specimen is grossly contaminated with blood, tests for globulin cannot be applied, as serum globulin may be present and result in a false positive finding. Increases in protein may occur in the absence of pleocytosis.

Urine dipsticks can be used to screen CSF for protein. Protein concentrations greater than 100 mg/dl can be detected. However, elevations (as determined spectrophotometrically) between 30 and 100 mg/dl will not give a positive reaction.

The simplest method for qualitative determination of globulin presence in CSF is Pándy's test. One ml of Pándy's reagent, which consists of 10 gm of carbolic acid crystals in 100 ml of distilled water, is placed in a test tube. A few drops of CSF are added, and the mixture is thoroughly shaken. If turbidity develops upon shaking, globulins are present. Normal CSF may produce a slight turbidity, whereas CSF with an increased globulin content will produce a definite white turbidity. The results should be graded from 1 to 4+ depending upon the intensity of turbidity.

A second screening test for qualitative estimation of globulin concentration is the Nonne-Apelt (Ross-Jones) test. In this technique, 1 ml of a saturated ammonium sulfate solution is placed in a small test tube, CSF is carefully overlaid, and the tubes are allowed to stand for a few minutes. In normal spinal fluid, no ring is formed at the junction of spinal fluid and reagent, but a white to grayish ring at the zone of contact indicates the presence of globulins.

The total protein concentration of CSF is readily determined using a trichloroacetic acid–turbidimetric procedure. In this technique, 0.5 ml of CSF is combined with 1.5 ml of 5 per cent trichloroacetic acid and allowed to react at room temperature for five minutes. The sample is agitated and the turbidity measured against a bovine serum albumin standard at 420 nm.

Increased globulin content is an indication of inflammation. Typical lesions causing protein increase and inflammation are encephalitis, brain or spinal cord abscessation, toxoplasmosis, and meningitis. Certain noninflammatory conditions such as pneumonia, convulsive states, and uremia may alter capillary permeability, resulting in the appearance of globulins in CSF. Globulins may be found in CSF as a result of hemorrhage.

If a considerable amount of tissue destruction resulting from congestion, hemorrhage, or edema occurs, there may be an increase in the quantity of protein. Repeated determinations of the protein content of CSF may give reliable information regarding the progress of an inflammatory condition. As the condition begins to subside, the quantity of protein decreases proportionally.

GLUCOSE CONCENTRATION

The concentration of glucose in CSF is approximately 60 to 70 per cent of the blood glucose level. In normal animals, glucose CSF values range from 40 to 80 mg/dl. The concentration of glucose in CSF is dependent upon: (1) the blood glucose level, (2) the selective permeability of the blood-cerebrospinal fluid barrier, and (3) the presence or absence of glycolytic microorganisms.

The technique for detection of glucose in CSF is the same as that utilized for determination of glucose in blood.

Urine dipsticks can be used to screen CSF samples. In normal CSF there is a trace to one plus reaction. If glucose is decreased the test is negative, while an increase will give a two plus or stronger reaction. If the dipstick test is negative, a quantitative analysis may be indicated. As the CSF glucose level is directly related to that of serum, a serum sample should be collected at the same time as CSF and submitted for glucose analysis.

Decreased CSF glucose levels (hypoglycorrhachia) may occur in association with a systemic hypoglycemia or as the result of acute pyogenic infection. The decreased level associated with acute pyogenic infections is chiefly the result of the glycolytic activity of the infection microorganisms.

Increased CSF glucose concentration (hyperglycorrhachia) is seen in association with any disease having a hyperglycemia. Perhaps the most common cause of this alteration is diabetes mellitus. A slight hyperglycorrhacia may be seen in association with encephalitis, spinal cord compression, brain tumors, or brain abscesses.

OTHER CHEMICAL EXAMINATIONS

Occasionally, nonprotein nitrogen determinations may be performed using CSF. Most of the nonprotein nitrogenous constituents of blood are also found in CSF. However, their relative concentration will differ from that found in blood, primarily owing to differences in diffusibility. In cases of uremia, the urea nitrogen level in CSF will increase at about the same rate that it does in blood.

Cholesterol concentration increases occur in association with hemorrhages of the central nervous system, tumors, meningitis, and brain abscesses. The normal level for cholesterol in the CSF of domestic animals varies from none to minute traces. Therefore, any increase may be indicative of one of the conditions mentioned.

The values for a variety of electrolytes—including phosphate, sodium, calcium, potassium, and magnesium—have been estimated in CSF. However, little information is available concerning alterations in these electrolyte levels in disease states in domestic animals.

Enzyme determinations have not been extensively studied. In humans, it has been found that lactic dehydrogenase activity was markedly increased in individuals having lymphoid tumors that involved the brain. The concentrations of CSF-AST and ALT are increased in dogs with distemper that exhibit signs of a CNS disturbance.[7]

Measurement of creatine phosphokinase (CK) activity may be of value. Plasma CK does not normally enter CSF; thus, any CK activity in this fluid is probably derived from the CNS or occurs because of leakage of serum into CSF. CK activity increases have been reported in a variety of neurologic diseases.[8] When there was an increase in CSF-CK activity there was poor response to therapy with progression of the disease and death.

CEREBROSPINAL FLUID ALTERATIONS IN DISEASE

Many of the changes that occur in CSF are nonspecific; the results of CSF analysis are seldom diagnostic except in cases in which a specific infectious agent—bacterium, fungus, or protozoa—can be demonstrated or if there is an exfoliating neoplasm that has invaded the subarachnoid space. Therefore, one must always interpret CSF findings in light of history and clinical findings. It is almost impossible to interpret CSF changes in samples that are contaminated with peripheral blood. If fresh blood is aspirated during collection and laboratory results are equivocal, the sampling procedure should be repeated in a few days. Laboratory findings in CSF from animals with CNS disturbances are summarized in Table 15–1.

SPECIFIC GRAVITY. The specific gravity of normal CSF is 1.003 to 1.006. Increases above 1.006 may occur in animals with CNS disturbances but this is not common. It will be increased if protein concentration has increased greatly. Large increases in CSF-glucose will also add to the specific gravity. The specific gravity is increased if there is a significant amount of peripheral blood contamination.

CSF GLOBULINS. The presence of globulins in CSF is determined using the Pándy or Nonne-Apelt (Ross-Jones) tests. Normal CSF contains little, if any, globulin and these tests are negative. Increases occur with inflammatory processes such as bacterial, viral, fungal, or protozoal infections. The results are variable with traumatic, neoplastic, and vascular lesions. If there is significant contamination with peripheral blood these tests will be positive.

TOTAL PROTEIN. The total protein concentration in normal CSF is less than 25 mg/dl. Increases occur in inflammatory reactions resulting from bacterial, viral, fungal, and protozoal infections and are usually increased in neoplastic diseases. Total protein can be normal or increased in traumatic, degenerative, or vascular lesions. Peripheral blood contamination will increase total CSF protein at the rate of approximately 1 mg/dl for each 400 RBC/μl.[9]

CELLS. Normal CSF is almost cell free, having less than five nucleated cells/μl. Cell numbers are increased in bacterial, viral, fungal, and protozoal infections. With bacterial diseases the increase is almost exclusively in neutrophils, but with fungal infections there is also an increase in macrophages. Occasionally fungal organisms can be demonstrated in these phagocytic cells. An increase in eosinophils has been reported in cryptococcosis.[5] In protozoal infections, macrophages predominate although there is also an increase in neutrophils. Lymphocytes are increased in viral infections. With traumatic lesions of the CNS the total cell count is normal to increased. The increase is usually in neutrophils and lymphocytes but is variable. If vascular lesions are present the cell count can be normal or increased. Hemorrhage is accompanied by an increase in erythrocytes and protein as well as leukocytes. Differentiation between hemorrhage that has occurred prior to sampling and that during sampling is

TABLE 15–1. Laboratory Findings in CSF in CNS Diseases[9,10]

Condition	Appearance	Specific Gravity	Total Protein	Globulins	Cells Total	Cells Principal Type	Glucose	Enzymes
Inflammation:								
Bacterial	Turbid	I-N	I	I	I	Neutrophils	D	I
Canine Distemper	Clear or turbid	I-N	I-N	I	I-N	Lymphocytes	N-D	I-N
FIP	Clear or turbid	I	I-N	I	I-N	Lymphocytes	N-D	—
Fungal (Cryptococcosis)	Turbid, Xanthochromic	I	I	I	I	Macrophages, neutrophils	N-D	N-I
Toxoplasmosis	Xanthochromic	I	I	I	I	Macrophages, neutrophils	N-D	N-I
Granulomatous meningoencephalitis	Clear or turbid	I	I-N	N-I	I	Macrophages, lymphocytes	—	—
Degenerative	Clear	N-I	N	N	N	N	N	N
Neoplasia:								
Cerebral	Clear	I-N	I	N-I	N	Rare neoplastic cells	N-D	N-I
Spinal cord	Clear	I-N	I	N	I	N	N	N-I
Trauma (vascular)	Xanthochromic	I-N	I-N	I-N	I-N	Macrophages, erythrophagocytosis	N	N-I
Congenital and Familial:								
Hydrocephalus (congenital)	Clear	N	N	N	N		N	N
Hydrocephalus (postnatal)	Turbid	I	I	—	I	Neutrophils		
Globoid leukodystrophy	Turbid	I	I	I	I	Globoid cells, macrophages		
Blood contamination	Red, turbid	I	I	I	I	Intact RBC	N	I

N = Normal
I = Increased
D = Decreased

based on the presence of xanthochromia. If hemorrhage occurred before sampling, the fluid is xanthochromic, and erythrophagocytosis and some crenated erythrocytes may be seen.

Peripheral blood contamination of CSF makes interpretation of total cell counts and cytologic examination difficult. Utilizing the ratio of 400 RBC to 1 WBC as a method for eliminating the artefactual results in contaminated samples leads to overestimation of the number of leukocytes and protein concentration introduced by such hemorrhage.

GLUCOSE. The normal CSF-glucose concentration is 60 to 70 per cent of that in serum. Decreased CSF-glucose is observed consistently with bacterial infections and may be normal to decreased with viral, fungal, protozoal, and neoplastic diseases. The decrease in glucose occurs because of increased utilization of glucose by bacteria or tissue cells present in CSF.

ENZYMES. Nerve tissue has high activity of CK, LDH, and AST. Changes in CSF activity of these enzymes can occur, not only as a consequence of destruction of nervous tissue, but also will occur when there is a disease that causes increased leakage of blood or plasma into CSF. If there is an increase of serum levels of these enzymes, even a small amount of leakage into the CSF will cause a remarkable increase in CSF activity. In normal animals only a slight increase in CSF enzymes will occur even though there is a massive elevation in serum enzyme activity. If there is an increase in CSF proteins, enzyme increases must be interpreted accordingly. Peripheral blood contamination will increase CSF enzyme activity.

Bovine. The most exhaustive study of CSF alterations in diseases involving the central nervous system of the cow was completed in 1953.[1] Progressive tuberculous meningitis was characterized by CSF that (1) had turbid flakes; (2) exhibited xanthochromia; (3) showed the presence of fibrinous nets; (4) was increased in pressure; (5) contained between 500 and 5000 cells/μl, including lymphocytes, endothelial cells, neutrophils, and histiocytes; (6) had a total protein level between 300 and 1500 mg/dl; (7) showed highly positive results in the Pándy and Nonne-Apelt tests; (8) had a glucose level between 27 and 59 mg/dl; and (9) had chloride values near 650 mg/dl.

CSF removed from animals having purulent meningoencephalitis was usually whitish yellow, contained fibrinous strings, and was turbid, and CSF pressure was normal to slightly elevated. Total neutrophil counts were dramatically increased, being as high as 6000/μl. Total protein values were also elevated, with increases up to 200 mg/dl reported. Bacteriologic examination of the fluid easily established the presence of microorganisms.

In nonpurulent meningoencephalitis and meningomyelitis, the following observations were made[11]: (1) the fluid was usually clear and colorless but occasionally turbid with fibrinous strings; (2) the total cell count varied from 30 to 400 cells/μl and contained up to 30 per cent neutrophils, with the remainder of the cells being lymphocytes and mononuclear cells; (3) glucose levels were as low as 34 mg/dl; and (4) total protein values up to 300 mg/dl were demonstrated.

Diseases causing severe inflammatory reactions in tissues that are in contact with the CSF may result in the escape of blood proteins into the fluid and cause marked reactions in Pándy's tests.[12] However, with bacterial infections that are limited to deep brain tissues, proteins are filtered by surrounding tissues and the Pándy reaction is reduced in intensity or negative. Thus, with listeriosis and other focal bacterial encephalitides, the result in Pándy's test could conceivably be negative or only weakly positive. Lesions that do not affect blood vessel contiguity may not result in a positive Pándy's test result. Examples of such lesions include polioencephalomalacia, coccidial encephalopathy, idiopathic myelopathy, and viral infections.[12] Total cell counts in viral, degenerative, and toxic conditions ranged from less than 25 to 100/μl. Cell counts in listeriosis and streptococcosis ranged between 100 and 200/μl. Mononuclear cells accompanied viral infections, polioencephalomalacia, idiopathic myelopathy, coccidial encephalopathy, and listeriosis.[12] Neutrophils accompany purulent diseases such as thromboembolic meningoencephalitis and encephalitis and meningitis caused by organisms of the genera *Staphylococcus, Corynebacterium,* and *Pseudomonas.*[12]

Porcine. The cerebrospinal fluid in animals experimentally infected with enzootic polioencephalomyelitis was studied.[13] The degree of pleocytosis paralleled the severity of clinical signs. Total cell counts as high as 3000/μl were reported and consisted of mononuclear cells and neutrophils. The total protein levels were increased up to 192 mg/dl. Cerebrospinal fluid from swine with Teschen disease or hog cholera is clear and has a lymphocytic pleocytosis and a marked increase in protein concentration. The degree of pleocytosis paralleled the severity of clinical signs in both diseases.

Equine. In a case of severe purulent basilar meningitis that originated from an alveolar periostitis, the cerebrospinal fluid was turbid, contained blood cells, and had highly positive Pándy and Nonne-Apelt test results. The CSF clotted a short time after collection, and on bacteriologic examination staphylococci were isolated.[1]

Varying results were obtained in studies on horses with encephalopathy.[1] Some of the horses affected with signs of central nervous system disorder had pathologic changes of cerebral edema at autopsy. Cerebrospinal fluids from these animals were clear, had 2 to 4 cells/μl and had a total protein value of 40 to 75 mg/dl. Findings in Pándy's test were positive, and the sugar concentration was 50 to 54 mg/dl. In one animal, xanthochromia and pleocytosis were observed. A slightly elevated cholesterol level (1.2 mg/dl) was present.

In a case of purulent meningitis, the cerebrospinal fluid appeared yellow and stringy and had a cell count of over 1000/μl, most of which were neutrophils; the screening tests for globulin were highly positive; and the glucose level was 27 mg/dl. *Spherophorus necrophorus* and *Staphylococcus aureus* were both isolated on culture.[14]

Canine. Fankhauser[1] divided canine cerebrospinal fluids into three groups as follows:

1. Fluids that have only minor variations in composition, such as a pleocytosis of up to 30 cells/μl with only slightly elevated protein levels. This type of fluid was found in association with serous meningitis, spinal cord trauma from herniated intervertebral protrusion, intraspinal tumors, tetanies, and congenital hydrocephalus.
2. Fluids that have xanthochromia and total protein values of up to 500 mg/dl, with highly positive globulin screening tests. Erythrocytes are present. This type of fluid is usually found in an inflammatory process with endothelial disruption and subsequent diffuse meningeal bleeding.
3. Fluids that are clear or slightly turbid with total cell counts between 30 and 3000/μl. Fibrinous flakes may be present. Total protein levels are increased up to 150 mg/dl, but the glucose level remains unchanged. Such changes are found generally in nonpurulent meningoencephalitides.

In general, disease of the meninges produces greater changes in CSF than do lesions of the parenchyma of the central nervous system. Thus, if neutrophil counts, protein values, and total cell counts are increased, meningitis is most likely present.

The following alterations were reported in cerebrospinal fluid in various clinical conditions of dogs in California[15]:

1. Lymphosarcoma. Pleocytosis was marked, with 1250 cells/μl. These cells were distributed as 81 per cent large mononuclear, 8 per cent small mononuclear, and 11 per cent neutrophils. The total protein level was 57 mg/dl.
2. Brain tumor with spondylitis. Xanthochromia was evident, the total cell count was 55/μl, of which 78 per cent were neutrophils and 22 per cent small and large mononuclear cells. Erythrocytes were present at a concentration of 4800/μl, and the total protein value was 200 mg/dl.
3. Chronic encephalomyelitis. The CSF from a patient with this condition was clear and colorless and had 107 cells/μl, of which 3 per cent were neutrophils and 97 per cent small mononuclear cells. The total protein concentration was 320 mg/dl.
4. Distemper. The CSF was slightly turbid. Leukocytes numbered 17/μl, and were composed of 13 per cent neutrophils and 87 per cent small

mononuclear reels. Erythrocytes were present and numbered 480/μl, and the reaction in Pándy's test was 2+ with a total protein level of 51.3 mg/dl.
5. Hypertrophic spondylitis. The fluid was pink and cloudy and had a xanthochromia. Neutrophils were present at a concentration of 32 cells/μl, erythrocytes numbered 12,000/μl, and the total protein value was 79.8 mg/dl.
6. Chronic disseminated nonsuppurative meningoencephalitis. Cerebrospinal fluid was clear and colorless and had 30 cells/μl, of which 9 per cent were neutrophils and 91 per cent were large mononuclear cells. Erythrocytes were present at a concentration of 24/μl, and the total protein was 51 mg/dl.

CSF of dogs was xanthochromic in cases of icterus resulting from long-standing infections with *Leptospira icterochaemorrhagiae*. The CSF in most experimental cases of leptospirosis was free from pleocytosis and elevation in albumin content.[16]

CSF in association with rabies in the dog has marked alterations. The reaction is primarily that of a meningeal response. A marked pleocytosis with 30 to 1200 cells/μl, 60 to 98 per cent of which were lymphocytes has been recorded.[17]

Cerebrospinal fluid alterations in distemper were studied.[18] In 17 dogs with distemper there was only a slight decrease in glucose levels; however, these animals had elevated CSF total protein and uric acid concentrations. Another paper[19] described the CSF alterations in dogs with distemper. These fluids exhibited the following characteristics: the CSF was clear to opaque, there was an increase in globulin values, the total protein levels increased up to 50 mg/dl, and there were increases in cell counts. In the CSF of animals with distemper the predominant cell types were small lymphocytes, degenerated forms, and large lymphocytes.[20]

Cerebrospinal fluid cytology associated with neurologic disease in the dog has been studied.[5] The authors compared the results of CSF analysis with the results of histopathologic examination of the CNS in 93 dogs. They concluded that CSF examination is a significant aid in obtaining a neurologic diagnosis and that a good correlation exists between CSF alterations and pathologic changes observed in the CNS. CSF examination facilitates the diagnosis of encephalitis and assists in the differentiation between viral and other causes of this disorder. Such examination also aids in the distinction between congenital malformations and congenital degenerative disease. In addition, CSF examination assists in the idenfication of physical spinal cord damage and the differentiation of this condition from muscular, neurogenic, or functional disorders that were clinically presented as spinal ataxia.

In the CSF of all dogs with encephalitis there was a high protein content and a marked pleocytosis. Mitotic figures were occasionally observed in the encephalitides, especially in dogs that had a marked pleocytosis. Pleocytosis in viral infections was due largely to an increase in mononuclear cells. Bacterial and mycotic infections were characterized by an increase in polymorphonuclear cells. Eosinophils were more often seen in nonviral inflammatory diseases, although in one dog with cryptococcosis, eosinophils formed 80 per cent of the cell population. Eighty per cent of the CSF specimens from dogs with canine distemper showed moderate pleocytosis, usually not exceeding 25 cells. The incease in leukocytes was predominantly due to lymphocytes.

In dogs with central nervous system trauma (for the most part spinal cord trauma), the CSF changes were not severe. In spinal cord compressions of a prolonged duration there was a moderately high CSF protein content. There was a slight increase in cell number, and the differential cell count usually showed a high number of neutrophils. There was marked pleocytosis in the CSF of dogs with compression lesions in the cervical area close to the puncture site. Such an observation might indicate that in spinal cord lesions located more caudally, a lumbosacral puncture might be of more value than a traditional occipital puncture. The authors did not feel that it was possible to relate CSF changes to the extent of spinal cord damage; thus the diagnostic and prognostic value of CSF was limited.

Cerebrospinal fluid findings in congenital and degenerative diseases were not constant. The cytologic features of CSF associated with cerebrovascular diseases of the dog included an increase in protein associated with vasculitis, and infarcts. The increase in CSF leukocytes was predominantly mononuclear cells. In dogs with nontraumatic hemorrhage in the CNS, there were many erythrophagocytes.

The cytologic findings in CSF from animals with neoplastic disease of the CNS were not constant. The total protein concentration was slightly increased in most cases, and the total nucleated cell count was variable. Neoplastic cells were demonstrated in dogs with lymphosarcoma.

Feline. The cerebrospinal fluid in cats with cerebellar ataxia varied from normal to a fluid exhibiting marked changes.[1] One cat had a positive Pándy test and a pleocytosis of 2600 cells/μl. In a cat with trauma to the head that resulted in a liquefaction of the hypothalamus, the fluid contained 30,000 erythrocytes/μl, and 358 total leukocytes/μl and reacted positively to the Pándy test. Cerebrospinal fluid samples obtained from two Siamese cats with congenital tremor were found to be normal. Meningeal infections produced by the injection of *Aerobacter aerogenes* resulted in a neutrophil increase of up to 22,400/μl, total protein values up to 1.7 gm/dl.[21]

REFERENCES

1. Fankhouser, R.: Der Liquor cerebrospinalis in der Veterinärmedizin. Zentralbl. Veterinaremed., 1:136, 1953.
2. Mayhew, I.G.: Collection of cerebrospinal fluid from the horse. Cornell Vet., 65:500, 1975.
3. Wilson, J. W., and Stevens, J. B.: Effects of blood contamination on cerebrospinal fluid analysis. J.A.V.M.A., 171:256, 1977.
4. Roszel, J. F.: Membrane filtration of canine and feline cerebrospinal fluid for cytologic evaluation. J.A.V.M.A., 160:720, 1972.
5. Vandervelde, M., and Spano, J. B.: Cerebrospinal fluid in canine neurologic disease. Am. J. Vet. Res., 38:1827, 1977.
6. Mayhew, I.G., and Beal, C. R.: Techniques of analysis of cerebrospinal fluid. Vet. Clin. North Am., 10:155, 1980.
7. Hibbs, C. M., and Coles, E. H.: Transaminases in blood, urine and cerebrospinal fluid of normal and unilaterally nephrectomized dogs. Proc. Soc. Eptl. Biol. Med., 118:1059, 1965.
8. Wilson, J. W.: Clinical application of cerebrospinal fluid creatine phosphokinase determination. J.A.V.M.A., 171:200, 1977.
9. Greene, C. E., and Oliver, J. E., Jr.: Neurologic examination. In *Textbook of Veterinary Internal Medicine. Diseases of the Dog and Cat*, edited by Ettinger, S. J., W. B. Saunders Company, Philadelphia, 1983.
10. Chrisman, C. L.: Cerebrospinal fluid evaluation. In *Current Veterinary Therapy VIII. Small Animal Practice*, edited by Kirk, R. W., W. B. Saunders Company, Philadelphia, 1983.
11. Schmid, G.: Uber Liquorbetunde bei Rindern mit bosartigem Katarrhalfieber. Bull. Schweiz. Akad. Med. Wiss., 9:270, 1953.
12. Howard, J. R.: Neurologic disease differentiation. J.A.V.M.A., 154:1174, 1969.
13. Fischer, K., and Starke, G.: Liquoruntersuchungen bei der Poliomyelitis der Schweine. Exp. Vet. Med., 5:38, 1951.
14. Schultz, J.: Meningitis purulenta beim Pferde. Monatsh. Veterinaermed., 8:165, 1953.
15. Cornelius, C. E.: Canine cerebrospinal fluid. Calif. Vet., 12(2):18, 1958.
16. Monlux, W. S.: Leptospirosis. Rep. N.Y. State Vet. Coll., 27:144, 1949.
17. Durand, P.: Cerebrospinal fluid cytology: Cell counts during animal rabies. Arch. Inst., Pasteur Tunis, 30:55, 1941.
18. Croft, P. G.: Biochemistry of the cerebrospinal fluid of the dog. Vet. Rec., 67:872, 1955.
19. Nigge, K.: Der normale und pathologische Liquor cerebrospinales bei Hund. Inaug. Diss. Giessen, Indexed in Dtsch. Tieraerztl Wochenschr./Tierärztl. Rundschau, 52:50:26, 1944.
20. Bindrich, H., and Schmidt, D.: Liquordiagnostik bei experimenteller Staupe des Hundes. Arch. Exp. Vet. Med., 6:162, 1952.
21. Felton, L. D.: Bull. Johns Hopkins Hosp. 30:241, 1919 quoted by Cornelius, C. E. and Kaneko, J. J., *Clinical Biochemistry of Domestic Animals*, Academic Press, New York, 1963.

16

AVIAN CLINICAL PATHOLOGY

TERRY W. CAMPBELL *and* E. H. COLES

As the number of pet birds has increased, the veterinarian is frequently involved in caring for their health. In order to arrive at a more accurate diagnosis and establish a reasonable regimen of treatment, the veterinarian has begun to use the clinical laboratory. Although there are few controlled studies correlating the pathophysiology of diseased birds and corresponding hematologic and biochemical responses, information has accumulated that may be of value. The following discussion is a summary of some of the information available.

AVIAN HEMATOLOGY

Methods of Blood Collection. As many pet birds are small, one should be familiar with the volume of blood that can be safely removed. The total blood volume in birds varies from 6 to 12 ml/dl of body weight (approximately 10 per cent of body weight).[1] Thus the total blood volume of a 30-gm parakeet would be about 3 ml. A normal healthy bird can lose 10 per cent of its total blood volume without any detrimental effects. Because of the rapid re-establishment of total blood volume, as much as 20 to 30 per cent of the blood volume can be removed without causing too much harm to the patient, but this much is not usually needed. Healthy birds are better able to tolerate blood loss than ill or stressed birds. In sick birds the blood volume collected should be less than 20 per cent of the total blood volume.

Equipment Required. A number of different micro-collection devices can be used. When only a small sample is required it is easiest to collect blood using a Becton-Dickinson I.M.-1 thin-walled needle. This needle makes a 23-gauge puncture but has a 21-gauge lumen. After the needle is inserted into an appropriate vein, blood is collected from the hub of the needle directly into microhematocrit tubes—micro-Nattleson blood collecting tubes (Sherwood Medical Industries, St. Louis, Missouri) or Microtainer tubes (Becton-Dickinson, Rutherford, New Jersey). We have found that collecting blood into EDTA and plain Microtainer capillary blood collection tubes simplifies blood collection (Fig. 16–1). In collecting blood from a vein it is better to permit it to flow through a needle rather than being pulled through a syringe. Hemostasis problems are minimal if this method is used. Blood can also be collected from the needle hub to fill a Unopette pipette (Becton-Dickinson, Rutherford, New Jersey) for total leukocyte or erythrocyte counts. Samples collected by use of microhematocrit tubes separate quickly, and once this has occurred it is difficult to reconstitute the sample. If microhematocrit tubes are utilized, blood can be carefully blown into another container such as a Wintrobe sedimentation tube. Gentle inversion of these tubes will permit adequate mixing of cells and plasma. These tubes can be centrifuged if plasma is required for additional testing. If serum is needed, blood in the microhematocrit tube should be permitted to clot and the sample spun in a microhematocrit centrifuge. Once separation has taken place the tube is broken just above the red cells and both ends of the broken tube containing

TABLE 16–1. Normal Hematology and Serum Chemistry Values for Some Avian Species*

	Parrots	Budgerigars	Cockatiels	Cockatoos	Lovebirds	Macaws
RBC × 10⁶/μl	2.4–4.5	2.5–4.5	2.5–4.7	2.2–4.5	3.0–5.1	2.5–4.5
PCV (%)	43–55	45–57	45–57	40–55	44–57	45–55
Leukocytes × 10³/μl	5–11	3.0–8.0	5–10	5–11	3–8	6–13.5
Heterophils × 10³/μl	1.5–8.3	1.4–5.6	2.0–7.0	2.3–8.3	1.2–6.0	2.7–9.5
Lymphocytes × 10³/μl	1.2–7.2	0.6–3.6	1.3–5.5	1.0–5.5	0.6–4.4	1.2–6.8
Monocytes × 10³/μl	0–0.3	0–0.4	0–0.2	0–0.4	0–0.2	0–0.4
Eosinophils × 10³/μl	0–0.2	0–0.1	0–0.2	0–0.2	0–0.1	0–0.3
Basophils × 10³/μl	0–0.6.6	0–0.44	0–0.6.6	0–0.6	0–0.5	0–0.7
Total Protein (g/dl)	3.0–5.0	2.5–4.5	2.0–5.0	2.0–5.5	2.2–5.1	3–5.05
Glucose (mg/dl)	190–350	200–400	200–450	190–350	200–400	200–350
Calcium (mg/dl)	8.0–13		8.5–13	8.0–13	9.0–15	9.0–13
Potassium (mEq/l)	2.6–4.5		2.5–4.5	2.5–4.5	2.5–3.5	2.5–4.5
Sodium (mEq/l)	134–152		132–150	131–157	137–150	136–155
Uric acid (mg/dl)	4.0–10	4.0–14	3.5–11	3.5–11	3.0–11	2.5–11.5
AST (IU/l)	100–350	150–350	100–350	150–350	100–350	100–280
LDH (IU/l)	150–450	150–450	125–450	225–650	100–350	75–425

*Veterinary Reference Laboratories, Anaheim, California.

serum or plasma are sealed with sealing clay. Several such tubes may be required depending upon the number and types of tests to be performed. Tubes containing plasma or serum should be placed in an empty test tube and the tube stoppered. Samples can then be placed into an appropriate container and forwarded to a laboratory for analysis. Before samples are submitted the veterinarian should check with the reference laboratory to determine what quantity of serum is required for the tests requested.

SITES FOR BLOOD COLLECTION

MEDIAL METATARSAL VEIN. The medial metatarsal vein is found on the lower leg just above the tarsal joint on the medial aspect of the tibiotarsus in front of the Achilles tendon (Fig. 16–2). This vein is the site of choice for blood sampling in most birds. As the vein is surrounded by muscles of the leg, hematoma formation is minimized.[2] A 21- to 25-gauge needle is inserted into the vein and blood collected into a heparinized syringe (large birds only) or a micro-collection tube held to the hub of the needle (Figs. 16–3 and 16–4).

WING VEIN. The cutaneous ulnar or brachial vein (wing vein) crosses the ventral surface of the humeral-radial-ulnar joint (elbow) directly beneath the skin (Fig. 16–5). The vein is penetrated with a 21- to 25-gauge needle and blood collected into a heparinized syringe (large birds only) or a micro-collection tube held to the hub of the needle. A hematoma frequently results from the use of a sy-

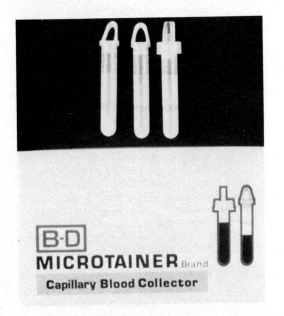

Figure 16–1. These Microtainer capillary blood collectors are routinely used in collecting blood from birds. They are available with several different anticoagulants.

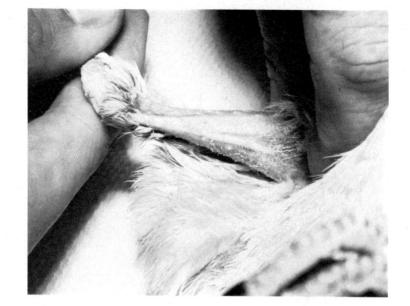

Figure 16–2. The medial metatarsal vein is found on the lower leg just above the tarsal joint on the medial aspect of the tibiotarsus.

ringe but it can be minimized by collecting blood directly into a micro-collection device.

Jugular Vein. The right jugular vein is used because many species of birds have no left jugular vein or only a small one (Fig. 16–6). A featherless tract of skin overlies the right jugular vein in most birds and permits ready location of it. The feathers should be moistened and a 21- to 25-gauge needle used to penetrate the jugular vein. Blood should be collected into a syringe because of the great blood flow and volume. The jugular vein is the site of choice for small birds (e.g., parakeets, canaries, and finches) if a maximum quantity of blood is required. A large hematoma frequently forms because the jugular vein is movable and there is a large subcutaneous space at this site.

Toenail Clipping. Many veterinarians prefer clipping a toenail for the collection of blood. The toenail is cleaned and cut back into the quick, which will allow blood to flow freely from the toe. If blood does not flow freely, do not "milk" blood from the nail because this will have a significant effect on cell population in the blood sample.[2] Hemostasis is accomplished by applying silver nitrate or Monsel's solution to the cut nail. It has been our observation that this method can be painful and result in permanent damage to the nail. In addition, the crushing action used to cut the nail may contaminate the blood with variable amounts of tissue fluid. This method of blood collection is not recommended unless all other methods of collection are impossible.

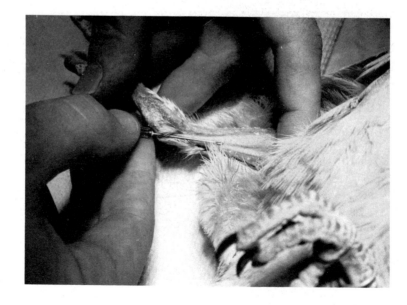

Figure 16–3. A hypodermic needle is inserted into the medial metatarsal vein and blood is collected as it flows from the hub of the needle. Permitting blood to flow freely minimizes hematoma development. Hematomas frequently occur when blood is collected using a syringe.

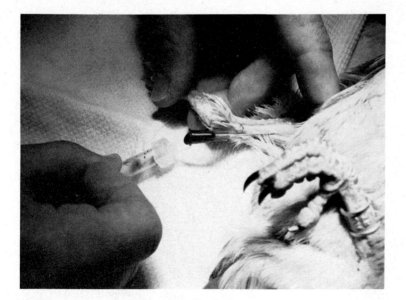

Figure 16–4. A Microtainer tube (Becton-Dickinson Co., Rutherford, N.J.) is used to collect the blood.

SKIN PUNCTURE. This technique is used on small birds with vessels too small for venipuncture. The skin overlying the vessel to be punctured is cleaned with an alcohol swab and allowed to dry. The vessel is punctured through the skin using a sharp needle or scalpel blade. Blood is collected as it leaves the puncture site. Commonly used vessels include the wing vein, medial metatarsal vein, and the external thoracic vein, which runs dorsally on either side of the rib cage just behind the shoulder.[3]

HEART BLEEDING. This method should be reserved for obtaining blood prior to necropsy as it is extremely dangerous and stressful to the bird. The heart may be approached anteriorly by inserting the needle along the ventral floor of the thoracic inlet, being careful to avoid the crop. The needle is inserted near the V formed by the furcula and directed toward the dorsum of the bird as it is passed caudally toward the heart. Once the heart is penetrated, its vibration can be felt and aspiration results in a rush of blood into the syringe. A lateral approach can also be used. The bird is positioned in lateral recumbency and the needle, with syringe attached, is inserted in the fourth intercostal space near the sternum. The heart can usually be located by digital palpation.

OCCIPITAL VENOUS SINUS. The venous occipital sinus is located at the junction of the dorsal base of the skull and the first cervical vertebra (atlas).[4] This procedure is useful in birds weighing 400 gm or more. Evacuated glass tubes with appropriate needles (usually 22 gauge) and needle holders are used. The space between the skull and atlas is

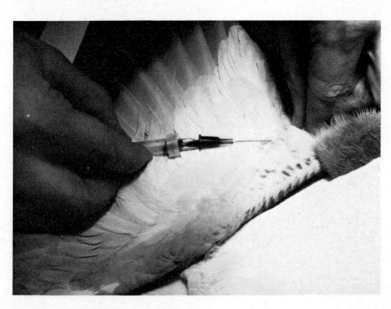

Figure 16–5. The cutaneous ulnar or brachial (wing) vein is a commonly used site for blood collection in birds. This vein crosses the ventral surface of the elbow directly beneath the skin.

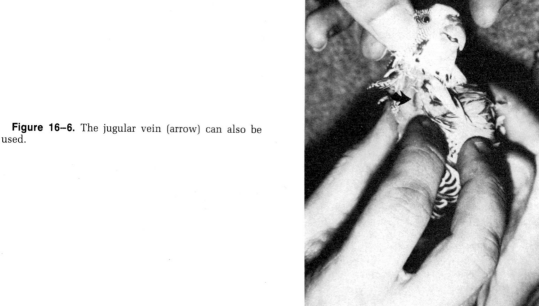

Figure 16–6. The jugular vein (arrow) can also be used.

located by digital palpation while the bird's head is flexed and held in a straight line with the cervical vertebrae. As soon as the skin is penetrated, the rubber stopper of the evacuated tube is perforated and the needle slowly advanced until the sinus is reached. Penetration of the sinus will result in a rapid flow of blood into the tube. This procedure has been successfully used with large raptorial birds, ducks, geese, and chickens. A 0.5 per cent fatality has been experienced using this technique in pigeons. This method of blood collection should be reserved for birds to be necropsied.

AVIAN VS. MAMMALIAN HEMATOLOGY

Although mammalian and avian hematology are similar in many ways, there are differences that must be considered. The important differences are:

1. Birds have nucleated mature erythrocytes.
2. Birds have nucleated thrombocytes instead of platelets.
3. Birds have heterophils instead of neutrophils.
4. Birds do not have a storage spleen so that splenic contraction does not cause an increase in erythrocyte parameters.[1]
5. The initial pathways for blood coagulation in birds are different from those in mammals.[1,5]

The avian system relies primarily on the extrinsic pathways.
6. Avian blood has a lower concentration of plasma albumin than mammalian blood.

AVIAN ERYTHROCYTES

PACKED CELL VOLUME. The quickest and most practical method of establishing the status of a bird's erythron is to do a microhematocrit determination. Most caged birds have a PCV of 35 to 55 per cent. A PCV less than 35 per cent indicates anemia, while one greater than 55 suggests dehydration. Hemoconcentration is also associated with hypothermia. Birds respond to hypoxia by increasing PCV and total erythrocyte counts. In an acute response to hypoxia, PCV's of 60 to 80 per cent can sometimes be observed.

TOTAL ERYTHROCYTE COUNT. A total RBC count can be completed using an electronic particle counter or by use of a hemacytometer. The erythrocyte Unopette (Becton Dickinson, Rutherford, New Jersey) is the best method for preparing a dilution for total RBC counting. Many factors influence the total erythrocyte count in birds. The count may vary among individual birds of the same species as well as among birds of different species. The number of erythrocytes varies with age, sex, hormonal influence, hypoxia, and environment. Generally the RBC count and PCV increase with age and are higher in males than in females.[5] Estrogens decrease erythrocyte counts and PCV while androgens and thyroxine have an erythropoietic effect.[1] The total erythrocyte count is also affected by season, time of day, environmental temperature, and laying cycle. Because of these variations, a total erythrocyte count has its greatest value for following the course of disease in a single animal.

Erythropoiesis takes place in the yolk sac and secondarily in the marrow in the embryo; in the adult bird central erythropoiesis occurs in the lumen of the medullary sinuses of the bone marrow.[5] Peripheral erythropoiesis occurs in young chickens but is more extensively observed in some species of wild birds.[5] New erythrocytes can also arise directly as nuclear membrane buds from young mature circulating erythrocytes. These clone cells are most frequently seen in the blood of recently hatched birds.[5]

HEMOGLOBIN. Hemoglobin can be measured by the same methods used for mammalian blood, but because avian erythrocytes are nucleated the lysed cell solutions must be centrifuged to remove the nuclei. The red blood cell indices (MCV, MCHC and MCH) can be calculated using standard formulas (see Chapter 2).

RETICULOCYTES. A reticulocyte count is completed using vital stains just as it is in mammalian species. Reticulocytes of birds resemble late polychromatophilic erythrocytes and have a cytoplasm that appears mature. These cells contain residual cytoplasmic RNA that appears as dark clumps in the cytoplasm of cells stained with a vital stain. Most avian erythrocytes contain dark clumps when stained in this fashion; it has been suggested that only cells with five or more clumps should be counted as reticulocytes.[6] Others have suggested that only those erythrocytes with a complete reticulum ring around the nucleus should be counted as reticulocytes.[7] There is less nuclear chromatin condensation in reticulocytes than in mature erythrocytes. Reticulocytes represent 10 per cent or less of the total erythrocyte count in adult psittacine birds. As many as 7 to 20 per cent reticulocytes and 20 per cent reticulocytes have been reported in chickens and ducks, respectively.[5]

ERYTHROCYTE MORPHOLOGY. The stem cell for erythrocytes is the rubriblast (erythroblast), which is a large round cell with more cytoplasm in relation to its nucleus than in most blast cells.[8] It has a basophilic cytoplasm with mitochondrial spaces and the nucleus is round with coarse clumped chromatin and a large nucleolus. Prorubricytes resemble rubriblasts, but the nuclear nucleolar rings are indistinct or absent. Rubricytes or polychromatophilic erythrocytes can be divided into three groups: (1) the basophilic rubricyte (early polychromatophilic erythrocyte) is a round cell that is smaller than the erythroblast and has a basophilic homogeneous cytoplasm and a nucleus with clumped chromatin. (2) The early polychromatophilic rubricyte (middle polychromatophilic erythrocyte) is also round, smaller than its precursor, and has a gray (basophilic to slightly eosinophilic) cytoplasm. The nucleus is round, small in relation to its cytoplasm, and has clumped chromatin. (3) The late polychromatophilic rubricyte (late polychromatic erythrocyte) is a round to slightly oval cell with a cytoplasm of variable color but is more eosinophilic than its precursor. The nucleus is round or slightly oval and has irregularly clumped chromatin.

Peripheral blood smears often have as many as 1 to 5 per cent basophilic erythrocytes (polychromatic cells); these will increase dramatically with a regenerative anemia (Plate 16–1A).

The mature erythrocyte is an oval cell with an oval centrally placed nucleus. The nucleus has a uniform network of chromatin clumps while the cytoplasm is orange-pink with a uniform texture. Two types of erythrocyte nuclei have been described.[8] The leptochromatic type is oval with fine chromatin strands but no massive chromatin clumps and the pachychromatic erythrocyte, which is elongated and has thick chromatin strands with dense chromatin clumps. Nuclear appearance varies with cell age, becoming more condensed and darker staining as it ages. The nuclear hemoglobin is dispersed among the chromatin particles and is continuous with cytoplasmic hemoglobin at the nuclear pores.

Erythrocyte life span varies among species of birds just as it does among mammals. The erythrocyte life span for chickens is 28 to 35 days, for ducks 42 days, for pigeons 35 to 45 days, and for quail 33 to 35 days.[1] The short life span in comparison to mammals is due partly to high body temperature and metabolic rate of the bird. Developmental stages of erythrocytes are common in the circulating blood of birds and if present are not considered pathologic. Polychromatophilic erythrocytes are common. Variations from the typical erythrocyte are occasionally seen in the peripheral blood. The cell shape may range from round to elongated or irregular. The nucleus may vary in its location within the cell and have indentations, constrictions, or protrusions. Perinuclear rings are considered artifacts. In anemic birds, spherical forms with oval nuclei are often seen. Anucleate cytoplasmic fragments, called erythroplastids, are occasionally present. Nuclear abnormalities are sometimes observed and include achromatic bands and chromophobic streaks. Achromatic bands result when the nucleus fractures and the two portions pull away from each other. Chromophobic streaks in the nucleus represent chromatolysis. Smudge cells are commonly seen in avian blood films. Their numbers can be minimized by using the coverglass method for preparation of the blood film (see Chapter 3).

ANEMIA

Anemia in birds (a PCV less than 35 per cent) can result from hemorrhage, increased erythrocyte destruction, or decreased erythrocyte production. Most hemorrhagic anemias result from traumatic lesions. Blood loss can occur in association with blood-sucking ectoparasites, in coagulopathies, as a consequence of gastrointestinal parasitism, or in association with organic lesions such as an ulcerated neoplasm, gastric ulcer, and hepatic or renal rupture. Shock and stress may result in hemorrhage into the gastrointestinal tract.

Increased erythrocyte destruction may occur as a result of erythrocyte lysis. Certain blood parasites such as *Plasmodium* and *Aegyptionella* will cause RBC destruction. Hemolytic anemias may result from aflatoxicosis or toxic chemicals. Heinz body anemias have been reported after ingestion of some toxic plants (members of the mustard family) and with petroleum toxicity.[9]

Birds suffering from an infectious process seem to develop an anemia more easily than do mammals.[10] This may be related to the short life span of normal avian erythrocytes. Because of the short erythrocyte life span, a higher percentage of erythrocytes are destroyed on a daily basis than in mammals. If there is depression of erythropoiesis associated with infection, the effects of depression appear earlier in the disease than they do in mammals. A number of chronic infections such as tuberculosis, chlamydiosis, aspergillosis, and chronic liver disease produce a nonregenerative anemia. Nutritional deficiencies (iron and folic acid) will also decrease erythrocyte production. Some antibiotics such as chloramphenicol as well as toxins such as lead and aflatoxins depress erythropoiesis. Erythropoietic depression is seen in association with the avian leukosis complex. Chronic renal disease produces a nonregenerative anemia as it does in mammals.

Regenerative anemias are characterized by the appearance of polychromasia, macrocytosis, and anisocytosis. Reticulocytosis accompanies regenerative anemias.

LEUKOCYTES

Total Leukocyte Counts. The presence of nucleated erythrocytes precludes the use of common lysing solutions or electronic particle counters for determining the total leukocyte counts in birds. An indirect method for determining the total leukocyte count in avian blood eliminates some of the problems that have been encountered in the past.

The indirect method involves use of the eosinophil Unopette 5877 (Becton-Dickinson, Rutherford, New Jersey). The procedure is as follows:

1. Fill the Unopette pipette with blood.
2. Mix the blood with the phloxine B diluent and use the mixture to fill both chambers of an improved Neubauer hemacytometer.
3. Permit the loaded hemacytometer to stand for five minutes. Do not allow the hemacytometer to stand in the open longer than five minutes as the erythrocytes will stain and make counting difficult. A loaded hemacytometer can be held in a humidified chamber for several hours.
4. Count all granulocytes in both sides of the hemacytometer chamber. Only round cells that are distinctly red-orange and refractile are counted.
5. Complete a leukocyte differential count and calculate the per cent of heterophils + eosinophils.
6. Calculate the total count using the formula:

Total WBC/μl

$$= \frac{\text{Number of cells stained in chamber} \times 1.1 \times 16}{\text{Per cent heterophils} + \text{eosinophils}/100}$$

For example: You count 500 granulocytes in the 18 squares on both sides of the hemacytometer and a differential cell count reveals a total of 50 per cent heterophils + eosinophils. The formula would then be:

Total WBC/μl

$$= \frac{500 \times 1.1 \times 16}{50/100} = \frac{8,800}{.50} = 17,600 \text{ WBC}/\mu\text{l}$$

The accuracy of this method for estimating total leukocyte counts in birds depends on several factors. First, the cells must not be allowed to stand exposed to the diluent too long or erythrocytes will begin to take up the stain and cannot be easily differentiated from leukocytes. Care must be taken to count only the distinctly red-orange refractile cells. As the total count is also dependent upon the accuracy of the differential count, care must be taken to make sure that the blood film examined had good cell distribution and that the differential count is completed in an accurate fashion. If all of these factors are carefully controlled, relatively accurate and reproducible total leukocyte counts can be achieved.

Crude estimations of leukocyte counts can also be made from a well-prepared peripheral blood film, just as can be done with mammalian blood (see Chapter 3). The average number of leukocytes per five oil immersion fields is calculated and the following formula used to estimate total WBC count:

Estimated WBC/μl

$$= \frac{\text{Average No. WBC/5 fields}}{1000} \times 3,500,000$$

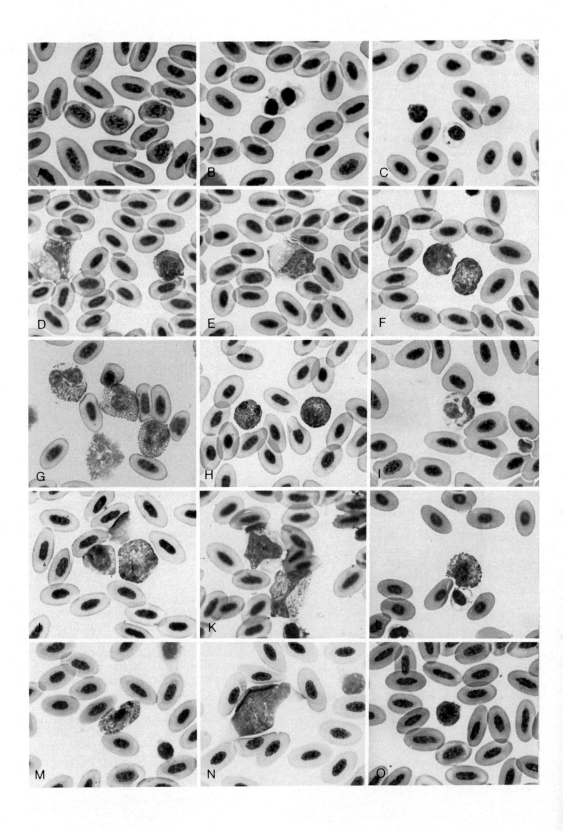

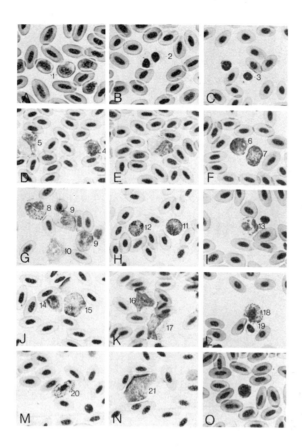

Plate 16–1 Key

A. Polychromatic erythrocytes (1) have a more basophilic cytoplasm and vesicular nucleus than the mature erythrocyte.

B. Avian thrombocytes (2) are nucleated cells that tend to clump in a blood smear.

C. Mature avian thrombocytes (3) have a densely clumped nuclear chromatin and a clear nonhomogeneous cytoplasm (reticulated appearance) that may contain red granules. The small mature lymphocyte contains clumped nuclear chromatin that is not as dense as the thrombocyte and a scant blue homogeneous cytoplasm.

D. Reactive lymphocytes (4) have a high nuclear to cytoplasm ratio but more abundant basophilic cytoplasm than the nonreactive lymphocyte. Monocytes (5) have an abundant blue-gray cytoplasm that is often vacuolated and a delicate reticular nuclear chromatin.

E. Avian monocytes may show occasional clumping of the nuclear chromatin but it is not as dense as in the lymphocyte.

F. Monocyte (6) nuclei are variable in shape and can be round to lobed. Heterophils (7) have a lobed nucleus with condensed chromatin and eosinophilic rod-shaped granules.

G. The cytoplasm of normal heterophils is colorless (8) whereas the cytoplasm of eosinophils (9) is a pale clear blue. Eosinophils usually have spherical granules that stain a dull red. The amorphous eosinophilic cellular debris (10) is a smudge cell. Such cells are commonly found in avian blood films.

H. Heterophil myelocytes (11) are round cells with a light blue cytoplasm and less than half the definitive number of mature heterophil granules. Primary granules and rings are present and the nucleus is round to oval with condensed chromatin. The presence of heterophil myelocytes and metamyelocytes indicates a left shift. (12) Mature heterophil.

I. This is a toxic heterophil (13). Toxic changes include a gray to blue cytoplasm, partial or total degranulation, cytoplasmic vacuolation, dark cytoplasmic (toxic) granules, and karyolysis.

J. A reactive lymphocyte (14) and a 2+ toxic heterophil (15).

K. A monocyte (16) and a 2+ toxic heterophil (17).

L. Avian basophils (18) have strongly basophilic cytoplasmic granules and usually a round to oval nucleus. A thrombocyte can be found just below the basophil (19).

M. The erythrocyte in the center contains a *Haemoproteus* gametocyte (20).

N. The large organism (21) is a *Leukocytozoon.*

O. A late polychromatic rubricyte that should not be confused with a lymphocyte.

The number 1000 is the average number of erythrocytes in five oil immersion fields and 3,500,000 the number of erythrocytes per μl in birds with a normal packed cell volume. For example: You count 30 leukocytes in 30 adjacent oil immersion fields in a monolayer of a blood film. This means that there was an average of five leukocytes per five fields. This is then placed in the formula as

Estimated WBC/μl

$$= \frac{5}{1000} \times 3,500,000 = 17,500$$

It must be remembered that this is a crude estimation of the WBC count and depends on preparation of a good blood film with good distribution of leukocytes and a normal PCV. If the PCV is outside the normal range of 40 to 55 per cent, the estimated total count can be corrected for packed cell volume as outlined in Chapter 3 using the formula

Corrected WBC/μl

$$= \text{Estimated total WBC} \times \frac{\text{Observed PCV}}{\text{Normal PCV (47.7)}}$$

This method can be used to estimate total leukocyte counts without doing a direct total count or may be used as a check on previously done counts if they appear to be erroneous as one scans the differential blood film.

Although there are problems associated with any method of determining the total leukocyte count in birds, if one technique is selected and used consistently, a sufficient degree of accuracy can be developed so that the clinician is confident of the results.

Differential Leukocyte Counts. A blood film for differential leukocyte count on bird blood is prepared in the same fashion as it is for mammals (see Chapter 3). The coverglass method is preferred as there are fewer smudge cells. Romanowsky stains (Wright's, Giemsa, or May-Grunwald) are preferred but quick dipstains can be used. Heparinized blood samples should not be used, because poor staining quality will result. Blood smears should be prepared from fresh blood, although EDTA can be used. Before beginning a differential count, it is wise to examine the film for distribution of leukocytes. This should be done by first examining the margins and feathered edges of the blood film. If there is poor leukocyte distribution on the slide, it will be reflected by the appearance of many leukocytes in these two areas.

GRANULOCYTES

Heterophils. Heterophils are the avian equivalent of the mammalian neutrophils. They go through similar developmental stages beginning with the myeloblast (granuloblast), which is a large round cell with a narrow rim of intensely basophilic cytoplasm. There are no specific cytoplasmic granules; therefore this stage is common to all granulocytes. The nucleus has a delicate reticulum-chromatin pattern. The next stage of development is the progranulocyte (promyelocyte or metagranuloblast), which is a round cell with a light blue cytoplasm, dark magenta granules and rings (suggestive of heterophils), and orange spheres (primary granules). The nucleus has a delicate reticular chromatin and there is an indistinct boundary between the nucleus and cytoplasm. The next stage is the myelocyte (mesomyelocyte), which resembles the progranulocyte but has a condensed nuclear chromatin. A few primary cytoplasmic granules and typical heterophil rod-shaped granules (less than half the definitive number) begin to appear. Next follows the heterophil metamyelocyte; this is smaller than its precursor and contains eosinophilic rod-shaped granules (greater than half the definitive number). The nucleus of this cell is typically bean-shaped and has condensed chromatin. The band heterophil nucleus is elongated and has parallel sides, the cytoplasm is filled with eosinophilic rod-shaped granules, and the nuclear chromatin is condensed. The mature heterophil has many eosinophilic cytoplasmic rod-shaped granules and a lobed nucleus with condensed chromatin (Plate 16–1G).

Immature heterophils are rarely seen in the blood of birds and if seen represent a poor prognosis. Heterophils can exhibit toxic granulation as seen in mammalian neutrophils with partial or total degranulation. Toxicity is indicated by cytoplasmic basophilia, vacuolization, and degranulation. Severe toxic heterophils show karyolysis or karyorrhexis. Degrees of toxicity are reported on a scale of plus one to plus four.

Heterophils of some avian species may be difficult to differentiate from eosinophils.

Eosinophils. Eosinophils are round with a tendency toward irregular or oval shapes. They are variable in size (from 4 to 11 μ) on the same blood smear. The eosinophil cytoplasm is a clear, pale blue in contrast to the heterophil cytoplasm, which is colorless. In most species eosinophil granules are spherical, relatively large, and stain a dull red. These granules often stain uniformly, are homogeneous and refractile, and are evenly distributed throughout the cytoplasm. The nucleus of the eosinophil usually stains bluer than does that of the heterophil.

The eosinophil goes through the same stages of development as the heterophil with the typical eosinophilic granules first appearing in the eosinophil myelocyte. The eosinophil progranulocyte contains only orange primary granules and lacks the magenta granules and rings found in the heterophil progranulocyte.

Basophils. In some species of birds basophils are more numerous than are eosinophils.[8] The basophil progranulocyte has magenta bodies with less tendency for ring formation. The normal mature basophil is slightly smaller than the heterophil, and has a colorless cytoplasm containing strongly basophilic granules (Plate 16–1L). The nucleus is typically round, centrally located, and often hidden by cytoplasmic granules.

Lymphocytes. Difficulty may be encountered in differentiating between lymphocytes and monocytes. To further complicate matters, some small lymphocytes are difficult to distinguish from thrombocytes (Plate 16–1C).

The lymphocyte series begins with the lymphoblast, which is a large round cell with a narrow rim of dark blue cytoplasm. The nucleus has a fine reticular chromatin pattern and usually one nucleolus. The prolymphocyte resembles the lymphoblast but does not contain a nucleolus. Mature lymphocytes have a high ratio of nucleus to cytoplasm and a condensed chromatin pattern that may or may not be in large clumps.

In some birds lymphocytes are the most frequently occurring leukocyte. Lymphocytes can be divided into three groups according to cell size. Small (less than 7.8 μ), medium (7.9 to 10.3 μ) and large lymphocytes (greater than 10.4 μ) have been identified.[8] Most normal mature lymphocytes in peripheral blood are small or medium, while large lymphocytes are more likely immature cells and are infrequent in healthy birds. Lymphocytes occur in a variety of shapes varying from uniformly round or irregular to those that seem to mold around adjacent cells in the blood film or have cytoplasmic budding. The cytoplasm can be homogeneous or granular. The granular cytoplasm contains some flocculations of basophilic material. The lymphocyte cytoplasm is usually weakly basophilic and homogeneous. The quantity of cytoplasm varies from a narrow rim in small lymphocytes to a moderately wide band in medium lymphocytes. The nucleus is usually centrally placed, round, and sometimes indented. Indentations are not deep and lymphocyte margins move inward to a sharp angle in contrast to monocyte margins, which form a round base. The nucleus has dense chromatin clumping. The nucleoplasm is usually colorless in lymphocytes that have a delicate reticular chromatin pattern and dark in those that have dense chromatin clumping. Lymphocytes sometimes contain intensely staining spheres called azurophilic granules. Such cells are considered abnormal.[8] Cytoplasmic vacuolization sometimes occurs and is always considered to be an abnormality.

Monocytes. The developmental sequence of the monocyte includes the monoblast (not well defined), early promonocytes, late promonocytes, and mature monocytes.

Monocytes are larger than lymphocytes and usually are larger than heterophils. They are round or slightly irregular in shape and have more cytoplasm that lymphocytes. Cytoplasmic blebs or molding between adjacent cells on the smear may be seen. The cytoplasm stains blue-gray with a homogeneous "ground-glass" appearance and is often vacuolated. The cytoplasm may have two distinct zones.[8] The outer hyaline mantle is a light-staining area where the inner portion of the cytoplasm stains more deeply. The cytoplasm may have azurophilic granules or an azurophilic tinge of reticulum characterized by fine dust-like particles scattered throughout the cytoplasm. The nucleus has delicate lace-like reticular chromatin with a transparent nucleoplasm (Plate 16–1D). Chromatin clumps may be present (Plate 16–1E). The nucleus is usually eccentrically located in the cell and can be round, elongated, bean-shaped, or bilobed.

EVALUATION OF THE LEUKOGRAM

The usefulness of leukocyte counts in avian medicine is subject to controversy because of technical errors in counting and factors such as age, sex, environmental temperature, nutritional status, and the degree of stress that influence results. These variations have caused some veterinarians to question the usefulness of leukocyte counts.[1]

When the hemacytometer method for enumerating leukocytes is used, the sources of counting error include blood sampling technique, cell distribution on the hemacytometer, improper equipment calibration, cell distribution on the blood film, improper white blood cell differentiation, and technical error by the technician.

In spite of these problems, the effect that these errors have on total cell counts can be minimized with experience. The degree of technical error can be evaluated by completing multiple determinations on a single sample and calculating the mean, standard deviation, and confidence intervals.

Until recently, "normal reference values" for various avian species have not been available, making interpretation of a leukogram difficult. As improved techniques became available and somewhat standardized from laboratory to laboratory, baseline values for many species have been established. Through utilization of these "normals," avian hematology can be diagnostically useful.

Repeated sampling is often necessary when evaluating avian leukograms as there are wide variations between normal individuals of the same species and with repeated samplings from the same bird. Young birds generally have lower leukocyte counts than adults, while birds raised indoors tend to have a lower count than those raised outside. Certain B vitamin deficiencies affect the leukogram. Riboflavin and B_1 deficiencies will increase heterophils and decrease lymphocytes, whereas a folic acid deficiency causes leukopenia and anemia.[1] Glucocorticoid increases, whether endogenous or exogenous, cause leukocytosis, heterophilia, and lymphopenia.

Because of the variations in counts according to age, environment, and daily fluctuations, values from diseased birds must differ greatly from the normal reference value to be considered significant. Abnormal values would fall outside the range of the mean for the species plus or minus two standard deviations.

Leukopenias occur with viremia (usually a mild leukopenia due to a decrease in lymphocytes), overwhelming septicemias, and in birds that have been exposed to toxic drugs or chemicals. Overwhelming septicemias often result in marked heteropenia.

Leukocytosis is seen with acute and chronic inflammatory lesions, mycobacterial disease, pyogenic infections, and with massive tissue necrosis. As with mammals, focal inflammatory lesions (bacterial abscessation) cause a greater leukocytosis than generalized inflammations. Birds respond to bacterial infection with a leukocytosis that includes heterophilia and monocytosis.

Heterophilia occurs in acute and chronic inflammatory diseases. Toxic heterophils may appear with some inflammatory conditions and particularly with those that are septic. Toxic changes are indicated by the presence of cytoplasmic changes that include basophilia, vacuolization, degranulation, and the presence of deeply basophilic granules (toxic granulation) (Plates 16–1I to 16–1K). Severe toxic changes affect the nucleus, causing nuclear degeneration (karyorrhexis) or lysis (karyolysis). If toxic changes become severe, a poor prognosis should be given. A relative increase in heterophils will occur with lymphopenia but in these cases the total heterophil count may be within normal range. Immature heterophils may or may not be present with the appearance of toxic heterophils. If they are present, the prognosis is poor.

Lymphopenias are seen with acute viral diseases and with glucocorticoid excesses. Lymphocytosis suggests chronic viral infections, immune-mediated diseases (not well documented in birds), or lymphoid leukemia, or may occasionally occur in birds that have a high normal lymphocyte count.

Monocytosis is observed in chronic disorders or diseases that result in monocyte chemotaxis such as granulomatous lesions, mycobacterial infections, and chlamydiosis. Eosinophilia suggests parasitic infections, allergic states, or may occur in association with marked tissue damage.

A leukogram can be useful in assessment of the progress of an avian patient. For example, in a bird with a septic inflammatory lesion that resulted in a marked leukocytosis, heterophilia with toxic heterophils, and a lymphopenia, decreasing total leukocyte and heterophil counts with no toxic heterophils and an increasing lymphocyte count indicate a favorable response to therapy.

THROMBOCYTES AND BLOOD COAGULATION

Unlike mammalian platelets, which are cytoplasmic fragments of megakaryocytes, avian thrombocytes arise from mononucleated precursor cells. The thrombocyte series begins with the thromboblast, which is functional in the embryo. This cell is round or ameboid with a narrow rim of basophilic cytoplasm around the nucleus. The nucleus is round, has punctate chromatin, and contains a nucleolus. Embryo thrombocytes are classified according to their size as large, medium, or small. Definitive thrombocytes are classified as early-immature, mid-immature, late-immature, and mature thrombocytes. The early-immature thrombocyte is a large round or oval cell with a basophilic vacuolated cytoplasm and a nucleus with clumped chromatin. The mid-immature thrombocyte is slightly elongated or irregular and has a light blue vacuolated cytoplasm that may contain specific granules. The nucleus shows excessive chromatin clumping. The late-immature thrombocyte is oval and slightly smaller than an erythrocyte. The cytoplasm is pale blue and has vaguely defined rarified areas. The nucleus is usually round with closely packed chromatin clumping, resembling a lymphocyte nucleus. Eosinophilic-specific granules are usually at one pole of the cell.

Changes that occur between the stages of immature thrombocyte include a decreasing ratio of nucleus to cytoplasm, decreasing cytoplasmic basophilia, increasing vacuolation, and increasing density of chromatin clumping. Early-, late-, and mid-immature thrombocytes may be seen occasionally in peripheral blood smears of normal birds. Reactive thrombocytes are considered abnormal and are seen in sick birds. In such cells the cell membrane, which was originally pale blue, begins to turn red or orange and the nucleus of the cell becomes rounded.[8] The latter reaction is indicated by a narrow rim of cytoplasm so that the cell often resembles a lymphocyte. Thrombocytes may also show some disintegration when they are exposed to air.

The usual mature thrombocyte is an oval cell that is smaller and more rounded than the erythrocyte (Plate 16–1B). The nucleus is larger compared with the amount of cytoplasm and more rounded than an erythrocyte nucleus. Thrombocytes vary in size and shape among the various species. The nuclear chromatin is dense and clumped; the cytoplasm is clear but not homogeneous because it may have a reticulated appearance. The cytoplasm may contain one or more red granules at the poles (Plate 16–1C). Thrombocytes often clump in peripheral blood smears, which makes their identification somewhat easier.

Unlike mammalian platelets, avian thrombocytes have little involvement with initiation of clot formation.[5] When blood has been lost, thrombocyte-specific granules break down, thrombocytes clump, their nuclei become pyknotic, and the cells degenerate in the same manner as mammalian platelets.[5] The rate of thrombocyte clumping is much slower than platelet clumping. Avian thrombocytes contain a large quantity of 5-hydroxytryptamine (serotonin) but little thromboplastin.[1,5] Thrombocytes have pseudopods and are constantly moving. They have a phagocytic function, contain acid-phosphatase, and are able to phagocytose bacteria and viruses.

The normal thrombocyte count in most birds is from 20,000 to 30,000/μl of blood. The thrombocyte count can be estimated from a blood smear in a manner similar to that described for estimating a total leukocyte count. An actual thrombocyte count is difficult to achieve, because thrombocytes tend to clump. A subjective estimation of the number of thrombocytes on a blood smear is reported as "normal," "increased," or "decreased." Normally, one should expect to find one or two thrombocytes in an average monolayer oil immersion field. Thrombocytopenias may be seen with severe septicemias, diffuse intravascular coagulation (not well documented in birds), and leukemias.

Avian plasma contains little or no factor IX (thromboplastin), factor XII (Hageman factor), factor V, or factor VII.[1,11] Avian blood coagulation depends on the extrinsic clotting system involving release of tissue thromboplastin. Thus the common and extrinsic pathways of coagulation are more important in birds than the intrinsic system. The extrinsic and common pathways can be evaluated using a one-step prothrombin time (OSPT) test. This involves collecting blood into a tube containing sodium citrate to bind calcium. Blood and sodium citrate must be in the proper ratio (one part of sodium citrate to nine parts of blood). Plasma is collected and a solution containing thromboplastin and calcium added in the proper proportions (see Appendix). The time required for a clot to form is the prothrombin time. Avian brain thromboplastin is required for avian prothrombin time tests because mammalian sources (i.e., commercial rabbit brain thromboplastin) give unreliable results in birds. The normal prothrombin time for most birds is 13 seconds or less. Severe liver disease and any defect in the extrinsic or common system will produce a prolonged prothrombin time.

Capillary clotting time in birds is another test for coagulation. Capillary clotting time for birds is usually less than five minutes. Prolonged clotting times have been reported in psittacine birds with vitamin K-responsive hemorrhagic disorders.[10]

AVIAN CHEMISTRIES

Serum or plasma chemistry is routinely used for the detection of organ disease in domestic mammals. Veterinarians are just beginning to use this tool in the evaluation of avian patients. However, avian clinical chemistry has yet to achieve the same degree of critical evaluation that it has in domestic mammals.

Veterinarians are confronted with the problem of sample size when dealing with avian serum chemistries. The majority of birds seen in veterinary practices are too small to allow collection of the quantity of blood that is used for the routine chemistry profile in mammals. This problem has been somewhat alleviated by the development of accurate microtechniques. Many commercial veterinary reference laboratories now have the capability of performing avian chemistry panels on as little as 0.5 ml of serum. The development of dry reagent and reflectance photometric methods (Seralyzer, Ames Division, Miles Laboratories, Inc., Elkhart, Indiana) offers the avian veterinarian a reliable and clinically meaningful "in-house" serum chemistry capability. The small sample size (10 to 30 μl) required for each test, short testing time, and minimal technical skill needed to operate the instrument makes this a practical approach to avian chemistries.

At the present time the data base needed for accurately evaluating specific organ function in the avian species is not adequate to permit the same depth of discussion provided for mammals elsewhere in this book. Therefore, this section is designed to reflect some of the current knowledge in the hope that veterinarians and investigators will continue their interest in avian clinical pathology and provide sufficient information to permit a continued evaluation of the various tests available.

PROTEIN

The serum protein concentration of avian blood is lower than that of mammals. Most normal birds have serum (or plasma) total protein values between 3 and 6 gm/dl. A rapid estimation of the plasma protein status of the avian patient can be obtained by transferring plasma from a spun microhematocrit tube to a refractometer. A reading less than 3.0 gm/dl usually indicates hypoalbuminemia, because albumin is the largest individual protein fraction in avian plasma. Total protein values less than 2.5 gm/dl indicate a grave prognosis; birds with severe hypoproteinemia rarely survive.[12] Hypoproteinemia can occur with chronic renal or hepatic disease, malnutrition, malabsorption (e.g., intestinal parasitism), or chronic blood loss. Elevated total protein (greater than 6.0 gm/dl) occurs with dehydration or if there is an increase in total globulins. Hyperglobulin-emia may be associated with chronic diseases such as avian tuberculosis, aspergillosis, chlamydiosis, bacterial septicemias, or chronic bacterial infection. Hyperalbuminemia has been associated with pituitary neoplasms that produce an increased level of growth hormone.[13]

Lipemia, hemolysis, and cloudy plasma (plasma with fibrin clots) will artefactually elevate total plasma protein values when a refractometer is used. Therefore, this method is not reliable in measuring plasma proteins under such sample conditions. A total serum protein determination using the biuret method or a serum albumin determination would be indicated whenever lipemia, cloudy plasma, or hemolysis is encountered.

Serum protein fractions can be separated by electrophoresis. A method using a constant voltage of 200 volts, an amperage of 2.5 amps, cellulose polyacetate strips, a separation time of 25 minutes, and measurements using a densitometer has been used for avian serums.[14] Serum electrophoresis shows that albumin is the largest protein fraction in normal avian serum. Avian albumin is similar in structure to mammalian albumin.[15] Albumin binds and transports anions, cations, fatty acids, and thyroid hormones.[16] Seventy-five per cent of the plasma T_4 is attached to albumin (10 per cent is attached to alpha globulins and 15 per cent to prealbumin-2) and 50 per cent of plasma T_3 is associated with albumin (30 to 40 per cent is attached to alpha globulin) in chickens.[11] Therefore, hypoalbuminemia will affect the blood concentration of the albumin-transported compounds.

The globulin component of avian serum protein is composed of separate alpha, beta, and gamma fractions. The alpha globulins include glycoproteins, haptoglobin, ceruloplasmin, and alpha$_2$ macroglobulin.[16] Transcortin, an alpha globulin, is the primary transport protein for corticosterone in chicken plasma.[11] Infections produce marked increases in ceruloplasmin, fibrinogen, and haptoglobin.[11] Therefore, the alpha globulins increase with infections. Alpha globulins increase with tissue destruction such as following surgery or in birds with osteomyelitis and decrease with liver disease, malabsorption, or malnutrition.[16,17] In the domestic fowl, cholecalciferol and 25-hydroxycholecalciferol are carried by the beta globulins.[11] The beta globulins are usually elevated when there is an increase in beta-lipoprotein in chronic infectious diseases.[16] The gamma globulins include the circulating antibodies, which elevate with chronic inflammation. Phosvitin and other phospholipoproteins that transport iron during ovulation also migrate with the gamma globulin fraction.[16] Antibodies may migrate in both the beta and gamma globulin ranges. One study indicated that IgG migrates primarily in the gamma globulin range whereas IgM migrates in the beta globulin range.[17] In the domestic fowl IgA is structurally different from mammalian IgA but has a similar function.[11] Avian IgA is primarily found in external secretions, with only about 4 per cent located in serum.[11] Avian IgG and IgM are comparable to mammalian IgG and IgM.

GLUCOSE

The normal blood glucose level for most birds is 200 to 450 mg/dl, which is much higher than for any mammalian species. Chemical test strips for the determination of blood glucose using a drop of whole blood can provide a rapid estimation of blood glucose levels on a small sample. A pediatric diagnostic test for glucose in whole blood (Chemstrip G, Bio-Dynamics, Indianapolis, Indiana) provides sensitivity to varying glucose levels, ranging from 10 to 800 mg/dl. Such strips should be used as a screening test only because they are not as accurate as serum or plasma glucose assays. Birds with serum glucose concentrations less than 150 mg/dl should be given supplemented feedings with dextrose, and values less than 70 mg/dl are a grave sign.[12] Hypoglycemic convulsions may occur in birds of prey having glucose values less than 80 mg/dl.[18] Hypoglycemia in birds may occur with starvation, malnutrition such as hypovitaminosis A, high protein diets and urea-containing diets, hepatopathies such as acute hepatitis, Pacheco's parrot disease, and chronic liver disease, septicemias, and endocrinopathies.[17-23] Hypovitaminosis A, high protein diets, and urea-containing diets result in hypoglycemia due to malabsorption of glucose from degenerated intestinal brush borders, malreabsorption due to degenerating renal tubules or low glucose-6-phosphatase activity.[19] Small birds become hypoglycemic within 24 hours with starvation, whereas larger birds may maintain normal glucose levels for two to three days.[13] Artefactual hypoglycemia is seen if serum or plasma is left in contact with blood cells, which permits in vitro metabolism of glucose.

Hyperglycemia in birds occurs with stress, iatrogenic glucocorticoid excess, hyperthermia, and diabetes mellitus. Stress produces a borderline hyperglycemia. Migrating ducks have been shown to have an elevated blood glucose when compared with nonmigrating ducks.[24] Geese with lead poisoning have a slight hyperglycemia.[25] Diabetes mellitus in birds is characterized by glucose levels greater than 700 mg/dl.

Noncarnivorous birds have a predominance of alpha cells in their pancreatic islets, suggesting that glucagon rather than insulin is the dominant hormone.[26,27] The pancreas and plasma of noncarnivorous birds contain five to ten times more glucagon than mammals.[28] The pancreas of carnivorous birds resembles that of mammals and contains high levels of insulin.[26,27,29] Total removal of the pancreas of noncarnivorous birds does not alter blood glucose levels significantly and is not associated with hyperglycemia or glucosuria.[30-33] Pancreatectomy in ducks does not alter blood glucose; however, the procedure in great horned owls results in a dramatic hyperglycemia.[30,32] Since insulin is found in small amounts in the pancreas and serum of noncarnivorous birds and is released slowly in response to a high glucose challenge, it is considered to be of minor importance in the carbohydrate metabolism of these birds.[28] The splenic lobe of the pancreas contains a higher concentration of pancreatic islets than does the rest of the gland. Removal of the splenic lobe of the pancreas in noncarnivorous birds results in hypoglycemia due to removal of the majority of the alpha cells and glucagon.[34]

In spite of the observations that insulin seems to play a minor role in the carbohydrate metabolism of noncarnivorous birds, diabetes mellitus has been reported in a variety of caged birds.[12,17,21,35-37] The clinical signs of diabetes mellitus in avian patients include polyuria, polydipsia, polyphagia, and progressive weight loss. These birds often have hepatic fibrosis, necrosis, and lipidosis, but a normal pancreas.[29] Normal birds have a negative or trace urate glucose when examined using urinalysis reagent strips or tablets. Therefore, suspected diabetes in birds can be ruled out with negative urate glucose tests. Diabetic birds often have a four plus urate glucose test.

Treatment and control of the disease in diabetic birds can be difficult. Regular insulin given to birds shows a peak activity in two hours, as indicated by a lowered glucose, and glucose returns to preinjection levels after five hours, whereas NPH insulin activity peeks in 16 hours and glucose levels return to normal in 24 hours.[29] Further investigation is needed in the study of carbohydrate metabolism and diabetes mellitus in caged birds.

Uric Acid

Uric acid is the primary catabolic product of protein, nonprotein nitrogen, and purines in birds. The avian kidney excretes uric acid primarily by tubular excretion, unlike the mammalian system that excretes urea entirely by filtration.[38,39] The clearance of uric acid by tubular secretion surpasses the glomerular filtration by a factor of 8 or higher, representing 80 to 90 per cent of the total excretion.[39,40] The site of uric acid secretion in the nephron of birds has not been determined. In man, filtered uric acid is reabsorbed at the proximal tubule and secreted in the distal nephron, whereas in the dog it is reabsorbed but not secreted (except in the Dalmatian dog, in which reabsorption and secretion occur in the proximal tubule).[39] The rate of uric acid excretion is largely independent of the hydration status and rate of urine flow in birds.[40] The rate of uric acid excretion is primarily influenced by the plasma uric acid concentration and renal portal blood flow.[39,40] A bird in normal nitrogen and acid-base balance will excrete approximately 80 per cent of the total nitrogen as uric acid, 15 per cent as ammonia, and 1 to 10 per cent as urea.[40]

The normal blood uric acid value for most birds is 2 to 15 mg/dl. Uric acid values greater than 20 mg/dl are considered elevated. Hyperuricemia in birds occurs with starvation, gout (visceral and articular), massive tissue destruction, and renal disease.[16,18,19,21,35,39,42-44] Nephrocalcinosis due to high levels of dietary calcium or hypervitaminosis D_3 will result in an elevated blood uric acid level.[41] Plasma uric acid increases with loss of two thirds of the functional renal mass in birds.[45] Hyperuricemia due to renal disease is the result of decreased rate of tubular excretion plus the poor nutritional status, which increases uric acid production as body proteins are degraded.[42] Nephrotoxic drugs such as aminoglycoside antibiotics cause tubular necrosis, resulting in high serum uric acid levels. Hypovitaminosis A causes impaired renal function and is accompanied by hyperuricemia.[19] Diets high in protein and urea will elevate serum uric acid due to an increase in uric acid biosynthesis.[19] Blood uric acid is elevated with retroperistaltic movement of urates from the cloaca into the large intestine, where reabsorption can occur.[46] Excess ammonia absorption from the large intestine can elevate serum uric acid.[19] Renal neoplasms have also been associated with hyperuricemia.[12,21] Serum uric acid may be artefactually increased if the toenail clip method of blood collection is used and the nail is not properly cleaned of urates from the bird's droppings. Urates clinging to the toenail may contaminate the specimen.

Urea Nitrogen

Birds are uricotelic and produce uric acid as the major nitrogenous end product of metabolism, whereas mammals are ureotelic and produce primarily urea as the end product of nitrogen metabolism. Therefore, blood urea nitrogen is not a useful test of renal function in birds. Studies of birds of prey indicate that the blood urea nitrogen level will become elevated only after major kidney damage.[44] These birds are probably exposed to higher levels of dietary urea than are noncarnivorous birds and excrete absorbed urea through their kidneys. Poultry fed high urea-containing diets will show increased levels of blood urea nitrogen.[19]

CREATININE

Creatinine is not a major nonprotein nitrogen component of avian blood. Avian urine contains very little creatinine but much more creatine.[47] Therefore serum creatinine has questionable value in the evaluation of renal function in birds. A study with red-tailed hawks showed a lack of elevation in serum creatinine with severe renal tubular necrosis.[48] Other investigators think that serum creatinine may become elevated in birds with renal failure, but less reliably than uric acid.[17,18] The normal serum creatinine for most birds is 0.5 to 1.5 mg/dl.[18,21,49] High serum creatinine values may be seen in psittacine birds fed high levels of animal protein.[21]

CHOLESTEROL AND FATTY ACIDS

Lipids in avian blood are similar in quantity and quality to those of mammals.[50] Circulating lipids are derived from intestinal absorption of dietary lipids, hepatic synthesis, or mobilization from fat deposits. Dietary lipids absorbed from the intestines enter the systemic circulation via the portal vein as very low density lipoproteins (VLDL), whereas mammals use a more highly developed lymphatic system and transport dietary lipid in larger particles (chylomicra).[11] Plasma lipids are classified as neutral fats (triglycerides), phospholipids, cholesterol esters, free fatty acids, and fat-soluble compounds such as the fat-soluble vitamins.

Cholesterol levels in avian blood are affected by age, heredity, nutrition, and various diseases.[50] The normal serum cholesterol value for most birds is 100 to 200 mg/dl.[18,22,42] Hypercholesterolemia has been associated with starvation, high levels of dietary fat, hypothyroidism, and liver disease.[18,50,51] Increases in serum cholesterol have also been reported in birds with xanthomatosis, a condition in which cholesterol is deposited in the skin.[17] Low serum cholesterol has been associated with bacterial septicemias and liver disease.[17,22,49] A decrease in serum cholesterol and total lipids occurs in domestic fowl with *Borrelia anserina* infections. This occurs because of decreased intestinal absorption due to enteritis or decreased hepatogenic lipogenic activity.[42] Free fatty acid levels in the blood of young chicks will be elevated following starvation.[52] Lead poisoning in geese causes a decrease in plasma free fatty acids.[25] Iron deficiency anemia in chickens is accompanied by hyperlipidemia due to reduction of lipoprotein lipase activity, which is required for lipid deposition in adipose tissue.[53]

BILIRUBIN AND BILIVERDIN

It is generally considered that biliverdin is the primary end product of heme catabolism and the principal bile pigment of the domestic fowl.[54–56] Biliverdin is excreted into the bile as a bile acid complex of sodium biliverdinate in chickens and turkeys.[55] Birds lack the enzyme biliverdin reductase needed to reduce biliverdin to bilirubin.[57,58] Therefore, bilirubin accounts for only a small percentage of the total bile pigment in birds that have been studied.

Little, if any, biliverdin or bilirubin is detectable in the plasma of normal birds. In one study using chickens, biliverdin and bilirubin were found in nearly equal concentrations in gallbladder bile. Bile obtained from the hepatoenteric duct had 70 per cent more bilirubin than biliverdin.[59] Ligation of one bile duct was followed by no hyperbiliverdinemia and slight hyperbilirubinemia. Ligation of both ducts resulted in a trace hyperbiliverdinemia and a distinct hyperbilirubinemia (50 per cent direct reading). Avian bile bilirubin resembles canine bilirubin diglucuronide. This study suggested that either biliverdin formation occurs extrahepatically or biliverdin from the liver bile canaliculi is reduced to bilirubin in the extrahepatic biliary system in the chicken.

Total bilirubin in the serum of birds of prey increases following severe hemolytic disorders.[18] Therefore, elevation of serum bilirubin may occur with biliary obstruction or intravasular hemolysis in carnivorous birds. Clinical icterus is rare in psittacine birds, and plasma bilirubin determinations have not been useful in detecting liver disease in these birds. Psittacine birds with severe liver damage or suffering from starvation frequently have a greenish discoloration to their serum and urates. This is considered to be a consequence of hyperbiliverdinemia and biliverdinuria, as biliverdin is green. Occasionally, psittacine birds with chronic liver disease will have icteric-appearing tissues; this may be caused by nonspecific reduction of biliverdin to bilirubin. It should be emphasized that many normal birds have yellow plasma that results from dietary carotene pigment and not bilirubin.

SERUM ENZYMES

Research has provided some information concerning enzyme activities of various avian tissues involving a large number of avian species. Enzyme activities vary greatly among tissues and species of birds. It is important to realize that the activity of a particular enzyme may be high in one organ or tissue, or even specific for that tissue, but if it does not change significantly in the blood when that tissue is damaged, it has little clinical significance. A specific enzyme may have a high concentration per gram of an organ; however, if the organ is small, a serum increase may reflect damage to another organ with less activity per gram of tissue but a much greater total mass. Care must be taken in interpreting serum enzyme activity. Before significance can be given to increased serum enzyme activity, controlled research and clinical studies must be completed.

ASPARTATE AMINO TRANSFERASE (AST) (FORMERLY GOT)

The distribution of AST in avian tissue varies among the species. The highest AST activity in the chicken and goose occurs in heart muscle, followed by liver and skeletal muscle.[60] The highest AST activity in tissue of the turkey is in heart muscle, followed by liver, kidney, brain, and skeletal muscle.[16,61] The distribution in duck tissues, in descending order, is skeletal muscle, heart muscle, kidney, brain, and liver.[16] AST activity in the blood of ducks is higher in erythrocytes than in plasma or serum, suggesting that hemolysis will elevate serum activity.[62] Serum AST is not liver-specific in birds; however, increased activity has been associated with hepatocellular damage in chickens, turkeys, caged birds (primarily psittacine), and ducks.[12,16,18,21,26,42,63,64,66,68–70] The most common cause of elevated serum AST activity in caged birds is hepatic disease.[17] Birds with serum AST activity greater than 230 IU/l are considered abnormal.[12] A moderate increase in serum AST activity (two- to fourfold increase) is seen with soft tissue injury, whereas liver necrosis causes a more marked elevation.[16,70] Moderate increases in serum AST activity occur following intramuscular injections. Slight elevations in serum AST may be associated with glucocorticoid excess.[65] Stress-induced increased serum AST activity would be accompanied by a stress leukogram.

ALANINE AMINO TRANSFERASE (ALT) (FORMERLY GPT)

The ALT activity of various avian tissues varies with the species. In turkeys ALT activity is highest in skeletal muscle and low in the liver and heart.[65] The highest ALT activity occurs in the kidney of the mallard duck, which also has a higher ALT content in erythrocytes than in serum or plasma.[62] Heart and skeletal muscle and liver and lung tissues have low ALT activity in chickens and geese.[65] There is little ALT activity in normal chicken plasma.[62] Some authors report elevations in serum ALT activity in raptors, chickens, and ducks with hepatic insult.[18,62,66] Others believe that ALT is not a useful diagnostic test for liver disease in birds.[17,60,63]

LACTATE DEHYDROGENASE (LDH)

LDH activity of various avian tissues varies among the species. The highest LDH activity in chickens and geese occurs in skeletal muscle followed by heart muscle, liver, and lung.[60] In turkeys LDH activity is highest in heart muscle, followed by skeletal muscle, liver, spleen, and lung.[61] In the duck the highest LDH activity is in the liver. The five LDH isoenzymes found in mammalian tissues also occur in birds but with different distribution, For example, pigeon LDH_1 and LDH_2 are highest in heart muscle and $LDH_{2,3,4}$ are highest in the liver.[16] Psittacine birds apparently have only one LDH isoenzyme, and hemolysis does not increase serum LDH activity.[17] Serum LDH activity will increase with hemolysis in other avian species.[18] Elevated serum LDH activity will usually indicate hepatic disease in psittacine birds, but it is not specific for liver disease. Soft tissue injury results in moderate elevations of serum LDH.[16–18]

ALKALINE PHOSPHATASE (AP)

Serum alkaline phosphatase does not appear to be an important test for hepatic disease in noncarnivorous birds. However, it does appear to be associated with intestinal and bone activity. In the domestic fowl, serum AP activity does not become elevated with severe cholestatic liver disease.[65] In the chicken the intestinal isoenzyme of alkaline phosphatase makes the largest contribution to plasma alkaline phosphatase activity and is affected by intestinal disturbances and inappetence.[65,71] Serum AP also appears to be associated with bone activity, because increased levels occur with bone fractures, osteomyelitis, primary and secondary hyperparathyroidism, and somatic growth.[13,16,18,72] Normal serum AP activity is less than 10 IU/l in noncarnivorous birds. If serum AP activity is greater than 40 IU/l, bone involvement should be considered.[72] Serum AP activity usually returns to normal in five days following calcium supplementation in cases of nutritional secondary hyperparathyroidism.[72]

Serum AP may be a useful test for liver disease in carnivorous birds. Increases in serum AP have been reported in raptors with severe liver disease such as herpes inclusion-body hepatitis and cholestasis.[18] The serum AP activity was five to six times normal with hepatic insult compared to a two- to threefold increase with osteoblastic activity in raptors. In chickens, serum AP activity is reduced with magnesium and zinc deficiencies, hypovitaminosis D_3, and coccidiosis.[62,73,74] Ducks with lead poisoning have lowered serum AP values because lead inhibits alkaline phosphatase activity.[62]

GAMMA GLUTAMYLTRANSPEPTIDASE (GGTP)

The usefulness of GGTP as a diagnostic test has not been well investigated in birds. In one study, young chickens with damage to the hepatobiliary system and pancreas showed elevated serum GGTP activity.[64] Elevated serum GGTP values have also been seen in caged birds, primarily psittacine, with liver disease.[17]

SORBITOL DEHYDROGENASE (SDH)

In the fowl, serum SDH is unstable and must be assayed immediately after sample collection. This limits its usefulness as a diagnostic test.[65] Storage under refrigeration will reduce serum activity in the fowl serum but freezing and storage ($-20°$ C for one week) of samples from geese did not reduce the activity.[75] Normal domestic fowl have low serum SDH activity.

CREATININE PHOSPHOKINASE (CK)

Serum CK activity for most birds is 100 to 200 IU/l. Elevated CK activity in avian serum may be seen with physical exercise, neuropathies, lead toxicity, chlamydiosis, and bacterial septicemias.[76] Plasma CK activity remained elevated in turkeys for 29 hours after physical exercise.[76] Intramuscular injections usually will not elevate serum CK activity unless the material is highly irritating (e.g., tetracycline).[77]

AMYLASE

The diagnostic use of serum amylase has not been well investigated in birds. Work with geese and chickens indicates that changes in the alpha amylase activity in pancreatic tissue is directly reflected in serum alpha amylase activity; therefore, the latter may be a useful indicator of pancreatic function.[78] The pancreas produces a specific quantity of alpha amylase that does not change, even during starvation. The rate of alpha amylase secretion from the pancreas is determined by the rate of carbohydrate metabolism; any excess is stored in pancreatic acinar cells and a small percentage diffuses into the peripheral circulation. Therefore serum alpha amylase activity reflects the degree of secretion or accumulation of pancreatic alpha amylase. Reduced carbohydrate intake causes decreased alpha amylase secretion from the pancreas and increased pancreatic tissue and serum alpha amylase activity.

CALCIUM

Serum calcium levels for most normal birds are 8 to 18 mg/dl. Hypercalcemia occurs with hypervitaminosis D_3, or as a normal physiologic occurrence in egg-laying hens.[79] An artefactual hypercalcemia may occur with calcium contaminated from the nail when the toenail clip method is used to collect blood.[21] Hypocalcemia is associated with advanced nutritional secondary hyperparathyroidism, renal failure, hypoalbuminemia, and excessive fat necrosis.[16,18,21] Nutritional secondary hyperparathyroidism is common with pet birds fed all-seed diets that are deficient in calcium and vitamin D_3. The calcium:phosphorus ratio of standard commercial seed diets for budgerigars and parrots is 1:37 and 1:10, respectively.[80] The dietary Ca:P ratio should be 1.5 to 2.5:1. Hypocalcemic seizures may occur with serum calcium levels less than 6 mg/dl.

PHOSPHORUS

Serum phosphorus levels for most normal birds is 2.0 to 4.5 mg/dl. Elevated serum phosphorus can be associated with renal disease, in which the phosphorus level can be 9.5 mg/dl or greater.[12] Avian renal disease is often associated with a hyperuricemia and hyperphosphatemia. Hypervitaminosis D_3 will increase serum phosphorus values. Low serum phosphorus levels are seen in enteric diseases when impaired intestinal absorption of phosphorus has occurred.[43] Starvation and anorexia will produce hypophosphatemia.[22]

THYROID EVALUATION

Thyroid hormone synthesis in birds is similar to that occurring in mammals. Iodide is concentrated in the thyroid glands and used in the production of the thyroid hormone. A lack of dietary iodine, goiter, is a common condition in budgerigars and results in a lack of thyroid hormone production, increased thyrotropin (TSH) production, and thyroid gland hyperplasia. Thyroxin (T_4), the primary secretory product of the avian thyroid gland, is converted to triiodothyronine (T_3) after it enters the cells. T_3 is the active hormone. Both T_3 and T_4 circulate in the plasma and show a diurnal rhythm with a T_3/T_4 ratio of 1.33 to 2.12.[81] In the domestic fowl, 75 per cent of the circulating T_4 is carried by albumin, 10 per cent by alpha globulin, and the remainder by prealbumin-2.[11] Therefore, hypoalbuminemia will lower T_4 concentration. The short half-life of thyroxine and triiodothyronine in birds ($T\frac{1}{2}$ of three to eight hours) creates an obvious diurnal variation in the resting plasma thyroid concentration that is not seen in mammals, which have a longer thyroxine half-life (two to six days).[81] Factors such as environmental temperature, photoperiod, molting, stress, disease, and drug administration can affect the resting plasma T_4 activity in birds.[81,82] For these reasons a diagnosis of hypothyroidism should not be based on a single low resting T_4 value. The ability of the thyroid gland to respond to TSH will not be affected by factors that influence resting T_4 levels. The diagnosis of hypothyroidism in the avian patient should be based on the lack of response to a TSH stimulation test. This test is performed by obtaining a baseline blood sample, giving the bird 1 or 2 IU of TSH (Dermathycin, Jensen-Salsbery Laboratories, Kansas City, Missouri; thyrotropic hormone, TS-10, Sigma Chemical Co., St. Louis, Missouri) in the pectoral muscle and obtaining a poststimulation blood sample between four and six hours after TSH administration. Both samples are assayed for T_4 activity. Normal birds will respond to TSH stimulation by at least doubling the baseline T_4.[82] Hypothyroidism is confirmed by a lack of typical response to TSH. Avian samples for hormone assay should be submitted to laboratories that have modified their radioimmunoassay procedures to quantitate avian hormones. The protein-bound iodine (PBI) test is insensitive in birds because avian blood has a large amount of nonhormonal iodine bound to protein.[81]

Other laboratory findings suggestive of hypothyroidism in birds include a slight normocytic normochromic anemia, persistent hypercholesterolemia, and hypertriglyceridemia.

Hyperthyroidism is rare in birds. However, the condition could be confirmed by demonstrating an elevated resting plasma T_4 or T_3 and an exaggerated response to TSH stimulation.

ADRENAL EVALUATION

Corticosterone and aldosterone are the primary adrenal corticosteroids in avian plasma. Hydrocortisone (cortisol), the principal glucocorticosteroid from mammalian adrenal glands, is relatively inactive in avian gluconeogenesis.[84] Research using domestic fowl indicates that these birds lose their ability to synthesize cortisol at 17 days of age.[85] This work, plus the observations of others, suggests that corticosterone is the predominant glucocorticosteroid in birds. Cortisol assays such as those used in mammals are not suitable for measuring corticosterone in birds. Aldosterone is the principal mineralocorticosteroid in both birds and mammals. Corticosterone is carried by an alpha globulin, while little is known about the transport of aldosterone.[11]

Plasma corticosterone in birds shows a normal variation and is affected by circadian rhythm, seasonal variation, stress, diet, and egg production.[85,86] Physical stimuli such as environmental temperature extremes, surgery, handling, housing conditions, noise, and dark photoperiod will elevate plasma corticosterone concentration.[85] A circadian rhythm was observed in pigeons, quail, and ducks exposed to a dark-light cycle with darkness triggering an increase in plasma corticosterone. Birds exposed to continuous light had a constantly elevated plasma corticosterone, increased

sensitivity to ACTH, and adrenal hypertrophy.[85] Deprivation of food and water, hypovitaminosis A, and moulting also elevate plasma corticosterone.[85]

Mammalian ACTH stimulates corticosterone and aldosterone synthesis and secretion in birds.[83–87] Therefore, an adrenal function test in birds is based on the ACTH stimulation. This test is performed by obtaining a baseline blood sample (50 μl of serum), administering 16 to 25 units of ACTH (Adrenomone, Burns-Biotec Laboratories, Omaha, Nebraska; Cosyntropin, Organon Inc., West Orange, New Jersey) intramuscularly and collecting a post-ACTH stimulation sample one to two hours later.[87] Normal psittacine birds show a variation in resting corticosterone concentration but exhibit an average eightfold increase following ACTH stimulation.[83] Birds with adrenal insufficiency, primary or secondary, have no increase in corticosterone after ACTH administration. Although hyperadrenocorticism has not been confirmed in birds, affected individuals should have a high baseline corticosterone and an exaggerated response to ACTH.

Hypoadrenocorticism in birds should be suspected when there is a decrease in the sodium:potassium ratio (Na:K less than 27), low fasting serum glucose, decreased urine specific gravity associated with polyuria, and a decreased serum calcium and inorganic phosphate.[85,87] This condition can be confirmed by a lack of response to ACTH.

EXAMINATION OF AVIAN DROPPINGS

Many birds produce two types of feces. Normal intestinal feces is formed, semisolid, composed of large particles, and is easily broken apart in water. The second type has a cecal origin, is thick, viscous, heterogeneous, composed of small particles, and is not easily broken apart in water.[88]

Examination of the intestinal component of avian droppings should include a direct fecal smear, wet mount examination, a fecal flotation, and examination of a Gram-stained smear. The urate portion of the droppings should not be a major component of the fecal examination unless one is checking for renal coccidia or flukes.

Direct smears are examined for parasite ova, protozoa, fungi, bacteria, and inflammatory cells. Commercial test reagent tablets can be used for detection of blood in the sample. A wet mount should be prepared and examined microscopically. The wet mount is allowed to dry and stained with Gram's stain. Normal psittacine droppings contain 100 to 200 organisms per oil immersion field. Sixty per cent of the bacteria are short to medium-size gram-positive bacilli and 40 per cent are gram-positive cocci.[89] One Candida-like yeast and one or two gram-negative bacilli per oil immersion field are accepted as normal. Large gram-positive bacilli (*Bacillus* sp.) are also considered normal. Droppings from carnivorous birds will have a larger number of gram-negative bacteria.

Abnormal findings in fecal smears from psittacine birds include absence of cocci, decrease in gram-positive rods, and the presence of many filamentous gram-positive bacteria, a large number of gram-negative rods, many yeasts, and a marked quantity of undigested food particles.[89] Any of these abnormal findings would be an indication for doing a cultural examination of the feces. A total absence of bacteria is abnormal and may be seen with overtreatment with antibiotics or if the urate portion of the droppings is the principal component of the smear.

A fecal flotation for avian droppings is performed in the same manner as a mammalian fecal flotation using $ZnSO_4$ or $NaNO_3$ with a specific gravity of 1.2 to 1.3. Coccidia oocysts, *Ascaris* ova, *Strongyloidea* ova, *Capillaria* ova, and *Syngamus* ova are most commonly observed. Tapeworms are usually identified by the presence of proglottids.

URINALYSIS

The urate portion of the droppings should be examined grossly for volume, consistency, color, and the frequency of deposition noted. Typical avian urine is a cream-colored, thick, mucoid semisolid that contains a high concentration of uric acid. Birds with polyuria have a watery urine that can be easily aspirated into a syringe or pipette from wax paper, plastic wrap, or aluminum foil placed under the perch. A routine urinalysis can be completed using the same urine dipsticks that are used for mammalian urine. The dipsticks can be cut in half lengthwise to provide smaller strips for use with small urine samples.

Normal urine for most birds varies from a clear to cream color. Dietary water intake will influence water content of urine. Birds fed a high moisture diet will have more liquid urine than those fed a low moisture diet. Greenish discoloration of urine is suggestive of hepatic disease and biliverdinuria. Green urates can be seen in birds suffering from starvation or anorexia and may indicate a fasting hyperbiliverdinemia. A yellow discoloration of urine may suggest hepatic disease caused by bilirubinuria.[90] Red to brown urine is suggestive of hematuria or hemoglobinuria (frequently associated with lead toxicity).

Urine specific gravity of noncarnivorous birds is 1.002 to 1.033 and will vary depending upon the state of hydration and osmolality.[47,90] It is difficult to obtain a specific gravity reading on semisolid urine, but this can be done on watery urine using a refractometer.

Urine pH of noncarnivorous birds is 5.0 to 8.0.[47] During metabolic acidosis with a decrease in serum bicarbonate, there is an increase in urine hydrogen ions and titratable acid.[34] Uric acid is the major component of the titratable urine acid. Excretion of ammonia is increased in an effort to conserve bicarbonate and results in an increase in urinary ammonia excretion and a decrease in uric acid excretion during acidosis.[34] Urine pH is acid (pH 5.3) during egg laying is hens but becomes alkaline (pH 7.6) with the cessation of egg production.[47] This is related to the excess of hydrogen ions produced during calcium deposition into the eggshell. Hypoxia in diving ducks also leads to an acid urine (pH 4.7) resulting from a respiratory acidosis and renal compensation.[47]

The majority of normal noncarnivorous birds have none to a trace of urine protein when tested with a dipstick. Elevated urine protein may occur with renal disease and urinary tract or cloacal infections.

Normal avian urine has a negative to trace dipstick glucose test. Birds with diabetes mellitus usually have a four plus urine glucose. Suspected hyperglycemia can be confirmed by glucosuria.

Although ketones are not normally present in avian urine, birds with diabetes mellitus or those having increased fat utilization associated with starvation may have a ketonuria.

Urine dipstick tests for occult blood are usually negative in normal birds. Positive readings suggest hematuria or hemorrhage from the gastrointestinal tract, reproductive tract, or cloaca. Normal avian urine is negative for bilirubin. Some birds with severe liver disease and an accompanying bilirubinuria will have positive results.[90] Birds with biliverdinuria will be negative on the bilirubin dipstick test, because biliverdin does not react with the dipstick reagents.

Microscopic examination of urine sediment is difficult with semisolid urine. This type of urine contains large quantities of urate crystals. These amorphous crystals are spherical, 2 to 8 microns in diameter, and consist largely of dihydrates of uric acid and urates with cations, sodium, and potassium, attached.[40]

A direct smear or a smear of centrifuged sediment can be used to examine the cytology of liquid urine. Normal urine has low cellularity. Epithelial cells of the urinary tract, reproductive tract, intestinal tract, or cloaca are often present. Bacteria are frequently observed because of urine contamination by fecal matter. An increase in heterophils indicates presence of an inflammatory lesion in the urinary tract, reproductive tract, intestinal tract, or cloaca. Bacterial phagocytosis indicates a septic lesion.

REFERENCES

1. Sturkie, P. D.: Blood: Physical characteristics, formed elements, hemoglobin, and coagulation. In: *Avian Physiology*, edited by Sturkie, P. D., Springer-Verlag, New York, 1976.

2. Dein, F. J.: Avian clinical hematology. *Proceedings of the Association of Avian Veterinarians*, 1982.
3. Arora, K. L.: Blood sampling and intravenous injections in Japanese quail (*Coturnix coturnix japonica*). Lab. Ani. Sci., 29:114, 1979.
4. Vuillaume, A.: A new technique for taking blood samples from ducks and geese. Avian Pathol., 12:389, 1983.
5. Hodges, R. D.: Normal avian (poultry) haematology. In: *Comparative Clinical Haematology*, edited by Archer, R. K. and Jeffcott, L. B., Blackwell Scientific Publications, London, 1977.
6. Christie, G.: Haematology and biochemical findings in an experimentally produced haemolytic anemia in eight-week-old brown leghorn cockerels. Br. Vet. J., 135:279, 1979.
7. DeEds, F.: Normal blood counts in pigeons. J. Lab. Clin. Med., 12:437, 1927.
8. Lucas, A. J., and Jamroz, C.: *Atlas of Avian Hematology*, U.S.D.A. Monograph No. 25, Washington, D.C., 1961.
9. Maxwell, M. H.: Production of a Heinz body anaemia in the domestic fowl after ingestion of dimethyl disulphide: A haematological and ultrastructural study. Res. Vet. Sci., 30:233, 1981.
10. Galvin, C. E.: Approach to the anemic patient, Calif. Vet., 2:12, 1978.
11. Butler, E. J.: Plasma proteins. In: *Physiology and Biochemistry of the Domestic Fowl*, edited by Freeman, B. M., Academic Press, London, 1983.
12. Altman, R. B.: Avian clinical pathology, radiology, parasitic and infectious diseases. *Proceedings of the American Animal Hospital Association*, A.A.H.A., South Bend, IN, 1979.
13. Leonard, J. L.: Clinical laboratory examinations. In: *Diseases of Cage and Aviary Birds*, edited by Petrak, M. L., Lea and Febiger, Philadelphia, 1982.
14. Mulley, R. C.: Haematology and blood chemistry of the black duck. *Anas. superciliosa*. J. Wildlife Dis., 15:437, 1979.
15. Schjeide, O. A.: Lipoproteins of the fowl—serum, egg, and intracellular. In: *Progress in the Chemistry of Fats and Other Lipids*, edited by Holman, R. T., Lindberg, W. O. and Malkin, T., Pergamon Press, Oxford.
16. Ivins, G. K., Weddle, G. D., and Halliwell, W. H.: Hematology and serum chemistries in birds of prey. In: *Zoo and Wild Animal Medicine*, edited by Fowler, M. E., W. B. Saunders Co., Philadelphia, 1978.
17. Galvin, C. E.: Laboratory diagnostic aids in pet bird practice. In: *Proceedings of the American Animal Hospital Association*, A.A.H.A., South Bend, IN, 1980.
18. Halliwell, W. H.: Serum chemistry profiles in the health and disease of birds of prey. In: *Recent Advances in the Study of Raptor Diseases*, edited by Cooper, J. E. and Greenwood, A. G., Chiron Publications, Ltd., West Yorkshire, England, 1981.
19. Chandra, M., Singh, B., Soni, G. L., and Ahuja, S. P.: Renal and biochemical changes produced in broilers by high-protein, high-calcium, urea-containing and vitamin A-deficient diets. Avian. Dis., 28:1, 1983.
20. Rosskopf, W. J., Jr., Woerpel, R. W., Howard, E. B., Holshuh, H. J., and Matsumoto, G.: Psittacosis in a parakeet. Mod. Vet. Pract., 62:540, 1981.
21. Rosskopf, W. J., Jr., Woerpel, R. W., Rosskopf, G., and VanDeWater, D.: Hematologic and blood chemistry values for common pet avian species. V.M./S.A.C., 77:1233, 1982.
22. Christie, G., and Halliday, W. G.: Haematological and biochemical aspects of an *E. coli* septicemia in brown leghorn chickens. Avian Pathol., 8:45, 1979.
23. Rosskopf, W. J., Jr., Woerpel, R. W., Richkind, M., and Howard, E. B.: Pathogenesis, diagnosis and treatment of adrenal insufficiency in psittacine birds. Calif. Vet., 36(5):26, 1982.
24. Driver, E. A.: Hematological and blood chemical values of Mallard, *Anasp. platyrhynchos*, drakes before, during and after remige molt. J. Wildlife Dis., 17:423, 1981.
25. March, G. L., John, T. M., McKeon, B. A., Sileo, L., and George, J. C.: The effects of lead poisoning on various plasma constituents in the Canada goose. J. Wildlife Dis., 12:14, 1976.
26. Ryan, C. P. Walder, E. J., and Howard, E. B.: Diabetes mellitus and islet cell carcinoma in a parakeet, J.A.A.H.A., 18:139, 1982.
27. Smith, H. A., Jones, T. C., and Hunt, R. D.: *Veterinary Pathology*, 4th ed., Lea and Febiger, Philadelphia, 1972.
28. Hazelwood, R. L.: The avian endocrine pancreas. Am. Zool., 13:699, 1973.
29. Altman, R. B., and Kirmayer, A. H.: Diabetes mellitus in the avian species. J.A.A.H.A., 12:531, 1976.
30. Nelson, N., Elgart, S., and Mirsky, A. I.: Pancreatic diabetes in the owl. Endocrinology, 32:119, 1942.
31. Hazelwood, R. L.: Carbohydrate metabolism. In: *Avian Physiology*, edited by Sturkie, P. D., Springer-Verlag, New York, 1976.
32. Mirsky, I. A., Nelson, N., Grayman, I., and Korenberg, M.: Studies on normal and depancreatized domestic ducks. Am. J. Physiol., 135:223, 1941.
33. Langslow, D. R., Kimmel, J. R., and Pollock, H. G.: Studies of the distribution of a new avian pancreatic polypeptide and insulin among birds, reptiles, amphibians and mammals. Endocrinology, 93:558, 1973.
34. Farher, D. S.: Some physiological attributes of small birds. In: *Diseases of Cage and Aviary Birds*, edited by Petrak, M. L., Lea and Febiger, Philadelphia, 1982.
35. Martin, S. L.: Diagnosis and management of common endocrine and metabolic diseases of pet birds. In: *Proceedings of 6th Kal-Kan Symposium*, 1982.
36. Spira, A.: Clinical aspects of diabetes mellitus in budgerigars. In: *Scientific Proceedings of 48th Annual Meeting American Animal Hospital Association*, A.A.H.A., South Bend, IN, 1981.
37. Douglass, E. M.: Diabetes mellitus in a Toco Toucan. Mod. Vet. Pract., 62:293, 1981.
38. Shannon, J. A.: The excretion of uric acid by the chicken. J. Cell. Comp. Physiol., 11:123, 1938.
39. Osbaldiston, G. W.: Diuresis and uric acid excretion in the fowl. Vet. Clin. Pathol., 2:235, 1968.
40. Skadhauge, E.: Formation and composition of urine. In: *Physiology and Biochemistry of the Domestic Fowl*, edited by Freeman, B. M., Academic Press, London, 1983.
41. Page, R. K., Fletcher, O. J., and Bush, P.: Calcium toxicosis in broiler chicks. Avian. Dis., 24:1055, 1980.
42. Rivetz, B., Bogin, E., Weisman, Y., Avidar, J., and Hadani, A.: Changes in the biochemical compo-

sition of blood in chickens infected with *Borrelia anserina*. Avian Pathol., 6:343, 1977.

43. Shane, S. M., Young, R. J., and Lutwak, L.: Avian nephrosis associated with high dietary calcium (abstr). Fed. Proc., 27:312, 1968.

44. Bauck, L. A., and Haigh, J. C.: Toxicity of gentamicin in great horned owls (*Bubo virginianus*). J. Zoo Ani. Med., 15:62, 1984.

45. Hartenbower, D. L., and Coburn, J. W.: A model of renal insufficiency in the chick. Lab. Ani. Sci., 22:258, 1972.

46. Bell, D. J., and Bird, T. P.: Urea and volatile base in the caeca and colon of the domestic fowl: The problem of their origin. Comp. Biochem. Physiol., 18:735, 1966.

47. Sturkie, P.D.: Kidneys, extrarenal salt excretion, and urine. In: *Avian Physiology*, edited by Sturkie, P.D., Springer-Verlag, New York, 1976.

48. Bird, J. E., Walser, M. M., and Duke, G. E.: Toxicity of gentamicin in red-tailed hawks. Am J. Vet. Res., 44:1289, 1983.

49. Black, D. G.: Avian clinical pathology. In: *Proceedings No. 55 Aviary and Caged Birds*, The Postgraduate Committee in Veterinary Science, Sidney, 1981.

50. Griminger, P.: Lipid metabolism. In: *Avian Physiology*, edited by Sturkie, P. D., Springer-Verlag, New York, 1976.

51. Lothrop, C. D.: Disease of the thyroid gland in caged birds. In: *Proceedings of the Association of Avian Veterinarians*, 1984.

52. Langslow, D. R., Butler, E. J., Hales, C. N., and Pearson, A. W.: The response of plasma insulin, glucose and non-esterified fatty acids to various hormones, nutrients and drugs in the domestic fowl. J. Endocrinol., 46:243, 1970.

53. Butler, E. J.: Role of trace elements in metabolic processes. In: *Physiology and Biochemistry of the Domestic Fowl*, edited by Freeman, B. M., Academic Press, London, 1983.

54. Sturkie, P. D.: Secretion of gastric and pancreatic juice, pH of tract, digestion in alimentary canal, liver and bile, and absorption. In: *Avian Physiology*, edited by Sturkie, P. D., Springer-Verlag, New York, 1976.

55. Cornelius, C. E.: Hepatic bilirubin 1X-alpha-glycosyltransferase activities in animals excreting primarily biliverdin into bile. Vet. Clin. Pathol., 10(1):27, 1981.

56. Colleran, E., and O'Carra, P.: Enzymology and comparative physiology of biliverdin reduction. *Fogarty International Center Proceedings No. 35*, Chapter VI, p. 69, 1977.

57. Tenhunen, R.: The green color of avian bile: Biochemical explanation. Scand. J. Clin. Lab. Invest., 27 (Suppl.) 116:9, 1971.

58. Lin, G. L., Himes, J. A., and Cornelius, C. E.: Bilirubin and biliverdin excretion by the chicken. Am. J. Physiol., 226:881, 1974.

59. Lind, G. W., Gronwall, R. R., and Cornelius, C..E.: Bile pigments in the chicken. Res. Vet. Sci., 8:280, 1967.

60. Bogin, E., and Israeli, B.: Enzyme profile of heart and skeletal muscle, liver and lung of roosters and geese. Zbl. Vet. Med. A., 23:152, 1976.

61. Bogin, E., Avidar, Y.,, and Israeli, B.: Enzyme profile of turkey tissues and serum. Zbl. Vet. Med. A., 23:858, 1976.

62. Rozman, R. S., Locke, L. N., and McClure, S. F.: Enzyme changes in mallard ducks fed iron or lead shot. Avian Dis., 18:435, 1974.

63. Lohr, J. E.: Fatty liver and kidney syndrome in New Zealand in chickens. N. Z. Vet. J., 23:167, 1975.

64. Pearson, A. W., Butler, E. J., and Fenwick, G. R.: Rapeseed meal and liver damage: Effect on plasma enzyme activities in chicks. Vet. Rec., 105:200, 1979.

65. Curtis, M. J., Jenkins, H. G., and Butler, E. J.: The effect of *Escherichia coli* endotoxins and adrenocortical hormones on plasma enzyme activities in the domestic fowl. Res. Vet. Sci., 28:44, 1980.

66. Bokori, J., and Karsai, F.: Enzyme-diagnostic studies of blood from geese and ducks, healthy and with liver dystrophy. Acta Vet. Acad. Scient. Hung., 19:269, 1969.

67. Al-Khateeb, G. H., and Hansen, M. F.: Plasma glutamic oxaloacetic transaminase as related to liver lesions from histomoniasis in turkeys. Avian Dis., 17:269, 1973.

68. Cornelius, C. E.: Liver function. In: *Clinical Biochemistry of Domestic Animals*, edited by Kaneko, J. J. and Cornelius, C. E., Academic Press, New York, 1970.

69. Molander, D. W., Sheppard, E., and Payne, A.: Serum transaminase in liver disease. J.A.M.A., 163:1461, 1957.

70. Cornelius, C. E., Law, G. R. J., Julian, L. M., and Asmundson, V. S.: Plasma aldolase and glutamic oxaloacetic transaminase activities in inherited muscular dystrophy of domestic chickens. Proc. Soc. Exptl. Biol. Med., 101:41, 1959.

71. Vertommen, M., VanDerLaan, A., and Veenendaal-Hesselman, H. M.: Infectious stunting and leg weakness in broilers. II. Studies on alkaline phosphatase isoenzymes in blood plasma. Avian Pathol., 9:143, 1980.

72. Altman, R., Montali, R., Kollias, G., and Harrison, G. J.: Avian clinical pathology evaluation panel. *Annual Proceedings of the American Association of Zoo Veterinarians*, 1975.

73. Chute, H. L., Zarkower, A., O'Meara, D. C., and Witter, R. L.: Acid and alkaline phosphatase levels in coccidiosis-infected chickens. Avian Dis., 5:107, 1961.

74. Schuster, N. H., and Hindmarsh, M.: Plasma alkaline phosphatase as a screening test for low zinc status in broiler hybrid chickens affected with "clubbed down." Aust. Vet. J., 56L:499, 1980.

75. Westlake, G. E., Bunyan, P. J., and Stanley, P. I.: Variation in the response of plasma enzyme activities in avian species dosed with carbophenothion. Ecotoxicol. Environ. Safety, 2:151, 1978.

76. Tripp, M. J., and Schmitz, J. A.: Influence of physical exercise on plasma creatine kinase activity in healthy and dystrophic turkeys and sheep. Am. J. Vet. Res., 43:2220, 1982.

77. Fudge, A.: IME 170. *Association of Avian Veterinarians Newsletter*, 3(1):14, 1982.

78. Rodeheaver, D. P. and Wyatt, R. D.: Effect of decreased feed intake on serum and pancreatic α-amylase of broiler chickens. Avian Dis., 28:662, 1984.

79. Wallach, J. D., and Flieg, G. M.: Nutritional secondary hyperparathyroidism in captive birds. J.A.V.M.A., 155:1046, 1969.

80. Arnold, S. A., Kram, M. A., Hintz, H. F., Evans, S.

H., and Krook, L.: Nutritional secondary hyperparathyroidism in the parakeet. Cornell Vet., 64:37, 1974.

81. Ringer, R. K.: Thyroid. In: *Avian Physiology*, edited by Sturkie, P. D., Springer-Verlag, New York, 1976.

82. Lothrop, C. D.: Diseases of the thyroid gland in caged birds. In: *Proceedings of the Association of Avian Veterinarians*, 1984.

83. Lothrop, C. D., Sr., Olson, J. H., and Loomis, M. R.: Endocrine diagnosis of feathering problems in psittacine birds. In: *Annual Proceedings of the American Association of Zoo Veterinarians*, 1983.

84. Ringer, R. K.: Adrenals. In: *Avian Physiology*, edited by Sturkie, P. D., Springer-Verlag, New York, 1976.

85. Freeman, B. M.: Adrenal glands. In: *Physiology and Biochemistry of the Domestic Fowl*, edited by Freeman, B. M., Academic Press, London, 1983.

86. Zenoble, R. D., and Kempppainen, R. J.: The influence of ACTH on plasma corticosterone and cortisol and influence of TSH on plasma T_4 and T_3 in psittacine birds. In: *Proceedings of the Association of Avian Veterinarians*, 1984.

87. Lothrop, C. D., Jr.: Diagnosis of adrenal diseases in caged birds. In: *Proceedings of the Association of Avian Veterinarians*, 1984.

88. Harrigan, K. E.: Parasitic diseases in birds. In: *Proceedings No 55 Avian and Caged Birds*, edited by Hangerford, T. G., The Postgraduate Committee in Veterinary Science, Sidney, 1981.

89. Harrison, G. J.: IME 3. *Association of Avian Veterinarians Newsletter*, 1(1):2, 1980.

90. Woerpel, R. W., and Rosskopg, W. J.: Clinical experience with avian laboratory diagnostics. Vet. Clin. North Am: Small Anim. Pract., 14:249, 1984.

17

IMMUNOLOGY

Few scientific disciplines have had an explosion in knowledge comparable to that occurring in the field of immunology. Classically, immunology is concerned with resistance to infectious diseases in association with natural infection or resistance that is induced by vaccines. Today it is evident that immune responses are not always beneficial and can be harmful to the host.

Immunologic processes are designed to defend against infectious agents, to remove outworn self-components, and to monitor recognition of abnormal cell mutants that arise constantly in the body.

The first function of defense against infectious agents is effective only if the cellular elements of the immune system are functioning properly. Undesirable effects such as hypersensitivity may occur if these elements are hyperactive. A host may have an increased susceptibility to infection if cellular elements are hypoactive. The second function, homeostasis, usually operates in a normal fashion but may become aberrant and result in autoimmune disease. The most recently recognized function of the immune system, surveillance, is essential in recognizing the appearance of mutant or aberrant T-lymphocytes, whether they arise spontaneously or are stimulated by infectious agents or chemicals.

It is not the purpose of the first part of this chapter to provide detailed information on immunology; this section is meant to provide sufficient background to assist the reader in understanding the role of immunologic processes in diseases and the use of the laboratory in their diagnosis.

CELLS INVOLVED IN IMMUNE REACTIONS

Although the principal cell in immunity is of lymphoid origin, other cells play an important role.

PHAGOCYTIC CELLS. Mononuclear phagocytes are distributed throughout the body. These cells include both the monocytes in blood and macrophages in tissues. They function in nonspecific and specific immunity. Their primary function in nonspecific immunity is to remove and destroy bacteria, damaged cells, neoplastic cells, colloidal material, and macromolecules. Phagocytosis can be enhanced by the presence of antibodies and complement. Macrophages, in addition to removing such material, also secrete substances that are important in specific immune responses, including complement components, lysozyme, enzymes, interferon, interleukin 1, and prostaglandins.

The principal function of macrophages in specific immunity is in antigen processing. Foreign substances are digested and destroyed but some material remains on the surface that can be presented to immune reactive lymphocytes. Because of their nonspecific and immune specific activities, macrophages often are the principal component of some inflammatory reactions, particularly those associated with cell-mediated immunity (CMI).

NEUTROPHILS AND EOSINOPHILS. Neutrophils function much as macrophages in nonspecific immunity, in which their principal action is phagocytosis with removal and destruction of foreign substances. Neutrophils have little function in specific immunity except as participants in response to an immune reaction. Eosinophils have little function in a primary immune response but play an important role in neutralizing the effects of inflammatory factors released by mast cells in a secondary response.

LYMPHOID CELLS. Lymphoid cells differ from those just considered because they have the ability to react specifically with an antigen and to elaborate cell products. Their origin can be traced to pleuropotential stem cells in the yolk sac, liver, and bone marrow in the fetus and in bone marrow of the adult. The lymphoid system consists of two compartments—central and peripheral. The central is composed of bone marrow, thymus, and bursa of Fabricius (birds), or marrow in mammals. The peripheral lymphoid compartment includes lymph nodes, spleen, and gut-associated lymphoid tissue.

There are two type of immunoreactive lymphocytes. B-lymphocytes are responsible for the production of immunoglobulins. They are processed by the bursa of Fabricius (in birds) or by bursal equivalent tissue in mammals. T-lymphocytes are responsible for cell-mediated immunity and are processed by the thymus gland.

Cells arising in the marrow that proceed to the bursa or its equivalent are processed through a series of developmental stages that lead to a B-lymphocyte that is committed to a specific antigen and to produce and secrete one type of immunoglobulin. Cells entering the thymus gland divide rapidly but not under the influence of an antigen. Most T-lymphocytes that enter the thymus die there, with only 5 to 25 per cent surviving to leave the gland. After leaving the thymus T-lymphocytes colonize secondary lymphoid tissue.

Morphologically it is impossible to differentiate between T- and B-lymphocytes. The characteristics that are used to differentiate them are summarized in Table 17–1.

CELL EVENTS IN ANTIBODY FORMATION

The immune response is initiated by exposure, natural or artificial, to an antigen. This response involves proliferation and differentiation of immunocompetent lymphocytes in lymphoreticular tissue that leads to antibody formation or the development of cell-mediated immunity.

In the primary antibody response there is an induction or latent period of variable duration followed by a four- to ten-day log phase of antibody formation. Next is a steady state in which the antibody level remains constant as production equals destruction. The steady state is relatively short and dependent upon immunoglobulin half-life and the amount of antibody production. The steady state will be longer if antibody production remains high. This is followed by a decline in antibody concentration as production wanes and immunoglobulins are destroyed.

The early response to antigen stimulation is the production of IgM. IgM production is transitory; within ten days to two weeks following antigen exposure IgM production is, in most cases, replaced by the formation of IgG. Antibodies produced early have a low affinity for antigen, while those produced later in the primary response have greater affinity as well as greater avidity for the immunogen.

A second exposure will elicit an enhanced immune response if an animal has been previously exposed to an immunogen. This secondary re-

TABLE 17–1. Differentiation between T- and B-Lymphocytes

Characteristic	T-Lymphocytes	B-Lymphocytes
Surface receptors for:		
Foreign RBC's	+ + +	—
Antigens	+ + +	+ + +
Ig Fc fragment	+	+ + +
Complement 3b	—	+
Antigen receptor	Immunoglobulin	Nonimmunoglobulin (unclear)
Cell surface antigens	Immunoglobulin	THY 1, LyT
Mitogen response	LPS, pokeweed mitogen	Phytohemagglutinin, Concanavalin A, BCG; pokeweed mitogen
Tissue distribution	Paracortex of lymph nodes; perioarterolar sheath—spleen, blood	Cortex of lymph nodes; follicles of spleen
Functions:		
Secrete IG	—	+ + +
Helper action	+ + +	—
Memory	+	+
Cell-mediated immunity	+	—
Tolerance	Long-lasting	Temporary

sponse is characterized by an accelerated appearance of sensitized immunocompetent T-lymphocytes and antibodies. This anamnestic response differs from primary response because the latent period is short, the rate of antibody synthesis is higher, the total quantity of antibody produced is greater, antibody titer persists longer, affinity and avidity of the antibody are greater, and cross-reactivity of the antibody is higher. There are many more memory cells than in the primary response. The predominating immunoglobulin is IgG, with little production of IgM, and the dosage of antigen necessary to elicit the immune response is low.

The B-lymphocyte antigen receptor is an immunoglobulin molecule attached so that the antigen-binding sites are exposed. Each B-lymphocyte contains 10^4 to 10^5 surface receptors. All receptor immunoglobulins on a single B-lymphocyte are identical and have the same specificity for a single molecular configuration. Therefore, B-lymphocytes can combine and respond only to the specific immunogen for which they have a receptor. B-lymphocytes of different specificity are generated in the bone marrow at random. This random generation appears to be genetically controlled.

Simple binding of the antigen to the receptor of a B-lymphocyte is not enough to stimulate antibody formation. Antibody formation will occur only if certain critical conditions are met. An antigen is processed by macrophages and presented to B-lymphocytes while fixed to the macrophage surface. At the same time, certain T-lymphocytes, called helper T-lymphocytes, respond to the same antigen. In addition to processing antigen and presenting it to the B-lymphocytes, macrophages elaborate a substance, interleukin 1, that stimulates or activates T helper cells. T-lymphocyte help occurs when helper T-lymphocytes encounter a macrophage-bound antigen and secrete helper substances such as interleukin 2, which acts in a nonantigen-specific fashion to enhance B-lymphocyte response to an antigen.

Once stimulated by an antigen on the surface of a macrophage in the presence of T helper cell substances, changes occur in the B-lymphocytes. The membrane-bound antigen becomes concentrated into a small cap on the cell surface; the B-lymphocyte enlarges and begins to divide rapidly. After a few days there are two distinct populations. Plasma cells have the ability to synthesize large quantities of antibody and morphologically unaltered memory B-lymphocytes. Memory cells are morphologically identical to their parent T-lymphocytes, contain immunoglobulin receptors identical to those of the parent, and live for months or years after first antigen exposure. These cells provide a mechanism of antigen recognition and are responsible for rapid initiation of the secondary response. Plasma cells are widely distributed in the body but have their greatest concentration in the red pulp of the spleen, in medulla of lymph nodes, and in bone marrow. Plasma cells are capable of synthesizing as many as 300 molecules of antibody per second. The antibody has specificity for the antigen that originally stimulated the B-lymphocyte.

CELLS IN CELL-MEDIATED IMMUNITY (CMI)

T-lymphocytes are heterogeneous. The following types are recognized: (1) Two types of effector cells that are capable of elaborating lymphokines or are able to destroy foreign cells; (2) T-helper cells that assist B-lymphocytes or other T-lymphocytes; and (3) T-suppressor lymphocytes that inhibit other T- or B-lymphocytes. Other lymphocytes that play a role in CMI are the killer (K) cells and the natural-killer (NK) cells. K cells are morphologically identical to small lymphocytes. They have an Fc receptor but no complement receptor. K cells have a cytotoxic effect on cells that are coated with IgG. No specific antigen stimulation of K cells is required in order for them to function. This reaction is called antibody-dependent cellular cytotoxicity (ADCC) and occurs whenever there is an IgG-coated cell. The antibody molecule on the cell appears to form a bridge between the target cell coated with antibody and the K cell. NK cells are large granular-appearing lymphocytes that have their origin in the bone marrow and effectively destroy tumors and virus-infected cells by direct cytotoxicity without prior antigen stimulation. NK cells have a receptor for the Fc end of IgG and therefore may participate in the ADCC reaction. However, antibodies are not necessary for these cells to produce their cytotoxic effects. NK cells produce interferon when the target cell is encountered. Interferon stimulates rapid differentiation of pre-NK cells and enhances T-lymphocyte activity and macrophage-mediated cytotoxicity.

When antigen binds to the receptor of a T-lymphocyte, the cell is stimulated to divide and differentiate. Interleukin 1 may assist in regulating this reaction just as it does for B-lymphocyte activation. T-helper cells aid in the activation of T-lymphocytes. T-lymphocytes respond to antigen determinants that are different from those that stimulate B-lymphocytes. T-lymphocytes react optimally to antigens presented in close association with histocompatibility antigens. Histocompatibility antigens are surface antigens on the cell that are characteristic for the individual. T-lymphocytes respond to antigens by dividing into effector cells and memory cells. Effector cells function to synthesize lymphokines. Lymphokines are nonimmunoglobulin factors that possess potent biologic activities. In addition to lymphokine-producing cells, some effector cells participate in direct cytotoxic reactions with target cells that have surface antigens identical to those that originally stimulated the T-lymphocytes.

Lymphokines are important in cell-mediated immune responses. Lymphokines are proteins with molecular weights between 25,000 and 75,000 daltons. They are released from activated T-lymphocytes; about 90 different functions have been identified. It has not been determined whether these are all different functions or whether they appear to be different because of the type of laboratory experiment used to identify them. Lymphokines are not antigen binding or antigen specific. Lymphokines act on macrophages, neutrophils, and lymphocytes. Their action is to attract macrophages to an area, activate them, and inhibit their migration. Lymphokines affect leukocytes by slowing their migration and by acting as a leukocyte chemotactic factor. Lymphokines affect T-lymphocytes by the production of interleukin 2, which stimulates them to divide. Evidence exists that there may be a T-lymphocyte–replacing factor that, when added to a culture of B-lymphocytes, will stimulate antibody production in the absence of T-lymphocytes. Some lymphokines suppress lymphocyte activity. Transfer factor is the most unique lymphokine because it acts on T-lymphocytes to specifically sensitize them to an antigen. Transfer factor is a small molecule, around 10,000 to 15,000 daltons. When transfer factor is administered to nonsensitized recipients, it will make them sensitive to a specific antigen within a few hours, as detected by a positive delayed-type hypersensitivity reaction.

REGULATION OF THE IMMUNE RESPONSE

Although both humoral and cell-mediated immunity are essential for protection, they have the potential to cause severe damage unless regulated. The production of autoantibodies is always a potential risk, while failure to mount an immune response can result in immunodeficiencies and increased susceptibility. Excessive immune response can cause disease while failure to control cellular divisions can cause neoplasia.

Immune tolerance (self-recognition) is essential. Without specific immune tolerance an animal would immunologically attack its own tissues. A breakdown in "self-recognition" may result in development of an autoimmune reaction.

The concept of immune tolerance was first established by experiments showing that nonidentical twin calves shared two sets of red cells: those of its own and those of its twin. These studies also showed that skin transplants could be made between the two animals without graft rejection. It was thought that this occurred because of a sharing of hematopoietic tissue while in utero. This concept was further strengthened by experiments in which lymphoreticular cells from one strain of mice were introduced into the developing embryo of a different strain. After birth the mouse that had received the lymphoreticular tissue while an embryo accepted a graft from the donor mouse. Immune tolerance can be experimentally established in embryos or very young animals. Unlike natural self-tolerance (self-recognition), induced tolerance is temporary.

A breakdown in self-tolerance can occur by a variety of means, including exposure of previously hidden antigens, development of new antigen determinants, cross-reactivity with microorganisms, development of previously suppressed immunologically competent cells, and as a consequence of viral infection.

Immune responses may be regulated by antibodies. It is known that antibodies or immune complexes exert a negative feedback on the immune response. Antibodies of IgG type can depress additional production of IgM or IgG. This is extremely important, as it is the reason that young animals with high antibody levels are not responsive to vaccination programs; they cannot respond. It was once thought that antibodies combined with the antigen to mask its determinants and thus reduce its immunogenicity. It has now been demonstrated that in order for immunoglobulins to exert negative feedback they must have intact Fc regions. It has been postulated that such antibodies combine with the Fc receptors on B-lymphocytes, causing the cells to "turn-off." As suppressor T-lymphocytes also have Fc receptors, it is possible that antibodies or immune complexes can attach to these cells, stimulating them to suppress immune reactions.

IMMUNOGLOBULINS

Antibodies (immunoglobulins) are complex protein molecules produced by plasma cells subsequent to an interaction between antigen-sensitive B-lymphocytes and an immunogen. Five different classes of immunoglobulins—IgG, IgM, IgA, IgE, and IgD—have been recognized. IgG, IgM, IgA, and IgE apparently occur in all animal species, while IgD has been found in humans, chickens, and laboratory animals. Once produced, immunoglobulins have the capacity to react specifically with the antigen that induced their production.

All immunoglobulin classes have the same basic structural unit. This monomer consists of two identical heavy chains and two identical light chains held together by disulfide bonds. Each class of immunoglobulin has a chemically different heavy chain, whereas the light chains are identical, irrespective of the type of heavy chain with which they are associated. Subclasses of immunoglobulins have been identified in most an-

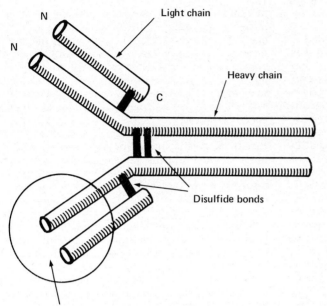

N

N

Light chain

Heavy chain

C

C

C

Disulfide bonds

The antibody combining site is in this region

Figure 17–1. A simple model of an IgG molecule. (From Tizard, I.: An Introduction to Veterinary Immunology. W. B. Saunders Company, Philadelphia, 1982.)

imal species.* Heavy and light chains of a given species of animal are identical for all animals of that species, but there is little similarity among the various species.

The most abundant immunoglobulin in plasma is IgG. The IgG molecule is a monomer consisting of two heavy and two light chains (Fig. 17–1). With a molecular weight of approximately 180,000 daltons, this immunoglobulin can easily escape from blood vessels. IgG provides the bulk of immunity to infectious agents by its ability to enhance phagocytosis and activate complement by agglutinating particulate antigens, and by precipitation of soluble antigens. It also has the capacity to neutralize viruses.

IgM is the largest immunoglobulin, having a molecular weight of approximately 900,000 daltons. It is a pentamer made up of five monomers (Fig. 17–2), each of which contains two heavy and two light chains. These monomers are linked by disulfide bonds in a circular fashion while a small polypeptide, called the *J chain*, links two of the units. This is the major immunoglobulin produced early in a primary immune response and is produced in lesser quantity than IgG in the secondary response. Although formed in a relatively small concentration, it is more efficient than IgG in opsonization, complement fixation, virus neutralization, and agglutination. Because of its large size, IgM is confined to the vascular system and provides little protective activity in tissue fluids or body secretions.

Immunoglobulin A is produced in high concentration by lymphoid tissue of gut, respiratory tract, and genitourinary tract. It is the major immunoglobulin in external secretions and is sometimes known as the secretory antibody. It usually occurs in the form of a dimer consisting of two units joined by a J chain. In secretions it has a secretory piece that apparently protects it from enzyme activities. This immunoglobulin does not activate the complement cascade by the classic pathway, nor can it act as an opsonin. It does have the ability to agglutinate particulate antigens and to neutralize viruses, and it can activate complement through the alternate pathway. It is thought

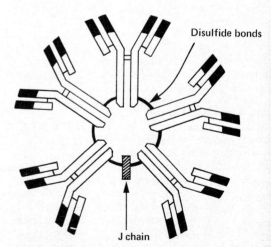

Disulfide bonds

J chain

Figure 17–2. The structure of IgM. (From Tizard, I.: An Introduction to Veterinary Immunology. W. B. Saunders Company, Philadelphia, 1982.)

---

* For more information on immunoglobulin subclasses see reference 1.

that its major action is to prevent adherence of antigens to body surfaces.

The fourth major immunoglobulin in animal plasma is IgE. IgE is produced chiefly in the linings of the respiratory and intestinal tract, binds easily to mast cells and basophils, and has the ability to attach to tissues and to initiate an allergic reaction. It is a typical four-chain immunoglobulin with a molecular weight of 196,000 daltons. IgE has an Fc portion that enables it to bind to mast cells and basophils. Together with an antigen, it mediates release of biologically active substances from these cells.

MEASUREMENT OF HUMORAL IMMUNE RESPONSE

Tests utilized to detect and measure humoral immune response fall into three main groups: (1) primary antibody-binding tests, which directly measure a reaction between antigen and antibody; (2) secondary binding tests, which measure the *in vitro* consequences of antigen antibody combinations; and (3) tertiary binding tests, which measure the *in vivo* consequences of antigen antibody combinations.

PRIMARY BINDING TESTS

Antigens and antibodies combine reversibly to form immune complexes. Primary tests permit the reactants to combine and then the amount of immune complex formed is measured. One or the other of the reactants in primary binding tests is labeled. After the reaction is permitted to proceed, immune complexes are separated from unbound material, and the amount of label in the immune complex is measured.

An example of this is the radioallergosorbent test (RAST). In this test, antigen-impregnated cellulose discs are immersed in test serum; any antibody present will combine with the antigen. The disc is washed and immersed in a radio-labeled solution of antiglobulin for the species being tested. This radio-labeled antiglobulin will combine with immunoglobulin that has attached to the antigen. The disc is washed and the amount of radioactivity present on the disc is evaluated to quantitate the antibody present in test serum. If the test is conducted using an antibody to a specific immunoglobulin class, the quantity of specific immunoglobulin against a particular antigen can be determined.

A commonly used primary-binding test is the radioimmunoassay for antigen. This technique is used for measuring substances such as hormones that are present in small concentrations. The general procedure for radioimmunoassay is: (1) Raise an antibody to a specific protein, such as a hormone, in a heterologous species. (2) Label some antigen with a radioactive label. (3) Add various concentrations of radio-labeled and unlabeled antigen to the antibody. (4) Incubate and permit the immunologic reaction to occur. The labeled and unlabeled antigens compete for antibody-combining sites. (5) After an appropriate incubation, the immune complexes are separated and the amount of radioactivity in the supernatant is measured. By utilizing different concentrations of labeled and unlabeled antigen, a curve can be constructed and used to determine antigen concentration in an unknown specimen.

An enzyme-linked immunosorbent assay (EIA) can be used for detection of antibody or antigen. For antibody detection, antigen is attached to a solid surface, tube, or microtiter tray; dilutions of serum are added and incubated with the antigen; the container is washed to remove unattached immunoglobulins; species-specific enzyme-labeled antiglobulin is added and the mixture is incubated and washed; the tube or microtiter tray is assayed for enzyme concentration.

EIA can also be used for detecting antigen by reversing the procedure. In this case unlabeled antibody is attached to the solid surface, various concentrations of antigen are added, an enzyme-labeled antibody to the antigen is added, and, following appropriate washes, the plate is assayed for enzyme activity. An alternative method for detecting antigen involves a similar procedure. Instead of labeled antibody for the antigen being tested, an unlabeled antibody prepared in a heterologous species (other than that used for surface coating) is added to the mixture of antibody and antigen. An enzyme-labeled antibody to the immunoglobulin of the second species is utilized and the material assayed for enzyme activity.

Another popular technique involves the labeling of antibody with an immunofluorescent substance such as fluorescein isothiocyanate or rhodamine.

Details of fluorescent microscopy are discussed in Chapter 18.

SECONDARY BINDING TESTS

Secondary binding tests are two-stage reactions. The first stage is union of the antigen and antibody; the second stage depends, in large part, on the physical state of the antigen. If antibody combines with an antigen in solution the result is precipitation. If antibody combines with a particulate antigen agglutination occurs.

PRECIPITATION. A variety of precipitation tests are used in clinical immunology. When increasing concentrations of antigen are added to a standard quantity of antibody, three zones can be identified according to the proportion of antigen to antibody. These are: zone of antibody excess, zone of optimal proportions, and zone of antigen excess. Maximum precipitation occurs in the zone of optimal proportions. The most widely used precipitation test is immunodiffusion. This method can be used to determine if two antigens or two antibodies are the same or different. A layer of agar is placed on a glass slide or in a small Petri dish. Wells are cut, using a template, and the agar is removed. The usual pattern is a variable numbers of wells around a center well. The antigen or antibody is placed in the center well and dilutions of the antigen or antibody in the peripheral wells. These reagents diffuse toward one another until the optimal proportion of antigen and antibody is achieved and at that point a precipitate forms. The lines produced and their location will make it possible to identify the antigen or antibody and to determine its specificity.

Radial immunodiffusion can be used to quantitate immunoglobulins. In this method a known concentration of antibody to an immunoglobulin is added to agar. Wells are cut and known concentrations of the immunoglobulin to be quantitated are added to the wells. This material will diffuse and a precipitate will form until the zone of antibody excess is reached; at that point, the ring of precipitation will stop. The size of the zone is measured and recorded for the various immunoglobulin concentrations (Fig. 17–3). A similar

procedure is conducted with an unknown sample and zone size compared with that achieved with known concentrations. This provides an accurate method for determining immunoglobulin concentrations in fluids.

An electric current can be used along with the precipitation test. Immunoelectrophoresis is completed by separating the antigen mixture using electricity and exposing separated antigens to an antibody (Fig. 17–4). Zones of precipitation appear where reactions occur. Electroimmunodiffusion (rocket electrophoresis) can be used to quantitate antigen. Antigen is driven into antibody-containing agar using an electric current; the length of the rocket formed by the precipitate reaction is proportional to the amount of antigen in each well. As with radial immmunodiffusion, this can be standardized and antigen concentration measured.

AGGLUTINATION. If an antigen is particulate, it will cross-link with antibodies to form aggregates that can be observed macroscopically. The agglutination test is usually used to demonstrate the presence of antibodies to particulate antigens. However, an indirect agglutination test can be used to detect soluble antigens. In this method soluble antigen is attached to a biologically inert particle such as a latex bead. Agglutination of the

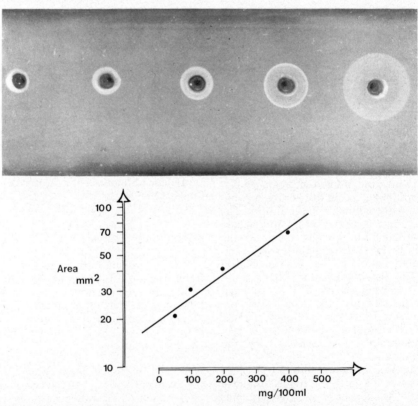

Figure 17–3. Radial immunodiffusion. In this case antiserum to bovine IgA is incorporated in the agar and is used to measure bovine serum IgA levels. (From Tizard, I.: An Introduction to Veterinary Immunology. W. B. Saunders Company, Philadelphia, 1982.)

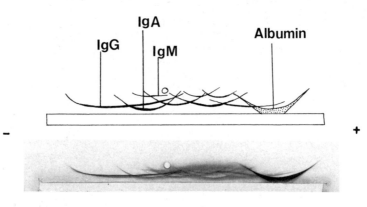

Figure 17–4. Immunoelectrophoresis of normal pig serum showing the precipitation lines produced by some of the major serum proteins. (From Tizard, I.: An Introduction to Veterinary Immunology. W. B. Saunders Company, Philadelphia, 1982.)

latex beads can be seen when these antigen-coated beads are added to a serum-containing antibody. In a similar fashion, antibodies can be attached to particulate matter and screening tests for antigen can be conducted.

COMPLEMENT FIXATION. Complement fixation tests are seldom used except in diagnostic and research laboratories. The complement fixation test consists of two superimposed antigen-antibody reactions. The first occurs among antibody, antigen, and complement to which is added a second mixture of RBC and antibodies to RBC. If complement is tied up because of the presence of antibody in the serum of the first test, no hemolysis will occur. If complement is not tied up because there was no antigen-antibody interaction in the first test, then complement will be available to unite with antibody-coated RBC and cause RBC lysis.

TERTIARY TESTS

These tests are conducted in living systems. The classic example is the neutralization test, which measures the ability of an antibody, when mixed *in vitro* with a living antigen, to neutralize its biologic activity. Antibodies to viruses are often detected in this manner. Protection tests can be used to assay antibody levels. These tests are carried out entirely *in vivo*. Various quantities of known antiserum are administered to a series of animals and the protective capacity determined by injecting these animals with the agent under study (virus, bacteria, toxin). Allergic sensitivities are also detected by *in vivo* tests and will be discussed later.

CONSEQUENCES OF IMMUNE RESPONSES

Immunologic reactions are designed to protect the animal and are primarily concerned with antigen removal. As a part of this activity, however, certain physiologic processes may be carried to extreme, producing lesions. The lesions themselves may hasten antigen removal but may, at the same time, cause harm.

When antibody molecules combine with antigen, their properties are altered. Immune complexes may serve as chemotactic agents for neutrophils, macrophages, and eosinophils, whereas an unattached antibody does not have this property. In addition, immune complex formation may initiate complement activation, cause platelet aggregation and degranulation, initiate degranulation of mast cells and basophils, promote lymphocyte division and differentiation, and generate K cell activity. In addition to these activities, the antigen-antibody complex may present a new molecular configuration to the immune system, which initiates an immune response.

Complexing of antigen with antibody makes it possible for the Fc region of the immunoglobulin to initiate some of its biologic activities, such as complement activation and opsonization.

THE COMPLEMENT SYSTEM

The complement system is composed of a series of proteins that are activated either by the classical (immunologic) or by the alternate (properdin) pathway. The classical pathway for complement activation is initiated by a combination of antigen with two closely spaced IgG molecules or a single IgM molecule. Active sites on the Fc region of immunoglobulin molecules combine with and activate the first component of complement, which in turn begins the activation cascade. As activation proceeds, several biologically active complement components are created. Completion of the cascade results in development of a complex that has the ability to damage cell membranes. Biologic activities of complement complexes are summarized in Table 17–2. Complement activation can also proceed by an alternate pathway in which antigen-antibody combination is not required. Substances known to activate complement by this alternate pathway include

TABLE 17–2. Biologic Activities of Complement

Activity	Responsible Complement Components
Cell lysis	C5678(weakly), C56789(strongly)
Chemotaxis	C3a, C5a, C567
Anaphylatoxin	C3a, C5a, C4a
Opsonization Immunoconglutinin Platelet adherence (thrombus formation) Lymphocyte adherence (regulate Ab)	C3b
Attach to mast cells (release histamine)	C3a, C5a, C4a
Kinin-like activity	C2b

bacterial endotoxins, some polysaccharides, and IgA.

As with other activation systems in the body, there are inhibitors to the complement system that prevent it from going out of control. Specific inhibitory molecules have been demonstrated and some complement complexes have a short half-life. Biologically, the complement system is closely linked to inflammation and the clotting process. The major activity of complement activation related to inflammation is production of chemotactic substances that attract leukocytes to the site. The release of vasoactive factors from mast cells and the aggregation and breakdown of thrombocytes will enhance the inflammatory reaction. Complement activation will initiate the coagulation cascade through activation of the Hageman factor (Factor XII, contact factor). Thrombus formation is enhanced by the enzyme complex C3b that promotes platelet aggregation.

INFLAMMATION

Inflammation associated with an immunologic reaction usually is the result of a hypersensitivity reaction. Hypersensitivity reactions are classified as immediate, cytotoxic, immune-complex, or delayed. Immediate hypersensitivity occurs when IgE and some subclasses of IgG attach to mast cells or basophils by sites on the Fc region. If antigen binds to the cell-associated antibody, the cell will immediately respond by releasing vasoactive factors present in cytoplasmic granules. Granular content release can also be stimulated by complement complexes C3a and C5a. Cytotoxic hypersensitivity is mediated through complement activation or by the action of cytotoxic cells. ADCC plays an important role. Cells that are de-

stroyed by either mechanism may initiate an inflammatory reaction. Immune complexes have the ability to fix complement, which in turn attracts neutrophils that attempt to remove the complexes. At the same time proteolytic enzymes released by neutrophils may produce tissue destruction. This is complicated by platelet aggregation, which causes the release of more vasoactive substances and mast cell degranulation produced by some complement complexes. The delayed type of hypersensitivity is a CMI response. Inflammation results from the release of lymphokines that have chemotactic and vasoactive properties.

IMMEDIATE (IgE-MEDIATED) HYPERSENSITIVITY

Immediate hypersensitivity (anaphylaxis) is mediated by IgE attached to mast cells through the Fc portion of the immunoglobulin. The antigen attaches to the Fab region of the cell-fixed IgE and cross-links two of these molecules. Mast cells respond by degranulating, but the mast cell is not destroyed. Mast cell granules loose their content of vasoactive substances into the tissue fluids. The combination of IgE molecules and antigen also stimulates mast cells to produce other vasoactive substances. Biologically active substances released include histamine, serotonin (5-hydroxytryptamine), leukotriene, eosinophilic chemotactic factors, platelet-aggregating factors, and prostaglandin. Histamine causes dilation of capillaries and venules, contracts specific vessels (species-dependent), increases permeability of microvessels, causes smooth muscle contraction (particularly in the bronchi, GI tract, uterus, and bladder), stimulates exocrine secretions (bronchial mucus, lacrimation, salivation) and is chemotactic for eosinophils. Serotonin is released from mast cells of larger domestic animals. It also exists preformed in platelets. It acts to stimulate the heart and causes vasoconstriction. Leukotrienes (formerly known as slow-reacting substance of anaphylaxis) are synthesized in the mast cells in response to antigen fixation. Leukotriene acts on smooth muscle to produce a slow, prolonged contraction, particularly of the bronchi. The eosinophil chemotactic factor exists preformed within mast cells and when released calls eosinophils to the area. The platelet-acting factor causes platelets to aggregate and release their contents and promotes prostaglandin synthesis. Some prostaglandins cause smooth muscle to contract, thereby promoting vasoconstriction, while others cause smooth muscle relaxation and vasodilation. Some inhibit platelet aggregation while others promote it. As each tissue of the body may synthesize different prostaglandins, the overall effect may be the sum of a large number of interactions.[1]

Measurement of Immediate Hypersensitivity.
The simplest method for measuring immediate hypersensitivity is a skin test. A very small amount of antigen is injected intradermally and if the animal is sensitized, a local reaction will occur at the site of injection, reaching its maximum in 30 minutes and disappearing in a few hours. This local reaction occurs as mast cells with attached IgE degranulate.

Sensitivity can also be determined indirectly by taking serum from a test animal. Serum is injected intradermally into a normal animal and 24 to 48 hours later suspect antigen is injected at the same site. If circulating IgE from the test animal has attached to localized mast cells, a typical wheal and flare reaction will occur in one or two minutes. A passive cutaneous anaphylaxis test can be conducted by injecting serum at several sites followed by an intravenous injection of antigen. If the test is positive, a wheal and flare reaction will develop at the sites of the serum injection. The RAST, previously described, can be utilized for screening a number of different antigens.

CLINICAL ENTITIES ASSOCIATED WITH IMMEDIATE HYPERSENSITIVITY

ACUTE SYSTEMIC ANAPHYLAXIS. If an antigen is absorbed rapidly in an animal that has been previously sensitized, it may result in a generalized mast cell degranulation. If the rate of release of vasoactive agents is greater than the capacity of the body to respond to the changes in the vascular system, the animal may develop anaphylactic shock and die.[1] In most animals the primary shock organ is the lung; therefore, pulmonary signs predominate in acute anaphylaxis. Dogs differ from other animals in that the primary shock organ is the liver, more specifically the hepatic veins. The intestinal tract may be involved in horses that sometimes develop edematous hemorrhagic enterocolitis. The massive release of histamine also will cause contraction of smooth muscles of the bladder and intestinal tract, producing urination and diarrhea.

LOCALIZED ALLERGIC REACTIONS. Most immediate hypersensitivities are not generalized but occur as allergic responses associated with the respiratory tract, intestinal tract, and skin.

CELL-CYTOTOXIC HYPERSENSITIVITY

The classic example of cellular cytotoxic hypersensitivity occurs in immune-mediated hemolytic anemias. This type of immunologic injury may also be associated with systemic lupus erythematosus (SLE), immune-mediated thrombocytopenia (IMT), and a variety of autoimmune diseases including autoimmune thyroiditis, pemphigus, one form of glomerulonephritis, and myasthenia gravis. Not all of these are simple cellular cytotoxic immunologic hypersensitivity; in these situations other types of immunologic reactions may occur simultaneously.

Cellular damage is the result of complement activation or initiation of ADCC. This type of hypersensitivity reaction may also be the result of an immune response to drugs. Drugs that bind firmly to cells modify them so they are recognized as foreign and are eliminated by an immune response.

IMMUNE COMPLEX HYPERSENSITIVITY

Damage produced by the deposition of immune complexes can occur as a local or generalized hypersensitivity reaction. The local type is known as the Arthus reaction and occurs when immune complexes are deposited locally. When an antigen is injected subcutaneously into an individual that has circulating antibodies capable of reacting with that antigen, an acute inflammatory reaction will develop. Initially, neutrophils adhere to the endothelium and escape into the tissues. These in turn cause vascular damage, and platelet aggregation produces thrombosis. Within a few hours mononuclear cells (macrophages) begin to accumulate and by 24 hours are the predominant cell type. Complement activation is important, because complement factors serve as chemotactic substances for neutrophils and are important in the accumulation and aggregation of thrombocytes. Immunoglobulins associated with the local type of hypersensitivity reaction are precipitating and complement fixing and usually of class IgG or, less frequently, IgM.

Systemic immune complex disease occurs when circulating immune complexes are deposited in various tissues. Most of the immune complexes formed in the body are removed by the reticuloendothelial system. Some complexes, however, are soluble and not easily phagocytosed. Such soluble complexes will fix complement and stimulate platelet aggregation, causing vascular damage. Immune complexes are then deposited within the walls of these vessels. Particularly affected are glomeruli and synovia. Immune complex–mediated lesions are most likely to occur when there is prolonged antigen circulation in the presence of antibodies. Therefore, lesions can be associated with chronic bacterial diseases, some viral infections, and administration of foreign serum. Complexes also play a role in SLE and rheumatoid arthritis.

CELL-MEDIATED HYPERSENSITIVITY

This hypersensitivity is the result of a reaction between an antigen and sensitized T-lymphocytes. The tuberculin reaction is typical of this type of hypersensitivity. When an antigen is introduced intradermally, an inflammatory response occurs that takes many hours to develop, reaching its maximum 24 to 72 hours after injection. The reaction may persist for several weeks. The lesion is characterized by the infiltration of macrophages, with very few neutrophils taking part. When an antigen contacts a sensitized circulating T-lymphocyte, the cell is activated and releases its lymphokines. These lymphokines, through their chemotactic activity, recruit cells into the area and, by the production of migration-inhibitory factor, inhibit their migration out of the area. In addition, some macrophages are activated by lymphokines and their ability to destroy the invading antigen is enhanced.

DISEASES ASSOCIATED WITH IMMUNOLOGIC DISORDERS

There are three types of diseases with an immune component: autoimmune diseases, immunoproliferative diseases, and immunodeficiencies.

AUTOIMMUNE DISEASES

Autoimmunity occurs when there is a breakdown in self-tolerance. As mentioned previously, the mechanisms involved include exposure of previously hidden antigens, development of new antigen determinants, cross-reactivity with microorganisms, development of suppressed immunologically competent cells, or as a consequence of viral infection.

EXPOSURE OF PREVIOUSLY HIDDEN ANTIGENS. Some antigens in the body are not normally in contact with immunocompetent cells. These include central nervous system tissue, testicular tissue, and the lens of the eye. If any of these tissues are damaged, either by infection or trauma, new antigens are released. These antigens enter the circulation, encounter immunologically competent cells, and stimulate an immune response. In a similar fashion, intracellular material may be released and initiate an immune response. The release of mitochondria from damaged cells is an example.

DEVELOPMENT OF NEW ANTIGEN DETERMINANTS. When new antigen determinants appear in a body fluid or tissue, the immune system will be stimulated. Rheumatoid factor is a good example. Rheumatoid factors are antibodies directed against antigen determinants on other immunoglobulins. They are found in the serum of animals with rheumatoid arthritis and SLE. Experimentally it has been possible to induce autoimmunity by the immunization of an animal with some of its own tissues suspended in Freund's complete adjuvant.

CROSS-REACTIVITY WITH MICROORGANISMS. Some antigens carried by infectious agents will stimulate antibodies that cross-react with animal tissues. Such has been reported with antibodies to *Mycoplasma hyopneumoniae* that react with pig lung and *Mycoplasma mycoides* antibodies that react with normal bovine lung. The exact role of such autoantibodies as a part of the disease-producing mechanism remains to be determined.

DEVELOPMENT OF PREVIOUSLY SUPPRESSED IMMUNOCOMPETENT CELLS. This probably is the most important phase in the development of autoimmune diseases. The precise mechanism by which these suppressed cells become active is not known. Three hypotheses have been proposed: the forbidden-clone theory, the sequestered-antigen theory, and the immunologic deficiency theory.

Any mechanism or combination of mechanisms that produce hypersensitivity may be responsible for tissue damage that occurs in autoimmunity.

ORGAN-SPECIFIC AUTOIMMUNE DISEASES

Autoimmune Thyroiditis. Dogs with thyroiditis resulting from autoimmunity have clinical and laboratory signs characteristic of hypothyroidism (see Chapter 12). The autoimmune character of the condition can be confirmed by histologic examination of a thyroid biopsy. The gland is infiltrated with lymphocytes, and plasma cells and lymphoid follicles are often present.

Antibodies to thyroglobulin can be demonstrated by use of a passive hemagglutination test employing erythrocytes that have been treated with tannic acid. For this test, tanned erythrocytes are prepared by washing them, adding a 1:25,000 dilution of tannic acid in PBS to a 4 per cent erythrocyte suspension, and allowing it to stand at room temperature for 30 minutes. These erythrocytes are washed and thyroid extract or purified thyroglobulin added, allowed to stand, and the cells are washed to remove unattached thyroglobulin. Various dilutions of patient serum are prepared and added to the tanned-coated erythrocytes. This mixture is incubated and examined for agglutination. Agglutination will occur if the serum contains antibodies to thyroglobulin.

An indirect immunofluorescence test can also be used to demonstrate antibodies to thyroglobulin. In this method dilutions of serum are added to sections of thyroid gland on a glass slide, incubated, washed, and a fluorescein-labeled species-specific anti-immunoglobulin is added. The result is examined with a microscope having an ultraviolet light source. If antibodies to thyroid antigens are present in patient serum, they will combine with thyroid tissue on the slide and are detected by the appearance of an apple-green fluorescence where labeled antibody has attached.

A lymphocyte blastogenesis test using thyroid extract as the antigen has been used to detect antigen-responsive lymphocytes in dogs with autoimmune thyroiditis.[3]

Autoimmune Skin Diseases. PEMPHIGUS.
Pemphigus is a group of autoimmune disorders that affect the skin or oral mucosa or both. Pemphigus arises as a result of the action of antibodies directed against intracellular cement in the skin. These antibodies are best detected by use of direct immunofluorescence. Skin biopsies are taken and immediately frozen for later sectioning or are placed in a special transport-holding medium (Michel's fixative). Tissue sections are prepared, species-specific fluorescein-labeled immunoglobulin is added, and the sample is examined using a microscope with an ultraviolet light source. Histologic examination is of value in distinguishing the various types of pemphigus.

DISCOID LUPUS ERYTHEMATOSUS.
Lupus erythematosus is an autoimmune disorder that can be divided into two categories. Systemic lupus erythematosus (SLE) is a multisystem disease, and will be discussed later in this chapter. Discoid lupus erythematosus is a cutaneous disorder with no systemic involvement. In this condition there are subepidermal deposits of immunoglobulin in skin lesions, and the animals are usually negative to ANA and LE cell tests. Presence of the disease can be detected by use of a direct immunofluorescence test. Immunoglobulin or complement can be demonstrated in the area of the basement membrane. Indirect immunofluorescence tests are negative.

IMMUNE-MEDIATED HEMOLYTIC ANEMIA.
Details of the various types of autoimmune reactions associated with immune-mediated hemolytic anemia are discussed in Chapter 2. Erythrocyte destruction results from removal of immunoglobulin-coated erythrocytes by macrophages or as a direct cytolysis of erythrocytes mediated through complement. The majority of the cases of immune-mediated hemolytic anemia are caused by antibodies of immunoglobulin class IgG. The presence of these immunoglobulins can be demonstrated by use of a Coombs' test conducted at 37° C. Most of the RBC destruction occurs by the action of phagocytes, because IgG does not fix complement with great efficiency. A good Coombs' reagent is a species-specific antiserum against IgG, IgM, and complement (component C3). A positive Coombs' test will result if any of these are on the surface of erythrocytes in sufficient quantity. A positive Coombs' test will ensue if blood parasites such as *Haemobartonella* or *Eperythrozoa* are present on the red cell membrane. Immunoglobulins will coat the erythrocyte if the animal has developed antibodies to these parasites. Likewise, it must be remembered that an erythrocyte membrane can be altered by certain infectious agents and drugs. When this occurs, the body recognizes the new determinant and produces antibodies to it; a Coombs'-positive immune-mediated anemia may result. If the principal antibody is of type IgM, the Coombs' test conducted at 37° C will be negative, while one conducted at 4° C will be positive. Immune-mediated anemias having IgM as their principal antibody are more likely to produce gross agglutination of red cells and intravascular hemolysis. A cold Coombs' test should be requested if the clinician suspects an IgM immune-mediated anemia.

The indirect Coombs' test, in which an attempt is made to identify circulating antibodies to erythrocytes, is of little value in the diagnosis of immune-mediated hemolytic anemias in dogs and cats.[3] Immune-mediated anemia is also seen in some animals with SLE.

In addition to the typical Coombs' reaction, dogs with immune-mediated anemia usually have a marked leukocytosis, neutrophilia, and left shift. If spherocytes are present they are highly suggestive of an immune-mediated anemia, but they are not found in all cases. Spherocytes are particularly difficult to detect in cats because of the small erythrocyte size. Icterus, hemoglobinuria, and hemoglobinemia are seen only in animals that have a significant amount of intravascular hemolysis. Other abnormal laboratory findings are dependent upon the amount of tissue damage that has accrued as a result of tissue hypoxia.

Immune-Mediated Thrombocytopenia (IMT).
Thrombocytopenia can be induced by the development of antibodies against them. These antibodies may be directed against the platelet membrane as the result of antigenic modification of the platelet or by antibodies that cross-react with them. It may occur in association with SLE.

Diagnosis of an autoimmune thrombocytopenia is dependent upon demonstration of a thrombocytopenia in animals that show clinical signs, including petechiation and ecchymoses in mucous membranes and skin. If there is an anemia, it can be regenerative or nonregenerative. The amount of regeneration is dependent upon the acuteness of hemorrhage, and the presence of antibodies to erythrocytes. The best test to confirm IMT is the platelet factor 3 release test. In this test platelets from a normal dog are incubated with plasma from the patient and plasma from a normal animal. If antiplatelet antibodies are present in the patient's serum, they will injure the membrane of the normal platelets, resulting in release of platelet factor 3. Following incubation of patient and normal plasma with normal platelets, coagulation tests are conducted on both. Clotting time in the tube containing patient serum will be shortened by at least 10 seconds in comparison to the clotting time of the tube containing normal plasma if platelet factor 3 has been released by action of antibodies to platelet membranes. This test should be conducted in a laboratory that specializes in coagulation studies.

Other tests for autoimmune disorders should be conducted simultaneously, because IMT often coexists with them. Suggested tests include ANA, LE cell test, and Coombs' test.

Myasthenia Gravis. This is a disorder of skeletal muscle characterized by weakness after moderate exercise. Weakness occurs because of a deficiency or blockage of acetylcholine receptors on motor end-plates of striated muscles mediated by the action of antibodies. Laboratory tests are seldom needed as the disease is clinically obvious and response to therapy often dramatic. Administration of a short-acting anticholinesterase leads to clinical improvement within a few seconds. Although antimuscle antibodies can be detected by immunofluorescence, the test is seldom used.

Sjögren's Syndrome. This condition has been reported concurrently with AIHA, SLE, hypothyroidism, rheumatoid arthritis, and polymyositis in man. A few cases have been reported in dogs with SLE. Autoimmunity develops against exocrine glands. The lacrimal gland is frequently affected, producing keratoconjunctivitis sicca. Laboratory tests, other than those routinely conducted for the diagnosis of autoimmune diseases, are of little help in arriving at a diagnosis.

Autoimmune Nephritis. There are two types of immune-mediated glomerulonephritis that occur in animals. The immune-complex type, which will be discussed later, is by far the most common. Antiglomerular basement membrane antibodies have been induced experimentally in animals; it is known that this occurs in Goodpasture's syndrome in man. Although a comparable condition has not been reported in dogs and cats, antibodies to glomerular basement membranes have been demonstrated in horses. Diagnosis is based on use of direct immunofluorescence on a kidney biopsy. The immunofluorescent pattern is an even coating of the membrane with a smooth deposit of immunoglobulin. This contrasts to the "lumpy-bumpy" immunofluorescence seen with glomerulonephritis produced by immune complexes.

AUTOIMMUNE DISEASES WITH WIDE ORGAN SPECIFICITY

Systemic Lupus Erythematosus (SLE). This is a generalized immunologic disorder involving many organ systems. It is characterized by the presence of antinuclear antibodies (antibodies to nucleic acids) and the concomitant occurrence of two or more of the following: IMT, AIHA, polyarthritis, and immune complex glomerulonephritis.[3]

The condition can be diagnosed by use of an LE cell test or an antinuclear antibody immunofluorescence (ANA) test. ANA is the test of choice for screening samples from animals suspected of having an immunologic disorder. Antinuclear antibodies are present in a number of immunologic disorders but are most frequently seen in SLE, rheumatoid arthritis, Sjögren's syndrome, mixed connective tissue disorders, scleroderma, polymyositis, and dermatomyositis.[5] Although these conditions are caused by injury resulting from antigen-antibody complexes, they may include injury occurring by any type of immune-mediated hypersensitivity.[5]

The ANA test can be conducted using a variety of substrates such as mouse or rat liver or kidney sections, tissue culture cells, or homologous leukocytes. The most commonly used method today employs cell cultures grown on a microscope slide. Serum from a patient is diluted, placed on the cells, and incubated. Following incubation the slide is washed and a fluorescein-labeled species-specific anti-immunoglobulin is added. The slide is washed, a coverslip is added, and the slide examined under a microscope with an ultraviolet light source. A number of different ANA patterns of fluorescence have been described (rim, speckled, nucleolar, homogeneous). These different patterns do not appear to have a great deal of significance in tests conducted on animal serum.[5] Interpretation of the results depends on the method by which the test is conducted. One immunologist[5] suggests that any reaction, even at a 1:10 dilution, with canine serum should be considered positive, while feline samples would need to be positive at 1:40 for the sample to be considered positive. ANA does not seem to be as severely affected by recent steroid therapy as does the LE cell test.

Although the ANA test is more sensitive and easier to perform, the LE cell test can be used. The LE cell test is probably the most reliable indicator of SLE; however, only about two thirds to three fourths of the SLE patients will have positive results. The ANA test is positive in approximately 90 per cent of dogs with SLE.[3] A positive ANA test is not specific for SLE.

Rheumatoid Arthritis. Rheumatoid arthritis is a chronic, recurrent systemic inflammatory disease primarily involving joints. Because systems other than joints are affected, the dog with rheumatoid arthritis may be depressed and anorectic in addition to being lame.

The antigen stimulus that initiates the immune response and inflammation in rheumatoid arthritis is unknown. No matter what the antigenic stimulus, the sequence of immunologic events leading to rheumatoid joint diseases has been fairly well described for man. Synovial lymphocytes produce IgG that is recognized as foreign and stimulates an immune response within the joint. IgM and IgG anti-immunoglobulins are produced and are known as rheumatoid factors. The presence of IgG aggregates or rheumatoid factor IgG complexes activates the classic complement system. The various factors produced during this activation procedure initiate and amplify the inflammatory response. Components of the inflammatory response include histamine release, production of factors chemotactic for neutrophils and mononuclear cells, and membrane damage with cell lysis. As the condition progresses, neutrophils are replaced, in part, by lymphocytes. In man this lymphocyte infiltrate is made up of both T- and B-lymphocytes. The immunologic interaction of these cells leads to the liberation of lymphokines responsible for an additional accumulation of macrophages within the inflamed joint, and continued immunoglobulin and rheumatoid factor synthesis.

Affected dogs also have secondary features that include the presence of subcutaneous nodules that contain lymphocytes and plasma cells. Disseminated arteritis, lymphatic hyperplasia, amyloidosis, and glomerulonephritis have been reported as complications.

Laboratory tests that may assist in a diagnosis include a synovial mucin clot test (see Chapter 14), the Rose-Waaler test, and a canine latex agglutination test.

With rheumatoid arthritis there is poor mucin precipitation of the synovial fluid. In normal animals the addition of acetic acid will produce a firm, hard, nonfriable clot, whereas with rheumatoid arthritis the clot is loose and friable, or only a flocculent precipitate forms.

The Rose-Waaler test is a form of antiglobulin test. The test is performed as follows: (1) Sheep RBC are collected in an anticoagulant and are washed three times to remove any globulin. (2) A subagglutinating concentration of anti-sheep RBC antibody prepared in a dog is added to the sheep RBC. (3) This mixture is incubated to permit attachment of the sheep RBC antibodies, and the cells are washed to remove any unattached antibodies. (4) Sensitized sheep RBC's are added to dilutions of the patient's serum and this mixture is incubated for one hour at 37° C, followed by an hour at room temperature. (5) Agglutination is read macroscopically and microscopically. A titer of 1:16 or greater is considered positive. Almost all dogs have a titer of 1:2 to 1:4. This, and other tests for rheumatoid factor, may be positive in dogs with other autoimmune or chronic infectious diseases.

Recently a commercial latex slide agglutination test has been made available (Synbiotics, San Diego, California). The correlation between clinical signs and positive tests by this method appears to be good, although some dogs without clinical signs of rheumatoid arthritis react positively.

IMMUNOPROLIFERATIVE DISEASES

Lymphoid neoplasia occurs in most species of domestic animals. It may involve a primary lymphoid proliferation in the nodes or lymphoid tissue only, or it may be manifested by peripheral blood changes. Such lymphoid neoplasia usually causes immunosuppression. It has been stated[1] that T-lymphocyte tumors interfere with the cell-mediated immune system and B-lymphocyte tumors with the humoral immune system. Most cases of lymphosarcoma of the dog, calf leukosis, feline leukemia, and Marek's disease are of T-lymphocyte origin. The adult forms of both bovine and ovine leukosis, alimentary forms of feline leukemia, and avian leukosis are usually of B-lymphocyte origin. In the adult form of bovine lymphosarcoma occasionally the neoplastic cell may be sufficiently differentiated to secrete immunoglobulin, and this is reflected by an increase in the amount of serum immunoglobulin.

Myelomas may develop as a result of malignant transformation of a single B-lymphocyte. This transformed cell then establishes a clone that begins to produce a single immunoglobulin. This immunoglobulin may be of class IgG, IgA, or IgM. Myelomas have been reported in dogs, cats, horses, cows, pigs, mice, rabbits, and man. A common clinical manifestation of myeloma in the dog is coagulopathy. This occurs as a result of hyperviscosity syndrome plus a loss of clotting components that bind to myeloma proteins. Because myeloma cells are also osteolytic, bone dissolution may occur and can be detected by radiography. Some animals with myeloma produce a preponderance of immunoglobulin light chains, which are rapidly excreted in the urine. These are known as Bence Jones proteins.

The diagnosis of gammopathies is based on laboratory findings. Animals with a gammopathy have an increase in total serum globulins and usually a decrease in serum albumin. Further differentiation of the immunoglobulins can be accomplished by the use of cellulose acetate electrophoresis, immunoelectrophoresis, and radial immunodiffusion. A bone marrow examination and a test for Bence Jones proteinuria may be of value.

Cellulose acetate electrophoresis is a method for quantitating the concentrations of various serum proteins (see Chapter 7). Examination of the electrophoretic pattern will reveal whether the increase in globulins is monoclonal or polyclonal. Most animals with myeloma have a monoclonal gammopathy. The monoclonal peak can occur anywhere in the electropherogram but most often is found in the gamma region. Occasionally two sharp peaks can be found, one of which is probably an aggregate or polymer of the other. Further determination of the type of immunoglobulin present in excess can be made by use of immunoelectrophoresis, as described earlier. This technique does not permit quantitation of the various immunoglobulins. The best test for determining the type of immunoglobulin is radial immunodiffusion. Slides containing animal anti-immunoglobulin antibodies are available commercially (Miles Scientific, Naperville, Illinois; VMRD Inc., Pullman, Washington; Cappel Laboratories, West Chester, Pennsylvania; Bethyl Laboratories, Montgomery, Texas; and other laboratories).

Plasma ("myeloma") cells are present in bone marrow, but similar cells are not usually present in large numbers in peripheral blood. Although careful examination of a blood film may reveal a few plasma cells, their presence is not diagnostic. An occasional patient will have plasma cell leukemia.

The test for Bence Jones proteinuria is performed by adjusting urine pH to 5 using acetic acid and heating the acidified urine slowly to boiling. Bence Jones proteins will precipitate between 50 and 60° C and redissolve on boiling. When urine is cooled the proteins reprecipitate. Albumin will not redissolve at high temperatures. As many animals with myeloma are Bence Jones protein negative, this is not a reliable test for ruling out the condition.

Polyclonal gammopathies are observed in a great number of disease conditions. Autoimmune diseases (SLE, rheumatoid arthritis, myasthenia gravis), some infections including ehrlichiosis, African trypanosomiasis, and chronic bacterial infections in which there is prolonged antigen stimulation may lead to an increase in immunoglobulins. IgG(T) levels are significantly elevated in horses heavily parasitized with Strongylus vulgaris. Similar polyclonal gammopathies can occur with virus infections such as feline infectious peritonitis or in conditions in which there is extensive liver damage.

IMMUNODEFICIENCIES

Immunodeficient animals, irrespective of the cause, have increased susceptibility to infectious diseases. Immunodeficiencies in domestic animals occur as the result of lack of adequate colostral intake by the newborn, inadequacy of T- or B-lymphocyte function, hereditary absence of T- or B-lymphocyte activity, or because of decreased macrophage activity that affects phagocytosis and antigen processing.

Methods for detecting inadequate intake of colostrum are discussed in Chapter 7.

Primary immunodeficiencies associated with T- and B-lymphocyte activity are hereditary. Secondary immunologic defects are acquired.

INHERITED T- AND B-LYMPHOCYTE DEFICIENCIES

Because of the greatly increased susceptibility of immunodeficient animals, most do not survive long enough to permit a complete assessment of the deficiency.

Hereditary Immunodeficiencies of Horses.

Hereditary deficiencies in horses have been well documented.[6-8]

COMBINED IMMUNODEFICIENCY (CID). The most severe immunodeficiency in horses is CID of the Arabian foal. These animals are born healthy but by two months of age are subject to a number of different infections with normally nonpathogenic organisms. This susceptibility is manifest after maternal IgG from the colostrum is gone. These foals do not have normal T- or B-lymphocyte production. Diagnosis of the condition is made on the basis of: (1) Absence of circulating lymphocytes or absolute lymphocyte counts that are constantly low (below 1,000/μl); (2) Absence of serum IgM. (IgG levels are not significant because their concentration depends upon the amount of colostrum and the age of the animal, whereas IgM is synthesized in response to an antigen.) (3) Presence of typical histopathology that includes a spleen devoid of germinal centers and no periarteriolar sheaths; no lymphoid follicles in nodes; and a small thymus gland. At least two of the three criteria should be present before CID is confirmed. Further confirmation can be achieved by studying the foal's ability to produce antibodies or to mount a CMI response.

The ability to produce antibodies can be tested by injecting the foal with an antigen such as RBC's from another species. Antibodies to such antigens would not normally be present in colostrum. Antibodies should appear within two to three weeks following antigen injection. Failure to respond supports a B-lymphocyte deficit. Cell-mediated immune response is best measured by use of a lymphoblast transformation test, in which culture lymphocytes are subjected to mitogens such as phytohemagglutinin. If T-lymphocyte activity is reduced or absent, there will be little or no response. Another test that has been used is inoculating a T-lymphocyte mitogen intradermally. A delayed-type hypersensitivity reaction will occur at the injection site if the foal is able to mount a T-lymphocyte response.

AGAMMAGLOBULINEMIA. This is a rare condition with only a few cases described. Affected animals were deficient in B-lymphocytes and there were no immunoglobulins in the serum. T-lymphocyte activity appeared to be normal as the peripheral lymphocytes responded to mitogens and the injection of a mitogen produced a delayed-type hypersensitivity reaction.

SELECTIVE IgM DEFICIENCY. The immune function in these foals appears to be normal except for very low serum IgM or the absence of IgM production.

SELECTIVE IgG DEFICIENCY. This is extremely rare with only one confirmed case. This was in a three-month-old foal that had normal IgM and IgA and a very low serum IgG concentration.

TRANSIENT HYPOGAMMAGLOBULINEMIA. Some foals have a temporary decrease in immunoglobulins at

TABLE 17–3. Normal Immunoglobulin Levels in Some Species of Domestic Animals*

Species	Immunoglobulin class – Mean values (mg/dl)					
	IgG	IgM	IgA	IgG$_1$	IgG$_2$	IgG(T)
HORSE, ARABIAN (SERUM)						
Foal						
1–20 days	814 ± 583	28 ± 11	21 ± 13			143 ± 88
21–40 days	480 ± 293	30 ± 10	17 ± 13			126 ± 41
41–60 days	264 ± 193	42 ± 12	20 ± 6			93 ± 33
61–80 days	252 ± 128	36 ± 12	25 ± 10			75 ± 17
81–140 days	248 ± 92	39 ± 15	64 ± 28			162 ± 126
7–12 mo.	1197	156				609
Mares—nonpregnant—thoroughbreds and Arabians (serum)						
	1640	156				619
Mares—pregnant—thoroughbreds and Arabians (serum)						
	1622	192				714
Shetland ponies (serum)						
Mature	1334 ± 350	120 ± 31	153 ± 86			821 ± 301
2–4 yrs	1065					705
Thoroughbreds (serum)						
1–14 days	1335 ± 652					
2–3 yrs	1227					162
Mixed breed						
3–5 months	380 ± 188	61 ± 22	38 ± 14			211 ± 148
DOGS (SERUM)						
Adult	1500 ± 500	150 ± 50	100 ± 60			
Puppy						
2 wks	36–70	70–370	0			
2 mo	50–170	68–130	0			
Dog (colostrum)	1453	70–370	170–520			
CATTLE (SERUM)						
Adults	1890	260	50	1100	790	
Calf—postcolostral						
2–7 days		30 ± 20		3700 ± 1330	50 ± 30	
8–15 days		80 ± 20		2500 ± 1000	40 ± 20	
30 days		60 ± 20		2200 ± 700		
60 days		120 ± 50		1000 ± 50	100 ± 100	
90 days		250 ± 70		1300 ± 300	110 ± 100	
Calf—precolostral	16	11				
Cattle—colostrum	5050	420	390	4760	290	

* Values cited by Miles Laboratories, Elkhart, Indiana and V.M.R.D. Inc., Pullman, Washington.

two to three months of age and may be susceptible to infection at that time. Such animals may have recurrent infections during this period. The hypogammaglobulinemia is transient and if affected foals survive infection, the immune response returns to normal.

Immunodeficiencies in Cattle. As with foals, the most significant clinical immunodeficiency results from the lack of colostrum. However, a few genetic immunodeficiencies have been identified in cattle.

TRAIT A–46. This immunodeficiency occurs in Black Pied Danish cattle. Calves are born healthy but at four to six weeks of age suffer from skin infections. If untreated these animals die. Immunologically affected calves have a T-lymphocyte deficiency but a normal humoral response. The T-lymphocyte inactivity can be reversed by feeding zinc oxide. The exact mechanism is not known but it has been theorized that affected animals are unable to absorb zinc. Because T-lymphocytes need zinc to respond, this lack of absorption affects their function.

SELECTIVE IgG$_2$ DEFICIENCY. An IgG$_2$ deficiency has been reported in Red Danish cattle. Affected animals have an increased susceptibility to pneumonia and mastitis. Immunologically, there are subnormal levels of IgG$_2$. Approximately 1 to 2 per cent of this breed are completely deficient in IgG$_2$, and an additional 15 per cent have subnormal IgG$_2$ levels, although the latter do not have increased disease susceptibility.[1]

IMMUNODEFICIENCIES IN DOGS. Congenital immunodeficiencies in dogs are not frequently encountered. Thymic atrophy has been reported in some inbred lines of Weimaraners. Affected dogs have normal immunoglobulins, but T-lymphocyte activity is reduced.[1]

DEFICIENCIES IN ANTIGEN PROCESSING

In man, two types of congenital deficiency syndromes have been associated with phagocytic failure. One is a failure of macrophage ability to destroy substances they have phagocytized and the other is a failure in opsonization. Opsonization failure has not been confirmed in domestic animals. A few deficiencies in the bactericidal ability of their immune systems have been reported.

CHÉDIAK-HIGASHI SYNDROME. This syndrome occurs in cats, cattle, mink, tigers, and killer whales. There is a defect in cell structure that results in formation of large primary granules in the phagocytic cells and very large melanin granules in pigmented cells. Affected leukocytes have a deficient chemotactic response and a decreased killing ability. The condition can be confirmed by finding typical bodies in leukocytes or the presence of large melanin granules in hair.

CANINE GRANULOCYTOPATHY SYNDROME. This is an autosomal recessive condition observed in Irish setters. Affected dogs have periodic episodes of infection, especially of the lymph nodes, skin, and gums. The total neutrophil count is normal or very high, but the neutrophils lack phagocytic ability and are not bactericidal.

GRAY COLLIE SYNDROME. This condition is associated with abnormal skin pigmentation, eye lesions, and cyclic neutropenia. Diagnosis is based on cyclic decreases in neutrophils and occurs about every 11 days. During the periods of neutropenia, the animals become unusually susceptible to infections.

For additional discussion on these phagocytic deficiencies, see Chapter 3.

SECONDARY IMMUNE DEFICIENCIES

Although inherited immunodeficiencies are the most prominent, acquired immunodeficiencies are probably more important clinically.

Viral infections are perhaps the most important cause of secondary immunologic defects.[1] Viruses known to cause lymphoid tissue destruction include canine distemper, feline leukemia, bovine virus diarrhea, and equine herpesvirus I.[1] Immunosuppression may also accompany infection with *Demodex*, *Toxoplasma*, *Trypanosoma*, some helminths, and some bacteria. Environmental toxins may suppress the immune system and include iodine, lead, methyl mercury, polychlorinated biphenyls, polybrominated biphenyls, and DDT.

Protein-deficient animals are unable to manufacture immunoglubins in a normal fashion. Excess protein loss as seen with renal disease, protein-losing enteropathy, and heavy parasitism will affect the immune capacity. Protein malnutrition will have the same effect.

Laboratory findings are not constant. Lymphopenia may be associated with viral diseases and all conditions may be accompanied by a hypoglobulinemia.

LABORATORY PROCEDURES IN DIAGNOSIS OF IMMUNODEFICIENCIES

Deficiencies in Humoral Immune Response. Methods for quantitating immunoglobulins have been discussed previously in this chapter. Confirmation of a deficiency in humoral immune response can be made by injecting these animals with an antigen and following development of antibodies to that antigen. This is the ultimate test for the ability of an animal to mount a humoral immune response.

Deficiencies in Cell-Mediated Immunity. Confirmation of a T-lymphocyte system deficiency is more difficult than that of a B-lymphocyte deficiency. A large number of laboratory tests have been used to identify T-lymphocyte activity, but these *in vitro* tests may not represent what is happening *in vivo*.

A total lymphocyte count may be of value because the majority (60 to 80 per cent) of the circulating lymphocytes are T-lymphocytes. A significant reduction might suggest CMI deficiency, but it must be remembered that a number of other conditions may produce lymphopenia. Lymphopenia resulting from excess glucocorticoids is of particular significance, as most sick animals are stressed. Normal or high absolute lymphocyte counts do not guarantee adequate CMI response.

It has been suggested[3] that the most reliable and simplest *in vivo* method to evaluate adequate cell-mediated immune capability in dogs and cats is a skin allograft transplant. Normal rejection time in dogs and cats is 10 to 14 days. A delay of one week or more is significant and reflects an impairment of T-lymphocyte function.

Intradermal injection of a mitogen to induce a delayed-type hypersensitivity reaction has been fairly successful in horses but apparently is not a good measurement of CMI in dogs and cats.[3]

LYMPHOCYTE BLASTOGENESIS. This is the most popular *in vitro* test for assessing T-lymphocyte function. The precise technique must be standardized for each laboratory. Once optimal conditions have been established, this provides a good immunodiagnostic method. Basically the test is conducted as follows:

1. Blood is collected in heparin.
2. Lymphocytes are isolated by centrifugation on a Ficoll-Isopaque gradient.
3. The lymphocytes are removed and cell suspension is adjusted to contain a specific number of cells.

4. Cells are placed in either a screw-cap vial or a microtiter tissue plate containing a supportive medium.

5. The mitogen of choice is added at a specified concentration.

6. Culture tubes and microtiter trays are incubated for 72 hours in 5 per cent carbon dioxide and air.

7. A radio-labeled substance, usually ^3H thymidine, is added to each cell culture a few hours before harvest.

8. The cells are harvested and the amount of radioactivity determined in a scintillation counter.

Samples should be run in duplicate or triplicate. (We run eight replicates for cattle.) Controls are run in a similar fashion except that no mitogen is added. The ability of lymphocytes to respond to mitogen is reflected by the amount of radioactivity present. Activity in mitogen-stimulated tubes is compared to activity in the controls. Radioactivity in mitogen-stimulated cultures should be two to three times that of controls if lymphocytes are capable of responding. The degree of stimulation considered to be normal must be established in each laboratory.

Decreased mitogen response has been reported in several conditions in dogs, including canine distemper, generalized demodectic mange, some nutritional deficiencies, some lymphosarcomas, and aspergillosis (uncommon). It has occurred in a percentage of dogs older than nine years, and animals treated with certain drugs.[3] Suppression in the cat has been associated with feline leukemia virus infection, panleukopenia virus infection, clinical leukemia, and occasionally in a cat that did not have a specific disease.[3] Cat lymphocytes generally respond more poorly to phytohemagglutinin than do lymphocytes of dogs or other species.

OTHER TESTS FOR CMI. The production of macrophage migration inhibition factor (MIF) can be studied *in vitro*. The technique involves placing peripheral blood cells in a capillary tube or a well in an agarose plate. Antigen or mitogen is added to the cells and if MIF is produced there is little or no migration from the tube or well. If lymphocytes do not produce MIF, normal migration will occur. The clinical interpretation of this test is not well defined.[3] Cell cytotoxic tests are also available but have not been widely used on a clinical basis.

SPECIFIC ASSAY FOR T- AND B-LYMPHOCYTES. These are primarily research techniques and involve the use of immunofluorescent antibodies to detect immunoglobulin receptors on B-lymphocytes or the erythrocyte rosette-forming assay for T-lymphocytes. The development of monoclonal antibodies for certain determinants on T-lymphocytes may make the immunofluorescence test available for identification of T-lymphocytes as well as B-lymphocytes. (For additional discussion on these techniques, see reference 3.)

REFERENCES

1. Tizard, I.: *An Introduction to Veterinary Immunology*, 2nd ed., W. B. Saunders Company, Philadelphia, 1982.
2. Schwartz, A., and Kehoe, J. M.: Fundamental principles of immunology. In: *Textbook of Veterinary Internal Medicine. Diseases of the Dog and Cat*, 2nd ed., edited by Ettinger, S. J., W. B. Saunders Company, Philadelphia, 1983.
3. Schultz, R. D.: Laboratory diagnosis of immunologic disorders. In: *Current Veterinary Therapy VII. Small Animal Practice*, edited by Kirk, R. W., W. B. Saunders Company, Philadelphia.
4. Bigazzi, P. E., and Rose, N. R.: Tests for antibodies to tissue-specific antigens. In: *Manual of Clinical Immunology*, 2nd ed., edited by Rose, N. R. and Friedman, H., American Soc. Microbiol., Washington, D. C., 1980.
5. Schultz, R. D.: ANA diseases. Calif. Vet., *7*:23, 1984.
6. McGuire, T. C., Poppie, M. J., and Banks, K. L.: Combined (B- and T-lymphocyte) immunodeficiency: A fatal genetic disease in Arabian Foals. J.A.V.M.A., *164*:70, 1974.
7. Perryman, L.: Primary and secondary immune deficiencies of domestic animals. Adv. Vet. Sci. Comp. Med., *23*:23, 1979.
8. Perryman, L., and McGuire, T. C.: Evaluation for immune system failure in horses and ponies. J.A.V.M.A., *176*:1374, 1980.

18

MICROBIOLOGY

Diagnostic medical microbiology is receiving increased emphasis as indicated by an awareness of the value of office microbiology as an aid in diagnosis of animal infections. Specific information can be learned about infective processes by applying microbiologic methods that can be performed with minimal effort and equipment. Diagnostic microbiology is concerned (1) with the etiologic diagnosis of infectious diseases by isolation and identification of infectious agents and demonstration of immunologic responses and (2) with the rational selection of antimicrobial agents to be utilized in treatment.

The results of microbial diagnostic tests in the study of infectious diseases are principally a function of the nature of the specimen, the care with which it is collected, the timing of its collection, and the technical proficiency of the individual performing the tests. A veterinarian should be competent to perform simple techniques that will assist in the diagnosis of infectious disease processes. The veterinarian dealing with infectious disease must know how and when to take a specimen, what examinations can be completed in the office laboratory, how to interpret the results, and how and when specimens should be submitted to a laboratory for confirmatory determinations.

COLLECTION OF SPECIMENS

Since results of many diagnostic tests in infectious diseases depend largely on the timing and method of collection, the veterinarian should be aware of certain rules for collecting and handling specimens. Specimens must be obtained from the site most likely to yield the infectious agent at a particular stage of illness and must be handled in a manner that will favor survival and growth of the infecting agent.

There are a few general rules for collection of samples for microbiologic examination that apply to all specimens:

1. The sample should be representative of the infectious process.
2. Care must be taken to avoid contamination of the specimen.
3. A sufficient quantity of material must be provided to permit a thorough examination.
4. Specimens must be secured prior to administration of antimicrobial drugs. If therapy is instituted prior to the collection of specimens, it may be necessary to discontinue treatment for a sufficient time to allow for disappearance of the drug. Microbial isolations from material containing a high concentration of antimicrobial drugs are difficult, if not impossible.
5. After collection, the specimen should be taken to the laboratory and examined promptly. If prompt examination is impossible, the sample should be refrigerated immediately.

The type of specimen is generally determined by the clinical signs or lesions observed at necropsy. If clinical signs point to the involvement of a specific portion of the animal body, specimens are obtained from that source. If pathologic lesions observed at necropsy are suggestive of the presence of a microbial agent, these lesions should be collected for examination. If the clinical signs indicate the possible existence of bacteremia or septicemia, blood cultures may be indicated.

In general, diagnostic tests in infectious diseases fall into the following categories:

1. The demonstration of the presence of a specific infectious agent (bacterial, viral, protozoal, or mycotic) in specimens obtained from the animal.

2. The demonstration of a skin reactivity as evidence of hypersensitivity to the antigens of a particular infectious agent.

3. The demonstration in the patient of a meaningful antibody response that involves positive information relative to an increase in specific antibody titer. This requires two serum specimens, the second of which is obtained after an interval of 10 to 21 days.

4. The demonstration of deviations in a variety of clinical pathology determinations, which may suggest or support a suspicion of infectious disease. These deviations are nonspecific but may provide evidence that could be of value in confirming a diagnosis.

ORGANS

The collection of an organ at the time of necropsy for subsequent microbial examination should be based upon the history, clinical signs, and necropsy lesions. If a bacteremia or septicemia is suspected, the selection of the organ for microbial examination should be based on the presence of lesions and should include samples of the organs through which much of the blood of the body normally passes. The organs most commonly selected include the kidney, liver, spleen, and heart.

In collecting organs for microbial examination during necropsy, care must be taken to avoid contamination by extraneous microorganisms. If material or tissues from the abdominal cavity are to be submitted for microbial examination they should be collected prior to opening the digestive tract. Exposure of organs to material in the intestine will cause excessive contamination, and the value of laboratory examination will be reduced. Tissues for microbial examination should be placed in a clean container and immediately refrigerated. If the animal has been dead for several hours, bacteriologic examination of the tissue will be less reliable than the examination of specimens obtained soon after death. In our laboratory, easily sealed plastic bags are used for collection of organs for microbiologic examination (Fig. 18–1).

In the collection of tissues for microbiologic examination, a sufficient quantity of material should be preserved to allow the technician to obtain representative samples. In smaller animals, the entire organ is collected, whereas in larger animals, representative specimens including the site of the lesion should be carefully removed and placed in a container. In collecting brain, one cerebral hemisphere should be preserved for microbial examination and the other half placed in 10 per cent formalin.

If immediate examination is impossible, the specimen should be refrigerated immediately or frozen if it is to be shipped to a laboratory.

BLOOD

Blood for microbiologic examination *must be collected under aseptic conditions.* The area over the vein should be shaved, scrubbed with soap and water, rinsed with clean water, and sterilized

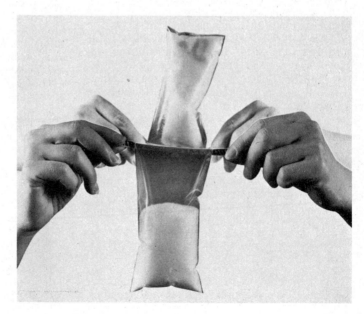

Figure 18–1. The Whirl-Pak bag is well adapted for use in collection and shipment of specimens for bacteriological examination. Photograph courtesy of Scientific Products Co. Division of American Hospital Supply Corp., Evanston, Illinois.

by placing a piece of cotton or gauze soaked in disinfectant over the entire shaved area. The skin is allowed to dry, and blood is removed with a sterile syringe and a needle. Care must be taken to avoid contamination by the skin. Depending upon the size of the animal, 5 to 10 ml of blood is removed. The blood is added to a flask containing 50 to 100 ml of a rich nutrient medium that will permit growth of fastidious organisms.

A specially designed blood culture tube is available containing supplemented peptone broth (Becton-Dickinson, Rutherford, New Jersey). Blood is drawn directly into the broth with a sterile disposable needle, and the tube is incubated and subcultured. Other commercially available blood culture sets are manufactured, and sterile blood collecting needle sets are also available (Difco Laboratories, Detroit, Michigan; Roche Diagnostics, Nutley, New Jersey; Baltimore Biological Laboratories, Baltimore, Maryland).

URINE

Urine secreted in the kidney is sterile unless the kidney is infected. Urine in the bladder is also normally sterile; however, the urethra has microbial flora. Consequently, voided urine may contain microorganisms in the absence of urinary tract infection.

The proper method for collection of urine specimens has been discussed in Chapter 9. In small domestic animals, urine is readily obtained for bacteriologic examination by means of cystocentesis. In larger animals, catheterization is the preferred method of collecting urine for microbiologic examinations, as it is almost impossible to obtain uncontaminated specimens by any other method. If the animal is catheterized, the operator must be careful to avoid contamination of the catheter, either by the skin of the animal or by the manipulation of the catheter.

When collected, urine should be placed immediately into a sterile test tube, and cultures prepared as soon as possible. If a delay of more than one hour must occur between the time of collection and culture examination, the urine may be refrigerated.

PUNCTURE FLUIDS

Exudates from the pleural, peritoneal, or synovial spaces must be aspirated, using the most careful aseptic technique. In all animals, the area should be prepared as described for obtaining blood for bacteriologic examination.

FECES

Fecal material to be examined microbiologically should be obtained directly from the rectum. In large animals, fecal material can be collected by placing a gloved hand in the rectum and obtaining a small quantity of material that is immediately placed in a sterile container. In smaller domestic animals, feces may be removed either with a finger covered with a sterile cot or by use of a sterile fecal spoon. Feces for microbiologic determination should be examined immediately or refrigerated if there is a delay in completing the examination.

WOUNDS, ABSCESSES, AND THROAT SWABS

Pus may be removed from closed, undrained abscesses by use of a sterile syringe and needle, provided the area over the infection has been carefully shaved, cleansed, and disinfected.

Sterile cotton-tipped swabs in test tubes offer the easiest method for specimen collection from open wounds or abscesses. Such swabs are prepared by inserting the stick end of the swab through a rubber stopper and inserting the swab into a test tube to fit the stopper. Swabs may be prepared and stored in the laboratory after sterilization in an autoclave or pressure cooker. In using a sterile swab, one should attempt to obtain fresh exudate. It is often difficult to recover the causative agent in an infected wound unless the specimen is taken from the deeper part of the lesion. Swabs taken from the wound surface often contain extraneous microorganisms. Extreme care must be taken to obtain the best specimen possible, and one must avoid touching any other part of the body. When swabbing has been completed, the swabs should be placed in the tube immediately and taken to the laboratory for examination. Care should be taken to prevent drying of the material. Some species of organisms are extremely susceptible to drying and will not survive long periods of time in the absence of moisture. This problem can be avoided by placing 0.5 to 1 ml of saline in the tube prior to sterilization. Tubes with a cotton swab and a special transport medium are available commercially.

Throat swabs must be carefully collected if the results are expected to reflect the true microbiologic status of the area. In making a throat swab for cultural examination, one must avoid, insofar as possible, contamination of the cotton swab with saliva. The swab should be extended to the immediate area to be examined without touching the teeth or allowing the cotton to become soaked with fluids. A myriad of organisms are present in the mouth and will interfere with proper evaluation if accidentally collected. Swabs from throat material should be soaked immediately in sterile broth to prevent drying if they are to be held prior to culturing. If the swabs are to be submitted to a central laboratory for examination, the swab may be placed in a sterile test tube containing 1 to 2 ml of sterile transport medium, and the cotton tip of the swab may be carefully broken and allowed to drop into the broth. Care must be taken to break the stick below the area that has been contaminated by handling the swab.

DIRECT SMEARS

The direct smear is a simple technique and should be used routinely as a part of any microbiologic determination. The expense of conducting such an examination and the time involved are negligible. The proper preparation of direct smears, their staining, and examination will often reveal information regarding the type of infection present and may enable the veterinarian to institute proper therapy. The direct smear technique for the detection of microorganisms is applicable in the examination of exudates, urine, cerebrospinal fluid, milk, and tissue.

PREPARATION OF SMEAR

Exudates. Exudates collected on a sterile swab can be placed on a microscope slide for examination by carefully rolling or swabbing the exudate on the surface of a precleaned microscope slide (Fig 18–2). It is recommended that two swabs be taken from the exudate, one of which is used for culturing and the other of which is used for a direct smear. If the exudate has been collected with a syringe, a small drop is placed on a clean microscope slide and carefully spread using an inoculating loop. After the slide has dried, it should be heat-fixed and stained by Gram's method.

Urine. If urine is grossly cloudy or opaque and direct microscopic examination has revealed the presence of large numbers of microorganisms, a small quantity of uncentrifuged urine can be placed directly on the slide, allowed to dry, heat fixed, and stained. However, it may be necessary to centrifuge clear urine specimens. An inoculating loop is used to remove a small quantity of sediment from the tube following centrifugation. The urine should not be spread too thinly on the slide.

Cerebrospinal Fluid. Direct smears are prepared from fresh uncentrifuged cerebrospinal fluid (CSF), which appears cloudy; otherwise smears should be prepared from sediment of centrifuged cerebrospinal fluid. These smears should be stained by Gram's method.

Milk. The direct examination of milk for detection of bacteria is discussed in the section on mastitis diagnosis later in this chapter. In general, measured quantities of milk are placed on a slide, evenly spread over a predetermined area, and stained with a methylene blue preparation.

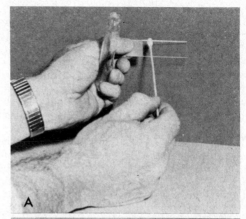
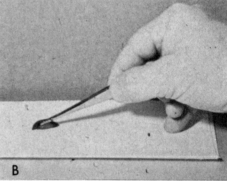
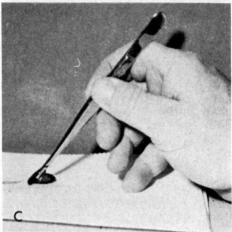

Figure 18–2. Methods for the preparation of direct smears.

A, A direct smear can be readily prepared by rolling a cotton applicator that has been used for collection of the sample over the surface of a clean glass slide. B, In the preparation of tissue impressions, the tissue should be blotted on a piece of paper towel or other absorbent surface. C, Several tissue impressions may be made by gently touching the tissue to the surface of a clean glass slide after excess blood has been removed by blotting.

Tissue. Direct microscopic examination of smears from tissue will sometimes reveal the presence of organisms with a morphology that provides a clue as to the immediate cause of death. Tissue smears for microscopic examination are easily prepared by cutting a small 1-cm square piece of tissue from an organ, blotting it carefully with cheesecloth or fine filter paper to remove excess blood, and carefully touching the cut surface of the organ to a precleaned microscope slide. Three or four such touch preparations may be made on a single slide. After the slide has dried it is heat fixed and stained by Gram's method.

If firm nodules are present, they should be crushed between two microscope slides, which are then gently drawn apart. If one suspects the presence of organisms of the genera *Actinobacillus, Actinomyces,* or *Nocardia,* the preparation should be examined unstained followed by staining with Gram's method.

In the diagnosis of certain diseases, smears should be examined in a fresh state. In addition to those already mentioned, the following diseases may be diagnosed by this procedure: coccidiosis, fungal skin diseases, trichomoniasis, trypanosomiasis, and *Balantidium coli* infection.

STAINS AND STAINING METHODS

Stained smears from fresh preparations or from bacterial colonies on a plate are routinely used in examination for the presence of bacteria. In addition, special stains may be employed to demonstrate viral inclusion bodies and to enhance the study of cellular morphology.

The most commonly used method for staining bacteria is Gram's stain. Details of the preparation of stains and the staining method are included in the Appendix. Inclusion bodies can be demonstrated by the use of a variety of different stains, including Wright's stain and Shorr's stain. Detailed techniques for preparing and using these stains are given in the Appendix.

DIAGNOSIS OF SPECIFIC BACTERIAL DISEASES BY EXAMINATION OF DIRECT SMEARS

ACTINOBACILLOSIS AND ACTINOMYCOSIS

Confirmation of a clinical diagnosis of actinomycosis is based upon the demonstration of the so-called ray fungus in a purulent exudate. The pus should be examined grossly for the presence of small calcareous granules. The presence of such granules is suggestive of this infection. Fresh smears are prepared by placing a small granule on a slide, adding a drop or two of a 1 to 5 per cent solution of sodium or potassium hydroxide, and crushing the granule by gently pressing a cover-

glass on it. This preparation is examined unstained, using low power of the microscope. Typical ray fungi appear as irregular, circular, disclike objects that have a higher refractive index than surrounding material. Examination with a ×40 objective will reveal the presence of club-shaped endings that appear as projections on the periphery of the discs.

Positive identification of the organism is dependent upon the Gram reaction. A smear stained by Gram's method is prepared and examined microscopically, using the oil immersion objective. An *Actinomyces* organism appears as a gram-positive rod that has a tendency to form heavily beaded chains or filaments. The club-shaped endings often stain poorly and may appear to be gram-negative. If the presence of the granules is a result of an infection with *Actinobacillus* organisms, the examination of the Gram-stained smear will reveal the presence of gram-negative short rods with rounded ends.

There are several other diseases in which these ray fungi bodies may occur, including botryomycosis (*Staphylococcus aureus*), coccidioidal granuloma, and nocardiosis.

ANTHRAX

A confirmatory diagnosis of anthrax *cannot be made by means of a direct smear alone but must be accompanied by animal inoculation, culture techniques, or both.* However, a direct smear prepared from blood and spleen impressions may provide evidence suggestive of the existence of anthrax.

Bacillus anthracis in blood and tissue occurs as a relatively large, square-ended, gram-positive rod, appearing in chains or sometimes occurring singly and in pairs. With the use of a methylene blue stain, a faint outline of a capsule may be noted. Correct interpretation of a direct smear is difficult, as the carcass is often contaminated with other gram-positive rods having an appearance similar to that of *Bacillus anthracis.* If typical gram-positive organisms are present in blood, edematous fluid, or tissues, the specimen should be prepared immediately for shipment to a diagnostic laboratory for confirmation (see Chapter 1).

JOHNE'S DISEASE

Cases of persistent and intermittent diarrhea in cattle should be suspected of being Johne's disease. Confirmatory diagnosis of this disease is dependent on the demonstration of acid-fast rods in feces or scrapings of the rectal mucosa or in scrapings from the thickened intestinal tract at the time of necropsy.

In preparing fecal specimens for examination, be sure to include particles of mucus or fibrin if they are present. Moderately thin smears should be prepared on slides, dried in the air, and heat fixed. The slide is stained by the acid-fast technique described in the Appendix. The specimen is examined with the oil immersion lens for the presence of acid-fast rods. *Mycobacterium paratuberculosis* appears as a bright red rod somewhat shorter than *Mycobacterium tuberculosis*. It may occur singly, in pairs, or in small clumps. A diagnosis of Johne's disease should be made if clinical signs of an intermittent and prolonged diarrhea are present and clumps of acid-fast rods can be demonstrated. These most commonly occur in epithelial cells. Similar findings may be observed in scrapings made from the rectal mucosa if that part of the digestive tract is affected.

Other acid-fast organisms not associated with disease may be observed in feces or rectal scrapings. These microorganisms are generally longer than *Mycobacterium paratuberculosis* and stain less intensely. The most common acid-fast organism present under these circumstances is the hay bacillus, *Mycobacterium phlei*. Since such contaminating organisms may be present, it is necessary to carefully evaluate fecal smears and rectal scrapings before making a positive diagnosis of Johne's disease.

A more reliable diagnosis is made by examination of slides prepared from intestinal mucosa. If a typical thickened, corrugated intestinal mucosa is present, principally in the ileum and colon, smears from this area are made. One must scrape deeply into the mucosa and prepare thin slides that are air dried, heat fixed, and stained by an acid-fast method. In smears made from infected intestinal mucous membrane, the organisms are sometimes found as single cells scattered throughout the preparation but more commonly occur in clumps. Most cells stain evenly; however, an occasional beaded form may be observed. The presence of acid-fast organisms in association with typical lesions is sufficient evidence for a positive diagnosis of Johne's disease.

Unfortunately, negative findings are never conclusive. Therefore, it behooves the veterinarian to render a diagnosis based on the combination of clinical signs, microscopic examination of smears, and, in particular, *in vivo* reaction to johnin or avian tuberculin.

LEPTOSPIROSIS

A laboratory diagnosis of leptospirosis cannot be based solely upon a direct microscopic examination of tissues, urine, or blood. However, it is possible, on occasion, to demonstrate a typical leptospiral organism in blood or urine. This microorganism is relatively resistant to most routine stains and is most readily demonstrated by darkfield examination.

In an attempt to demonstrate the presence of leptospirae, urine should first be centrifuged for a short time at a relatively low speed—1200 to 1600 revolutions per minute (rpm)—to sediment the organisms. The supernatant material is discarded, and a small amount of sediment is placed on a slide for darkfield examination.

Under darkfield illumination, the typical leptospira is a closely spiraled rod the ends of which are often bent into the shape of a hook. These organisms are actively motile, moving across the slide by means of a serpentine undulating motion.

An inexperienced individual will often make false positive diagnoses from urine preparations, mistaking rod-like or other spiraled artifacts for leptospirae. Extreme care should be taken in confirming a diagnosis of leptospirosis based solely on microscopic examination of urine.

Demonstration of an increasing titer by use of paired serum samples is the best method for confirming a diagnosis of leptospirosis.

PYELONEPHRITIS

The specific entity pyelonephritis, caused by *Corynebacterium renale*, can often be confirmed by microscopic examination of urine sediment. A Gram's stain preparation of urine sediment in cases of pyelonephritis will reveal the presence of gram-positive rods that tend to form aggregates in palisade-like clusters. This organism is a medium-sized rod-shaped bacterium having a tendency toward pleomorphism. When stained with methylene blue, the bacterium will show indistinct banding; however, this stain is not recommended as a routine procedure since it does not enable the veterinarian to differentiate gram-positive and gram-negative organisms. Methylene blue stain should be used only after a gram-positive rod has been demonstrated and is used only as a method for confirming the morphology of the organisms.

Care must be taken to differentiate between the *Corynebacterium* organism causing pyelonephritis and diphtheroids that may appear in urine as contaminants. Diphtheroids appear in small numbers, usually as individual organisms, whereas *Corynebacterium renale* appears in clusters in infected animals. Degenerate neutrophils are usually present in large numbers.

STAPHYLOCOCCAL INFECTION

Infections with *Staphylococcus aureus* in animals are characterized by the presence of purulent material. Smears made from purulent exudates may be stained by a variety of techniques including Gram's method, Wright's stain, Löffler's methylene blue, and new methylene blue. These purulent exudates are composed predominantly of neutrophils, many of which are degenerate, with the causative microorganism often present. In long-standing pyogenic infections, direct smears are frequently negative.

If the cause of the lesion is S. aureus, this organism appears as a gram-positive coccus arranged in irregular clusters. Occasionally, cocci will occur singly or in pairs, but the majority are clustered. Phagocytic cells may be seen that have a number of these coccoid organisms within the cytoplasm.

STREPTOCOCCAL INFECTION

Streptococcal infections are also characterized by the presence of a purulent exudate. As with staphylococci, streptococci can be demonstrated by several different staining techniques. In direct smears, streptococci appear as coccoid organisms occurring in chains of varying length with an occasional single coccus or diplococcus formation. Demonstration of this organism in purulent exudates is usually sufficient to confirm a diagnosis of streptococcal infection.

In open wounds, both streptococci and staphylococci are often demonstrated along with a myriad of other microorganisms. If a large variety of organisms is present, a culture examination should be completed and all isolates identified.

CLOSTRIDIAL INFECTIONS

Members of the genus Clostridium are anaerobic, spore-forming rods capable of producing a variety of diseases in domestic animals. These bacilli are extremely pleomorphic with rounded ends; however, some may appear as long, slender rods. Spores are present in all species but have a variable position, being located centrally, subterminally, or terminally. These microorganisms are generally gram-positive but are easily decolorized. With a methylene blue stain, granulation may be noted in the cells of some Clostridium species.

One of the most common clostridial infections in domestic animals is blackleg. Direct smears from affected muscle tissue will sometimes reveal the typical organism, which is a rod with rounded ends occurring either singly or in short chains. Swollen cells may be found that contain spores located terminally or subterminally, giving the organism its pear-shaped appearance. If a methylene blue stain is used, some cells may have granular material present in one or both poles. Similar microscopic observations can be made in malignant edema caused by Clostridium septicum.

In enterotoxemia, a disease produced by toxins of Clostridium perfringens, direct smears of intestinal contents of animals having succumbed to this intoxication will often reveal the presence of typical clostridial organisms. If death has resulted from such an infection, the organism is present in the intestinal contents in exceedingly large numbers and in almost pure culture. Other gram-positive organisms may be present in the intestinal contents, and a tentative diagnosis of clostridial enterotoxemia should be made only if typical organisms are abundant and are present in almost pure culture. Confirmatory diagnosis of clostridial enterotoxemia can be made only by demonstration of the toxin and its specific properties.

Clostridium haemolyticum, which causes bacillary hemoglobinuria, may be demonstrated in the liver of infected animals. Microscopic examination of a smear prepared from a characteristic liver infarct will reveal the typical gram-positive organism. The bacilli are rod-shaped with rounded ends if the organisms occur singly but may be truncate when they occur in chains. If spores are present, they appear to be heavy-walled and oval or slightly elongated, and are located terminally or subterminally.

EXAMINATION OF STOMACH CONTENTS OF AN ABORTED FETUS

A quick method for the direct examination of the stomach contents of an aborted fetus is the use of a modified acid-fast stain.[1] This staining technique is performed as follows:

1. Prepare a thin smear of stomach contents and lightly heat fix.
2. Stain 10 minutes with Ziehl-Neelsen carbolfuchsin diluted 1:10 in distilled water.
3. Wash with tap water.
4. Decolorize for 20 seconds with 1 per cent acetic acid.
5. Counterstain for 30 seconds with 1 per cent methylene blue.
6. Blot and examine with oil immersion objective.

Brucella species appear as extracellular red, coccobacillary rods usually occurring in clumps. Other bacteria will stain blue. Campylobacter fetus can be recognized by its characteristic "seagull" shape. Occasionally, some large rods will be stained red but are to be ignored. Chlamydia organisms also stain red and appear as coccoid bodies within a cell.

BACTERIAL CULTURE METHODS

GENERAL PRINCIPLES

Although much of the equipment used in the microbiology laboratory can be purchased in the form of sterile disposable plastics or glass, the veterinarian should be aware of methods for preparation of glassware to be used in microbiologic determinations. New glassware may be contaminated with spores from the surrounding packing material or may contain chemicals detrimental to the growth of certain microorganisms. Therefore, new glassware should be boiled with a detergent and well rinsed in tap water and distilled water prior to sterilization.

Sterilization of materials to be used in microbiologic determinations must be carefully conducted. Routine boiling is not sufficient for materials to be used in microbiologic work. Sterilization of glassware is best accomplished by heating in a hot-air oven. A temperature of 160° C for one hour will destroy all bacterial life, including spores. The oven of a kitchen stove is adequate for most dry-heat sterilization techniques. The temperature of such ovens should be carefully checked prior to use to determine the actual temperature in relation to the temperature indicated on the thermostatic control. Glassware should be packed loosely in the oven and covered with a material that will not ignite at the temperature used. A temperature of at least 160° C (320° F) is required for adequate sterilization. Glassware should remain at this temperature for a minimum of one hour and preferably two hours. After the glassware has remained in the oven for a sufficiently long period of time, the oven should be allowed to cool slowly. The doors should not be opened immediately, as a rapid temperature change may cause cracking of the glassware.

An oven is ideal for sterilization of flasks, Petri dishes, pipettes, and assembled all-glass syringes. Apparatus with rubber tubing, washers, or stoppers must not be sterilized in the hot air oven. Apparatus made with both metal and glass should not be sterilized by the hot-air method because of unequal expansion between glass and metal or melting of the solder or cement. The oven is not applicable for the sterilization of liquids or bacteriologic media.

Steam under pressure is an excellent method of sterilization. Sterilization by steam requires a pressure of 15 pounds per square inch at 121° C. The sterilization time required for most materials at this temperature and pressure is 15 to 20 minutes. Small autoclaves that are useful in the veterinary laboratory are commercially available. Large pressure cookers, such as those used in canning, may provide an economical method for steam sterilization. If a pressure cooker is to be used, one that indicates the pressure should be purchased. This method of sterilization is suitable for bacteriologic media, liquids, apparatus with rubber, and glass syringes that also contain metal. If liquids are being sterilized, the autoclave or pressure cooker must be allowed to return to normal pressure slowly in order to avoid boiling.

In the routine preparation of microbiologic cultures, an open flame may be utilized for the sterilization of spatulas, scissors, forceps, and inoculating loops. Care should be taken in utilizing an open flame that the material being flamed is free of excessive debris. If debris is present, it will often burst and spread contaminated material throughout the area. A small jar of disinfectant can be used for removal of such particles prior to sterilization in an open flame.

CULTURING METHODS AND TYPES OF CULTURE

Preparation of Culture Media. Most types of media useful in the isolation and identification of microorganisms may be purchased in a prepared form. Plastic disposable Petri dishes containing a variety of general and selective media are commercially available, as are disposable test tubes containing media useful in microbial identification. Such media are relatively expensive but are useful in the veterinary laboratory. If large numbers of bacteriologic cultures are done, it may be more economical to prepare media in the laboratory.

Media for bacteriologic isolation and identification are available in a dehydrated form. Such media are reconstituted by the addition of distilled water. If the manufacturer's directions are followed, these media provide an excellent nutritive source for microorganisms.

Several different types of media are used in bacteriology. Care must be taken to use the most suitable type for isolation and identification of microorganisms. Media may be either liquid or solid; the type most commonly used for isolation is solid. Types of media used in a microbiologic laboratory can be divided into four main groups: (1) simple media for use in the routine bacteriologic examinations of tissues, fluids, or swabs; (2) enriched media that are required for the growth of certain fastidious bacteria; (3) selective media that are designed to permit the growth of certain types of bacteria while either preventing or decreasing the growth of other microorganisms; and (4) media used for detecting biochemical functions.

The simplest medium utilized in microbiologic determinations is usually nutrient agar, which consists of beef extract, peptones, agar, and water. This medium is generally used for the maintenance of microorganisms and is seldom used for original isolation. Simple broths may be used to support the growth of bacteria after the original isolation has been made on a solid medium. Cultures to be used for antibiotic sensitivity determinations are grown in such a medium.

The most common enriched medium used in veterinary practice is blood agar. Blood agar is prepared by adding 5 to 10 per cent sterile blood to a base medium. The base medium is usually a form of nutrient agar containing the essentials required for bacterial growth. In the preparation of blood agar, the base medium is melted and cooled to about 45° C. Sterile blood is added aseptically and mixed by careful swirling of the flask in a circular fashion. Every attempt should be made to avoid shaking, which will create air bubbles. As soon as mixing is completed, the medium is poured into sterile Petri dishes and allowed to solidify. This medium serves as a base for the isolation of most aerobic microorganisms.

Selective media are important, as they contain deterrents to the growth of bacteria other than those under examination. Several different types of deterrents are employed: for example, bile salts in a medium prevent growth of nonenteric organisms, and sodium chloride prevents the growth of organisms other than staphylococcus. The use of selective media for the isolation of specific microorganisms will be discussed later.

Technique of Plate Inoculation. Only the proper technique of streaking a Petri dish containing a solid medium will ensure isolated colonies (Fig. 18–3). It is a waste of time and material to simply smear a specimen over a plate and expect to arrive at a bacteriologic diagnosis. Every attempt should be made to streak a plate in such a manner that isolated colonies will be present. If no isolated colonies are obtained, a fresh specimen should be cultured or the original plate should be subcultured. The method found to be most useful in our laboratory is performed as follows: (1) Have available a Petri dish containing the nutrient medium in which the bacteria will multiply. Blood agar is routinely used. (2) If a liquid such as milk is to be cultured, pick up a loopful of material and rub it across the surface of a small area next to the edge of the plate. Be careful to just touch the surface of the medium and do not dig into the agar (Fig. 18–4). If isolation is to be attempted from tissues, a small piece of tissue is aseptically removed from the organ and carefully swabbed over a small area of the plate. If the material to be cultured is on a swab, the swab

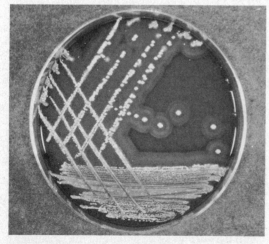

Figure 18–3. A plate should be streaked so that single well-isolated colonies are present.

should be rubbed across the surface in a gentle manner, and care taken not to break the surface of the agar. The lid of the plate is opened just wide enough to admit the loop, forceps, or swab. If the plate is opened widely it may result in contamination from the air. (3) Flame an inoculating loop and allow it to cool or cool it by stabbing it once or twice in the medium in an area that has not been streaked. (4) Turn the plate at right angles and streak over approximately one fifth of the plate. Be careful not to streak into the previously inoculated area. Several streaks approximately $\frac{1}{4}$ inch from each other should be made. (5) Again flame the inoculating loop and cool it. (6) Turn the plate at right angles and streak into the second area. (7) Flame the inoculating loop and cool it. (8) Turning the Petri dish at right angles, again streak, being sure that you do not enter the area of original inoculation. (9) Turn the plate upside down and incubate it for a minimum of 24 hours at 37° C or until a good growth has been obtained.

Blood Cultures. Although blood cultures are not routine, they may be indicated for detection of bacteremia or septicemia. The technique for collecting blood for culture examination has been previously discussed.

Perhaps the simplest method of blood culture is to utilize a special Vacutainer (Becton-Dickinson, Rutherford, New Jersey) designed specifically for this purpose. If such equipment is not available, the technique described as follows is acceptable.

Addition of blood to a flask containing nutrient medium must be carefully completed. The rubber top of the bottle is disinfected with alcohol and flamed. A needle other than the one used for collecting the blood should be used to introduce blood into the culture flask. The medium utilized in the flask may vary. One medium that has proven successful is brain-heart infusion with agar and para-aminobenzoic acid (PABA) (Difco Laboratories, Detroit, Michigan) to which penicillinase may be added if the animal has been under treatment. This medium will support both aerobic and anaerobic microorganisms, and the PABA and penicillinase neutralize the bacteriostatic effect of sulfonamides and penicillin, respectively. The medium most commonly used to detect the presence of anaerobes is thioglycollate broth. After inoculation, the broth is incubated at 37° C for periods of up to three weeks. The collecting bottles are examined for bacterial growth every 24 to 48 hours by inspection, subcultures, and smears. Strict aseptic precautions should be observed in obtaining material for subculturing or preparation of smears. The rubber stopper in the blood flask must be sterilized with alcohol and flaming, and a sterile syringe and needle must be used to remove a small quantity of material.

If bacteria grow from blood cultures, it is necessary to determine their significance by ruling out any technical error. The following criteria

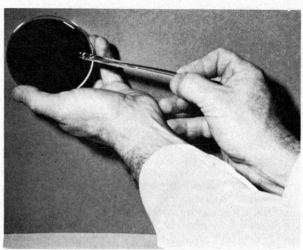

Figure 18–4. Care must be used in streaking an agar plate to avoid digging into the agar. The inoculating loop is a piece of glass tubing that has a Nichrome wire loop placed into the hole in the tube and then secured in place by heating and crushing the heated end with a pair of forceps. This provides an economical and light-weight inoculating loop.

may be used in differentiating a true positive from a contaminated specimen: (1) growth of the same type of organism in repeated cultures indicates a bacteremia; (2) growth of a large number of a single type of organism will also indicate the presence of a bacteremia; (3) small numbers of several different types of organisms is suggestive of contamination; (4) the isolation and identification of common skin flora such as *Staphylococcus epidermidis* or diphtheroids are usually suggestive of contamination.

For cultural examination, a single blood specimen taken at the height of the illness is usually meaningless, unless a microbial type is identified that may commonly be encountered as a problem in the species of animal being examined. Any type of pathogenic microorganism isolated from the blood is a significant diagnostic finding. If repeated culture examination of the blood continues to reveal the presence of this microorganism, the therapy being used should be carefully evaluated. *In vitro* antibiotic sensitivity determinations may be of assistance in selecting the proper therapeutic agent for treatment.

Urine Cultures. In the examination of urine cultures, attempts should be made to quantitiate the number of bacteria present. Properly collected urine is best cultured by adding a measured quantity onto the surface of a solid medium such as blood agar. The number of colonies and the type of organism present are both of significance. If the majority of colonies present represent a single bacterial type, it may be assumed that this organism is present in the urinary tract. If only a few colonies appear on the plate and they appear to have different colony characteristics, it may be assumed that they exist in the specimen as a result of contamination. All urine cultures should be incubated for 48 to 72 hours prior to being discarded. Bacteria most commonly encountered in diseases of the urinary tract grow well on blood agar, and the use of selective or enrichment media is seldom indicated.

If the animal from which urine was obtained has been treated with an antimicrobial agent, isolation is difficult. Some antimicrobial activity may be counteracted by washing the urine sediment prior to culturing. Urine to be cultured is centrifuged for 15 to 30 minutes in order to sediment the bacteria. The supernatant urine is carefully poured from the tube, and sterile saline is added. The sediment is resuspended by agitating the tube, and centrifugation is repeated. This washing procedure should be repeated two or three times, and following the final centrifugation, the sediment is carefully streaked onto a blood agar plate. This washing procedure has the effect of diluting the antimicrobial agent to a point at which it no longer prohibits microbial multiplication.

Cerebrospinal Fluid Cultures. Cerebrospinal fluid should be cultured whenever the results of a laboratory examination of this material indicate the possible existence of a bacterial infection. The presence of large quantities of protein, decreased glucose concentration, and large numbers of leukocytes may suggest bacterial infection. Approximately 1 ml of cerebrospinal fluid that has been aseptically removed should be spread over the surface of a blood agar plate, and the plate should be incubated at 37° C for 24 to 96 hours. As in the case of urine culture examination, the presence of relatively large numbers of colonies of an identical type is suggestive of bacterial infection. The finding of only a few colonies having varying characteristics is usually a sign of contamination. It is important, however, to examine microscopically any colony found on a plate that has been prepared from cerebrospinal fluid.

Oxygen Requirements. The majority of the pathogenic microorganisms encountered are aerobic and grow well when placed in an incubator.

However, certain bacteria require an increased carbon dioxide concentration in order to grow well upon original isolation. A simple method for creating a high carbon dioxide atmosphere is to place the culture plates in an airtight container with a candle. The candle is lighted and the lid securely tightened. As the candle burns, it reduces the concentration of oxygen, and the concentration of carbon dioxide will be increased to satisfactory proportions. A small pressure cooker that will easily fit into the incubator provides an excellent container for carbon dioxide incubation. A large-mouthed gallon jar is also an adequate container if it can be tightly closed.

Although anaerobic culture methods are not generally used, techniques for creating an anaerobic atmosphere are relatively simple. Prepackaged chemicals are commercially available (Gas-Pak, Baltimore Biological Laboratories, Baltimore, Maryland) as are anaerobic jars and disposable anaerobic systems.

In our laboratory, three-pound peanut butter jars (content 1.5 liters) are used and an anaerobic atmosphere is created as follows:

1. Place 22.5 ml of 15 per cent sulfuric acid in a small beaker (50 to 100 ml).
2. Add 2.25 gm of powdered chromium metal.
3. Place beaker and contents in jar.
4. Put preinoculated plates on or beside the beaker.
5. Screw lid on firmly and place in incubator at 35 to 37° C.

This technique can be modified to produce a carbon dioxide atmosphere by adding a gelatin capsule containing 0.75 gm of sodium carbonate to the mixture of sulfuric acid and chromium. The acid will destroy the gelatin to release sodium carbonate, and carbon dioxide will be generated.

BACTERIAL IDENTIFICATION

COLONY CHARACTERISTICS

The examination of a culture plate should be carefully conducted, and the characteristics of the colonies present noted. Considerable information concerning identification can be ascertained from the colony type.

Contaminants commonly encountered in veterinary bacteriology fall into two categories, bacilli and diphtheroids. The typical bacillus colony is relatively large, often hemolytic on blood agar, and dry in appearance; it has a rough surface and irregular edges. Diphtheroids produce colonies that are smaller (1 to 3 mm in diameter), white to tan, and usually nonhemolytic.

The majority of the pathogenic microorganisms have a colony size that will vary from less than 1 mm to 5 mm; characteristically they are smooth, moist, entire, and slightly raised, and their hemolytic properties vary according to the genus and species. There are certain exceptions, however, as colonies of *Bacillus anthracis* are typical for that genus and the colonies of *Corynebacterium pseudotuberculosis* and *Nocardia asteroides* are small but rough in character.

MORPHOLOGY

In the identification of bacteria, single isolated colonies that are characteristic of the growth should be examined by preparing a smear on a glass microscope slide for Gram's stain. Correlation of the findings with colony characteristics may enable the veterinarian to make a tentative identification. Absolute information concerning the genus and species can be obtained only by the use of additional tests.

Morphologically, bacteria appear as either cocci or rods that are gram-positive or gram-negative. Cocci are further divided into those appearing in clumps (staphylococci) or those occurring in chains (streptococci). Pathogenic cocci are almost universally gram-positive. Rods, on the other hand, may appear as large or small gram-positive organisms or as gram-negative organisms whose morphology may vary from a very small, almost coccoid rod to a comma-shaped or spiral organism.

SEROLOGIC IDENTIFICATION

Bacteria are chemically composed of a variety of compounds that have the ability to serve as antigens. Because of the specificity of these antigens in the production of antibodies, serologic tests may be used as a method for identification of bacteria. Such identification is dependent upon the availability of antisera that are either group specific or genus and species specific. The specific application of these serologic determinations will be discussed later in the chapter in the description of methods for the identification of specific microorganisms.

In general, either group or specific antisera are added to a pure culture of the organism, and the reaction is observed. The type of test utilized may vary from the microscopic agglutination test to the refined fluorescent antibody technique. Although veterinary practitioners probably will not use fluorescent microscopy as a diagnostic technique in bacteriology, they should be familiar with the basic principles involved.

Fluorescent Microscopy. The conjugation of specific antibodies with fluorescein and the application of such a conjugated antibody to bacteria or tissues for the identification of specific infectious agents has become an important diagnostic tool. Fluorescent antibody (FA) methods may replace some serologic methods for making a final identification of a specific bacterium. Diagnosis of some virus-induced diseases is now routinely made by use of FA.

The fluorescent antibody technique depends on the combination of a specific antibody with its antigen. In the direct FA method, the antibody coats the antigen (bacteria, viruses, or protozoa, for example) and is not easily removed. If the antibody has been rendered fluorescent by conjugation with a dye such as fluorescein isothiocyanate and all nonantibody globulin is removed by washing, all remaining antibody is firmly attached to the antigen. If the antigen is a bacterial cell and is viewed with the appropriate optical system, the bacterial cell is outlined with fluorescent material.

An important consideration in fluorescent microscopy is the availability of correctly designed special equipment. Important to the success of a fluorescent microscopy determination are the light source, microscope, and various heat-absorbing exciter and barrier filter combinations. It is advisable to use a darkfield condenser for routine work, although fluorescence microscopy with a brightfield microscope can be used for certain preparations. A number of light sources are available commercially, and care should be exercised in the selection of a unit. The most expensive units feature a closed system that can be set up more permanently than the less expensive types. A variety of filters are employed between the lamp and the object and between the object and the observer so that only wavelengths that are characteristic of fluorescence are seen. A variety of filter combinations are used, depending upon the type of material examined. Other than the special lenses, filters, and light source that are required, little in the way of additional equipment is necessary.

In order to reduce nonspecific fluorescence, special glass slides and an oil with low fluorescence index are required.

Two basic techniques are used in fluorescent microscopy. These are the direct FA method and the indirect FA technique (Fig. 18–5). In the direct method, smears of the material to be examined are fixed, and the smear is flooded with the conjugated globulin reagent containing a specific antibody. The flooded smear is incubated in a moist chamber at 37° C for 30 to 60 minutes. The smear is washed twice, first in buffered saline for five to 10 minutes, then in tap water for an additional five to 10 minutes. This washing removes all uncombined conjugated globulin. A drop of buffered glycerol is placed on the smear, and a nonfluorescing coverslip is added. The smear is then ready for examination under the fluorescent microscope.

In the indirect method, the smear is first treated with unlabeled antiserum. This is sometimes referred to as the primary combining action and is carried out in a manner identical with that for the direct test. Following incubation and washing, fluorescein-labeled antiglobulin homologous to the globulin of the animal species whose serum is used in the primary reaction is added, and the smear is again incubated and washed. Treatment

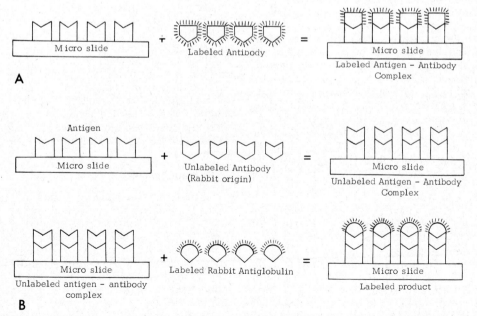

Figure 18–5. Schematic representation of: *A*, Direct staining with fluorescein-labeled antibody specific for the antigen. *B*, Indirect fluorescent antibody technique using unlabeled specific antibody of rabbit origin and labeled rabbit antiglobulin.

of the preparation with this fluorescein-labeled antiglobulin will result in a specific attachment of the antiglobulin to the globulin that is already specifically attached to an antigen. When this preparation is examined under the microscope, fluorescence will indicate a reaction between the antigen and the unlabeled specific antibody employed in the first stage. If no combination between antigen and specific antibody has occurred, then no fluorescence will be seen subsequent to the addition of the fluorescein-labeled antiglobulin.

The indirect method has the advantage of reducing the number of labeled antisera needed. If all diagnostic antisera are produced in a single animal species, such as the rabbit, one needs only a fluorescein-labeled antirabbit globulin. Such sera are produced by the inoculation of rabbit globulin into another species of animal.

Many labeled antisera can be purchased commercially, as can antirabbit globulin and nonlabeled specific antisera. Since the production of labeled antisera is complicated and time consuming, commercial preparations should be utilized when available.

The EIA Technique (Chapter 17) is rapidly replacing immunofluorescence.

BIOCHEMICAL PROPERTIES

Identification of an unknown organism is dependent not only on its morphologic characteristics and antigenic content but also on its biochemical properties. Determining the genus, species, or both of an unknown organism may require identification of a variety of biochemical activities.

The ability or inability of a particular organism to utilize a given sugar or other carbohydrate is often of value in identification. Such biochemical activity is determined by testing for the production of acid, gas, or both. Acid and gas are most readily produced by preparation of a liquid growth medium incorporating the specific carbohydrate to be studied. A small glass vial is inverted in the liquid medium in order to trap any gas produced. An indicator is incorporated in the medium, and a color change demonstrates the production of an acid as a result of fermentation of the carbohydrate.

In addition to their activity on a specific carbohydrate, bacteria may be characterized on the basis of the production of specific metabolic products. Metabolic products that may be identified and serve as a method for characterization of the organism include indole, acetylmethyl carbinol, hydrogen sulfide, and ammonia. In most of these tests, a specific medium is used so that the bacterium will have an opportunity to produce such an end product as a result of its metabolic activity on a specific substrate.

Some microorganisms have the ability to produce specific changes in milk. Alterations that may be observed in milk containing litmus include pH balance alteration, the production of a variety of curds, peptonization, and reduction.

Bacteria may also exhibit a variety of reducing capacities that are relatively simple to observe. One of the reduction tests most commonly used is detection of the ability of a bacterial species to reduce nitrate or nitrite to ammonia or gaseous nitrogen. The reduction of dyes such as methylene blue or litmus to a colorless form may also be used.

Detection of the ability of a bacterial species to produce an exoenzyme may also be of significance in identification. Included among such enzymes are digestive enzymes that are capable of breaking down gelatin, serum, casein, albumin, or starch. Some organisms produce an enzyme that is capable of coagulating serum or one that may dissolve red blood cells. It is a well-recognized fact that some exoenzymes produced by bacteria are capable of acting as potent toxins, and the identification of the presence of a specific toxin may be an indication of the presence of a specific bacterial species.

CHARACTERISTICS OF PATHOGENIC BACTERIA

GRAM-POSITIVE COCCI

Gram-positive cocci pathogenic to domestic animals belong to two genera, *Streptococcus* and *Staphylococcus*. In the clinical laboratory, members of these two genera can be differentiated by microscopic examination.

Blood agar is the medium of choice for isolation of gram-positive cocci. Some species are fastidious in their growth requirements, and one important identifying characteristic is their effect on blood. Specialized media may be used for isolation and identification of organisms within this group, and these will be discussed when appropriate.

Streptococcus

Streptococci are spherical bacteria characteristically arranged in chains and widely distributed in nature. Some species are part of the normal animal flora, whereas others are associated with disease. These bacteria may produce a variety of extracellular substances and enzymes. One of the important methods of classification is dependent upon their ability to hemolyze red blood cells.

MORPHOLOGY. Individual cocci are ovoid or spherical and are arranged in chains. Cocci forming a chain may have a striking diplococcic appearance and the length of the chains varies widely, depending on environmental factors (Fig. 18–6).

ANTIGENIC PROPERTIES. Hemolytic streptococci can be divided into serologic groups. The basis for such typing is the precipitation reaction using a specific carbohydrate substance as the antigen. This grouping, called Lancefield typing, divides the streptococci into the following groups: group A, which is composed of the more virulent human strains as typified by *Streptococcus pyogenes*; group B, which includes the bovine mastitis streptococci typified by *Streptococcus agalactiae*; group C, which is made up of human and animal strains that produce hemolysis on blood agar, such as *Streptococcus equisimilis*; group D, which includes the enterococci and strains isolated from dairy products; group E, which includes strains isolated from milk and from abscesses in swine; group F, which is composed of a streptococcus that produces a minute colony and is isolated from the respiratory tract of humans; group G, which contains both a minute colony type and a large colony type, the small colony having been isolated from the respiratory tract of humans and the large colony from dogs; group H, which is composed of strains isolated from the respiratory tract of humans but are of questionable virulence; group K, which includes strains isolated from the respiratory tract of humans but are of doubtful virulence; group L, which includes strains isolated from the genital tract of the dog; group M, which is composed of strains isolated from respiratory tissues of the dog; and group N, which includes streptococci found in milk, such as *Streptococcus lactis* and *Streptococcus cremoris*. This method for typing streptococci is used in the confirmation of strain identification that cannot be made by other methods. It is not a procedure widely used in a practice laboratory for the identification of streptococci.

CULTURE. Most streptococci grow well on a solid medium such as blood agar as discrete, transparent, dewdrop-like colonies approximately 1 to 2 mm in diameter. The degree and type of hemolysis produced may vary from none to the alpha (green) hemolysis or beta (complete) hemolysis. This variation in hemolytic abilities may serve as an identifying characteristic. The degree of hemolysis produced by the various species of streptococci in animals is shown in Table 18–1.

LABORATORY IDENTIFICATION. Members of the genus *Streptococcus* are readily identified in the laboratory by streaking all specimens suspected of containing this organism on blood agar. Growth of a bacterium producing a characteristic small, glistening, dewdrop-like colony capable of varying degrees of hemolysis is suggestive of the presence of the genus. Positive identification of the genus can be made by means of Gram's stain, which will reveal the presence of cocci arranged in chains. In slides prepared from solid medium, the chains may be short, being composed of two to 16 organisms (Fig. 18–6). If the organism is grown in broth, some species will produce extremely long chains.

Species identification is dependent upon activity on a variety of carbohydrates, production of alterations in milk containing litmus, and ability to hemolyze blood. An isolate may be further categorized by use of Lancefield typing (Table 18–1).

Staphylococcus

Staphylococci are coccoid cells usually arranged in grape-like clusters, although short chains and pairs are frequently seen in liquid media. Staphylococci grow readily on a variety of media, are metabolically active, and produce pigments that may vary from white to orange. Pathogenic staphylococci usually hemolyze blood and produce the enzyme coagulase, which has the ability to coagulate plasma. These organisms are found ubiquitously in nature, occurring as part of the normal flora, but may on occasion be quite

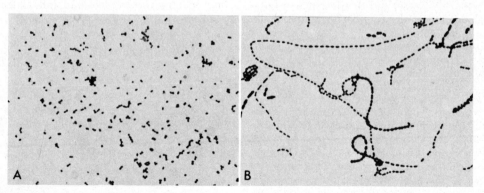

Figure 18–6. Gram stain of *Streptococcus* sp. *A*, From a colony grown on an agar plate. When smears are made from such a source, chain formation is minimal and the organisms may be mistaken for diplococci, micrococci, or staphylococci. *B*, Typical chain formation of streptococci grown in broth.

TABLE 18–1. Some Distinguishing Characteristics of Animal Streptococci*

Bacterial Species	Hemolysis	Lancefield Group	Litmus Milk			Animal Species Infected
			ACID	COAGULATION	REDUCTION	
Str. pyogenes	Beta	A	+	−	±	Cow
Str. zooepidemicus	Beta	C	+	−	−	Horse, cow, pig
Str. equi	Beta	C	−	−	−	Horse
Str. equisimilis	Beta	C	+	−	±	Horse, cow, pig, dog, birds
Str. agalactiae	Gamma, alpha, or slight beta	B	+	+	±	Cow
Str. dysgalactiae	Gamma, alpha, or slight beta	C	+	−	+	Cow
Str. uberis	Gamma, alpha, or slight beta	?	+	±	+ +	Cow
Str. canis	Beta	C	+	−	+	Dog

* Carbohydrate fermentation will result in more positive identification.

virulent. In general, *Staphylococcus aureus* is found in association with suppurative processes.

MORPHOLOGY. As previously indicated, the typical organism is a spherical cell that is approximately 1 micron in diameter and arranged in irregular clusters, although single cocci, pairs, and chains may be seen in liquid media. Young cocci stain strongly gram-positive; however, as the culture ages many cells may become gram-negative. Staphylococci do not form spores and are nonmotile.

ANTIGENIC CHARACTERISTICS. Staphylococci contain antigenic proteins and polysaccharides, which permit limited grouping of the strains. These organisms are not easily differentiated into antigenic strains. Strain identification of staphylococci has been more readily accomplished by testing their susceptibility to bacteriophages.

TOXIN PRODUCTION. The pathogenic *Staphylococcus aureus* produces potent culture filtrates for which several terms are employed; dermonecrotoxin, hemotoxin, lethal toxin, leukocidin, enterotoxin, coagulase fibrinolysin, and hyaluronidase. These toxins undoubtedly play a role in the production of disease, and the presence of coagulase is an important criterion for classification as a pathogen.

LABORATORY IDENTIFICATION. *Staphylococcus aureus* can be tentatively identified in the laboratory on the basis of its characteristic colony (Plate 18–1D). On blood agar *Staphylococcus aureus* appears as a hemolytic organism often producing a "double zone" hemolysis. The colonies are smooth, round, glistening, and opaque, and the color ranges from white through yellow to orange. Identification of this organism as a pathogen may be made by use of the coagulase test conducted either as a rapid plate method or by means of the tube technique. (Details of these techniques are presented in the Appendix, pp. 452–453.) Gram's staining of a typical colony will reveal the presence of cocci arranged in clusters (Fig. 18–7).

Use of a selective medium such as Staphylococcus 110 medium containing 7.5 per cent sodium chloride may enhance growth of the organism in pure culture, as few other species grow at this high salt concentration. Glycine tellurite agar may also be used as a selective medium on which staphylococci produce a black shiny colony.

Some strains of *Staphylococcus aureus* of animal origin can be identified by the use of bacteriophage typing. This technique is particularly applicable for use in epidemiologic studies of staphylococcal infection. *Staphylococcus epidermidis* is a nonpigmented, coagulase-negative staphylococcus (Table 18–2). This organism is considered to be a normal inhabitant of the skin and mucous membranes and the animal environment. This organism does not produce toxins and is not thought to be a frequent cause of disease.

GRAM-POSITIVE RODS

A number of genera are gram-positive bacilli: *Listeria, Erysipelothrix, Corynebacterium, Bacillus, Actinomyces, Nocardia,* and *Clostridium.*

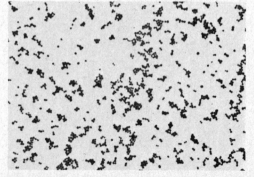

Figure 18–7. Typical arrangement of staphylococci when the smear is made from an agar plate.

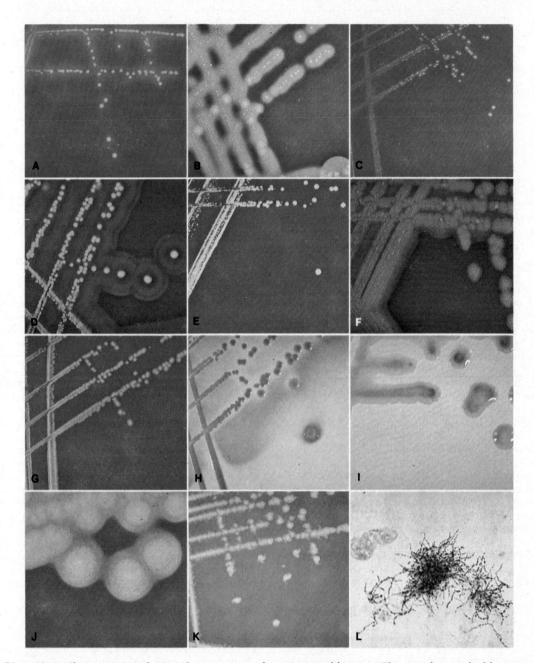

Plate 18–1. Characteristic colonies of some commonly encountered bacteria (Photographs supplied by courtesy of Dr. Wayne Bailie, Kansas State University). *A*, Alpha hemolytic streptococcus, *B*, Beta hemolytic streptococcus; *C*, Nonhemolytic streptococcus; *D*, *Staphylococcus aureus* with double-zone hemolysis; *E*, Nonhemolytic *Staphylococcus epidermidis*; *F*, *Pseudomonas aeruginosa* showing the characteristic hemolytic rough colony; *G*, Typical appearance of a nonhemolytic gram-negative rod on blood agar; *H*, *Escherichia coli* colonies on MacConkey agar; *I*, Mucoid colonies of *Klebsiella* sp. on MacConkey agar; *J*, *Bacillus cereus*, a common soil microorganism on blood agar. Such hemolytic bacilli are frequently encountered in contaminated specimens. *K*, *Bacillus anthracis* on blood agar; *L*, A modified acid-fast stain of a *Nocardia* organism in an exudate. Note the beaded appearance.

TABLE 18–2. Differentiation of *Staphylococcus Aureus*, *Staphylococcus Epidermidis*, and *Micrococcus* Organisms

Property	S. AUREUS	S. EPIDERMIDIS	MICROCOCCUS
Hemolysis	+	–	–
Coagulase produced	+	–	–
Pigmented	White, golden to orange	No pigment	No pigment
Mannitol fermented	+ (usually)	– (usually)	– (usually)
Gelatin liquefaction	+ (usually)	– (usually)	–
Anaerobic fermentation of dextrose	+	+	–

With the exception of the genus *Clostridium*, all of these ogranisms are aerobes, although *Actinomyces* grows best upon primary isolation under anaerobic or microaerophilic conditions. These bacteria have varying morphologic and growth characteristics that will be discussed.

Listeria

The single species within this genus is *Listeria monocytogenes*. This organism is widely distributed in a number of different hosts in which it may produce various types of disease that are collectively called listeriosis. In ruminants and swine, lesions are usually confined to the central nervous system, producing a meningitis and monocytic infiltration and focalization. This organism has been isolated from an aborted fetus, and in laboratory animals such as the guinea pig, rabbit, and chinchilla, it produces liver necrosis. It may occasionally be associated with meningitis and uterine infections in humans.

MORPHOLOGY. *Listeria monocytogenes* is a small gram-positive rod with rounded ends. In some cultures, filamentous forms as long as 4 microns have been observed. It may occur singly or in short chains of three to six organisms. It is motile and non–spore-forming and does not produce a capsule.

CULTURE. Examination of tissues for the presence of *Listeria* organisms may be difficult. In fresh brain tissue there apparently is an inhibitory substance that may prevent growth. The organism is more easily isolated from brain tissue that has been refrigerated for a few weeks. Isolation may be enhanced either by swabbing large quantities of brain tissue over the surface of a blood agar plate or by grinding the tissue prior to inoculation of the culture medium. The utilization of a 0.05 per cent concentration of potassium tellurite in tryptose agar may assist in isolation. Colonies of *Listeria* organisms appear on this medium as black with a green peripheral color.

LABORATORY IDENTIFICATION. On blood agar, this organism appears as a minute colony that is smooth, transparent, and circular. The typical colony is surrounded by a zone of beta hemolysis on blood agar.

Listeria monocytogenes can best be identified in the laboratory by the presence of a typical colony and its characteristic morphology. Positive identification is dependent upon the fermentation of carbohydrates, action on litmus milk, and motility. This organism produces an umbrella pattern in motility medium after incubation at 25° C.

Erysipelothrix

Bacilli classified in this genus are gram-positive slender rods. The single species is *Erysipelothrix insidiosa*. This organism is capable of producing in swine a disease that may exist in an acute, chronic, or urticarial form. Sheep infected with this organism may exhibit clinical signs of a chronic polyarthritis. In addition to causing diseases in swine and sheep, this organism has been isolated in sporadic infections of dogs, cattle, and horses. Natural infection may occur in chickens, pigeons, geese, ducks, and turkeys, in which it produces a peracute septicemia.

MORPHOLOGY. *Erysipelothrix insidiosa* is variable in form, appearing either as short rods, thickened filaments, or bent and tangled filaments resembling mycelium. Branching is not common but has been observed. In smears from tissue, it usually appears as a short, straight, or bent, slender rod 1 to 2 microns in length. A greater variety of shapes are observed in liquid media.

CULTURE. The presence of serum is usually required for adequate growth. The typical colony is small, round, discrete, and translucent; it has entire edges and is seldom more than 1 mm in diameter. Larger opaque, uneven-surfaced colonies that tend to become confluent are sometimes observed and are referred to as the R, or rough, form. This organism produces hemolysis that may vary according to the age of the culture, tending to be green at first and later becoming a clear zone of beta hemolysis. Blood agar containing sodium azide and crystal violet may be advantageously used in isolating this organism from contaminated tissues.

LABORATORY IDENTIFICATION. Isolation of the gram-positive rod with typical morphology and a characteristic colony may be sufficient for identification of this organism. Demonstration of the typical slender gram-positive rods in smears of tissue is suggestive of infection with *Erysipelothrix insidiosa*. Serologic tests are of value in the living animal only in chronic infections. Most strains of *Erysipelothrix insidiosa* produce hydrogen sulfide following 48 to 96 hours incubation at 37° C. This characteristic may be used as an aid in identification.

Corynebacterium

This genus is composed of bacteria found in both animals and humans, and many of these organisms are nonpathogenic, being found on normal mucous membranes. A few species are pathogenic and may be associated with acute and chronic diseases of animals. Included in the strictly animal species are *Corynebacterium pyogenes*, *Corynebacterium renale*, *Corynebacterium pseudotuberculosis*, and *Corynebacterium equi*. A few other species have been described and named but are not important to animal health.

MORPHOLOGY. Members of the genus *Corynebacterium* are small, coccoid, pleomorphic gram-positive bacilli. *Corynebacterium pyogenes* is characteristic of this genus, which is sometimes referred to as the diphtheroid genus. The organisms are usually single but show a tendency to form clumps, sometimes in a palisade arrangement. *Corynebacterium pseudotuberculosis* may have filamentous forms. It also has a tendency to clump together in a palisade formation. In smears from infected tissue, the organism is quite pleomorphic but on artificial media is uniformly coccoid. Metachromatic granules are observed in the bacillary or filamentous forms but are absent from coccoid cells. *Corynebacterium renale* is a very pleomorphic rod, and palisade formations are common in direct smears from kidney exudate. If smears from urine or kidney exudate are stained with methylene blue, the organisms stain unevenly and cells with swollen ends commonly occur. *Corynebacterium equi* is extremely pleomorphic, and in a fluid medium, large swollen bacillary shapes are common. Metachromatic granules are not numerous.

CULTURE. Culture examination for the genus *Corynebacterium* is best completed on blood agar. On blood agar *Corynebacterium pyogenes* forms minute pinpoint colonies that resemble those of streptococci but often are smaller. Typically, it produces a zone of beta hemolysis following 24 hours' incubation on blood agar. Occasionally, the colony is so small that only the hemolysis is evident unless the plate is carefully examined.

The colony of *Corynebacterium pseudotuberculosis* is characteristically dry and concentrically ringed. Some colonies may have a rosette-like appearance. Coloration of the colonies may occur, varying from cream to orange, depending on the strain. Hemolysis is present on blood agar.

Corynebacterium renale forms a small dewdrop-like colony that may become enlarged after 48 hours' incubation and has an opaque ivory appearance. In young growth, colonies are moist but later may become dry, although not as dry as colonies of *Corynebacterium pseudotuberculosis*. No hemolysis is produced on blood agar.

Corynebacterium equi grows readily on any laboratory medium, producing a colony that is large, moist, viscid, and has an entire edge. After 24 hours, the culture is creamy white, but as the colony ages it becomes pink. When the colony is touched with an inoculating loop it is quite viscid. It is nonhemolytic on blood agar.

LABORATORY IDENTIFICATION. Laboratory identification of *Corynebacterium* organisms is dependent upon the demonstration of typical colony formation by a gram-positive diphtheroid bacillus. Absolute identification is dependent on the biochemical properties of the species.

Corynebacterium pyogenes produces a characteristic alteration in litmus milk. The milk is first coagulated and acidified; subsequently, the clot is dissolved, and within one week the medium is clear. *Corynebacterium pseudotuberculosis* is identified by its colony formation and morphology, although fermentation of carbohydrates may be required for positive identification. *Corynebacterium renale* has little ability to utilize carbohydrates, and this is characteristic of the species. In litmus milk, some strains produce no change, whereas others may digest casein, producing alkalinity. This species of *Corynebacterium* degrades urea, producing ammonia. *Corynebacterium equi* is limited in its ability to ferment carbohydrates but does differ from other members of this group by being able to reduce nitrates to nitrites (Table 18–3).

Bacillus

Only one species, *Bacillus anthracis*, is pathogenic. This genus includes aerobic spore-forming bacilli that are ubiquitous in nature, being found in the soil and on decaying vegetation and often encountered as air contaminants. Differentiation of the various species of *Bacillus* can be made on the basis of size, shape, position of spores, motility, tendency for chain formation, and by differences in culture and physiologic characteristics. *Bacillus anthracis* can be differentiated from some nonpathogenic species only by animal inoculation, serologic tests, susceptibility to a species-specific bacteriophage, and use of the "string of pearls" test.

MORPHOLOGY. *Bacillus anthracis* is a cylindrical rod, having spores that are ellipsoidal and situated centrally. Spores are not formed in the animal body, but a capsule is present in tissues. In tissue smears, the organism appears in short chains and has square ends.

ANTIGENIC CHARACTERISTICS. It appears that there are two antigenic substances in *Bacillus anthracis*. A protein-like material is found in the capsule, and the somatic antigen is a polysaccharide.

TABLE 18–3. Differentiation of Species within the Genus *Corynebacterium*

Organism	Hemolysis	Gelatin Liquefaction	Nitrate Reduction	Litmus Milk	Animal Species Infected
C. pyogenes	+	+	–	Coag. reduction, digestion	Cow, pig, sheep, goat
C. renale	–	–	–	Alkaline, digestion	Cow, pig
C. equi	–	–	+	No change	Horse, pig
C. pseudotuberculosis	±	–	–	No change	Sheep, horse, goat

Both antigens will act specifically with precipitating sera and may be of value in identifying the organism. The presence of these antigenic substances has resulted in the development of adequate control measures that utilize either the entire organism, its spore, or a variant organism for the production of immunity.

CULTURE. *Bacillus anthracis* grows readily on most laboratory media, appearing on the surface of an agar plate 12 to 18 hours following inoculation. The colonies have a dull, opaque, grayish-white appearance with an irregular border. If the border is examined under the low power of the microscope, long strands of cells may be seen in a parallel arrangement, giving the typical "medusa head" appearance. This organism loses its capsule when grown on artificial medium unless incubated in an atmosphere containing 10 per cent carbon dioxide. Other members of the genus *Bacillus* produce a similar colony, and differentiation between pathogenic and nonpathogenic species is difficult. Many of the nonpathogenic species are capable of hemolyzing blood, but *Bacillus anthracis* is not.

LABORATORY IDENTIFICATION. Positive identification of *Bacillus anthracis* may be made by animal inoculation. A guinea pig is inoculated subcutaneously in the abdomen with the suspected material or organism suspended in saline. If *Bacillus anthracis* is present, death usually occurs in 40 to 42 hours, although death may occur earlier, and if the animal has been treated with antibiotics prior to collection of the sample, death may be delayed for several days. Typical postmortem lesions include subcutaneous edema that may be blood-tinged occurring at the site of inoculation. The spleen is enlarged, dark red, and soft.

If typical lesions are produced in the laboratory animal, direct smears should be prepared from heart blood and the surface of the liver, and an impression smear should be prepared from the spleen. Gram-positive bacilli that contain no spores but have a capsule halo and are arranged in short chains with square ends are suggestive of infection caused by *Bacillus anthracis* (Fig. 18–8). Subcultures on a good nutrient medium should be made from the heart blood and spleen.

Prior to animal inoculation, suspect material should be suspended in saline and heated for 10 minutes in a water bath at 80° C. This procedure reduces the number of non–spore-forming contaminants. The only danger encountered in this pasteurization process occurs if one is dealing with fresh specimens. Fresh specimens may not contain spores of *Bacillus anthracis* and therefore are sometimes negative following such treatment. Fresh specimens should be streaked directly onto a nutrient medium or injected into a laboratory animal without pasteurization. Occasionally, animals injected with nonpasteurized material will succumb to infection caused by contaminating organisms. Whenever possible, the specimen should be dried to enhance spore formation and to permit the use of the heating process to eliminate non–spore-forming contaminants.

Isolation of a bacteriophage specific for *Bacillus anthracis* has improved the identification of this organism, and its use provides a reliable method for differentiating this pathogen from other aerobic, spore-forming bacilli. Suspected material is

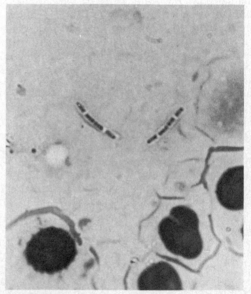

Figure 18–8. *Bacillus anthracis* is an impression smear from the surface of the liver of an inoculated guinea pig. Note the halo that surrounds the organisms and the typical short chains of square-ended rods.

generously swabbed over the surface of a plate of nutrient agar, and a drop of the phage is placed on the surface after the plate has dried. The site of inoculation of the phage should be marked on the Petri dish with a ring. If the organism present is *Bacillus anthracis*, a cleared area will appear where the phage was added. Errors may be encountered in this technique if a few viable organisms of another species are present, resulting in overgrowth of the lysed area. It is therefore advisable to use a light saline suspension of the organism from an agar slant to swab the agar plate.

Additional criteria that may be used for identification are lack of motility and the "string of pearls" test. Details of the latter method are presented in the Appendix, p. 452.

Actinomyces and Nocardia

The genera *Actinomyces* and *Nocardia* include organisms that form a branched mycelium and that often break up into bacillary or coccoid segments that may function as conidia. Species of the genus *Actinomyces*, of which *Actinomyces bovis* is the most typical member, grow best on primary isolation under anaerobic conditions. However, when adjusted to artificial media, they will grow aerobically. Species of the genus *Nocardia* are aerobic. Three species, *Nocardia asteroides*, *Nocardia caprae*, and *Nocardia farcinica*, have been described as producing lesions in domestic animals.

MORPHOLOGY. *Actinomyces bovis* is a long, filamentous, branching organism when grown on artificial media. The filaments contain small coccoid forms. In infected tissues, the organism produces typical sulfur granules composed of a mass of club-like processes that originate in the center of the granule. If a smear is prepared by crushing one of these sulfur granules, typical branching filamentous gram-positive organism can be demonstrated.

Members of the genus *Nocardia* are gram-positive organisms that appear in exudates as long, filamentous, branching organisms that have a tendency to break into typical segments, forming small coccoid cells. If tissue smear preparations are stained by the Ziehl-Neelsen method, some filaments appear to be acid-fast. This acid-fast property is only partial, and care should be taken in performing such a stain to avoid prolonged decoloration with acid alcohol. The modified acid-fast stain previously described may be used to advantage.

CULTURE. *Actinomyces bovis* is difficult to culture from tissues, as original growth is slow. Several days are required for a colony of any significant size to form under anaerobic conditions. This organism commonly occurs in association with pyogenic infections and is frequently associated with other species of bacteria, making isolation of a pure culture difficult.

Nocardia organisms grow readily on blood agar under aerobic conditions. Colonies appear slowly, requiring four to eight days to become visible. The typical colony is irregular, raised, and usually wrinkled or granular with a pigmentation ranging from light tan to orange to bright red. When grown on artificial media, *Nocardia* organisms usually lose their acid-fast properties.

LABORATORY IDENTIFICATION. Laboratory identification of both *Actinomyces* and *Nocardia* organisms is probably best accomplished by examination of the typical sulfur granule and demonstration of the characteristic morphology. Since culture identification of *Actinomyces* species is difficult, it is not suggested as a method for clinical laboratory diagnosis. However, *Nocardia* can be grown readily on blood agar if the plate is incubated for a longer period of time. During long incubation, dehydration of the medium may be prevented by sealing the plate with a clear cellulose tape or a wide rubber band or by incubating the plate in a closed chamber containing a small piece of wet filter paper or cotton. Production of the typical colony and determination of the morphology are usually sufficient for identification of *Nocardia* organisms.

Clostridium

The genus *Clostridium* incorporates the spore-forming anaerobic bacilli. These organisms are commonly present in the soil, and diseases caused by this group of bacteria are often referred to as soil-borne infections. Anaerobic microorganisms are studied by specialized techniques that are beyond the scope of the usual clinical pathology laboratory. Our discussion of this genus, therefore, will be principally concerned with the identification of the organism by methods other than culturing.

Clostridia produce a variety of disease entities in a number of animal species. Characteristically, the diseases are manifested first as an acute toxemia, such as in botulism and tetanus, and second as a gas edema in which edema is the general rule and gas formation is inconstant. The members of the genus that are of significance in animal disease include *Clostridium chauvoei*, *Clostridium septicum*, *Clostridium novyi*, *Clostridium perfringens*, *Clostridium sordellii*, *Clostridium botulinum*, *Clostridium tetani*, and *Clostridium haemolyticum*.

MORPHOLOGY. These bacilli vary in size but are usually plump with rounded ends, although some may appear as long slender rods. Spores develop in all species with a variable position—central, terminal, subterminal. These organisms are gram-positive in young cultures but may easily be decolorized when older.

Clostridium chauvoei, the etiologic agent of blackleg, is characteristically a rod with rounded ends occurring singly or in short chains. Long filaments are relatively common, and swollen cells are often found. Spores are elongated and oval, being located subterminally or terminally and are wider than the cell, giving it a typical "tennis racket" appearance. *Clostridium septicum* closely resembles *Clostridium chauvoei*, being a cylindric rod with rounded ends arranged singly, although it may be filamentous and may be found in long chains. *Clostridum novyi* is one of the largest members of the genus *Clostridium*, with parallel edges and rounded ends. It may occur in long jointed filaments or singly and in pairs. *Clostridium perfringens* is a rod, usually with rather square ends. This organism differs from other members of the genus in being nonmotile. *Clostridium sordellii* is also nonmotile, forming a bacillus that is rather long and has spores that are located either centrally or subterminally. *Clostridium botulinum* is a large bacillus with rounded ends, occurring in short chains occasionally but more often occurring singly or in pairs. The oval spores have a diameter usually greater than that of the cell and are located terminally. *Clostridium tetani* is a long slender rod that may sometimes assume a filamentous form. It usually occurs either singly or in short chains and has rounded ends. The spores found in this species are two or three times the diameter of the cell and are located terminally giving the bacterium a "drumstick" appearance. *Clostridium haemolyticum* has a morphology characteristic of the genus, occurring as a rod-shaped organism with rounded ends, but if it appears in chains it may be truncate. The spores are heavily walled, usually oval or elongated, and situated subterminally or terminally.

CULTURE. Isolation of members of the genus *Clostridium* is difficult, and this procedure should be restricted to a central diagnostic laboratory.

LABORATORY IDENTIFICATION. Absolute laboratory confirmation of the species of *Clostridium* should be made in a central diagnostic laboratory. Tentative identification of clostridial infection may be made in the routine laboratory. Demonstration of a typical spore-forming, rod-shaped organism in tissues or fluids is suggestive of a clostridial infection. This is particularly true if tissue impressions are prepared from patients suspected of having blackleg, malignant edema, or other muscular clostridial infections. In infections with *Clostridium perfringens*, the organism can be demonstrated in almost pure culture in the intestinal tract of animals have succumbed to the toxins produced by this species. *Clostridium haemolyticum* infections can be tentatively confirmed by demonstration of the organism from liver impressions.

GRAM-NEGATIVE RODS

The Enterobacteria

The enteric organisms are a large group of gram-negative, non–spore-forming rods whose natural habitat is the intestinal tract of animals and hu-

mans. Some species form a part of the normal intestinal flora, whereas others are regularly pathogenic. These bacteria are aerobes; they ferment a wide variety of carbohydrates and have a complex antigenic structure.

Included in the Enterobacteriaceae family are the genera *Escherichia*, *Enterobacter* (*Aerobacter*), *Klebsiella*, *Proteus*, *Salmonella*, *Shigella*, *Edwardsiella*, *Arizona*, *Citrobacter*, and *Serratia*.

Coliform Bacteria. Included in the coliform group are a number of species of *Escherichia*, *Enterobacter*, and *Klebsiella*. Also included are the so-called paracolon bacilli, *Citrobacter* and *Arizona*.

MORPHOLOGY. The typical coliform bacterium is a short gram-negative rod that may form chains. Capsules are rarely produced in *Escherichia coli*, are more frequent in occurrence in *Enterobacter*, and are large and occur with regularity in the genus *Klebsiella*. *Escherichia coli* and some strains of *Enterobacter* are motile, although *Klebsiella* organisms are not. If these bacteria are grown under unfavorable conditions, such as exposure to antibiotics, long filamentous forms may appear.

CULTURE. *Escherichia coli* forms a circular, convex, smooth, wet-appearing colony that is white to yellowish-white and somewhat translucent. Some strains are hemolytic on blood agar. Colonies grown on eosin methylene blue agar have a blackish center and produce a metallic sheen. The colony of *Enterobacter* organisms is similar in appearance but may be somewhat more mucoid and tends to coalesce if incubation is prolonged. No metallic sheen is observed. *Escherichia*, *Enterobacter* and *Klebsiella* organisms grow well on MacConkey agar, producing a red or pink colony.

LABORATORY IDENTIFICATION. Laboratory identification of the coliform organisms depends on biochemical tests. The indole production and urea utilization tests can be used to differentiate among *Escherichia*, *Enterobacter*, and *Klebsiella* organisms as follows:

	Indole	Urea
Escherichia	+	−
Klebsiella	−	+
Enterobacter	−	−

Additional tests include (1) methyl red test: this test indicates the pH of a culture in 0.5 per cent glucose broth after four days' incubation. *Escherichia coli* is methyl red positive, and the pH is less than 4.5. (2) Voges-Proskauer reaction: this reaction depends on the ability of the organism to produce acetylmethyl carbinol from dextrose. *Enterobacter aerogenes* is capable of producing this chemical compound. (3) Citrate test: in this assay the organism is tested for its ability to utilize citrate as the sole source of nitrogen. *Escherichia coli* is unable to grow on such a medium, whereas *Enterobacter aerogenes* may do so. *Escherichia coli*, *Enterobacter aerogenes*, and *Klebsiella* organisms are capable of fermenting lactose rapidly, whereas the paracolon bacilli ferment it only slowly. This ability to ferment lactose will separate the coliform organisms from the salmonellae.

Proteus. *Proteus* is a gram-negative, motile, non–spore-forming, aerobic bacillus. Species within this genus are most commonly associated with urinary tract infection in small animals, although they have been isolated from animals with other conditions, including prostatitis in the dog, endocarditis in the pig, bacteremia in the turkey, pneumonia in the dog, and skin wounds in the dog and cow. *Proteus* organisms have also been isolated from dogs exhibiting a variety of abnormalities, including peritonitis, omphalitis of newborn puppies, acute bloody diarrhea, chronic dysentery, and nervous disorders.

MORPHOLOGY. *Proteus mirabilis* and *Proteus ammoniae* are closely related and considered to be identical by some authors. Morphologically, this organism is a plump rod that is motile, non–spore-forming, noncapsulated, and gram-negative. In smears prepared from solid media, the organism is exceptionally pleomorphic, ranging from short coccoid rods to long slender rods.

CULTURE. *Proteus* species grow well on nutrient media, forming colonies that are thin and transparent and have a tendency to swarm over the surface of the agar. This ability to form a swarming colony results in a confluent growth that covers the surface. Because of this microbe's ability to produce ammmonia from urea, a rather typical ammoniac odor is associated with its growth. This organism grows well on MacConkey agar, producing colorless colonies.

LABORATORY IDENTIFICATION. Identification of this genus is most readily accomplished by inoculating a swarming colony into a medium containing urea. If urea is utilized, a typical color change occurs. Hydrogen sulfide is characteristically produced, and some strains produce indole. Members of the genus *Proteus* do not ferment lactose but usually produce acid and gas in other carbohydrates. Because of its lack of ability to ferment lactose this microbe may be confused with salmonellae, and the use of the urea decomposition test will give positive differentiation.

Salmonellae. As are other enterobacteria, the salmonellae are non–spore-forming gram-negative rods closely related physiologically and morphologically to other genera in this family. The salmonellae are usually motile, although nonmotile forms can occur. These organisms do not ferment lactose. They are parasitic in both animals and humans, usually producing an inflammatory reaction in the intestinal tract.

There is increasing evidence that food products of animal origin are often contaminated with salmonella and may cause extensive outbreaks of enteric infections in humans. All species of domestic animals are susceptible to salmonella infection; consequently, the organism is one that is encountered in all phases of veterinary practice.

MORPHOLOGY. The salmonellae are gram-negative non–spore-forming bacilli that vary in length. With the exception of *Salmonella pullorum* and *Salmonella galinarum*, most species are motile.

ANTIGENIC CHARACTERISTICS. There are three main antigens found in the salmonellae: (1) H or flagellar antigens, (2) O or somatic antigens, and (3) the Vi antigen. Utilizing the existence of these antigens, a serologic typing system has been established for identification of species within the genus *Salmonella*. As a result of this technique, many serotypes have been identified. This method of identification is useful in epidemiologic studies of salmonella infections.

CULTURE. Since the salmonellae are most commonly encountered in the intestinal tract, it may be necessary to use enrichment or selective media, or both, for isolation of this organism. On the surface of nutrient agar, colonies of salmonellae are homogeneous, smooth, glistening, and grayish in appearance and either transparent or translucent. Colorless colonies are produced on MacConkey agar.

LABORATORY IDENTIFICATION. Identification of the members of the genus *Salmonella* is originally made on the basis of their lack of ability to ferment lactose, although other techniques must also be used. Salmonellae can be differentiated from *Proteus* species by their inability to utilize urea.

Group antisera have been developed that are useful in the preliminary identification of salmonellae. A saline suspension of the organism is prepared by suspending colonies from a plate or agar slant, being careful to break up all clumps and aggregates. A drop of this heavy suspension of organisms is placed with a drop of antiserum. If the suspected organism is a salmonella, agglutination will occur. Nonspecific reactions may be observed, and this tentative identification must be followed by biochemical tests.

Shigella. Members of the genus *Shigella* are nonmotile gram-negative rods that may be associated either with dysentery in humans (*Shigella dysenteriae*) or with purulent nephritis, septicemia, and joint infections in foals (*Shigella equirulis*).

MORPHOLOGY. *Shigella equirulis* is a small, nonmotile rod that is notably pleomorphic, with long filaments, streptococcus-like chains, and single cells appearing in a smear.

CULTURE. This organism grows readily in media containing meat infusion, producing a characteristically rough, dry, irregular, mucoid colony. These colonies are opaque and raised and sometimes hemispherical. The colony may appear radially striated in transmitted light. It grows well on MacConkey agar, producing a colorless colony.

LABORATORY IDENTIFICATION. *Shigella* organisms are most readily identified by their characteristic colony formation and action on a variety of carbohydrates. Growth in broth is also characteristic, as shigellae appear first as a collection of small masses along the sides of the tube and floating in the medium near the surface. The sides of the tube may become covered with bacteria, and a thin pellicle develops. As the culture ages, a viscid sediment forms.

Another characteristic that may be used for differentiating shigellae from most species of Salmonella is shigellae's lack of motility. In addition, shigellae ferment lactose with the production of acid but no gas.

Other Gram-Negative Rods

Pseudomonas. Members of the genus Pseudomonas are found principally in soil and water. Only one species, Pseudomonas aeruginosa, is pathogenic for animals. This typical non–spore-forming, motile, gram-negative rod may be associated with a variety of diseases, being found particularly in wound infections and producing a pyogenic reaction. In addition, it has been isolated from mastitis, urinary tract infections in small animals, and inner ear infections.

MORPHOLOGY. Pseudomonas aeruginosa is a motile, slender, gram-negative rod with rounded ends. Pleomorphism may be observed.

CULTURE. The organism will grow on any nutrient medium under aerobic conditions. The colony produced on the agar surface is translucent, large, and irregular and has a tendency to spread. A blue-green water-soluble pigment will diffuse throughout the medium, although the ability to produce this pigment is not characteristic of all strains, as some produce small quantities and others large amounts. Growth of this organism results in a characteristic sickly sweet odor. The organism will produce hemolysis on blood agar and a colorless to pigmented (green, blue, brown) colony on MacConkey agar.

LABORATORY IDENTIFICATION. Pseudomonas organisms may be recognized in culture by the appearance of a greenish pigment that readily disperses in the medium. This characteristic plus the heavy sweet odor that accompanies growth is often sufficient for identification. The color of the purulent exudate associated with Pseudomonas aeruginosa is suggestive of the infection. The exudate is blue-green.

Brucella and Bordetella. Microorganisms of the genus Brucella are gram-negative, minute, coccoid rods. On initial isolation, Brucella abortus requires an increased concentration of carbon dioxide. There were originally three species in the genus Brucella: Brucella abortus, Brucella suis, and Brucella melitensis. Two additional species, Brucella ovis and Brucella canis, have been identified. The organism now identified as Bordetella bronchiseptica was once identified as a brucella.

Since the Brucella species are closely related and produce brucellosis, they will be discussed as a group.

MORPHOLOGY. The species of the genus Brucella are essentially identical in size and shape. They are coccobacillary, nonmotile, and gram-negative. It is often difficult to distinguish between this small rod and a gram-negative coccus. Only careful microscopic examination will reveal them to be rod-shaped and not coccoid.

ANTIGENIC CHARACTERISTICS. The main species of Brucella (abortus, melitensis, and suis) have common major antigens, but the agglutination-absorption tests reveal some minor antigenic differences. A common antigen is utilized as a method for detecting infections in animals and humans. Brucella canis does not cross-react with any other species except Brucella ovis.

CULTURE. As previously indicated, Brucella abortus will grow on nutrient medium only if the atmospheric content of carbon dioxide has been increased. The optimum concentration of carbon dioxide is 10 per cent. Although Brucella suis and Brucella melitensis normally require no more carbon dioxide than is found in the air, it is often desirable to place initial cultures of the organisms in containers with a 5 to 10 per cent carbon dioxide content. On original isolation, the colonies are small, delicate, and semitransparent and have a light bluish tinge by transmitted light. It may require several days for growth to appear on the surface of agar. Brucella canis grows aerobically on Albimi Brucella or tryptose medium. Growth is slow, and colonies appear in 48 to 72 hours. The colonies become very mucoid after several days' incubation. Growth is inhibited by carbon dioxide.

LABORATORY IDENTIFICATION. Guidelines for differentiation among the species of Brucella are presented in Table 18–4. In original culture, it may be necessary to use a selective medium that will prohibit growth of contaminants. For original isolation, the addition of gentian violet at a concentration of 1:200,000 does not inhibit growth of Brucella microbes but will delay or prevent growth of many gram-positive organisms.

On this medium, the colonies have the same

TABLE 18–4. Differentiation of *Brucella* Species by the Use of Dyes

	Crystal Violet		Thionin			Basic Fuchsin
	1:50,000	1:100,000	1:30,000	1:50,000	1:75,000	1:50,000
B. abortus	–	±	–	–	–	+
B. suis	–	–	+	+	+	–
B. melitensis	+	+	–	+	+	+

general characteristics observed on nutrient agar but have a bluish-violet color. Positive identification of these organisms as members of the genus *Brucella* will be dependent upon their ability to produce hydrogen sulfide, their utilization of urea, and the fact that they are catalase positive. If there is a doubt as to the identification of the organism, bacteria may be suspended in a small quantity of saline by removing a loopful of growth from an agar plate. A heavy suspension is prepared and well stirred to break down any aggregates. A drop of this suspension is mixed with a drop of known positive serum containing brucella antibodies, and agglutination will occur.

Bordetella bronchiseptica has a slightly different morphology, being a short slender rod usually occurring singly, but chains may be observed in fluid media. This organism grows slowly on primary isolation, but at the end of 48 hours, small dewdrop-like circular colonies may appear scattered over the surface. As the culture ages, the colonies increase in size and become flat, glistening, and translucent, having a smoky tinge when examined by transmitted light. Colorless, opaque colonies are produced on MacConkey agar. This organism is often encountered as a secondary invader in canine distemper and can be identified in the laboratory by its inability to ferment carbohydrates. In litmus milk, after 24 hours a blue ring appears that extends about $\frac{1}{2}$ inch from the surface of the medium. In 72 hours, this ring is a deeper blue, and the remainder of the litmus milk has assumed a deeper blue color. In five to 10 days, the medium becomes typically blue-black. This organism does not form hydrogen sulfide but is urea and oxidase positive.

Pasteurella, Yersinia, and Francisella. Microorganisms within these genera are commonly short, plump coccoid rods, although elongated cells may be observed. These organisms are gram-negative and stain more distinctly at either pole, resulting in the characteristic bipolar staining property. Members of the genera are usually encapsulated, but noncapsulated forms have been isolated. The genera are divided into three subgroups.

1. Members of this group cause pneumonia and/or hemorrhagic septicemia. The species are *Pasteurella multocida* and *Pasteurella haemolytica*.

2. Members of this group cause acute, subacute, or chronic infections in rodents that are transmissible to humans. The two species are *Yersinia pestis* and *Francisella tularensis*.

3. This group consists of a single species, *Yersinia pseudotuberculosis*, that causes a chronic localized caseation necrosis in rodents.

MORPHOLOGY. *Pasteurella multocida* and *Pasteurella haemolytica* are both small coccoid rods that show a marked pleomorphic appearance when grown in broth for prolonged periods of time. These organisms usually possess a capsule when freshly isolated. *Yersinia pestis* is also a short nonmotile rod appearing in body fluids singly, in pairs, or in short chains.

Francisella tularensis is a small, pleomorphic, nonmotile, gram-negative rod, and in young cultures both ovoid and bacillary forms may be found. *Yersinia pseudotuberculosis* closely resembles *Francisella tularensis*.

CULTURE. *Pasteurella multocida* and *Pasteurella haemolytica* grow best on original isolation if blood agar is used. *Pasteurella multocida* may have varying colony characteristics. The fluorescent colonies are moderate in size, opaque, whitish, and often iridescent. An intermediate colony varies in appearance between the fluorescent and blue forms. The blue colonies are small and dewdrop-like and may have a rough appearance. Many strains recovered from chronic processes are composed principally of mucoid variants. The mucoid colonies are large and have a wet, slimy appearance. *Pasteurella* species and *Yersinia* species grow poorly on MacConkey agar.

LABORATORY IDENTIFICATION. A tentative diagnosis of pasteurellosis may be made by the demonstration of typical bipolar rods in smears made from infected tissue. This is not a dependable criterion for diagnosis, as other gram-negative rods may be bipolar in tissue smears. Growth of an organism with typical colony characteristics and morphology on direct smear is suggestive of *Pasteurella* organism infection, although positive identification of the bacteria can be made only by utilization of biochemical reactions. The typical biochemical reactions used to make such an identification are presented in Table 18–5.

Moraxella and Haemophilus. The genera *Haemophilus* and *Moraxella* are both classified in the family Brucellaceae. The species within these genera are coccobacilli but have varying characteristics in terms of their growth requirements. Members of the genus *Haemophilus* require growth-promoting substances known as the X factor and the V factor. Members of the genus *Moraxella* do not require these factors for growth.

Moraxella. MORPHOLOGY. The most significant species within this genus is *Moraxella bovis*, which consists of short diplococcoid rods usually found in pairs, although short chains may be observed. In young cultures, a definite capsule is present but will disappear upon prolonged incubation. Pleomorphism may be present in older cultures.

CULTURE. Blood agar is the most satisfactory medium for isolation. The typical colony of *Moraxella bovis* is a medium small, round, grayish-white, translucent colony that develops in 24 hours. A narrow zone of beta hemolysis is present. If incubation is prolonged, colonies will enlarge and often develop a small raised area in the center. There is no growth on MacConkey agar.

LABORATORY IDENTIFICATION. Isolation of *Morax-*

TABLE 18–5. Biochemical Reactions Characteristic of *Pasteurella* Organisms

Reaction	P. Multocida	P. Haemolytica	Y. Pseudotuberculosis
Hemolysis	–	+	–
Motility	–	–	+
Indole formation	+	–	–
Litmus milk	Neutral	Acid	Alkaline
Glucose	+	+	+
Saccharose	+	+	–
Lactose	–	+	–

ella bovis may be made from the lesions of infectious keratoconjunctivitis in cattle, and these organisms have been isolated from a similar condition in sheep. Demonstration of the typical colony on blood agar should be followed by studies of the biochemical features of the isolate. This organism is incapable of producing acid in any carbohydrate, the medium usually becoming more alkaline. The reaction in litmus milk is typical. The milk becomes alkaline and three zones develop: the bottom zone is composed of coagulated white casein upon which is superimposed a middle zone containing a soft curd that is lighter in color than is normal; the upper zone is a deep blue fluid that results from increased alkalinity.

Haemophilus. Morphology. Members of the genus *Haemophilus* are characteristically small, slender, gram-negative rods occurring occasionally as curved thread-like shapes. If the culture is allowed to age, coccoidal forms appear, and by the time the culture is 48 hours old, the majority of the organisms have this morphology. It may occasionally occur as an extremely large club-shaped coccoid bacillus.

Culture. The most outstanding growth characteristic of this genus is the requirement for X and V growth factors. The X factor is present in hemoglobin of any animal, whereas the V factor is found in many vegetable and fruit juices and is also present in red blood cells recently collected. On the surface of a solid medium such as blood agar prepared from freshly drawn blood, the organism produces a semitranslucent, flattened, circular, grayish, small colony that has a sharply contoured edge.

Some species within this genus do not require both X and V growth factors. *Haemophilus canis* requires the X factor but not the V factor; *Haemophilus gallinarum* does not require the X factor.

Laboratory Identification. Positive identification of the members of the genus *Haemophilus* can be made only by an assessment of the growth requirements plus the use of biochemical tests such as carbohydrate fermentation.

Actinobacillus. Only one species, *Actinobacillus lignieresii*, is of significance in animal health.

Bacteria in the genus are medium-sized rods that are pleomorphic, aerobic, and gram-negative.

Morphology. The pleomorphism of *Actinobacillus lignieresii* is characteristic. This organism varies in size from coccoid forms to elongated filaments. It is nonmotile, noncapsulated, and non–spore-forming. An outstanding morphological characteristic is the tendency to form clumps within infected tissue. The demonstration of such accumulations, which appear as small brownish-white granules, may be suggestive of the presence of the organism, although the organism must be differentiated from *Actinomyces bovis* and *Nocardia asteroides*. This differentiation may be readily accomplished, as *Actinobacillus lignieresii* is a gram-negative rod as compared with the filamentous branched cells of *Actinomyces bovis* and *Nocardia asteroides*.

Culture. Although *Actinobacillus lignieresii* is aerobic, growth on original isolation is enhanced by the presence of an increased concentration of carbon dioxide. On the surface of blood agar, growth is usually scant, the colonies being flat, transparent, and slightly bluish.

Laboratory Identification. Identification of this organism is most easily accomplished by demonstration of the typical "sulfur granules" composed of gram-negative coccoid to filamentous rods. If the organism is isolated, it can be partially identified by carbohydrate studies.

Campylobacter. There are several species within this genus. Many occur in water, and there are several pathogenic species, including *Campylobacter jejuni*, the cause of enteritis in calves and mature cattle, and *Campylobacter coli*, associated with swine dysentery. *Campylobacter* (previously *Vibrio*) *fetus* causes abortion in mature cattle and sheep.

Characteristically, members of the species have short cells and bent rods that may be single or united into spirals. The organisms are motile and are either aerobic or facultative anaerobic. These organisms are generally gram-negative.

Campylobacter fetus. Morphology. *Campylobacter fetus* is a comma-shaped to S-shaped organism in young cultures. A number of these short cells may cling together, forming long spirals in older cultures. Granules may be demonstrated in either young or old cultures by use of a polychrome stain such as Wright's. The organism is characteristically gram-negative and may be intensely stained by crystal violet or alkaline methylene blue.

CULTURE. This organism grows best under microaerophilic conditions with an atmosphere of 10 per cent carbon dioxide. The medium of choice for original isolation is thiol medium, although the organisms will also grow on blood agar. Thiol is a semisolid agar medium and is superior to blood agar for original isolation. In thiol medium, the organism grows profusely within 0.5 mm of the surface. On blood agar, the organism has a colony that is bluish and pinpoint in size, being slightly raised above the surface.

LABORATORY IDENTIFICATION. Tentative identification may be accomplished by demonstrating the organism in stomach contents from an aborted fetus, using dark-field microscopy (Fig. 18–9). Confirmatory diagnosis is made only by isolation from an aborted fetus or the vaginal discharge of an infected cow. Isolation is most readily accomplished from stomach contents of an aborted fetus or from such organs of the fetus as the liver, lungs, and kidney. Thiol medium is recommended for initial isolation attempts, and these are followed by subculturing on blood agar. If the organism is present, a typical colony will be seen, and the demonstration of the comma-shaped gram-negative organism with a certain amount of pleomorphism is considered to be a presumptive identification of the bacterial species.

Other techniques used for identification of an infection with *Campylobacter fetus* include the agglutination test using both serum and vaginal

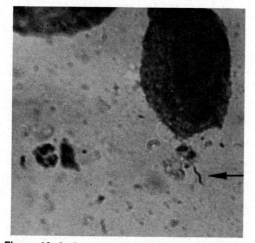

Figure 18–9. Smear prepared from the stomach contents of an aborted fetus. The *Campylobacter fetus* organism is typical, having a shape resembling that of a flying gull.

mucus or only one of the two. Under these circumstances, the antigen used is prepared in such a manner that the H antigen is preserved. A positive reaction in a 1:200 dilution is considered suspicious, and in a 1:400 dilution is positive evidence of infection.

Campylobacter jejuni. MORPHOLOGY. This species is notably pleomorphic, having three forms in a single preparation: one form is completely nonmotile and has a long convoluted appearance; the second form is slightly motile and has two or more complete coils; the third form is very actively motile, slightly convoluted, and relatively short. The organism is gram-negative.

CULTURE. Isolation of this organism is complicated by the fact that it occurs most commonly in the intestinal tract and therefore is almost always accompanied by many other enteric organisms. Some coliform organisms can be eliminated by obtaining a small quantity of intestinal mucosa, washing it thoroughly, and grinding it to be inoculated onto condensate of a blood agar plate. This organism is microaerophilic; therefore, all culture plates should be sealed. Inoculation of blood agar is usually made in the condensation fluid, which becomes cloudy in four to five days. Later, thin veil-like delicate lines become visible at the border of the agar.

LABORATORY IDENTIFICATION. Positive identification can be made only by the isolation and differentiation of *Campylobacter jejuni* from other species by use of an agglutination test. This organism is seldom isolated in the veterinary hospital laboratory.

Campylobacter coli. MORPHOLOGY. This organism is similar in size and shape to *Campylobacter fetus*, being comma-shaped, although long chains may be found in old cultures.

CULTURE. *Campylobacter coli* may be grown on blood agar containing tryptose, usually in a chamber containing an atmosphere of 15 per cent carbon dioxide. The colonies are dewdrop-like and round, and grow sparsely.

LABORATORY IDENTIFICATION. Positive identification of *Campylobacter coli* may be made only by the isolation and use of carbohydrate fermentation.

A SIMPLIFIED SCHEME FOR IDENTIFICATION OF BACTERIA

Most genera of bacteria can be tentatively identified by use of a few simple biochemical tests, observation of their growth characteristics, and determination of their morphology and Gram's reaction.

The following outline is adapted from Bailie and Coles[2] and can be used for tentative identification of the most commonly isolated bacteria.

I. Media for Primary Isolation
  A. Blood agar plates (5 per cent ovine or bovine red blood cells)
    1. Inoculate to ensure separate colonies (4-flame streak method)
    2. Interpretation
      a. Hemolysis of red cells
        (1) No action
        (2) Complete (beta) destruction of hemoglobin
        (3) Incomplete (alpha) destruction: cell modified, discoloration around colony
        (4) Double zone: combination of alpha and beta forming target patterns
      b. Additional characteristics evident with experience (see genus descriptions)
        (1) Colony size
        (2) Shape
        (3) Color
        (4) Consistency
  B. MacConkey agar, a selective and differential medium
    1. Inoculation same as for blood agar
    2. Interpretation
      a. No growth—bile salts prevent growth of gram-positive and some gram-negative microorganisms
      b. Slow growth—bile salts inhibit but do not prevent growth of gram-negative organisms
      c. Rapid growth—gram-negative microorganisms
      d. Colorless colonies—no fermentation of lactose
      e. Red to pink colonies—fermentation of lactose
      f. Colonies other colors—pigment produced by microorganism

II. Differential Media, Determination of Morphology, and Reactions Used for Identification
  A. Gram's reaction. This is the first characteristic that should be determined in an identification scheme. It immediately divides organisms into one of two groups and determines morphology.
    1. Gram's stain. A thin film of the microorganism is stained by one of a variety of methods
    2. Gram's reaction using 3 per cent potassium hydroxide (KOH)
      a. Place 1 drop of 3 per cent KOH on a clean microscope slide
      b. With the inoculating loop, mix a moderately large amount of the microorganism in the KOH
      c. Gram-positive microorganisms will either clump or form a uniform suspension
      d. Gram-negative microorganisms will form a viscous solution that strings out when teased with the loop
  B. Determination of morphology
    1. Shape, arrangement, and internal structure
      a. Cocci
        (1) Clusters
        (2) Packets
        (3) Pairs
        (4) Chains
      b. Large rods
        (1) Chains
        (2) Spores
        (3) Pairs
        (4) Individually arranged
      c. Small rods
        (1) Chinese letters
        (2) Palisades (picket fence)
        (3) Individually arranged
        (4) Granules (beaded)
        (5) Bipolar
      d. Filaments
        (1) Branched
        (2) Not branched
        (3) Beaded
    2. Methods for observation
      a. Wet mount (may also determine motility)
      b. Stained smear
  C. Triple sugar iron (TSI) agar
    1. Inoculation method: streak slant and stab butt
    2. Active ingredients
      a. Glucose 0.1 per cent
      b. Lactose 1 per cent
      c. Sucrose 1 per cent
      d. Ferrous sulfate
      e. Amino acids, including those containing sulfur
    3. Interpretation of reaction for slant method/butt method: Alkaline (Alk) = red; Acid (A) = yellow
      a. No change/no change (NC/NC): No growth or no action on substrates
      b. Alkaline/no change (Alk/NC): Amino acid degradation on slant surface
      c. Alkaline/acid (Alk/A): Glucose fermentation with amino acid degradation on slant surface
      d. Alkaline/acid with hydrogen sulfide (Alk/A + H_2S): Same as Alk/A, but H_2S produced from

sulfur-containing amino acids blackens the medium

   e. Acid/acid (A/A): Lactose and/or sucrose and glucose fermentation

   f. Acid/acid + gas (A/A + gas): Same as A/A, but carbon dioxide or other gas produced from carbohydrate

   g. Acid/acid + hydrogen sulfide (A/A + H$_2$S): Same as A/A, but H$_2$S produced from sulfur-containing amino acids blackens the medium.

D. Indole production
1. Medium—1 per cent tryptone broth
2. Reagents
   a. Xylene or chloroform [Solvent]
   b. Ehrlich's reagent
     (1) Ethyl alcohol, 95 per cent 95 ml
     (2) Hydrochloric acid concentrate 20 ml
     (3) p-Dimethylaminobenzaldehyde 1 gm
3. Method
   a. Add solvent and shake
   b. Add Ehrlich's reagent to layer between medium and solvent
4. Positive reaction = red color in ring of Ehrlich's reagent

E. Utilization of citrate (Simmons citrate medium)
1. Medium: sodium citrate as the sole source of carbon—a slant
2. Inoculation: streak slant and stab butt with small amount of culture
3. Positive reaction = citrate utilized, sodium released with alkaline reaction and change from green to blue

F. Degradation of urea
1. Medium: broth stored in refrigerator in presence of thymol crystals
2. Positive reaction = urea degraded to ammonium ions with alkaline reaction and change to brilliant red

G. Test for cytochrome oxidase
1. Reagents (use either a or b, plus c)
   a. Tetramethyl-p-phenylenediamine dihydrochloride (Eastman Chemical Co., Rochester) 1 per cent aqueous solution
   b. p-Amino-dimethylaniline oxalate (Difco Laboratories, Detroit, Michigan) 1 per cent aqueous solution
   c. Use 0.2 per cent solution of ascorbic acid as solvent
2. Smear culture from blood agar plate on filter paper with sterile swab

3. Add one drop of reagent
4. Positive reaction = blue or pink color (depending on reagent) within one minute

H. Determination of motility at 25° C
1. Microscopic wet mount preparation—motile organisms move across field
2. Motility medium
   a. Semisoild (0.3 percent agar)
   b. Stab in center with wire
   c. Positive reaction = growth out from stab

I. Catalase production (enzyme that attacks peroxidases)
1. Reagent: 3 per cent hydrogen peroxide (H$_2$O$_2$)
2. Method: a few drops on surface of TSI slant
3. Positive reaction = bubbling off of O$_2$

J. Coagulase production
1. Reagent: rabbit plasma
2. Rapid slide test
   a. One drop rabbit plasma on slide
   b. Loopful of culture
   c. Positive reaction = clumping
3. Tube test
   a. Rabbit plasma (0.5 ml) in tube
   b. Loopful of culture
   c. Incubate at 37° C for four to 12 hours
   d. Positive reaction = coagulation

K. Growth in 6.5 per cent sodium chloride (NaCl)
1. Add 6.5 per cent NaCl to Todd-Hewitt broth
2. Growth of streptococci indicates fecal origin

L. Casein hydrolysis
1. Medium
   a. Ten per cent powdered milk in water
   b. Double strength blood agar base
   c. Autoclave separately
   d. Mix in equal quantities
   e. Long slants in tubes
2. Inoculate slant heavily
3. Positive reaction = clearing of medium

III. Genera of Gram-Positive Organisms Possibly Isolated (Fig. 18–10)
A. *Staphylococcus* and *Micrococcus*
1. Colonies
   a. White to yellow
   b. Circular and smooth
   c. Hemolytic or nonhemolytic; possible double zone hemolysis

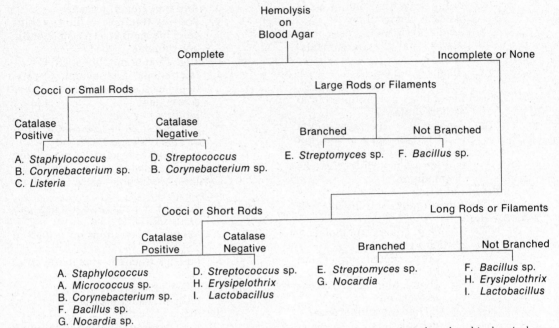

Figure 18–10. The identification of various genera of gram-positive microorganisms based on biochemical reactions and morphology.

2. Organisms
   a. Gram-positive cocci
   b. Arranged in clusters or packets (see Fig. 18–9)
3. Differentiation (Table 18–6)

B. *Corynebacterium* sp.
   1. Colonies—variable
   2. Organisms
      a. Gram-positive, small rods to coccobacilli
      b. Arranged in "Chinese letters" or palisades
   3. Differentiation (Table 18–7)
   4. Other organisms of similar morphology occasionally isolated are not classifiable and are referred to as diphtheroids

C. *Listeria monocytogenes*
   1. Colonies
      a. Complete narrow zone hemolysis
      b. Pale white
      c. Tiny
   2. Organisms
      a. Gram-positive small rods
      b. Arranged in palisades or individually
   3. Differentiation—only organism that is a small gram-positive rod that is motile at 25° C and has an umbrella pattern in motility medium

D. *Streptococcus*
   1. Colonies
      a. Transparent to pale white
      b. Smooth and glistening to rough
      c. Most are tiny (*Streptococcus zooepidemicus* moderately large)
      d. Hemolysis varies from complete (beta), incomplete (alpha), to none (gamma)
   2. Organisms
      a. Gram-positive cocci
      b. Arranged in chains (seen better from broth; see Fig. 18–6)

TABLE 18–6. Distinguishing Characteristics of Some *Staphylococcus* and *Micrococcus* Species

	Hemolysis	Acid Butt in TSI*	Coagulase
Staphylococcus aureus	+(−)	+	+
Staphylococcus epidermidis	−	+	−
Micrococcus sp.	−	−	−

* Triple sugar iron agar.

TABLE 18-7. **Distinguishing Characteristics of Some *Corynebacterium* Species**

	Hemolysis	Consistency	Casein	Urea	Catalase
Corynebacterium pyogenes	+	dry	+	−	−
Corynebacterium pseudotuberculosis	+	crumbly	−	+	+
Corynebacterium renale	−	dry	−	+ +	+
Corynebacterium equi	−	wet	−	−	+

3. Differentiation
  a. Catalase negative
  b. Hemolysis
    (1) Beta—likely pathogen
    (2) Alpha—questionable pathogen
    (3) Gamma (none)—most likely not a pathogen
  c. Growth in 6.5 per cent NaCl—fecal streptococcus (Lancefield group D)

E. *Streptomyces* sp. (isolated as contaminants rarely associated with disease, confused with *Nocardia* organisms)
  1. Colonies
    a. White to gray
    b. Adherent to agar
    c. Very rough
    d. Odor of dry soil
    e. Hemolytic or nonhemolytic
  2. Organisms
    a. Gram-positive
    b. Filaments to long rods
    c. Branching
    d. May be beaded
  3. Differentiation—produce clearing of casein agar

F. *Bacillus* sp. (usually isolated as contaminants, only pathogen of animals is *Bacillus anthracis*)
  1. Colonies
    a. White to gray
    b. Smooth or rough
    c. Hemolytic or nonhemolytic
  2. Organisms
    a. Gram-positive
    b. Large rods
    c. Form spores
  3. Differentiation
    a. *Bacillus anthracis* string of pearls test positive, all others negative
      (1) Make one streak of suspect on Mueller-Hinton agar plate
      (2) Place coverslip on streak
      (3) Place 10-unit penicillin disc on streak next to coverslip

      (4) Incubate two to four hours
      (5) Observe under high dry objective of microscope
      (6) Chains of spherical cells indicate positive results

G. *Nocardia*
  1. Colonies
    a. Form after three to five days of incubation
    b. Gray to brown
    c. Dry
    d. Adherent to surface of or pit into agar
  2. Organisms
    a. Gram-positive
    b. Modified acid-fast—decolorize with 1 per cent sulfuric acid (H_2SO_4) (Plate 18–1L)
    c. Filaments to small rods
    d. Beaded
    e. May see branching
  3. Differentiation—most strains do not clear casein agar

H. *Erysipelothrix rhusiopathiae*
  1. Colonies
    a. Tiny on blood agar after 48 hours
    b. Narrow zone of incomplete hemolysis
  2. Organisms
    a. Gram-positive
    b. Thin rods of variable length
  3. Differentiation—produces A/A + H_2S in TSI agar slant (only Gram-positive rod that does this)

I. *Lactobacillus* sp. (isolated as part of normal flora)
  1. Colonies
    a. Tiny after 48 hours (Streptococci-like)
    b. May have narrow zone of incomplete hemolysis
  2. Organisms
    a. Gram-positive
    b. Short rods, often in chains to filaments
  3. Differentiation
    a. Catalase-negative
    b. H_2S negative in TSI

IV. Genera of Gram-Negative Organisms Possibly Isolated (Fig. 18–11)
   A. *Escherichia coli*
      1. Colonies
         a. Usually red on MacConkey agar
         b. May be colorless (rare)
         c. May be hemolytic on blood agar
      2. Organisms
         a. Gram-negative
         b. Small rods to coccobacilli
         c. Arranged singly
         d. Usually motile
      3. Differentiation—see Branch 1 reactions (Table 18–8)
   B. *Klebsiella* (rarely isolated from small animals)
      1. Colonies
         a. Usually red-pink on MacConkey agar
         b. May be colorless
         c. Very wet consistency
      2. Organisms
         a. Gram-negative
         b. Small rods to coccobacilli
         c. Arranged singly
         d. Capsule present
      e. Nonmotile
      3. Differentiation—see Branch 1 reactions (Table 18–8)
   C. *Enterobacter* (rarely isolated from small animals)
      1. Colonies
         a. Usually pink on MacConkey agar
         b. May be white and opaque to colorless
         c. May be wet in consistency
      2. Organisms
         a. Gram-negative
         b. Small rods to coccobacilli
         c. Arranged singly
         d. Capsule may be present
      3. Differentiation—see Branch 1 reactions (Table 18–8)
   D. *Salmonella*
      1. Colonies
         a. Colorless on MacConkey agar
         b. Rare strains are pink-red
      2. Organisms
         a. Gram-negative
         b. Small rods
         c. Arranged singly

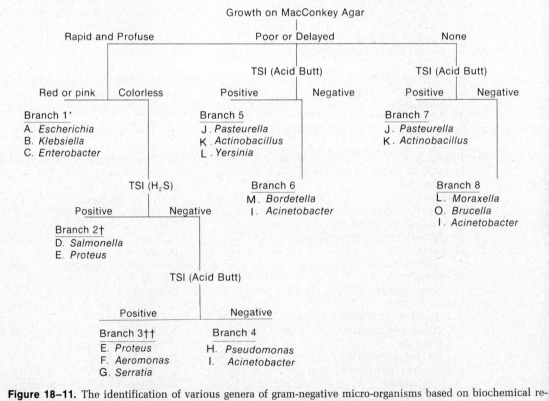

Figure 18–11. The identification of various genera of gram-negative micro-organisms based on biochemical reactions and morphology.

* *Serratia* (pigmented), *Citrobacter*, and *Arizona* (Paracolon) may appear in this branch.

† *Edwardsiella*, *Citrobacter* and *Arizona* (Paracolon) may appear in this branch.

†† *Escherichia*, *Klebsiella*, *Enterobacter* (rare isolates), *Shigella* (from animals) and *Citrobacter* (paracolon) may appear in this branch.

TABLE 16–6. Selected Typical Reactions of Gram-Negative Bacteria

Genus	Reaction						
	TRIPLE SUGAR IRON AGAR	HYDROGEN SULFIDE PRODUCTION	INDOLE PRODUCTION	UREA DEGRADATION	OXIDASE PRODUCTION	CITRATE UTILIZATION	MOTILITY
Branch 1*							
A. *Escherichia*	A/A	–	+	–	–	–	+
B. *Klebsiella*	A/A	–	–	+	–	+	–
C. *Enterobacter*	A-Alk/A	–	–	–	–	+	+
Branch 2†							
D. *Salmonella*	Alk/A	+	–	–	–	±	+
E. *Proteus*	Alk/A	+	±	+	–	±	+
Branch 3‡							
E. *Proteus*	Alk/A	–	+	±	–	±	+
F. *Aeromonas*	A/A	–	+	–	+	±	+
G. *Serratia*	Alk-A/A	–	–	–	–	+	+
Branch 4							
H. *Pseudomonas*	Alk/NC	–	–	–	+	+	+
I. *Acinetobacter*	Alk/NC-Alk	–	–	–	–	–	–
Branch 5							
J. *Pasteurella haemolytica*	A/A	–	–	–	+	–	–
K. *Actinobacillus*	A/A	–	–	+	+	–	+
L. *Yersinia*	Alk/A	–	–	+	–	–	±
Branch 6							
M. *Bordetella*	Alk/NC	–	–	+	+	+	+
I. *Acinetobacter*	Alk/NC-Alk	–	–	+	±	±	–
Branch 7							
J. *Pasteurella multocida*	A/A	–	+	–	+	–	–
Pasteurella gallinarum	A/A	–	–	–	+	–	–
Pasteurella pneumotropica	A/A	–	+	+	+	–	–
K. *Actinobacillus*	A/A	–	–	+	+	–	–
Branch 8							
N. *Moraxella*	Alk/NC	–	–	–	+	±	–
O. *Brucella*	Alk/NC	–	–	+ +	±	±	–
I. *Acinetobacter*	Alk/NC-Alk	–	–	–	±	–	–
Other Gram-negative Rods							
Citrobacter	Alk/A	±	±	±	–	±	+
Arizona	Alk/A	+	–	–	–	+	+
Edwardsiella	Alk/A	+	+	–	–	–	+
Shigella	Alk/A	–	–	–	–	–	–

* *Serratia* (pigmented), *Citrobacter*, and *Arizona* (paracolon) organisms may appear in this branch.

† *Edwardsiella*, *Citrobacter*, and *Arizona* (paracolon) organisms may appear in this branch.

‡ *Escherichia*, *Klebsiella*, *Enterobacter* (rare isolates), *Shigella* (rare from animals), and *Citrobacter* (paracolon) organisms may appear in this branch.

3. Differentiation—see Branch 2 reactions (Table 18–8)

E. *Proteus*
1. *Proteus vulgaris* and *mirabilis*
   a. Colonies
      (1) Colorless on MacConkey agar
      (2) Irregular filmy edges
      (3) Swarms on blood agar
      (4) Characteristic fetid odor
   b. Organisms
      (1) Gram-negative
      (2) Small rods
      (3) Arranged singly
   c. Differentiation—see Branch 2 reactions (Table 18–8)
2. *Proteus morganii, rettgeri,* and *inconstans*
   a. Colonies colorless on MacConkey agar
   b. Organisms
      (1) Gram-negative
      (2) Small rods
      (3) Arranged singly
   c. Differentiation—see Branch 3 reactions (Table 18–8)

F. *Aeromonas* (seen in fish and rabbits)
1. Colonies colorless on MacConkey agar
2. Organisms
   a. Gram-negative
   b. Rapidly motile
3. Differentiation—see Branch 3 reactions (Table 18–8)

G. *Serratia* (related to *Enterobacter*)
1. Colonies
   a. Usually colorless on MacConkey agar
   b. May be red pigmented, especially at room temperature
2. Organisms
   a. Gram-negative
   b. Motile
3. Differentiation—see Branch 3 reactions (Table 18–8)

H. *Pseudomonas*
1. Colonies
   a. Colorless to pigmented (green, blue, brown) on MacConkey agar
   b. Characteristic fruity odor
   c. Wide-zone complete hemolysis (may be delayed)
2. Organisms
   a. Gram-negative
   b. Arranged singly
   c. Motile
3. Differentiation—see Branch 4 reactions (Table 18–8)

I. *Acinetobacter* (*Herellea*) (rarely isolated)
1. Colonies opaque on MacConkey agar
2. Organisms
   a. Gram-variable (some gram-positive; some gram-negative)
   b. May be rods or cocci
   c. Often arranged in pairs
3. Differentiation—see Branch 4 reactions (Table 18–8)

J. *Pasteurella*
1. *Pasteurella haemolytica*
   a. Colonies
      (1) Small and usually red on MacConkey agar
      (2) Narrow zone of complete hemolysis on blood agar
   b. Organisms
      (1) Very small coccobacilli
      (2) May stain bipolar
   c. Differentiation—see Branch 5 reactions (Table 18–8)
2. *Pasteurella* (*multocida, gallinarum,* and *pneumotropic*) (commonly to rarely isolated from small animals)
   a. Colonies smooth to mucoid on blood agar
   b. Organisms
      (1) Small coccobacilli
      (2) May stain bipolar
   c. Differentiation—see Branch 7 reactions (Table 18–8)

K. *Actinobacillus*
1. Colonies
   a. Small and usually red if grown on MacConkey agar
   b. One species, *Actinobacillus suis,* is hemolytic
2. Organisms
   a. Small to pleomorphic rods
   b. May stain bipolar
3. Differentiation—see Branch 5 reactions (Table 18–8)

L. *Yersinia* (*Pasteurella*) *pestis* and *pseudotuberculosis*
1. Colonies
   a. Small and colorless on MacConkey agar
   b. Possible slight incomplete hemolysis on blood agar
2. Organisms
   a. Short rods to filaments
   b. May stain bipolar
3. Differentiation—see Branch 5 reactions (Table 18–8)

M. *Bordetella bronchiseptica* (common in upper respiratory tract of dog)
1. Colonies
   a. Colorless, opaque colonies on MacConkey agar
   b. May produce hemolysis on blood agar
2. Organisms
   a. Small coccobacilli
   b. May stain bipolar

3. Differentiation—see Branch 6 reactions (Table 18–8)
N. *Moraxella*
   1. Colonies
      a. Small
      b. May produce narrow zone complete hemolysis
   2. Organisms—bacilli arranged in pairs
   3. Differentiation—see Branch 8 reactions (Table 18–8)
O. *Brucella canis*
   1. Colonies small and smooth on blood agar
   2. Organisms very thin coccobacilli
   3. Differentiation—see Branch 8 reactions (Table 18–8)
P. *Citrobacter, Arizona, Edwardsiella,* paracolon group, and *Shigella*
   1. Enteric species of bacteria
   2. Colonies and organisms similar to other Enterobacteria
   3. Differentiation (Table 18–8)

ACID-FAST ORGANISMS

The most consistently acid-fast organisms belong to the genus *Mycobacterium*. Acid-fast organisms are widely distributed in nature. Some are pathogenic for humans and animals, whereas others are parasitic for cold-blooded animals or are found in the soil. The species pathogenic for humans and animals include *Mycobacterium tuberculosis, Mycobacterium bovis, Mycobacterium avium, Mycobacterium paratuberculosis,* and *Mycobacterium leprae.*

Tuberculosis-Causing Mycobacteria

The organisms *Mycobacterium tuberculosis, Mycobacterium bovis,* and *Mycobacterium avium* are capable of producing tuberculous lesions in humans and animals and will be discussed as a group.

MORPHOLOGY. *Mycobacterium tuberculosis* is a slender rod that is acid-fast and gram-positive. *Mycobacterium bovis* is shorter and thicker than the human form, but this is not a positive diagnostic criterion because pleomorphism may exist in both species. The organism may be uneven in size with forms ranging from coccoid to filamentous within the same culture. *Mycobacterium avium* is morphologically similar, although it is somewhat more pleomorphic.

CULTURE. Growth of *Mycobacterium tuberculosis* is slow, requiring several days to weeks for the appearance of colonies. Several specialized media have been developed for use in studying *Mycobacterium tuberculosis*. Colony characteristics on the these media may assist in differentiation. On Petragnani's medium, the human type produces a luxuriant, dry, crumbly growth that causes a yellow coloration in the medium. On this same medium, the bovine type produces a more delicate glistening light yellow growth that may become green upon prolonged incubation. The avian type grows rapidly, producing a moist slimy growth that is occasionally yellow. In a liquid medium, Besredka bouillon, the human organism produces a crumbly deposit as does the bovine type. In this medium, the avian organism produces a slimy, tuft-like growth.

LABORATORY IDENTIFICATION. A tentative diagnosis of tuberculosis can be made if typical acid-fast organisms are demonstrated from direct smears prepared from a characteristic lesion. Differentiation of the various types can be made only by use of laboratory animals for a determination of susceptibility (Table 18–9).

The most common method for demonstration of infection with the tubercle bacillus is use of the skin sensitivity technique. If a tuberculous lesion is demonstrated, specimens should be submitted for positive confirmation to the National Animal Disease Center, Ames, Iowa.

Mycobacterium Paratuberculosis

MORPHOLOGY. This organism is a short, thick, acid-fast rod. In smears from infected mucous membrane, the organism is most commonly found in clumps, although single cells may be scattered throughout the preparation.

CULTURE. This bacillus is extremely difficult to grow on artificial media and is seldom successfully isolated in the laboratory.

LABORATORY IDENTIFICATION. Laboratory identification of infection caused by *Mycobacterium paratuberculosis* (Johne's disease) is probably best made by demonstration of the organism in direct smears from the intestinal mucous membrane. As previously described, demonstration of the rod in scrapings from the rectal mucosa or in the feces may be suggestive of the disease.

In the affected animal, the use of johnin or avian tuberculin as an intradermal sensitivity test may also be helpful.

LEPTOSPIRA

Many different serovars of leptospirae have been incriminated as the cause of disease in domestic animals. These organisms are of particular significance because of their ability to produce disease in humans.

TABLE 18–9. Laboratory Animal Susceptibility to Mycobacteria

Type	Guinea Pig	Chicken	Rabbit
Bovine	+	−	+
Avian	±	+	+
Human	+	−	±

MORPHOLOGY. Morphologically, the various serovars of *Leptospira* are indistinguishable. The organisms are closely spiraled rods possessing many wavy curves and having ends that are often bent into the shape of a hook. These organisms resist staining with aniline dyes. However, they may be demonstrated by use of Giemsa or silver impregnation techniques. The organism is most readily demonstrated by use of dark field microscopy.

CULTURE. These organisms are difficult to grow in the laboratory, although a variety of media containing serum have been successfully used. The most common media used are Stuart and Fletcher liquid media. It is questionable whether the veterinarian should attempt to make such isolations, as they are difficult and time consuming, even in a well-equipped laboratory.

LABORATORY IDENTIFICATION. In the veterinary laboratory, attempts to identify the existence of leptospiral infections will usually be limited to the use of the agglutination test on serum from suspected animals. Commercially available antigens are used, and directions for conducting the agglutination test should be carefully followed. Positive identification of leptospiral infection can be made from serologic tests only if an increase in antibody is demonstrated. If leptospirosis is suspected, a serum sample should be obtained, followed by a second sample 10 days to two weeks later. Demonstration of an increase in antibody titer is evidence of exposure to the leptospiral organisms.

VETERINARY MEDICAL MYCOLOGY

The general term *fungus* is used to indicate a group of organisms characterized by the existence of vegetative filaments known as hyphae. These hyphae may become divided into a chain of cells by formation of transverse walls called septa. Such fungi are said to have septate hyphae. As hyphae grow and branch, a mat of tangled growth develops called a mycelium. Part of the growth will project above the surface of the substrate and is referred to as aerial mycelium. Another part of the growth will penetrate the supporting medium and absorb food. This is known as the vegetative mycelium.

Spores of various types serve as the reproductive mechanism for fungi. If spores are produced on the aerial mycelium, it is referred to as reproductive mycelium. Asexual spores occur when there is no fusion of the nuclei prior to or during their formation. If fusion does take place, they are sexual spores. The majority of the fungi of importance in veterinary medicine have no known sexual spore development.

The types of spores most commonly produced in fungi of interest in veterinary medicine are: (1) blastospores, which are simply asexual spores that develop by budding and subsequent separation of this bud from the parent cell; (2) chlamydospores, which are formed by the cells in the hyphae enlarging and developing thick walls; (3) arthrospores, which are asexual spores resulting from a hyphae fragmenting into individual cells; and (4) conidia, which are spores produced on specialized hyphae by a pinching off at the point of attachment.

SUPERFICIAL MYCOSES

The dermatomycosis complex (ringworm) is caused by the invasion of the keratinized epithelial cells and hair fibers by fungi of two genera, *Trichophyton* and *Microsporum*.

Confirmatory diagnosis of dermatomycosis is dependent upon a close observation of the lesion accompanied by the fluorescence test, microscopic examination, and culturing.

Fluorescence Test. An animal suspected of ringworm should be examined in a darkened room using Wood's light, which gives off ultraviolet rays. Infected hairs glow with a bright yellow to yellow-green fluorescence. In cats, care should be taken to check the nails for presence of fluorescence. The principal value of Wood's light is for recognition of infection with *Microsporum canis* or *Microsporum audouini*, as only these two fungi produce fluorescence. Fluorescence may be masked or confused with a bluish-white fluorescence that occurs normally from mud, nails, skin scales, or substances having a petrolatum base. If no fluorescence is observed, ringworm may be present as the result of infection with one of the nonfluorescing dermatophytes.

Microscopic Examination. Microscopic examination must be conducted on carefully selected hairs and skin scrapings. Fluorescing hairs seen under Wood's light should be plucked out for subsequent microscopic examination. If no fluorescing hairs are seen in the lesion, the broken dull hairs or those that have a whitish gray color at their base should be selected for microscopic examination. Properly selected hairs, skin scrapings, or both should be placed on a glass slide in a few drops of 10 per cent potassium hydroxide (Fig. 18–12). A coverslip is applied, and the slide is gently heated for a few seconds with a flame from a Bunsen burner or warmed by placement adjacent to a light bulb. Potassium hydroxide serves as a clearing agent so that under the high power dry objective of the microscope, details of spores and hyphae on or in the hairs may be observed. Arthrospores appear as small spherical refractile bodies occurring in chains or as a complete sheath surrounding the infected hair. Hyphae are seen as filaments occasionally fragmenting into arthrospores and occur on the infected hairs. Hairs may be stained with lacto-

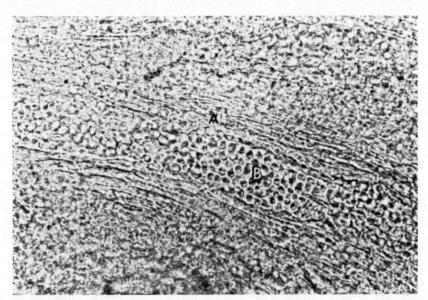

Figure 18–12. In animals with ringworm, fungal spores can sometimes be observed clinging to the hairs removed from the edge of the lesion. This specimen has been cleared with 10 per cent potassium hydroxide. The hair is located at *A*, the fungal spores at *B*. Note the arrangement of the fungal spores.

phenol cotton blue to demonstrate these spores more clearly.

Culture. Positive identification of a fungus may be established by the inoculation of culture media and study of the morphologic characteristics of growth. The standard medium for isolation of dermatophytes from clinical material is Sabouraud-dextrose agar. The problem encountered in utilization of this medium is that hair and skin scrapings are often contaminated with saprophytic fungi and bacteria, which may make isolation difficult. The addition of antibiotics and other inhibitory substances such as cycloheximide may assist in controlling these contaminants. Such media are available commercially (Mycosel agar, Baltimore Biological Laboratories, Baltimore, Maryland; Mycobiotic agar, Difco Laboratories, Detroit, Michigan).

Large test tubes containing the medium to be used are inoculated by placing the hairs or skin scrapings on the surface and pushing them partly into the agar. Inoculated slants are incubated at room temperature and examined every few days for the presence of growth. Slants should be maintained for at least one month before being reported as negative; however, most commonly isolated fungi will grow rapidly. Colonies produced are somewhat characteristic for the genus. Positive identification can be made only by microscopic examination of the growth.

Trichophyton mentagrophytes is associated with lesions in a variety of domestic animals. This organism grows on Sabouraud agar in one week to 10 days, producing a colony that is white, often turning tan with age, and has a downy or granular pigment. Microscopically, this organism is char-

acterized by the presence of numerous microconidia, with only rare occurrence of macroconidia. Macroconidia are often produced on specialized sporulating agar such as potato-dextrose agar. Microscopic examination of fungi may be enhanced by preparing the mounts in lactophenol cotton blue. A few drops of stain are placed on a slide, and a small portion of the filamentous growth is placed in the dye and gently separated with teasing needles.

Microsporum canis, another rather commonly isolated dermatophyte, requires only three to four days to grow on Sabouraud agar. This fungus produces a flat downy colony that is white but may appear yellow in the early stages of development. Microscopically, only a few, if any, micronconidia are observed. If microconidia are present, they are borne laterally. Macroconidia are numerous, being large, spindle-shaped, multiseptate, thick-walled bodies having a knob at the tip (Fig. 18–13).

DEEP SYSTEMIC FUNGI

Included in this group are several species that are unrelated but are all capable of producing disease. The most commonly encountered fungi producing deep-seated mycoses in domestic animals include *Aspergillus fumigatus* (in poultry), *Candida albicans, Blastomyces dermatitidis, Cryptococcus neoformans, Histoplasma capsulatum,* and *Coccidioides immitis.*

Aspergillus Fumigatus. This fungus is most commonly encountered as a factor in lung infections in poultry. In mammals, it has also been ob-

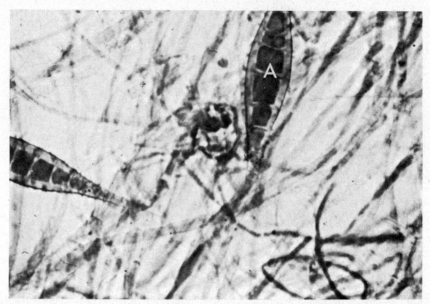

Figure 18–13. A new methylene blue-stained specimen of *Microsporum canis*. Note the large multiseptate macroconidia (*A*).

served to occur in the horse, cow, sheep, and dog. If smears are made from infected tissues, these slides may have fragments of hyphae accompanied by small rounded spores. On Sabouraud medium, the organism grows quickly at room temperature, yielding a white colony growth that may subsequently become green. A microscopic mount from such a culture will have a typical swollen conidiophore supporting flask-shaped processes that bear spores in short chains.

Candida Albicans. This organism produces a disease characterized by persistent erosive lesions on the skin and mucous membranes. It may also result in a generalized systemic infection. When observed in tissues, *Candida albicans* is a small, oval, budding, yeast-like organism. It grows readily on Sabouraud agar either at room temperature or at 37° C. The typical colony on Sabouraud agar is soft and cream colored and has a characteristic yeasty odor. If contaminants are present, a variety of selective media may be used to isolate this organism. Positive identification of the organism may be made by studies of its ability to ferment carbohydrates.

Blastomyces Dermatitidis. Blastomycosis occurs in the dog and horse. The organism produces a granulomatous lesion that commonly occurs in the lungs and skin. In infected tissues, the organism occurs as large round cells having a so-called "double-contoured" cell wall. Buds may be observed (Fig. 18–14). The organism can be cultured on Sabouraud agar at room temperature, producing a white colony that turns brown as it ages. Identification of this organism in culture should not be attempted in the small veterinary laboratory. If typical cells are present in lesions, a sam-

ple should be submitted to a central diagnostic laboratory for confirmatory diagnosis. The organism produces branching septate hyphae containing lateral oval conidia.

Blastomyces dermatitidis must be differentiated in tissue from *Cryptococcus neoformans*, which has a conspicuous capsule. The cells of *Blastomyces dermatitidis* must be differentiated from the cells of *Coccidioides immitis*. *Coccidioides immitis* cells do not bud. Positive identification of any of the diseases caused by these fungi, however, can be obtained only by cultivation and identification of the organism by a reference laboratory.

Cryptococcus Neoformans. Cryptococcus organisms have been isolated from the udder of cattle with mastitis. In addition, these fungi have been isolated from meningitis in the horse, pulmonary abscesses in horses and goats, localized lesions of the oral and nasal mucosa of dogs and cats, and in generalized infections in these species. In tissue, *Cryptococcus neoformans* is a thick-walled, oval to spherical budding cell. It is surrounded by a gelatinous capsule. The organism will grow readily on laboratory media designed for the cultivation of pathogenic bacteria. Growth is slow on such media, requiring 10 days to two weeks for the appearance of colonies. On Sabouraud agar, white, glistening, mucoid colonies appear that may become brownish as the culture ages.

Histoplasma Capsulatum. Histoplasmosis in animals is manifested by a wide range of clinical conditions. This organism has been recovered most commonly from infections in dogs but also has been isolated from cattle, sheep, swine, poul-

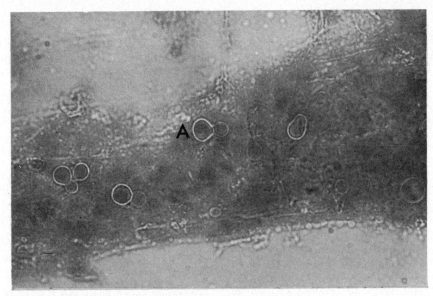

Figure 18–14. Direct smear prepared from an animal experimentally infected with *Blastomyces dermatiditis*. Note the budding yeast form (*A*).

try, and horses. This organism may appear as either a yeast or a mold. In lesions of the naturally occurring disease, small, oval, budding, yeast-like bodies are found in the cytoplasm of endothelial and mononuclear cells. The organism can occasionally be demonstrated in circulating monocytes (Fig. 18–15). On blood agar, this organism produces a smooth, white colony at 37° C. On Sabouraud dextrose agar incubated at room temperature, the colony is white and cottony and may become brown with age. In microscopic preparations made from such growth, the young cultures have definite branching septate hyphae that bear small microconidia. In older cultures, large thick-walled conidia (macroconidia) are present. Histoplasmin has been developed as a diagnostic test and, like tuberculin, is injected intradermally.

Coccidioides Immitis. *Coccidioides immitis* is capable of producing disease in cattle, horses, sheep, and dogs. In infected tissue, *Coccidioides immitis* forms spherical, thick-walled, double-contoured cells that are filled with a large number of ellipsoid spores. Occasionally these cells (spherules) rupture, and minute endospores are found in the surrounding tissue. When this organism is grown on common laboratory media or on Sabouraud dextrose agar, a fluffy white colony develops. The hyphae contain rectangular ar-

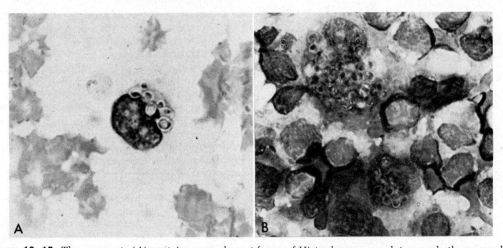

Figure 18–15. The monocyte (*A*) contains several yeast forms of *Histoplasma capsulatum* as do the macrophages (*B*). These macrophages containing yeast forms were demonstrated in an impression smear from the spleen of a dog with histoplasmosis.

throspores. These spores are light in weight and float readily in the air. Because of this danger of air contamination, isolation attempts should be confined to a central diagnostic laboratory and should not be undertaken in the veterinary hospital.

ANTIMICROBIAL SENSITIVITY TESTING

The choice of antimicrobial therapy is based first on the clinician's impressions of the disease to be treated. This choice is often dictated by the experience of the clinician in treating similar conditions and often such a choice proves efficacious. However, with the increasing number of antimicrobial agents and their promiscuous use, a number of strains have developed resistance to one or more of these drugs, and proper therapy is more difficult to select based solely on clinical observations. Often it is advisable to identify the organism prior to institution of therapy, as some species of organisms are uniformly susceptible to antibiotics, whereas others are known for their antibiotic resistance. The addition of *in vitro* antibiotic sensitivity determination will often enable the clinician to make a more appropriate choice of therapy.

The commonly performed disc test is a practical method for the determination of the spectrum of susceptibility or resistance of an organism to a variety of antimicrobial agents. This test must be used judiciously and interpreted with some restraint. The choice of antimicrobial agents to be used in the test must be left to the judgment of the clinician, but, in general, gram-negative organisms should be tested for their sensitivity to streptomycin, chloramphenicol, tetracycline, neomycin, penicillin, polymyxin, or other broadspectrum antibiotics. For gram-positive organisms, the polymyxin disc is omitted, but erythromycin may be added. For staphylococci, methicillin, oxacillin, vancomycin, novobiocin, and bacitracin may also be employed. Nitrofurantoin (Furadantin) discs are useful only in urinary tract infections, as this drug is active only in the urine and not systemically. Testing with sulfonamide discs is rarely indicated and is meaningless unless a para-aminobenzoic acid (PABA)–free medium is employed.

Procedure. Antimicrobial sensitivity testing is best done on pure cultures of isolated organisms, but occasions may arise when exudates, transudates, or other material may be used for an estimation of the spectrum of antimicrobial sensitivity or resistance. For a pure culture the test is conducted as follows:

1. Prepare a suspension of the pure culture in a small quantity of nutrient broth (1 to 2 ml).
2. Using a sterile cotton-tipped wooden applicator, soak the cotton in the suspension of organisms.
3. Carefully swab the entire surface of an agar plate (preferably blood agar) with the organism suspension. Be sure to cover the entire surface by streaking in one direction over the surface and performing a second streaking at a 90-degree angle from the first.
4. Allow the plates to dry completely. If wet plates are used, the antimicrobial agents may be removed from the disc and diluted beyond their scope of activity.
5. After the plate has completely dried, add the selected discs containing the antimicrobial agents. If an accurate estimation of sensitivity is desired, both high and low concentrations of the antibiotic discs should be used.
6. Prior to incubation, each disc should be gently but firmly pushed onto the surface of the agar, using a sterile applicator stick.
7. Invert the plate and incubate. If a 10 per cent blood agar is used, the sensitivity can be estimated following six to eight hours of incubation. It is recommended, however, that the plate be allowed to incubate overnight at 37° C prior to assessment of the sensitivity. The rapid method should be used only when rapid results are needed for institution of therapy.

Interpretation. Interpretation of results must be made after careful examination of the plates following incubation. The sizes of the zones of antimicrobial activity will vary with the molecular characteristics of the different drugs. In contrast to interpretation of results with the Kirby-Bauer technique, zone size cannot be correlated with the therapeutic efficacy of the drug. In most instances, only the presence or absence of a significant zone is recorded. The presence of single colonies within the zone of inhibition may be an indication of either the presence within the total population of a few organisms resistant to the antimicrobial agent or the presence of a contaminant. If such colonies are present, the possibility of contamination can be eliminated by microscopic examination of the colony or a more complete identification of the specific microorganism. If colonies present within the zone of inhibition are of the same genus and species as the organism being tested, they may represent antimicrobial-resistant mutants within the population.

If commercial discs of low and high concentration are used in the test, the results may be interpreted as follows:

1. Significant zone around the high-concentration disc: organism susceptible.
2. Significant zone around the high-concentration disc, no zone around the low-concentration disc: organism slightly susceptible.
3. No significant zone around either the high- or low-concentration discs: organism resistant.

The antibiotic sensitivity test as conducted on the agar plate is an indication of the ability of the drug to prevent growth of the organism when an optimum contact between drug and organism is present. This reaction is, in general, an indication that the drug may be effective *in vivo*. However, the clinician must remember that it is sometimes difficult to obtain this optimum relationship between drug and organism within the animal body. Therefore, practicing veterinarians should not expect to achieve dramatic and sudden success simply because they have instituted therapy with the drug that has proved to be effective against the invading organism when tested *in vitro*. A second consideration must be based on the level of the antimicrobial drug in the blood that can be expected to be achieved. If the expected blood level is much below the level used in the *in vitro* test, the results of the therapy may be disappointing. In spite of these inherent faults in the technique, it should be used as an aid in the selection of therapy in infectious conditions caused by bacteria.

Kirby-Bauer Technique. The standard technique now being used for a more accurate estimation of the antibiotic sensitivity of bacteria is that described by Bauer et al.[3] It attempts to standardize the paper disc method mentioned earlier and permits a more accurate assessment of the degree of antibiotic sensitivity. The test is conducted as follows:

1. Large (150 mm. × 15 mm) Petri dishes are prepared with Mueller-Hinton agar 5 to 6 mm in depth. (For fastidious organisms add 5 per cent blood.)
2. Plates are allowed to dry for a minimum of 30 minutes before inoculation and are used within four days of preparation.
3. A suspension of the test organism is prepared by either of the following methods:
   a. Select a few colonies from the original culture plate and place in a tube containing 4 ml of tryptose phosphate or trypticose-soy broth. Incubate the tube for two to five hours. The suspension is then diluted with sterile water or saline to a density visually equivalent to a standard prepared by adding 0.5 ml of a 1.175 per cent barium chloride to 99.5 ml of 1 per cent sulfuric acid.
   b. Dilute an overnight broth culture to the density of the opacity standard.
4. Streak the suspension of the test organism evenly in three planes onto the surface of the medium with a cotton swab. Surplus suspension is removed from the swab by gently rotating the swab against the sides of the tubes prior to inoculation of the plate.
5. Permit the inoculum to dry for five to 30 minutes, and place the discs on the agar with flamed forceps or a disc applicator. Space the discs so that there is no overlapping of the zones. Discs should be located 10 to 15 mm from the edge of the plate.
6. Gently press each disc with sterile forceps to ensure contact with the agar surface.
7. Incubate the plates overnight at 37° C.
8. Measure zone diameters on the underside of the plate using a metric ruler or with calipers held near the surface of the medium. The end point is taken as complete inhibition as determined by the naked eye. If several individual colonies develop within the zone of inhibition, the culture should be checked for purity and retested. If such colonies are still present, they should be regarded as significant growth. With sulfonamides, the organisms will grow through several generations before inhibition takes place; therefore, slight growth is ignored and the margin of heavy growth is read to determine zone size.
9. Record the zone diameters and interpret them according to Table 18–10.

The standards outlined in Table 18–10 are acceptable for fast-growing organisms, but larger zones of inhibition may be observed with slow-growing, fastidious strains.

Although more complicated to perform than the simpler test that was described first, results with this method are reproducible, and use of a standardized inoculum and medium depth provide a standardization not possible with simpler techniques.

MASTITIS DIAGNOSIS

Clinical diagnosis of acute bovine mastitis does not usually present a problem to the practicing veterinarian. Detection of subclinical mastitis may be more difficult but is an important part of any herd survey to establish disease incidence. Increasing emphasis on the detection of abnormal milk has resulted in the development of a large number of indirect tests utilized to recognize the presence of inflammatory exudates and cells in market milk. Veterinarians are seldom called upon to participate in these evaluations of market milk, as their problem is to detect, treat, and prevent disease in dairy herds under their supervision.

The various laboratory tests used in the diagnosis of mastitis may be divided into chemical, microscopic, and culture. Some tests may be conducted in the field, whereas others must be made in the laboratory. Our discussion will be confined to those tests that are used principally for the detection of clinical or subclinical mastitis. Many of the screening tests that have been developed primarily for laboratory detection of mastitic milk in bulk samples are not included.

TABLE 18–10. Interpretation of Zone Sizes in Antibiotic Sensitivity Testing of Bacteria Cultures*

Antibiotic	Disc Content	Diameter (millimeters) of Zone of Inhibition		
		RESISTANT	INTERMEDIATE	SUSCEPTIBLE
Ampicillin[1] when testing gram-negative microorganisms and enterococci	10 μg	11 or less	12–13	14 or more
Ampicillin[1] when testing staphylococci and penicillin G–susceptible microorganisms	10 μg	20 or less	21–28	29 or more
Ampicillin[1] when testing *Haemophilus* sp.	10 μg	19 or less	—	20 or more
Bacitracin	10 units	8 or less	9–12	13 or more
Carbenicillin when testing *Proteus* sp. and *Escherichia coli*	50 μg	17 or less	18–22	23 or more
Carbenicillin when testing *Pseudomonas aeruginosa*	50 μg	12 or less	13–14	15 or more
Cephalothin when reporting susceptibility to cephalothin, cephaloridine, and cephalexin	30 μg	14 or less	15–17	18 or more[2]
Cephalothin when reporting susceptibility to cephaloglycin	30 μg	14 or less	—	15 or more
Chloramphenicol	30 μg	12 or less	13–17	18 or more
Clindamycin[3] when reporting susceptibility to clindamycin	2 μg	14 or less	15–16	17 or more
Clindamycin when reporting susceptibility to lincomycin	2 μg	16 or less	17–20	21 or more
Colistin	10 μg	8 or less	9–10	11 or more
Erythromycin	15 μg	13 or less	14–17	18 or more
Gentamicin	10 μg	12 or less	—	13 or more
Kanamycin	30 μg	13 or less	14–17	18 or more
Methicillin[5]	5 μg	9 or less	10–13	14 or more
Neomycin	30 μg	12 or less	13–16	17 or more
Novobiocin	30 μg	17 or less	18–21	22 or more[6]
Oleandomycin[7]	15 μg	11 or less	12–16	17 or more
Penicillin G when testing staphylococci[8]	10 units	20 or less	—	21 or more
Penicillin G when testing other microorganisms[8]	10 units	11 or less	12–21[9]	22 or more
Polymyxin B	300 units	8 or less	9–11	12 or more[4]
Rifampin when testing *Neisseria meningitidis* susceptibility only	5 μg	24 or less	—	25 or more
Streptomycin	10 μg	11 or less	12–14	15 or more
Tetracycline[10]	30 μg	14 or less	15–18	19 or more
Vancomycin	30 μg	9 or less	10–11	12 or more

* Reprinted from the Federal Register, 37:20527, 1972.

[1] The ampicillin disc is used for testing susceptibility to both ampicillin and hetacillin.

[2] Staphylococci exhibiting resistance to the penicillinase-resistant penicillin class discs should be reported as resistant to cephalosporin class antibiotics. The 30-μg cephalothin disc cannot be relied upon to detect resistance of methicillin-resistant staphylococci to cephalosporin class antibiotics.

[3] The clindamycin disc is used for testing susceptibility to both clindamycin and lincomycin.

[4] Colistin and polymyxin B diffuse poorly in agar and the accuracy of the diffusion method is thus less than with other antibiotics. Resistance is always significant, but when treatment of systemic infections due to susceptible strains is considered, it is wise to confirm the results of a diffusion test with a dilution method.

[5] The methicillin disc is used for testing susceptibility to all penicillinase-resistant penicillins; that is, methicillan, cloxacillin, dicloxacillin, oxacillin, and nafcillin.

[6] Not applicable to medium that contains blood.

[7] The oleandomycin disc is used for testing susceptibility to oleandomycin and troleandomycin.

[8] The penicillin G disc is used for testing susceptibility to all penicillinase-susceptible penicillins except ampicillin and carbenicillin; that is, penicillin G, phenoxymethyl penicillin, and phenethicillin.

[9] This category includes some organisms, such as enterococci and Gram-negative bacilli, that may cause systemic infections treatable with high doses of penicillin G. Such organisms should be reported susceptible only to penicillin G and not to phenoxymethyl penicillin or phenethicillin.

[10] The tetracycline disc is used for testing susceptibility to all tetracyclines; that is, chlortetracycline, demeclocycline, doxycycline, methacycline, oxytetracycline, rolitetracycline, minocycline, and tetracycline.

SAMPLE COLLECTION

Since absolute diagnosis of mastitis and identification of its causative agent are based on the isolation and identification of bacteria, all specimens for laboratory examination should be collected with as little contamination as possible. Samples should consist of foremilk taken at least six hours following a regular milking. Foremilk is preferred, as the first few milliliters of milk will usually have the greatest change if the udder is in any way abnormal. Samples should be collected methodically as follows:

1. Clean the udder well by brushing off any dirt, loose straw, or mud that is clinging to the skin.

2. Wash the udder thoroughly with a clean cloth soaked in a disinfectant solution of your choice.

3. Allow the udder to dry, and treat the teat orifice with tincture of iodine solution and allow it to dry.

4. While the tincture of iodine is drying, label the tubes as to cow and quarter from which the sample will be taken. One procedure commonly used is to label the tubes by the symbols RH, LH, LF, RF. Test tubes used for collecting specimens should be sterilized by autoclaving. Small screw-cap vials with a frosted area that can be used for labeling are preferred.

5. The cap of the sterile tube is carefully removed and held between the fingers in such a manner that the inside of the cap is facing downward. The tube should be held at a slight angle to prevent contamination of the sample by falling particles. In order to avoid contamination of the teat orifice, the specimens should be collected in the following order: LF, LH, RH, RF.

6. Immediately following collection, refrigerate the samples for transportation to the laboratory.

In herd surveys, it may not be necessary to collect individual quarter samples, and composite samples may be used. In collecting a composite sample at least 5 ml of milk should be collected from each quarter, the collector being careful to avoid contamination.

CHEMICAL METHODS OF DIAGNOSIS

The majority of the chemical methods for diagnosing mastitis depend upon the demonstration of abnormalities in milk composition and thus are indirect tests for mastitis. Since the use of the indirect test is based on the demonstration of abnormal substances in the milk, samples from animals with clinical mastitis will usually react positively. However, abnormal changes may not appear with regularity in the milk of all cows having an udder infection. In most instances, a positive test indicates an infected quarter, but a negative test does not indicate that the quarter is not infected. The only positive method for detecting udder infection is bacteriologic examination of a properly collected sample.

The most commonly used indirect tests for the existence of mastitis include pH determination and chloride, catalase, and Whiteside tests and the California mastitis test or a variation of this technique.

pH Determination. Milk from affected udders is abnormally alkaline, with the degree of alkalinity depending upon the severity of inflammation. Abnormal milk may have a pH as high as 7.4, whereas normal milk has a pH of 6.4 to 6.8.

The reaction of milk may be determined by several different methods, the most common of which is the use of indicators that change color at or near the normal pH. The pH should be determined on freshly drawn milk, although milk held at refrigerator temperatures for 24 to 48 hours may be used. Contaminated milk samples or samples containing a large number of bacteria are not suitable for testing after being exposed to a warm temperature for a few hours, as lactose-fermenting microorganisms alter pH.

Several commercial tests have been devised for detecting the pH of milk by impregnating absorbent heavy filter paper with an indicator. These test blotters are used in the field by placing a small quantity of milk on the spot of indicator and noting the color change. These tests are not as accurate as those in which small quantites of the dye are placed in a test tube and the milk added. With the latter technique, alterations in color are more easily discernible. Both bromthymol blue (BTB) and bromcresol purple (BCP) have been widely used for the detection of pH alterations in mastitic milk.

Bromthymol Blue Test. Several types of solutions may be used in the bromthymol blue test for detecting alterations in pH. The method for preparation of these solutions is presented in the Appendix, p. 453.

One milliliter of bromthymol blue solution is pipetted into a test tube having a capacity of 8 to 15 ml. Five milliliters of milk from a sample bottle is added with a pipette, or, more conveniently, tubes may be marked to the 6-ml level and filled to that mark directly from the udder. If tubes are filled directly from the udder, care must be taken to avoid foaming.

When bromthymol blue is added to normal milk, a yellow color appears, but a sample containing abnormal milk from an infected quarter will be green to greenish-blue, depending upon the amount of alkalinity. This increase in alkalinity is due to the presence of exudate containing unusually large amounts of alkaline salts derived from blood and lymph. Care must be taken in interpreting pH alterations, as cows in late stages of lactation may give false-positive reactions, milk at this stage of lactation being normally more alkaline than during the other stages of lactation. This test will indicate alterations associated with most acute or subacute cases of mastitis, but in chronic conditions there may not be sufficient pH change to be detected. In chronic mastitis, there is so little active inflammation that exudate is not produced in a quantity sufficient to cause a pH change.

Bromcresol Purple Test. Bromcresol purple is used in the same manner as bromthymol blue for determining milk pH. Bromcresol purple has the advantage of becoming yellow in a pH range below 5.2, and thus abnormally acid milk may be detected. In addition, this indicator is used in the Hotis test so that a pH determination using bromcresol purple and the Hotis test may be conveniently combined. The method for preparation of bromcresol purple indicator is presented in the Appendix, p. 453.

In both the test for pH and the Hotis determination, 0.5 ml of bromcresol purple solution is added to 9.5 ml of milk. If the Hotis test is to be conducted, the bromcresol purple should be sterilized in the test tube prior to the addition of milk. With normal milk, the addition of bromcresol purple produces a pale grayish-purple color, whereas abnormal milk becomes a deep purple with increased alkalinity, the intensity of color varying with the degree of alkalinity.

Determinations of pH are of limited value in detecting the existence of udder inflammation, and other screening tests have, for the most part, replaced the pH determination.

Chloride Test. The chloride test is dependent upon the determination of an abnormal quantity of chloride in the milk. Details for preparation of the solutions for the chloride test are presented in the Appendix, p. 453.

Normal milk contains 0.08 to 0.14 per cent chloride. Abnormal milk contains a greater quantity of chloride because of the presence of an inflammatory exudate. These exudates contain a considerable quantity of chloride, and even a small amount of exudate in milk will result in a positive chloride test. The test is conducted by adding 5 ml of a silver nitrate solution to 1 ml of milk, followed by the addition of two drops of a potassium chromate solution and mixing by inversion of the tube. The appearance of a yellow color indicates that more than 0.14 per cent chlorides are present in the sample, and a brownish red color indicates that the sample contains less than that amount. Cows in either early or late lactation may give a false-positive reaction to the chloride test because of normal physiologic processes of the udder.

Whiteside Test. The modified Whiteside test[4] is quick, simple, and inexpensive. The equipment needed includes:

1. A dark, smooth surface on which the test can be conducted. Black sheets of Bakelite or ordinary window glass on a black background make a suitable working area.

2. Sodium hydroxide, 4 per cent solution, should be stored in either flint glass or Pyrex containers in order to preserve the proper concentration.

3. Medicine droppers should be of good quality and designed to deliver approximately the same quantity of milk per drop as for the sodium hydroxide from its dropper bottle. Separate droppers must be used for the reagent and milk.

4. Slim wooden applicator sticks 6 inches long are used for stirring the milk–sodium hydroxide mixture.

5. Paper cups or small containers are required. One is filled with clean water and the other is used for discharging the water, as the medicine dropper is rinsed between samples.

6. A good light source is essential for proper interpretation. Reflected light from a lamp seems to be the most suitable, but the lamp should be kept far enough from the test to prevent warming of the test area.

7. A picture guide for interpretation may be found advantageous in correlating test results.

The test is conducted as follows:

1. Thoroughly mix each individual milk sample, being careful to avoid violent shaking. If the cream has separated, the sample must be sufficiently mixed to ensure an even distribution of cream throughout the sample.

2. Place five drops of milk on a glass plate with a dark background or on a Bakelite sheet. Care must be taken to avoid spreading the milk over too great an area, as proper mixing with reagent may prove difficult.

3. Two drops of 4 per cent sodium hydroxide solution are added to the milk and the mixture stirred rapidly with an applicator stick for 20 to 25 seconds. The drop should be gradually spread over a circular area about the size of a half dollar.

4. Milk from normal animals will have no change after the addition of the sodium hydroxide. Milk from a cow suffering with acute or subacute mastitis will become thick and viscid, but that from an animal with a chronic case may have only a few white flakes. Accurate interpretations in terms of the reaction can be made only by comparing the test results with a standard chart. Estimates can be made if the following ratings are used:

Negative (N). The mixture is milky and opaque and entirely free of precipitant. In such animals, the leukocyte count is generally under 500,000/ml.

Trace (T). The mixture is opaque and milky, but fine particles of coagulated material are present. These particles of coagulated material may be few or many but have no tendency toward clumping. In such milk, the total leukocyte count is usually between 500,000 and 1.5 million.

1+   The background is less opaque but still somewhat milky, with larger particles of coagulated material being present and thickly scattered throughout the area. A slight degree of clumping is observed. The leukocyte count is usually between 1 and 2 million.

2+   The background is more watery, and large clumps of coagulated material are present. If the stirring has been rapid, fine threads or strings may be present. In such specimens the total leukocyte count is usually over 2 million.

3+   The background is very watery and whey-like, with large masses of coagulated material forming into strings and shreds. The total leukocyte count in such samples is usually several million. Milk with extremely high total leukocyte counts will often thicken shortly after the addition of sodium hydroxide and the stirring is started and may have the tendency to follow the applicator stick in a gummy mass.

Milk from fresh cows and cows in late lactation will often have a positive Whiteside test reaction. Milk is not considered to be normal until the fifth day after calving.

California Mastitis Test. The California Mastitis Test (CMT)[5] is a rapid, easy, simple test that, like the Whiteside test, has a specificity for leukocytes in milk. The reagent used consists of an anionic surface active reagent and an indicator, bromcresol purple. In this test, a white plastic paddle with four receptacles into which milk may be drawn is used (Fig. 18–16). Test solution is added in an estimated equal quantity to milk in each cup by squirting reagent from a polyethylene wash bottle. Reactions occur immediately and are graded as the milk and reagent are mixed by a gently circular motion of the paddle. The total cell count of milk is reflected by the degree of precipitation or gel formation that occurs. The pH change associated with abnormal milk is indicated by a color reaction with bromcresol purple in the formula.

The CMT may be used with foremilk or strippings from individual glands. It is also applicable to bucket milk for rapid screening of herds for mastitic cows and to bulk milk as delivered to the processor for selection of herds that have a high degree of udder irritation.

CMT reactions are scored as follows:

Negative. The mixture remains liquid with no evidence of formation of a precipitate.

Trace. A slight precipitate that tends to disappear with continued movement of the paddle.

1+   A distinct precipitate but no tendency toward gel formation.

2+   The mixture thickens immediately, with a suggestion of gel formation. As the mixture is

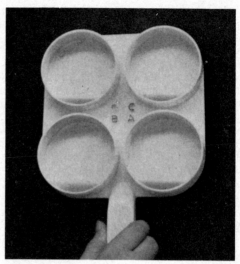

Figure 18–16. Paddle used in performing the California mastitis test.

caused to swirl, it tends to move in toward the center, leaving the bottom of the outer edge of the cup exposed. When the motion is stopped, the mixture levels out again, covering the bottom of the cup.

3+   A distinct gel forms that tends to adhere to the bottom of the paddle, and during swirling a distinct central peak forms. Alkaline milk is indicated by a plus sign, which is used when the mixture is distinctly purple as indicated by a contrasting deep purple color. The symbol Y for acid milk is used when bromcresol purple becomes yellow.

Following the original development of the CMT, a variety of other tests having the same general basis for their use have been developed. Included in this group are the milk quality test (MQT), the Michigan mastitis test (MMT), the Lye mastitis test (LMT), the Wisconsin mastitis test (WMT), and the Feulgen-DNA test. Any or all of these tests may be of value for evaluating the amount of irritation present in the bovine udder.

MICROSCOPIC EXAMINATION

Although microscopic inspection of milk does have limitations, it remains one of the more efficient techniques for rapid examination of milk for the presence of both leukocytes and bacteria. Because of the necessity for a microscope, these methods are limited to the laboratory. With microscopic techniques, the total leukocyte count can be more accurately estimated than with the screening methods previously described. In addition, the operator may determine the morphology of bacteria in the specimen. If the sample is incubated prior to microscopic examination, the type of organism in the specimen is more easily determined. However, such a procedure may be misleading, since it provides an opportunity for multiplication of any contaminants.

Direct Leukocyte Count. In estimations of the number of leukocytes in a milk sample, care should be taken to prepare the slide and complete the examination as accurately as possible. It is possible to give a rough estimate as to the number of leukocytes present on a slide by a quick scanning of the slide; however, accurate interpretations are possible only if a total cell count is completed. A direct leukocyte count is completed as follows:

1. Mix the samples thoroughly, being sure to disperse the cream throughout the specimen.

2. Using either a pipette or a standard 4-mm loop, spread 0.01 ml of milk over an area of 1 sq cm. Ordinary 1 × 3 inch microslides are employed. A card should be prepared or purchased that outlines 1 sq cm over which the milk must be spread. In spreading the milk, care must be taken to ensure even sample distribution over the entire area. Milk that is thicker in one part of the slide than another may lead to erroneous results, particularly if care is not taken in examination of the slides.

3. Dry the slide on a flat surface. Do not heat the slide, as cracks appear in the milk film if drying occurs too quickly. Stain the slide, using a stain acceptable for the demonstration of leukocytes. The Newman-Lampert stain provides an excellent method for demonstrating both leukocytes and bacteria (Fig. 18–17). The method for preparation of this stain is presented in the Appendix, p. 453. This stain has the advantage of fixing the milk film on the glass slide, removing the fat, and staining both bacteria and leukocytes. The slide is stained by being dipped into the stain and allowed to dry before being dipped into water

to remove excess stain. Drying is important, as the solvent used to extract fat does not mix with water. The slide should be washed carefully in water to remove all excess stain and air dried.

4. Microscopic examination should be done carefully, with the number of fields examined depending upon the numbers of leukocytes observed. If a large number of leukocytes are present in each field, only a few fields (20 to 30) need to be examined. If only an occasional cell is observed, 50 or more fields should be counted. For optimum accuracy, a minimum of 50 fields should be counted. The final result is calculated by multiplying the cells per field (average) by the microscopic factor by 100, which will give the number of leukocytes per milliliter.

The calculation of the microscopic factor is conducted as follows:

1. Using a stage micrometer ruled in 0.1 to 0.01 mm, measure the radius of the field to the third decimal place.

2. Calculate the microscopic factor using the formula:

$$MF = \frac{10,000}{3.1416} \times r^2$$

With field diameters measuring approximately 0.26 mm, 0.178 mm, 0.160 mm, and 0.146 mm, microscopic factors of 300,000, 400,000, 500,000, and 600,000 respectively, will be calculated.

In addition to counting the leukocytes in a specimen, bacterial morphology should be noted. In evaluating the bacteriologic status, the entire smear is examined under the high dry objective, and if bacteria are observed, the oil immersion objective is used to determine morphology. It is possible by this examination to demonstrate the presence of streptococci, staphylococci, and rods.

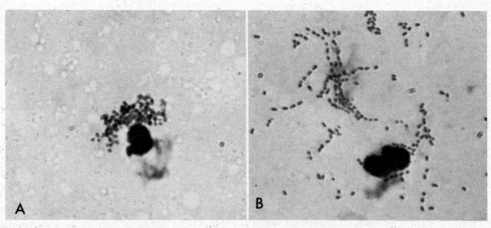

Figure 18–17. *A*, A single leukocyte and a clump of staphylococci in a smear prepared from fresh milk. *B*, Streptococci and a leukocyte in a smear from fresh milk. Newman-Lampert stain.

If rods are present, the sample can be smeared and stained by the Gram method.

If the sample is incubated for 18 to 20 hours and then smeared and stained, the bacterial population will have increased greatly, and it is possible to obtain more accurate information regarding bacteriologic population with such a sample than with an unincubated sample. The number of microorganisms in an incubated sample is of no significance. However, less accurate estimations of the number of leukocytes are made on incubated samples, as some cells undergo degeneration, making identification more difficult. In examinations of incubated specimens, it is impossible to distinguish pathogens from nonpathogens on the basis of morphology alone. Therefore, the presence or absence of leukocytes must be used as a guide. If streptococci are observed in a smear, and no leukocytes are present, it is probably a contaminant nonpathogen. If, however, both leukocytes and streptococci are present, a diagnosis of streptococcic mastitis may be warranted (Fig. 18–18). If the sample has been badly contaminated with airborne organisms, they usually appear as large, rather square-ended rods containing spores. These bacilli often occur in long chains and must be differentiated from streptococci. Such bacilli are not usually accompanied by an increase in leukocytes and, therefore, are ignored, as their only significance is that they indicate that the sample has been contaminated.

CULTURE METHODS

Although many of the tests discussed are of value in detecting the presence of acute to subacute mastitis, many chronic mastitis cases are detected only by culture methods. Isolation and identification of a specific microorganism from milk is usually considered to be evidence that the quarter is infected. This statement is true only if the sample has been collected in such a manner as to avoid contamination with skin microorganisms or airborne bacteria. Cultural examination of milk from an infected udder will usually reveal several colonies of the same organism on the agar plate.

A nutrient medium containing blood is recommended for isolation of bacteria from milk samples. Dehydrated blood agar base is commercially available and requires only the addition of distilled water for preparation. This agar should be sterilized by autoclaving or heating in a pressure cooker at 121° C for 20 minutes. Following sterilization, the agar is cooled to 45 to 48° C and sufficient sterile citrated or defibrinated blood is added to provide a concentration of 5 per cent. The most commonly used blood is from sheep, although it has been found in our laboratory that human blood obtained from blood banks after it has become outdated provides an economical and adequate source of blood cells. Following addition of the blood and careful mixing in such a manner as to avoid foaming, the agar is poured directly into sterile Petri dishes and allowed to harden before the material is streaked. Sufficient medium should be placed in each dish to provide an even $\frac{1}{4}$ to $\frac{3}{8}$ inch thick layer of agar. Disposable plastic Petri dishes containing sterile blood agar are commercially available and, unless large numbers of specimens are to be examined, are recommended.

In order to conserve media, the plate is divided into quarters by marking on the back of the Petri dish with a wax crayon. Milk samples are mixed by inverting several times in order to distribute cream throughout the sample. The sample should not be shaken vigorously, as foaming should be avoided. In most instances, freshly collected milk or milk that has been preserved by refrigeration is preferred. Incubated milk samples are employed for culture examination only if the specimen had been previously examined and no bacteria were present but the clinical diagnosis indicated that mastitis was a problem. In milk incubated for any length of time, the relationship between the presence of a potentially pathogenic organism and mastitis is more difficult to establish. For example, a few staphylococci from the skin multiply rapidly in an incubated sample, and when the sample is cultured, large numbers may be present, leaving the investigator with the impression that staphylococci are present in numbers sufficient to create a problem. If the same sample is streaked onto blood agar prior to incubation, the chances are that none or one or two colonies will appear. It is, however, a good procedure to incubate all samples overnight following initial culturing.

In streaking milk onto agar, a wire inoculating loop having a diameter of approximately 4 mm is preferred. The loop should be sterilized in an open flame of a Bunsen or alcohol burner and allowed to cool, and a loopful of the well-mixed milk should be streaked onto one quarter of the blood plate. These plates are allowed to dry, inverted, and incubated overnight at 37° C. The plate is examined for bacterial colonies. Any colonies found should be examined and Gram's stain should be performed to assist in positive identification. If no colonies are present, plates should be incubated for an additional 24 hours. If, following this additional incubation, no colonies are present, it may be wise to streak the incubated specimen on a new blood agar plate.

Any aerobic organisms, either saprophytic or pathogenic, produce colonies if present in the original sample. Mastitis streptococci appear as small colonies having varying degrees of hemolysis classified as alpha, beta, or gamma. Since saprophytic streptococci have much the same colony characteristics as well as a similar morphology, it

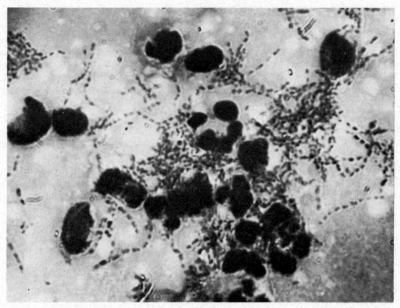

Figure 18–18. A stained smear of mastitic milk that was incubated overnight. Many leukocytes and streptococci are seen.

may be necessary to complete the differentiation by use of carbohydrate fermentation reactions. Colonies of *Corynebacterium* organisms may resemble streptococcic colonies but are differentiated by their characteristic morphology and Gram's stain reaction. Staphylococci normally produce a larger colony than streptococci and usually are hemolytic or have double zone hemolysis.

Since contaminating microorganisms may create a problem in identification of types of organisms on a blood agar plate, differential media may be employed that inhibit many of the more common contaminants. Although every attempt to avoid contamination should be made in the collection of the samples, these bacteria may still present a problem in diagnosis. The following media are suggested for use in mastitis diagnosis.

Edward's Medium. The formula for Edward's medium is presented in the Appendix, p. 453. This medium inhibits staphylococci, and coliform bacteria are readily distinguished by their characteristic black colonies. The various species of mastitis streptococci produce characteristic colonies as follows:

Streptococcus agalactiae, gray-blue colonies; *Streptococcus dysgalactiae*, gray or grayish-blue colonies; *Streptococcus uberis*, brown colonies. If, by experience, the veterinarian knows that streptococci are a problem in a herd, Edward's medium may be used for original isolation.

Sodium Azide–Crystal Violet Blood Agar. This medium inhibits the growth of almost all organisms except streptococci and is particularly adapted to culturing badly contaminated samples. The formula for preparation of this medium is pre-

sented in the Appendix, p. 453. In addition to streptococci, certain species of micrococci will also grow on this selective medium. Staphylococcal colonies are usually larger than those of streptococci and frequently have a fairly large zone of alpha hemolysis. Streptococcus colonies are quite small and have a varying amount of hemolysis characteristic for their species. It is not possible to differentiate pathogenic from saprophytic streptococci, so that isolation and subsequent identification of the organism using carbohydrate fermentation is necessary.

Salt Agar. Sodium chloride added to any of the common media at a concentration of 7.5 per cent makes a selective medium for the isolation of staphylococci. Specialized media such as Chapman's 110 or mannitol-salt agar may also be utilized. Staphylococci are not inhibited by a concentration of salts as high as 7.5 per cent, but most other organisms fail to grow. Any colonies appearing on salt agar must be identified by staining, hemolysis, and coagulase production before a positive diagnosis of staphylococcal infection can be made.

Glycine-Tellurite Agar. This is also a selective medium that will allow staphylococci to grow but inhibits many other organisms. On the surface of glycine-tellurite agar, staphylococci appear as black colonies, whereas other organisms produce a clear to colorless colony.

HOTIS TEST

The Hotis test provides a considerable amount of information regarding the condition of a milk sample. Milk (9.5 ml) for the Hotis test should be collected in a sterile test tube containing 0.5 ml of bromcresol purple. The following observations may be made.

1. The pH of the milk may be determined by noting the color produced after addition of milk.
2. A portion of this milk sample may be used for the isolation of pathogenic microorganisms.
3. The milk may be utilized for examination as an incubated sample.
4. A direct leukocyte count may be made.
5. The Hotis test itself is useful in determining the presence of streptococci and staphylococci.

Following the collection of 9.5 ml of milk in 0.5 ml of bromcresol purple, the sample is incubated at 37° C for 24 hours. The appearance of canary yellow colonies of organisms along the sides of the tube or on the bottom indicates the presence of *Streptococcus agalactiae* in the sample. This color change is due to the production of acid from the milk lactose by the action of these microorganisms, which grow in colony form on the sides or bottom of the tube. If the sample is incubated for 48 additional hours, the entire sample often turns yellow.

Staphylococcus aureus produces a characteristic change in some, but not all, tubes. The organism grows in small agglutinated colonies, producing a rust-brown color. This organism may also digest the milk. If the presence of *Staphylococcus aureus* is suspected, the sample may be incubated for 72 hours. Such prolonged incubation yields a higher percentage of positive reactions with this organism.

If more than one type of organism is present, or if the sample has become contaminated, a combination of changes may obscure the typical Hotis test reaction. If such a change occurs, other techniques such as direct smear examination or culture examination must be used in order to make an accurate diagnosis.

REFERENCES

1. Stamp, J. T., McEwen, A. D., Watt, J. A. A., and Nislet, D. I.: Enzootic abortion in ewes. I. Transmission of the disease. Vet. Rec., 62:251, 1950.
2. Bailie, W. E., and Coles, E. H.: Diagnostic microbiology and basic techniques and interpretation. *Proceedings 42nd Annual Meeting American Animal Hospital Association*, American Animal Hospital Association, South Bend, IN, 1975.
3. Bauer, A. W., Kirby, W. M. M., Sherris, J. C., and Turck, M.: Antibiotic susceptibility testing by a standardized single disc method. Am. J. Clin. Pathol., 45:493, 1966.
4. Murphy, J. M., and Hanson, J. J.: A modified Whiteside test for the determination of chronic bovine mastitis. Cornell Vet., 31:47, 1941.
5. Schalm, O. W., and Noorlander, D. O.: Experiments and observations leading to development of the California mastitis test. J.A.V.M.A., 130:199, 1957.
6. Spencer, G. R., and Simon, J.: The catalase, California and cell count tests for detecting abnormalities in milk. Am. J. Vet. Res., 21:578, 1960.

CHAPTER

19

TOXICOLOGY

The practicing veterinarian may be faced with the problem of attempting to explain sudden, unexpected illness or death to an owner who is convinced that an animal has been poisoned. Although many sudden deaths or illnesses may be explained as having resulted from other causes, occasionally poisoning must be ruled out as the cause. Toxicologic analysis of material should be performed by experts. It should be undertaken only by those having specialized experience and training. This is particularly true if there is any possibility that the case will culminate in the courtroom. "Rough qualitative testing, sometimes attempted by those with little or no experience in forensic chemistry, is most unwise, for at best it consumes irreplaceable material and at worst it may lead to miscarriage of justice."[1]

It remains, however, that the veterinarian may be called upon to make a diagnosis in poisoning cases in which several animals are involved. Under such circumstances, certain toxicologic screening tests can be completed in the veterinarian's laboratory. In all cases of suspected poisoning, material should be collected in duplicate, and if a part is utilized for testing in the clinical laboratory, the remainder should be forwarded to a laboratory equipped to complete toxicologic examinations.

Selection of material to be tested or submitted to a laboratory for confirmation will depend in large part on the type of poisoning suspected and on the lesions observed at necropsy. For details regarding the fluids and tissues required see Chapter 1. If the indications are that the poison has been absorbed and its nature is known or suspected, portions of organs in which it is most

likely to be found should be retained for analysis. Generally, it is wise to submit kidneys, spleen, a portion of the liver, urine, whole blood, serum, and possibly brain. If toxic material has been taken orally, the stomach of small animals may be removed unopened. The esophagus and duodenum should be tied with a double ligature prior to removal of the stomach. In larger animals or ruminants, the contents can be removed and a representative portion placed in a chemically clean container for shipment or delivery to the laboratory. All specimens for toxicologic examination should be submitted without any preservative. Tissues should be frozen prior to shipping and shipped to arrive frozen. Blood should not be frozen but should be shipped under refrigeration.

All specimens should be adequately labeled with the veterinarian's name, owner's name, samples submitted, history of the case, and special directions as to the poison or poisons suspected. Samples should be carefully packed in either glass jars or plastic containers, with not more than one organ placed in a single container. If litigation is anticipated, it is wise to have the labels signed by a witness and to make sure that no unauthorized person has access to the unsealed containers. Care must be taken to ensure that the containers in which these samples are submitted do not contain contaminating chemicals that might interfere with the toxicologic examination. If glass jars are used, they should be chemically cleaned with chromate and rinsed six to eight times in tap water, followed by two or three rinses in distilled water.

In addition to submitting fresh specimens, small sections from all organs having gross disease should be placed in 10 per cent formalin, and a histopathologic examination should be requested. Some types of poisoning produce histologic alterations of significance.

TESTS FOR DETECTION OF TOXIC SUBSTANCES

A complete history is essential and should include a description of physical signs, necropsy lesions, and any other relevant information.

Tests for the presence of the following substances may be conducted in the clinical pathology laboratory with a minimum of equipment and reagents: cyanide; heavy metals, including arsenic, mercury, bismuth, antimony, and silver; nitrate and nitrite; and possibly strychnine. Other tests that may be conducted include those for detection of the presence of barbiturates, lead, fluoride, thallium, phosphorus, carbon monoxide, phenothiazine compounds, sulfonamide derivatives, aspirin, phenol, and aflatoxins. These tests are screening procedures and should be interpreted accordingly. Information gained from use of these techniques may be useful in selecting appropriate therapy, but the results should be confirmed by a reputable toxicology laboratory. Failure to utilize the resources of such a laboratory could result in an embarrassing case in a law court.

Cyanide. Clinical observations are often sufficient to detect the presence of cyanide poisoning, but occasionally a chemical test may be necessary to confirm the diagnosis. For the detection of cyanide in gastrointestinal contents, fluids, and body tissues, the copper-guaiac test may be used. The copper-guaiac test is conducted as follows:

1. Place approximately 50 gm of finely ground tissue or stomach contents in a 100-ml flask.
2. Acidify the flask contents with tartaric acid.
3. In the neck of the flask, suspend a strip of filter paper that has been moistened in turn with 10 per cent alcoholic solution of guaiac and 0.1 per cent aqueous copper sulfate solution.
4. Stopper the flask and warm the contents a little and allow the flask to stand for approximately 30 minutes. If a blue or green color does not develop, the presence of cyanide is excluded. If a blue color does develop, cyanide may be present; however, a blue color is also produced by chloride; hydrogen; ammonia gas; and oxides of nitrogen, bromine, chlorine, and hydrogen peroxide.

The veterinarian may be faced with the unenviable task of attempting to predict whether a

---

TABLE 19–1. Laboratory Tests and Anticipated Results That May Aid in Diagnosis of Some Common Poisonings

Poison	Animal	Tests	Results
Dicumarol	All species	OSPT, APTT, ACT, platelet count	Increased OSPT, APTT, ACT platelets normal in number
Organophosphate	All species	Cholinesterase	Cholinesterase activity < 25% normal activity
Oxalate	All species	Chemistry profile	Azotemia, hypocalcemia in ruminants
Mercury	All species	BUN, creatinine	Azotemia
Ethylene glycol	Dogs, cats	BUN, creatinine, urinalysis	Azotemia, oxalate crystals in urine
Thallium	Dogs, cats	CBC, chemistry profile, UA	Stress leukogram, azotemia, glycosuria
Sodium fluoroacetate	Dogs, cats	Chemistry profile	Hyperglycemia
Salt	Pigs	Serum electrolyte	Sodium >160 mEq/l
Iron	Pigs	Serum iron, liver enzymes	Hyperferremia, increase in enzyme activity
Lead	Dog	CBC	Many NRBC with little or no anemia; basophilic stippling of RBC
	Ruminants	CBC	Basophilic stippling is not constant—must be differentiated from regenerative anemia
Urea	Ruminants	Rumen pH, blood ammonia	Rumen pH >7.5, increased blood ammonia
Nitrate	Ruminants	Methemoglobin	Increased
Selenium (chronic)	Ruminants	CBC, liver enzymes	Anemia, increased enzyme activity
Bracken fern	Herbivores	CBC, OSPT, APTT	Nonregenerative anemia, leukopenia, thrombocytopenia, normal OSPT, APTT
Molybdenum (Cu deficiency)	Ruminants	CBC	Microcytic, hypochromic anemia
Copper (acute)	Ruminants	CBC	Hemolytic anemia
Polybrominated biphenyls	Ruminants	Chemistry profile	Increased liver enzymes, azotemia, hypocalcemia, hypoalbuminemia

CBC = complete blood count; UA = urinalysis; OSPT = one-step prothrombin time; APTT = activated partial thromboplastin time; ACT = activated clotting time.

given field of green feed such as Sudan grass or sorghum may contain hydrocyanic acid. A test that has proved to be of value in plant materials is the Steyn test. This test for hydrocyanic acid in plant materials is conducted as follows:

1. Prepare picric acid test strips by dipping strips of filter paper in a solution that contains 5 gm of sodium carbonate and 0.5 gm of picric acid in 100 ml of water. Allow the strips to become almost dry.

2. Add 2 to 3 gm of moistened shredded plant material to a test tube and add four drops of chloroform. Plant samples should be collected from several areas of the field and tested separately.

3. Place one end of a picrate strip in a split cork stopper and insert carefully into a test tube without letting the strip touch the side of the container.

4. Incubate the test tube for at least 24 hours at 37° C.

5. A positive test is indicated by a red to reddish-brown color on the filter paper strip. If the change occurs within a few minutes, it is significant, but a mild reaction, as indicated by faint color changes in one to several hours, is of less importance.[2] It is possible to complete this same test using rumen contents, but this is not an adequate assay for testing animal tissues for the presence of cyanide.

Heavy Metals. A fairly rapid and easily conducted test for the detection of heavy metals, including arsenic, mercury, bismuth, antimony, and silver, is Reinsch's test. This test may be confusing, since several elements may react to produce false positives with Reinsch's test.[2] All positive tests should be confirmed by a qualified toxicology laboratory. This test is conducted as follows:

1. Place approximately 25 gm of finely diced liver, stomach, or other tissue to be tested in a chemically clean Pyrex beaker.

2. To the material being tested, add 10 ml of concentrated hydrochloric acid diluted in 90 ml of distilled water.

3. Introduce into the flask a strip of bright pure copper foil or copper wire that has been brightened with nitric acid or burnished with steel wool. Copper wire can be cleaned with alcohol, then with ether, and dried.

4. Place a flask filled with cold water over the opening in the container and boil the material gently for 30 to 45 minutes.

5. Remove the copper, wash it thoroughly with distilled water, and allow it to dry on a piece of filter paper. A dark discoloration indicates the presence of either arsenic or bismuth. The presence of a silver deposit may indicate that mercury is present. Antimony will also produce a dark color that may have a purple to blue-violet sheen.

The black arsenic deposit may be confirmed by placing the copper in 1 to 2 ml of 10 per cent potassium cyanide. If the black deposit is due to the presence of arsenic, it will dissolve. If the deposit is due to bismuth or antimony, it will persist.

Absolute confirmation of the presence of arsenic may be accomplished by utilizing Gutzeit's test, which is conducted as follows:

1. Fit a suitable flask with a rubber stopper carrying a drying tube that has been plugged with absorbent cotton moistened with lead acetate solution.

2. Into the upper part of the drying tube, but not in contact with the cotton, place a strip of filter paper that has been freshly impregnated with a 5 per cent solution of mercuric bromide in 95 per cent alcohol.

3. Place a few pieces of pure zinc in the flask, add a few drops of dilute stannous chloride solution, acidify with dilute sulfuric acid, and add the material to be tested. The material to be tested may be either the copper used in Reinsch's test, an acid digest of tissue, or stomach contents.

4. Allow the apparatus to stand for one hour. The development of a canary yellow color on the impregnated strip indicates the presence of either arsenic or antimony. To eliminate the possible interference of antimony, expose the strip to hydrochloric acid fumes from an empty bottle. If the yellow color is due to the presence of antimony, it will completely fade, whereas with arsenic the yellow color persists.

If the color of the deposit on the copper is suggestive of mercury, the presence of this metal can be confirmed as follows:

1. Dissolve 5 gm of cupric sulfate and 3 gm of ferrous sulfate in 10 ml of water. Slowly add 7 gm of potassium iodide in 50 ml of water while stirring. Filter and wash the precipitate with water (by decantation) to free all of the excess iodide. The cuprous iodide is transferred to a brown bottle with approximately 10 ml of water and may be stirred and used in the form of a suspension.

2. Completely wash the copper wire or strip and place on it several drops of the suspended cuprous iodide.

3. Cover with a watch glass and allow it to stand for about one hour. If mercury is present, the cuprous iodide will turn light pink, the intensity of the color being proportional to the concentration of mercury present.

Strychnine. Detection of strychnine in stomach contents or tissues is extremely difficult to accomplish in the clinical pathology laboratory with any degree of certainty. A screening test that may be used is conducted as follows:

1. Add 5 ml of concentrated sulfuric acid to 3 ml of filtered stomach contents in a test tube.

2. A control using 5 ml of sulfuric acid and 3 ml of distilled water should be used.

3. Drop a few crystals of potassium dichromate into each tube and shake gently.

4. Examine in front of a light. Falling streamers of blue, violet, red, and orange from a falling crystal indicate the possible presence of strychnine.

A biologic test can be conducted by adding the stomach contents from the animal suspected of being poisoned or a solution of the suspected toxic material to 10 per cent sodium hydroxide of sufficient quantity to alkalinize the preparation. This mixture is extracted several times with ether, and the extracts are pooled and evaporated to dryness. The residue is resuspended in 1 ml of water, neutralized, and injected into the abdominal sac of a live frog. If the sample is positive, typical tetanic spasms will develop within 10 minutes. A young mouse injected intraperitoneally will react similarly if strychnine is present.

Neither test is sufficient for positive identification of strychnine, and it is recommended that if this chemical is suspected, the stomach contents be submitted to a toxicology laboratory for confirmation.

Nitrate. Nitrates per se are not usually toxic, and their importance as a cause of poisoning is due to their conversion into nitrite either in the food material or within the digestive tract. This conversion is of particular importance in ruminant animals, as nitrite is an intermediary product in the reduction of nitrate to ammonia in the rumen.

A diagnosis of nitrite poisoning may be suggested by the color of the blood. Blood taken from an animal poisoned with nitrite is chocolate brown and will remain that color upon exposure to air. This is due to the presence of methemoglobin.

A simple test for detecting the presence of this substance in blood is the "cooking test." Draw a sample of blood from the animal suspected of being poisoned and a second sample from a known normal animal. This blood should be collected with no anticoagulant. After the samples have clotted, they are placed in a boiling water bath for 45 minutes or longer. After cooking and cooling, a normal blood sample is chocolate brown, pulls away from the side of the tube, and has a convex surface. After cooking and cooling, a blood sample containing nitrite will be salmon pink. These clots do not pull away from the side of the tube, and the surface will be either level or concave. The intensity of color and the difference between the positive cooked blood clot and the negative will depend upon the concentration of the chemical present.

In addition to the diagnosis of poisoning in an animal that has become affected, the veterinarian is occasionally faced with the task of attempting to detect the presence of either nitrate or nitrite in water or feed.

A simple nitrate test is conducted as follows:

1. Dissolve 0.5 gm of diphenylamine in 20 ml of distilled water.

2. Add sulfuric acid to bring the total volume to 100 ml.

3. Cool the solution and store it in a brown bottle. This represents the full-strength solution and may be diluted with equal parts of 80 per cent sulfuric acid to obtain a half-strength solution.

4. To test a plant for the presence of nitrate, put one drop of the test reagent on the cut surface of a plant.

5. A green to blue color indicates the presence of nitrates.

6. A green to blue color with a half-strength solution indicates a 2 + nitrate, which is the danger point for feed.

A nitrite field test may be conducted as follows:

1. Dissolve 0.5 gm of sulfanilic acid in 150 ml of 20 per cent glacial acetic acid.

2. Dissolve 0.2 gm of alpha-naphthylamine hydrochloride in 150 ml of 20 per cent glacial acetic acid by gently heating.

3. Add to a clean test tube 2 ml of the unknown solution. The solution may be prepared by soaking some of the suspected feed material in distilled water.

4. Add 2 ml of sulfanic acid solution.

5. Add 2 ml of the alpha-naphthylamine solution and mix well. A pink to red color is positive for the presence of nitrites.

Corn stalks may be tested for the presence of nitrites by adding three to four drops of sulfanilic acid solution to a freshly cut surface and allowing it to soak in. Three or four drops of alpha-naphthylamine solution are then added, and a pink to red color is positive for nitrites.

OTHER TESTS

Lead. There is no simple test for the presence of lead in biologic materials. Therefore, tissues from the majority of animals with suspected lead poisoning should be submitted to a toxicologic laboratory for a confirmatory diagnosis. The Grunwald test for lead can be used but is somewhat difficult to read and interpret. The test is conducted as follows:

1. Remove a small amount of scraping from stomach wall.

2. Add four drops of concentrated nitric acid and heat very gently until dry. Care must be taken not to overheat the sample, as it will turn black, making reading difficult.

3. Add a few drops of water and two drops of a 10 per cent solution of potassium iodide.

4. A positive test for the presence of lead is indicated by the presence of a marked yellow color.

Nitric acid has a tendency to produce a yellow color when evaporated, and this must be differentiated from the color observed following the addition of 10 per cent potassium iodide.

Fluorides. A simple test for the presence of fluorides is the Gettler test. This test utilizes either urine or stomach contents and is conducted as follows:

1. Alkalinize a sample of urine or stomach contents (as little as 1 to 3 ml) with several drops of sodium hydroxide solution.
2. Dry at low heat in a glass or porcelain dish.
3. After drying is completed, add a small amount of powdered glass to the dry residue and mix thoroughly.
4. Add several milliliters of concentrated sulfuric acid and cover the dish with a small glass plate from the undersurface of which is suspended a drop of 5 per cent sodium chloride solution. Place a small piece of ice on top of the plate to prevent evaporation of the drop.
5. Heat gently for three to five minutes, then carefully remove the glass plate and examine the drop.

If fluorides are present in the specimen, silicon fluoride is formed and appears as small, faintly pink, hexagonal crystals along the rim of the drop. These crystals are much smaller than the large sodium chloride crystals. Additional differentiation can be made on the basis of shape, as sodium chloride crystals are usually square. The crystals should be examined under low power of the microscope.

Thallium. Thallium salts have been used extensively as rodent poisons and will produce death when consumed by domestic animals. A simple test for the detection of thallium poisoning may be conducted as follows:

1. To one drop of weakly acidic urine add one drop of 10 per cent potassium iodide on a watch glass. This mixture should be observed with a dark background.
2. If a yellow precipitate appears, add one drop of 2 per cent sodium thiosulfate. Failure of the precipitate to dissolve is an indication of the presence of thallium.

An alternative method for detecting the presence of thallium in canine urine has been described.[3] The test is performed as follows:

1. Place three drops of the urine to be tested in a 10 ml screwtop vial.
2. Add three drops of bromine water and agitate until a permanent yellow color is present, adding more bromine water until the color persists.
3. Add a few drops of sulfosalicylic acid solution, prepared by dissolving 10 gm of reagent grade sulfosalicylic acid in 100 ml of distilled water and agitating until the yellow color is dissipated.
4. Filter to remove protein from the urine sample.

5. Add one drop of concentrated reagent grade hydrochloric acid and one or two drops of rhodamine B solution (0.05 gm rhodamine B dissolved in concentrated hydrochloric acid to make 100 ml) and mix well.
6. Add 1 ml of reagent grade benzene, cap the vial, and mix by shaking.
7. Centrifuge the specimen.

A positive reaction is indicated by a purple or bluish color in the benzene phase. The aqueous layer may retain some of the red of the rhodamine B, regardless of the reaction. The color is most easily detected by holding the tube against a white background.

To ensure accuracy of the test, distilled water samples and water samples containing thallium sulfate should also be tested.

Phosphorus. The Scherer test is of value in preliminary determinations, as it will, if negative, indicate the absence of phosphorus. The test is carried out as follows:

1. Mix a small portion of the finely divided material to be examined with distilled water in an Erlenmeyer flask. The specimen should be acidified with dilute sulfuric acid.
2. Suspend two strips of filter paper in the mouth of the flask over the suspected sample. One is impregnated with silver nitrate and the other with lead acetate.
3. Heat the contents to about 50° C in a water bath for approximately one hour.
4. If the silver nitrate paper turns black, either phosphorus or hydrogen sulfide may be present.
5. If both papers turn black, hydrogen sulfide is present, and phosphorus may also be present in the original specimen. The fact that the silver nitrate paper turns black is not conclusive proof that phosphorus is present, as any volatile reducing agent, such as formaldehyde, may give the same reaction. If the test results indicate the possible presence of phosphorus, the specimen should be submitted to a qualified toxicology laboratory for confirmation.

Carbon Monoxide. Although the veterinarian is not often called on to demonstrate the presence of carbon monoxide, such an examination may occasionally be required. A very simple procedure for detecting the presence of carbon monoxide poisoning is conducted as follows:

1. Dilute two drops of blood with approximately 15 ml of water so that the solution is a faint pink.
2. Add five drops of 20 per cent sodium hydroxide, shake quickly, and observe the color.
3. If the blood is normal or contains less than 20 per cent carboxyhemoglobin, the pink color will immediately become straw yellow on shaking. If the pink color persists for several seconds or more, it indicates the presence of carboxyhemoglobin in excess of 20 per cent. However, even

in high concentration this will also turn a straw yellow, usually within one to two minutes. The persistence of the pink color and its intensity before turning yellow give a rough approximation of the concentration. This test is specific for carbon monoxide. Less than 5 per cent is considered normal, 5 to 20 per cent subclinical, and 20 per cent or more may be toxic.

Phenothiazine Compounds. With the increasing use of drugs made from phenothiazine compounds, the veterinarian may be faced with the necessity of attempting to detect the presence of such drugs in animal patients. A simple procedure for detecting the presence of phenothiazine compounds in urine is conducted as follows:

1. Add six drops of sulfuric acid and two drops of 10 per cent ferric chloride to 2 ml of urine.
2. A light pink to purple color indicates a positive reaction for a phenothiazine compound.

Sulfonamide Derivatives. The veterinarian occasionally will be presented with an animal that has been previously treated by the owner or by another practitioner. Under such circumstances, the veterinarian may find it necessary to establish whether or not a sulfonamide has been used. A simple test can be conducted on urine or an unknown drug as follows:

1. Place a drop of urine or a small portion of the unknown drug on a piece of newspaper.
2. Place one drop of concentrated hydrochloric acid on the urine drop or drug. The appearance of an intense orange color indicates the presence of a sulfonamide.
3. As a control, place one drop of hydrochloric acid on a blank portion of the newspaper; only a straw yellow color should appear.

This same technique may be used to test medicaments for the presence of sulfonamides.

Aspirin. Toxicity resulting from the ingestion of aspirin may occur following large accidental doses or the use of improper therapeutic quantities in cats or young dogs. Salicylates can be presumptively identified by chemical examination of urine, whole blood, or serum. In tests of urine, 2 ml is added to 1 ml of a 10 per cent ferric chloride solution. If salicylates are present, a purple color will develop. Phenol derivatives will also give a positive result. If whole blood is tested, 5 ml is acidified with 0.2 ml of concentrated hydrochloric acid, which is then extracted with 10 ml of ethylene dichloride. Following extraction, the blood will separate into two layers. The upper layer is discarded, and four drops of 10 per cent ferric chloride and 2 ml of distilled water are added to the remaining layer. This is shaken, and if the sample is positive for salicylates, a purple color will develop. In testing serum samples, a porcelain dish is recommended. Two drops of serum are placed on the dish and one drop of 10 per cent ferric chloride added. A purple color is a positive reaction for salicylates.

Phenol. Phenols, such as those used in disinfectants, and phenolic derivatives used as wood preservatives, herbicides, fungicides, and photographic developers may produce severe intoxications. The presence of phenol can be tentatively identified by the addition of 1 ml of a 20 per cent aqueous solution of ferric chloride to 10 ml of urine. If the urine becomes purple, the test is positive. A second test utilizes Millon's reagent. This reagent is made by dissolving 10 gm of mercury in 20 ml of nitric acid, which is then diluted with an equal quantity of distilled water and allowed to stand for two hours, at which time the excess water is decanted. The test is conducted by boiling 10 ml of the suspected urine with 1 to 2 ml of Millon's reagent. A positive reaction results in the development of a red color.

Aflatoxins. A variety of aflatoxins have been identified as products of the growth of *Aspergillus flavus* and *Penicillium* spp. These metabolites are most likely to be identified in feeds. Absolute identification and quantification should be completed in a qualified toxicology laboratory. A rapid qualitative test for aflatoxin can be conducted.

Approximately 100 gm of feed material is placed in a blender with 300 ml of a solvent composed of seven parts methanol and three parts water. This material is blended for two to three minutes or up to five minutes if low levels of aflatoxin are suspected. The blended material is permitted to stand until a layer of noncloudy liquid forms on the surface. Eighty to 150 ml of the clear surface liquid is removed and placed in a 500-ml separatory funnel, and 30 ml of benzine is added. The funnel is shaken for 30 seconds, and 200 ml of water is added. This material is allowed to separate, and the lower layer is discarded. The upper layer is placed in a beaker and evaporated to dryness. Material remaining in the beaker is resuspended in 0.5 ml of benzine. A small quantity is spotted on No. 4 Whatman filter paper, allowed to dry, and placed under a long-wave ultraviolet light. If the spot on the filter paper gives a blue fluorescence, the sample is considered positive for aflatoxin.

REFERENCES

1. Kaye, S.: Toxicology. In *Gradwohl's Clinical Laboratory Methods and Diagnosis*, Edited by Frankel, S., and Reitman, S., 6th ed. C. V. Mosby Co., St. Louis, 1963.
2. Buck, W. B.: Laboratory toxicologic tests and their interpretation. J.A.V.M.A., *155*:1928, 1969.
3. Gabriel, K. L., and Dubin, S.: A method for the detection of thallium in canine urine. J.A.V.M.A., *143*:722, 1963.

20

EXAMINATIONS FOR PARASITES

S. A. EWING, B.S.A., D.V.M., M.S., PH.D.

The infectious diseases of vertebrates have been separated artificially into several categories, and those that are traditionally designated as parasitisms include a heterogeneous group caused by protozoans, helminths, arthropods, and a few organisms of uncertain or disputed classification, such as *Anaplasma marginale*. In this chapter, diagnostic aids are presented that may be used in determining which particular organisms are involved in producing disease in a given animal. All other infectious agents are discussed in appropriate chapters. This chapter deals with methods used to detect the presence of parasites or their generative products and the relation of these structures to specific identifications.

Techniques that are indispensable in diagnosing parasitisms have been described in other chapters. It should be emphasized that the methods discussed here are only of supplemental or, at best, confirmatory value. The mere presence of a parasite in or on an animal cannot be considered adequate evidence that it is the etiological agent of a disease syndrome that may exist. Therefore, the examinations described in this chapter as diagnostic aids should be considered to be only part of the resources to be used by the diagnostician in solving problems of differential diagnosis. They, like any laboratory techniques, are used to supplement, not supplant, clinical observations.

FECAL EXAMINATION

It is essential to have a fresh sample of feces uncontaminated in any way either by the feces of another animal or by the substrate. The sample should be placed in a properly labeled, clean container, and its subsequent manipulation should be determined by what is wanted from the sample. If feces are to be examined for the presence of trophozoite stages of protozoans, the sample must not be refrigerated and must be examined without delay. It also is inadvisable to incubate such samples; in other words, be prepared to look at the sample when it is collected. If the specimen is to be scrutinized for certain nematode larvae, it should be kept at room temperature. If it is to be examined for helminth eggs or protozoan oocysts, it may be refrigerated, within limits, until time is available to make the examination.

Spurious Parasites: When examining fecal smears or flotation preparations, a wide variety of extraneous material is encountered. The uninitiated may mistake these either for parasites or for generative products of parasites. Experience is needed to avoid such pitfalls, for one can never anticipate every type of pollen, fungal spore, or other debris that may be encountered. Figure 20–1 shows several of the most commonly observed artifacts that often confuse those examining fecal preparations.

DIRECT SMEAR

Reagent Needed: Water or Physiological Saline. A direct smear can be made utilizing either tap water or physiological saline, but saline is preferable, for trophozoites will remain intact and

Objects Sometimes Mistaken for Helminth Eggs and Protozoan Cysts

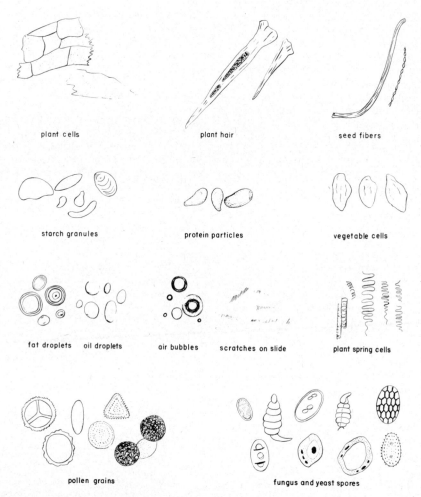

plant cells

plant hair

seed fibers

starch granules

protein particles

vegetable cells

fat droplets   oil droplets

air bubbles

scratches on slide

plant spring cells

pollen grains

fungus and yeast spores

Figure 20–1. Objects sometimes mistaken either for parasites or for generative products of parasites. (Courtesy of Dr. H. J. Griffiths, University of Minnesota.)

motile longer in this fluid than in tap water. The direct smear method is a rapid and easily completed procedure, but, unfortunately, eggs and oocysts are not concentrated. One must be alert, therefore, to "false-negative" examination results.

Place a drop of the dilution fluid on a glass microscope slide and thoroughly mix a bit of feces with it, using an applicator stick. Apply a coverslip with forceps or fingers and examine at low power and at high dry if necessary. A properly made slide should not contain enough feces to make it opaque but should remain an almost translucent preparation. It is also important that excess material does not accumulate to any extent around the margin of the coverslip; if excesses run over the edge of the slide, the microscope stage may be contaminated, and damage may be done to the condenser or even the objective, especially if high power is employed in the examination.

FLOTATION

Reagent Needed: Zinc Sulfate. The following zinc sulfate ($ZnSO_4$) and water (H_2O) solution is needed for this technique:

$ZnSO_4 \cdot 7H_2O$ 331 gm
Tap water   1000.0 ml
Specific gravity: 1.18–1.22

Comminute thoroughly a small quantity of feces, about 1 to 2 gm, with sufficient water in a beaker to make a fluid mixture. The feces must be thoroughly dissociated so that eggs or oocysts will be freed from the feces. Pour the comminuted preparation through cheesecloth, and discard the debris. Transfer the fluid promptly to pointed centrifuge tubes and spin for five minutes at 1000 revolutions per minute (rpm). Remove the tubes from the centrifuge, pour off the supernatant fluid, add zinc sulfate solution, and, using an applicator stick, thoroughly mix the contents. Centrifuge again at the same rate and time. Using a wire loop, remove fluid from the top of the centrifuge tube, place it on a glass microscope slide, apply a coverslip, and examine. Material should be sufficient to fill the area between the coverslip and slide.

A simple modification of the method described and one for which no centrifuge is needed is as follows: Comminute feces in zinc sulfate solution, strain through cheesecloth and discard fecal debris as described. Pour fluid into a straight-sided tube, such as a shell vial, until a convex meniscus appears at the top of the tube, and apply a coverslip immediately. Little or no fluid should escape from the container when the coverslip is applied and there should not be so little fluid as to permit air bubbles under the coverslip. Allow the preparation to stand on a level surface for eight to ten minutes, remove the coverslip, apply it to a glass microscope slide, and examine. It should be reemphasized that the amount of fluid in the shell vial should not exceed the quantity that will accommodate the coverslip without spilling and it should not be so small that an air bubble can be trapped under the coverslip when it is applied. It is important to examine slides soon after preparation, for the hypertonic solution eventually will cause distortion of the egg shell. Some flotation media* are more satisfactory than others, in that distortion of eggs and oocysts is slow to occur.

SEDIMENTATION

Reagent Needed: Water or Physiological Saline. Most operculated trematode eggs and a few nematode eggs are difficult or impossible to recover by flotation techniques, and sedimentation procedures must be used. Mix 1 gm of feces with 40 ml of water or saline in a beaker, making certain that the feces are thoroughly dissociated to free the eggs. Pour the mixture into centrifuge tubes and spin at a moderate rate of speed for five minutes. Pour off the supernatant fluid, collect a

small quantity of the sediment with a pipette, put it on a glass microscope slide, apply coverslip, and examine.

BAERMANN APPARATUS

Reagent Needed: Water or Physiological Saline. In some instances it is necessary to examine feces for the presence of nematode larvae. The Baermann apparatus is suitable for this purpose (Fig. 20–2). Equipment needed includes a funnel fitted with a rubber hose with a tight stopcock or clamp and a sturdy ring-stand to hold the funnel. Place a piece of hardware cloth in the top of the funnel and add fluid to cover the mesh. Put feces on a double thickness of gauze and place it carefully on the hardware cloth. The fluid in the funnel should be at a level to just cover the feces supported by the gauze and the hardware cloth. Warm water, not more than 37° C, usually stimulates activity of larvae for more rapid collecting. Allow the apparatus to stand for a period of time—15 minutes to hours—draw off the fluid in the rubber hose, and examine it in flat glass containers under low power or with a dissecting microscope. The nematode larvae are freed from feces by their activity and collect in the hose due to the effect of gravity. Use caution in drawing off the fluid, for the first material released contains the largest number of larvae and may be lost easily. If more magnification is needed, transfer the helminths to a glass microscope slide, apply coverslip, and examine; if necessary apply heat to inactivate them.

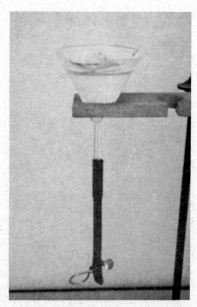

* Among other substances used for flotation (or levitation) procedures are solutions of sodium nitrate, sucrose, magnesium sulfate, and sodium chloride. Each of these has its own merits and what is used is largely a matter of personal preference.

Figure 20–2. Baermann apparatus used for recovering nematode larvae from feces or soil and for collecting parasites such as *Stephanofilaria* sp. from tissue.

QUANTITATIVE EVALUATION METHODS

Stoll Egg Counting Technique. **Reagent Needed: 0.1 N Sodium Hydroxide.** Fill a Stoll flask with 0.1 N sodium hydroxide (NaOH) to the bottom mark etched on the neck of the flask; this will be 56 ml. Use an applicator stick or teasing needle to add a sufficient amount of feces to raise the flask contents to the 60-ml level, which is etched on the flask. Add six to eight glass beads and firmly insert a rubber stopper into the neck of the flask. Shake the flask vigorously with a straight up and down motion for one minute or until a homogeneous suspension is secured. If the feces are very hard, allow the mixture to soak until it will dissociate when shaken. It is recommended by some that the flask be shaken in an inverted position. It is very important to avoid a circular motion since this will concentrate the eggs in a relatively small area and defeat the purpose of the shaking. Routinely, it is best to lay the sample aside at this point and to repeat shaking later. To secure material for examination, use a Stoll or other pipette calibrated to 0.15 ml and quickly withdraw a measured sample immediately after inversion of the flask several times. Insert the tip of the pipette into the center of the flask before withdrawing fluid. Expel the measured contents of the pipette onto a 2 × 3 inch glass microscope slide immediately, cover it with a 22 × 40 mm coverslip, and examine the preparation under the low power of the microscope, moving the slide methodically with a mechanical stage. Count all eggs on the preparation and multiply the number obtained by 100, which will give the total number of eggs per milliliter of formed feces. For mush stools, multiply this latter number by the correction factor 2 and for diarrheic stools by 4.

McMaster Technique. This technique has been modified slightly from the original introduced by Gordon and Whitlock.[42] Weigh 2 gm of feces into a shell vial, add 28 ml of water, and crush the feces as completely as possible. If the feces are in the form of pellets, set the sample aside for an hour or more and then comminute if necessary and mix thoroughly. Place 1 ml of the mixture in a test tube, add 1 ml of Sheather's sugar solution,* and again mix thoroughly. While keeping the mixture in motion, withdraw sufficient material with a pipette to fill a McMaster counting chamber. Let the preparation stand for a few minutes to allow the eggs to rise to the top, then place the slide on the microscope and count the eggs, all of which should be at the same focal level in the marked area. Multiply the number counted by 300 to calculate the number of eggs per gram of feces. In making the

---

* Sheather's sugar solution: Sucrose (ordinary cane or beet sugar) 500 gm. Distilled water 320 gm. Phenol (melted in water bath) 6.5 gm.

count, first focus on the line that marks the edge of the area to be counted and then move back and forth systematically across the entire marked area. Repeat the count by filling the chamber with additional material until the average number of eggs counted is within 10 per cent of the average obtained, omitting the last count.

PLASMA ENZYME ANALYSIS

Quantitative diagnosis of helminth infections is very difficult in part because egg production fluctuates from day to day. Furthermore, prepatent infections cannot be detected by fecal examination even though injury has already occurred. An attempt to diagnose prepatent fascioliasis and to quantitate adult liver fluke infections led Wyckoff and Bradley[105] to use of plasma constituent analysis. Cattle with experimental *Fasciola hepatica* infections had significant increases in aspartate aminotransferase (AST) and T-glutamyl transpeptidase (GGT) within four and nine weeks, respectively, of exposure. Although enzyme analysis alone did not give conclusive evidence of fascioliasis, liver damage was detected before fluke eggs were recoverable from feces, and analysis of GGT revealed fluke burden–related differences in the plasma activities of this enzyme. (See Chapter 7 for techniques for determining AST and GGT.)

There has not been adequate opportunity to evaluate this approach to quantitative diagnosis of fascioliasis. Nevertheless, plasma enzyme analysis may prove useful for evaluating this and other helminthiases.

CENTRIFUGATION TECHNIQUE

Reagents Needed: 1 Per Cent Aluminum Potassium Sulfate, Household Liquid Detergent. Since most trematode eggs do not float in the usual flotation media, it is necessary to use other methods to concentrate eggs for examination. Mix 5 ml of liquid household detergent with 995 ml of tap water to which a few drops of 1 per cent aluminum potassium sulfate (alum) have been added. Since this fluid becomes gelatinous on standing, it should be prepared at the time needed. Thoroughly mix 1 to 3 gm of feces with about 15 ml of the detergent solution in a large test tube or other container and strain the mixture through cheesecloth (or a sieve) into a 50-ml centrifuge tube. Wash the material retained in the cheesecloth with sufficient detergent solution to fill the centrifuge tube to the 50-ml mark. Allow the suspension to stand for five to 10 minutes and carefully decant the supernatant fluid, allowing 2 to 3 ml with the debris to remain in the centrifuge tube. Then wash the sediment by refilling the tube to the 50-ml mark with detergent solution, and allow it to stand for five to 10 minutes. Pour off the supernatant fluid as before. Transfer a small amount of the sediment to a slide and examine for fluke eggs. The eggs settle quickly in either water or detergent solution, but the latter floats off more of the debris.

ACID-ETHER TECHNIQUE

Reagents Needed: 5 Per Cent Solution of Acetic or Hydrochloric Acid, Ether. This is a centrifugal sedimentation method that may be substituted for direct sedimentation. Add 10 ml of a 5 per cent solution of acetic or hydrochloric acid to 1 gm of feces in a test tube, comminute thoroughly, and sieve or strain through three layers of cheesecloth. Place the strained suspension in a centrifuge tube, add an equal amount of ether, and shake thoroughly. Centrifuge for 1 to 1½ minutes at 2500 rpm. The tube contents will be in four distinct layers: (1) ether extract layer, (2) plug of fecal debris, (3) clear column of acid solution, and (4) a sediment at the bottom of the tube. Discard the first three layers; it is usually necessary first to loosen the second layer with an applicator stick in order to do this. Remove some of the remaining sediment (layer 4) with a pipette, place it on a glass microscope slide, apply a coverslip, and examine. This method is not suitable for recovering protozoan oocysts but is particularly good for fluke eggs.

CULTURE OF FECES FOR NEMATODE LARVAE

Reagents Needed: Granulated Wood or Animal Charcoal (Sand or Sandy Soil May Be Substituted for Charcoal), Water. Mix fresh feces thoroughly with an equal amount of charcoal; moisten, if necessary, to form a damp, but not wet, crumbly mixture. Store on filter paper in a covered container at room temperature for the period necessary for the development of larvae to the desired stage; maintain moisture content by adding water if necessary. The larvae may be separated from the culture medium with the use of the Baermann apparatus.

SPORULATION OF COCCIDIAN OOCYSTS

Reagent Needed: 2.5 Per Cent Potassium Dichromate Solution. In order to identify coccidia, it is sometimes necessary to retain them for development, i.e., sporulation to the infective stage. Mix a fresh sample of feces with several volumes of 2.5 per cent potassium dichromate solution and transfer thin layers of the mixture to Petri dishes or other glass containers. Oxygen is essential for oocyst development, and potassium dichromate prevents bacteria from exhausting the oxygen supply or destroying the oocysts. Therefore, the layer

of fluid must not be more than a few millimeters thick. If masses of oocysts are cultured in deep containers, an aquarium pump may be used to aerate the medium. Sporulation will occur in a few days to weeks, depending on the conditions and the species. The sporulated oocysts can be kept indefinitely in closed containers if refrigerated.

DIAGNOSIS OF COCCIDIOSIS BY MUCOSAL SCRAPINGS

Antemortem diagnosis of coccidiosis is usually confirmed by recovery of oocysts from feces by flotation. Diagnosis of porcine neonatal coccidiosis has proved difficult by this method, however, and diagnoses have been made most consistently by demonstration of parasites in histopathological sections taken at necropsy. A quicker and only slightly less dependable method involves staining mucosal scrapings from jejunum and ileum.

Open the gut and flush away ingesta. Select an area where lesions are present and scrape the mucosa with the edge of a glass slide or other suitable implement. Apply mucosal scrapings to a clean glass slide, air dry, and stain with a modified Wright's stain.

SEPARATION OF FREE-LIVING AND PARASITIC NEMATODE LARVAE

Reagents Needed: Hydrochloric Acid, Water. When using the Baermann apparatus to collect nematode larvae from contaminated samples, especially dog feces, one often encounters free-living nematodes as well as parasitic ones. The parasitic forms may be separated from free-living nematodes by the use of a solution of 1.0 ml concentrated hydrochloric acid added to 30 ml of water. After collecting larvae from the Baermann apparatus, simply place them in this solution. All stages of free-living nematodes will be killed almost instantly, but parasitic forms will survive for a period ranging from minutes to 24 hours.

DIAGNOSIS OF BOVINE GENITAL TRICHOMONIASIS

Reagents Needed: Physiological Saline and Perhaps Beef Extract-Glucose-Peptone Serum Medium. In heavy infections, particularly in females, the trichomonads may be seen by immediate direct examination of mucus or exudate from the vagina or uterus. Examine with ordinary light microscope at a magnification sufficient to distinguish organisms 10 to 20 microns long and 3 to 15 microns wide. These organisms also may be found in amnionic or allantoic fluids, fetal membranes, and stomach contents of the fetus. In bulls, they may be found in washings from the preputial cavity but are rarely in seminal fluid. If the organisms cannot be found by direct microscopic examination, the animal must not be declared negative until culturing has been attempted.

Examination of the Bull. Thoroughly clean the external genitalia and clip the hair from around the prepuce. Introduce saline into the preputial cavity using a long, plastic insemination tube and a rubber bulb. Wash the prepuce thoroughly and remove the fluid from it with the same instrument. Transfer the fluid to a suitable container and either allow it to settle for one to three hours or centrifuge prior to examination of the sediment.

Examination of the Cow. Obtain samples from the vagina by washing it with physiological saline and recovering fluid, using a bulb douche syringe. Allow the fluid to settle or centrifuge it before examining the sediment.

Organisms are more abundant in the vagina two to three weeks after infection than at any other time. In the bull, however, the numbers fluctuate and the interval between population peaks is five to 10 days. Since the recovery of organisms is somewhat problematic, it is perhaps wise to subject samples to a cultivation technique when direct microscopic examination proves negative.

There are a number of media that can be used. The following is the formula for beef extract-glucose-peptone serum (BGPS) medium:[60]

1. Mix the following in a 3-liter flask:

Difco beef extract	3	gm
Glucose	10	gm
Bacto peptone	10	gm
Sodium chloride	1	gm
Agar	0.7	gm
Distilled water	1000	ml

2. Dissolve compounds by subjecting mixture to boiling. After cooling to room temperature, adjust the pH to 7.4 with 1.0 N NaOH.
3. Cover the mouth of the flask with heavy paper and autoclave for 30 minutes at 15 pounds pressure.
4. After cooling, add 20 ml inactivated beef serum aseptically and mix thoroughly. Inactivation of the serum is completed by heating it to 56° C for 30 minutes.
5. Dispense 10-ml amounts in 15-ml cultures tubes. Check for sterility by incubating at 37° C for two days.
6. Just before inoculation add 500 to 1000 units of penicillin and 0.5 to 1.0 mg of streptomycin to each milliliter of medium and mix thoroughly.
7. Pipette the inoculum on top of the medium in such a way as to minimize mixing. Incubate at

39° C for three to five days. The trichomonads migrate toward the bottom of the tube, whereas yeasts and molds tend to remain at the top. To examine, remove a sample from the bottom of the tube with a pipette. Cultured organisms often exhibit considerable pleomorphism and are usually more varied in size and shape than are those recovered directly from cattle.

EXAMINATION OF URINE FOR NEMATODE EGGS

Collect a sample of urine free of contaminants, agitate, and transfer some or all to a centrifuge tube. Centrifuge at 1500 rpm for two minutes, pour off the supernatant fluid, and mount the sediment on glass microscope slides. Apply a coverslip and examine.

Eggs that may be recovered include *Stephanurus dentatus* from swine, *Dioctophyma renale* from dogs, and *Capillaria plica* from carnivores.

EXAMINATION OF BLOOD FOR PARASITES

Methods for preparing smears of blood have been described elsewhere in this book. The majority of protozoan parasites and rickettsia-like organisms that are found in the bloodstream can be identified by examining properly prepared blood films with an oil immersion objective. A preparation that is suitable for differential leukocyte counts is usually adequate for identification of blood parasites.

Anaplasma. In properly stained blood smears, *Anaplasma marginale* bodies appear as spherical granules 0.2 to 0.5 microns in diameter (Plate 20–1). The number of bodies in a single cell may vary from one to seven, depending upon the severity and state of the disease. The *Anaplasma* organisms are, in some forms, confused with artifacts or with Howell-Jolly bodies. In general, both Howell-Jolly bodies and *Anaplasma* organisms remain in focus as long as the erythrocyte edge is in focus, whereas artifacts usually appear light in the center when slightly out of focus. The differentiation between Howell-Jolly bodies and *Anaplasma* organisms is somewhat more difficult to make, but the two usually can be differentiated by position in the erythrocyte. *Anaplasma* organisms are usually located near the periphery of the cell and have a slight halo surrounding them. Howell-Jolly bodies may be located anywhere within the erythrocyte and usually are not surrounded by a halo. (*A. centrale*, which is usually found centrally located in the host cell, does not occur in the United States and is probably restricted to Africa.) Another criterion that may be utilized is the size var-

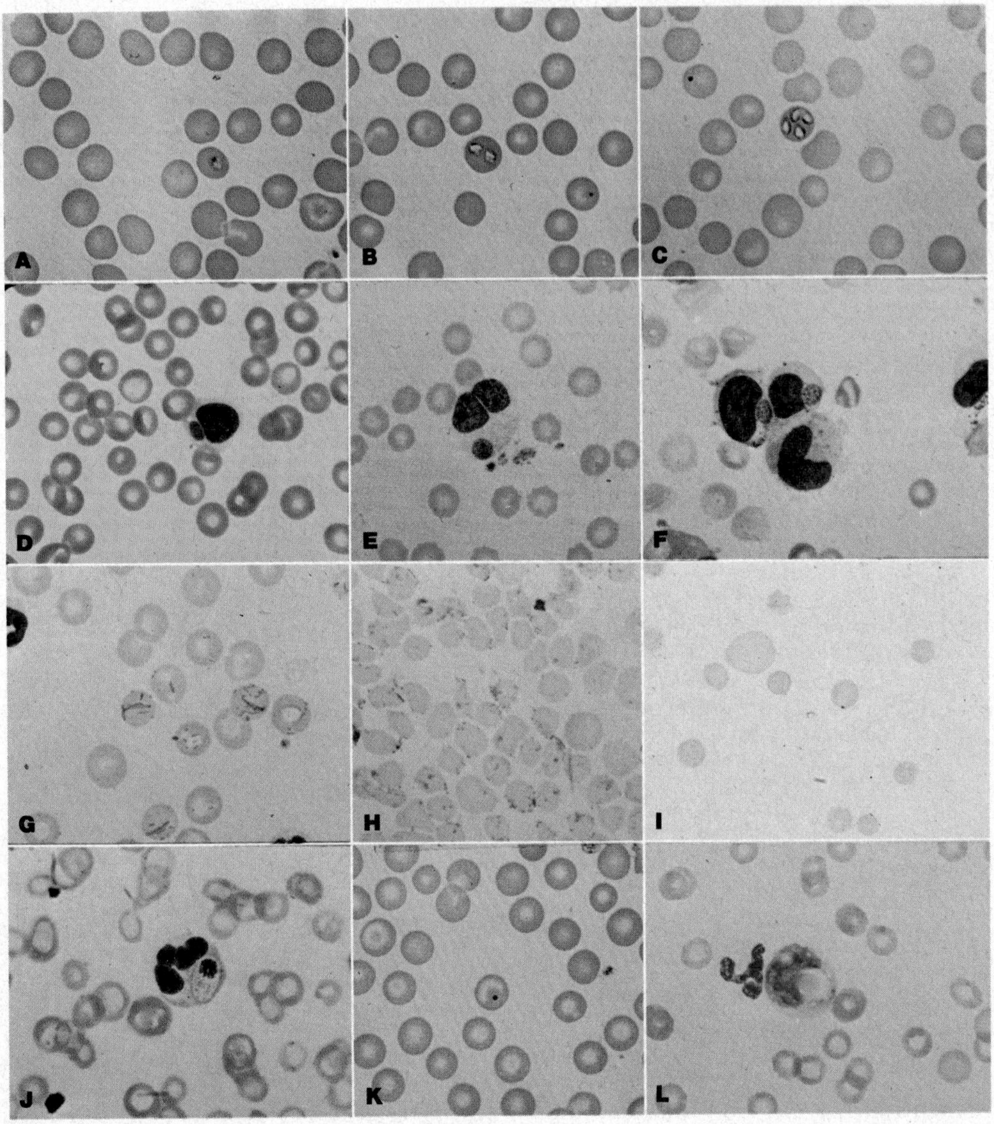

Plate 20–1. Hematozoon parasites, Howell-Jolly body, and erythrophagocytosis. *A, Babesia canis*, one trophozoite (Wright's stain). *B, Babesia canis*, two trophozoites (Wright's stain). *C, Babesia canis*, four trophozoites (Wright's stain). *D, Ehrlichia canis* in cytoplasm of a lymphocyte (Wright's stain). *E, Ehrlichia canis* in cytoplasm of a monocyte (Wright's stain). *F, Ehrlichia canis* in each of two lymphocytes (Wright's stain). This is an impression smear from the lung of an infected dog. *Ehrlichia canis* morulae are readily demonstrated in such impression smears. *G, Haemobartonella canis*. Coccoid, chain, and "violin bow" forms are present (Wright's stain). *H, Eperythrozoon suis* from an experimentally infected animal I, *Anaplasma marginale* (Wright's stain). Note the anisocytosis and polychromasia. *J. Hepatozoon canis* gametocyte (Romanowsky stain). *K*. Howell-Jolly body in a canine erythrocyte (Wright's stain). *L*, Erythrophagocytosis (Wright's stain).

iation that occurs routinely among Howell-Jolly bodies. The *Anaplasma marginale* inclusions are usually quite uniform in size.

In attempts to diagnose anaplasmosis, a thin film of blood on a clean slide is required in order to have an area with a single layer of erythrocytes to examine. If possible, freshly prepared blood smears should be utilized rather than smears prepared from a sample of blood containing an anticoagulant. *Anaplasma* inclusions do not stain well and they are not as readily observed in smears prepared from a blood sample containing an anticoagulant.

One of the few standardized immunodiagnostic tests available for parasitic infections is the complement fixation (CF) test for anaplasmosis. Production of CF antigen and certification of laboratories for performing the test are controlled by the United States Department of Agriculture through its National Veterinary Services Laboratory in Ames, Iowa.

Babesia. In the United States, babesiosis (piroplasmosis) is a problem mainly in dogs. Bovine babesiosis apparently was eradicated from the United States when its arthropod host, *Boophilus annulatus*, was successfully controlled. The periodic recurrence of the arthropod in the Southwest has fortunately not been accompanied by the recurrence of the protozoan parasite. Spread of equine babesiosis apparently has been limited since its introduction into the United States in 1961, a testimonial to the value of an effective disease-control program of national scope.

Babesia bigemina appear in cattle as pyriform to ovoid bodies in erythrocytes. They occur singly, in pairs, or as multiples, and they range from 2.5 to 5.5 μm by 2 μm.

Babesia caballi and *B. equi* are found in the horse. These organisms differ in size. *Babesia caballi* ranges from 2.5 to 4 μm and *B. equi* is less than 2 μm in length. *Babesia equi* often forms tetrads and the so-called "Maltese cross configuration" is characteristic.

The organisms are rather difficult to demonstrate in the peripheral blood from a horse. They are usually present in only 1 to 8 per cent of the erythrocytes. Watkins[98] described a concentration and staining technique for diagnosis of equine piroplasmosis. A blood sample to which ethylenediaminetetraacetic acid (EDTA) has been added is centrifuged at 1,500 to 2,000 rpm. A thin smear is made from the red blood cells (RBC's) just beneath the buffy coat and is fixed in methyl alcohol. This thin blood film is stained with Giemsa stain and examined for the presence of the organisms. If no organisms are demonstrated on this type of preparation, a fixed smear is made. These fixed smears of blood are then warmed at 45 to 50° C for 20 minutes and placed directly into buffered distilled warm water with the stain. Since fixation in methyl alcohol is eliminated in this procedure, the erythrocytes will be laked, and the

parasites may be seen free of cells. Watkins also described a plasma concentration technique in which blood treated with EDTA is allowed to stand for 30 to 60 minutes. The plasma is removed in its entirety, placed in a centrifuge tube, and centrifuged at 2,500 to 3,000 rpm for five to 10 minutes. The plasma is removed; and the small button of cells remaining in the bottom of the tube is mixed and placed on a glass slide so that there are thick and thin areas. This smear is stained by the Giemsa method, and the cells are examined for the presence of parasites. Comparative studies indicated that the organism could be detected by this technique, whereas in using the thin smear technique on blood from the same animal, parasitized cells were not demonstrated. This technique may be superior to the thick smear technique.

Babesia canis is seen in the dog. The *B. canis* trophozoites are larger than those of other species, ranging up to 6 or 7 μm (Plate 20–1). Erythrocytes usually contain one, two, or exponential multiples of two parasites. Sixteen appears to be the maximum number accommodated by a host cell, and one rarely sees more than four in a given erythrocyte. *B. gibsoni*, also parasitic in dogs, is a smaller parasite (1.1–2 × 1.2–4 μm) that has been imported to North America, probably from Okinawa. The diseases produced by the two parasites are similar, usually characterized by regenerative anemia.

Ehrlichia. *Ehrlichia canis* is found in the dog. Ewing[27] described an inclusion body of undetermined origin that appeared in leukocytes of dogs infected with *Babesia canis*. Subsequently, this inclusion was identified as the morula stage of an *Ehrlichia* organism, probably *E. canis*.[28]

Ewing and Buckner[31] described the manifestations of babesiosis, ehrlichiosis, and combined infections in the dog. Animals experimentally infected with *E. canis* developed a parasitemia approximately two weeks after exposure. The numbers of *Ehrlichia*-infected leukocytes varied considerably; in some animals, they disappeared entirely, whereas in others, they increased and at the time of death were plentiful.

Anemia developed soon after inoculation and increased in intensity until the dogs died. The anemia was of the normocytic normochromic type. There was no marked increase in reticulocytes, suggesting that erythropoiesis was impeded. In two infected dogs, no reticulocytes were present in the peripheral blood within a five-day period, during which time the number of total erythrocytes, packed cell volume (PCV), and hemoglobin values reflected a severe anemia. Leukopenia and thrombocytopenia are often severe in naturally occurring cases of ehrlichiosis.

The mulberry or morula form of *E. canis* is readily visible in the cytoplasm of infected leukocytes (Plate 20–1) stained by Wright's method. Ewing and Buckner[30] found that morulae were not present as frequently in monocytes and neutrophils as they were in lymphocytes. Subsequently, Ewing and co-workers[32] reported a milder form of canine ehrlichiosis in which neutrophils were the major host cells that contained morulae.

In recent years, serological techniques have been developed for diagnosing ehrlichiosis. Carter and associates[10] described a direct immunofluorescence test, and Ristic and colleagues[76] have developed serological techniques to check for both humoral and cellular immune responses. Antigens are not available commercially, however, and the indirect fluorescent antibody test (IFAT) must be made in research laboratories or in selected animal disease diagnostic laboratories.

Clinical signs of ehrlichiosis include fever and depression; bilateral, mucopurulent ocular discharge accompanied by photophobia; nasal discharge that is first serous and later purulent; and splenomegaly. A few dogs developed a transient pustular dermatitis on the abdomen during the early part of the febrile period. Canine ehrlichiosis is often masked by or confused with other diseases; differentiation from Rocky Mountain spotted fever is probably best done serologically.

Ehrlichia equi, horse: A syndrome characterized by edema of the legs and leukopenia has been recognized in California horses. Inclusions in neutrophils are morphologically very similar to those of *E. canis*.

A condition known commonly as Potomac horse fever (PHF) and as acute equine diarrhea syndrome (AEDS) has been shown to be caused by an *Ehrlichia*-like organism. The organism has considerable serological affinity for *E. sennetsu*, a pathogen of human beings, and it can be cultured in canine monocytes. The disease has been designated equine monocytic ehrlichiosis to distinguish it from the usually milder condition caused by *E. equi*.

Eperythrozoon. Members of the genus *Eperythrozoon* may produce clinical disease in swine, cattle, sheep, and certain laboratory animals. Morphologically, organisms of this genus are similar in all host species affected. Under light microscopy, the most common form observed is a ring-like structure located on the erythrocyte; it may also be seen in the intercellular spaces (Plate 20–1H). Other forms that may be observed include larger rings, discoid forms that appear as flat chromatin masses, cocci, rods, and budding forms.

Eperythrozoon suis causes infection in swine.[88-90] In experimental infections produced in splenectomized animals, the blood picture is typical. When parasites become numerous in the peripheral blood, clinical signs may be evident. The total erythrocyte count begins to decline at this time, and nucleated erythrocytes appear. The total red blood cell count may reach a low of one to two million cells, which is accompanied by a continual fall in packed cell volume. As the anemia becomes more acute, the number of parasites demonstrable in a smear may decrease.

Splitter and Williamson[90] developed a method by which the degree of infection may be designated. Their rating is based on the number of parasites demonstrated in a peripheral blood smear. The classification is as follows: (1) rare—one parasite in five or more microscope fields; (2) scarce—one parasite in one to five microscope fields; (3) occasional—approximately 10 to 20 per cent of the erythrocytes with at least one parasite; (4) frequent—approximately 50 per cent of the erythrocytes parasitized; (5) numerous—approximately 80 to 90 per cent of the erythrocytes affected; (6) very numerous—all erythrocytes affected and some completely covered with parasites; and (7) extremely numerous—all erythrocytes infected and many completely covered with parasites, and parasites may be observed in intercellular spaces.

Eperythrozoon wenyoni produces eperythrozoonosis in cattle. The acute disease probably has not been observed in normal susceptible cattle, because only a very mild anemia and accompanying fever usually occur. It may, however, become a problem in splenectomized animals. Although this surgical procedure is not done often in the practice of veterinary medicine, it may be used in research animals.

Eperythrozoon ovis causes eperythrozoonosis in sheep. This condition may be very widely distributed and possibly responsible for some undiagnosed disease conditions. However, at the present time, it is not recognized as a disease of great importance. Routine splenectomy of apparently normal sheep may result in the appearance of a disease condition closely resembling eperythrozoonosis in cattle. Blood findings in sheep closely resemble those in other animals with eperythrozoonosis and include a decrease in the total erythrocyte count, a lowered PCV, decreased hemoglobin values, and the appearance of morphological alterations in erythrocytes typically associated with anemia.

Haemobartonella. Haemobartonellosis occurs in the dog and cat as a distinct clinical entity. The typical haemobartonella organism is present on the erythrocyte (Plate 20–1G) and may take one of several forms including chains of cocci, rods, bows, and rings, or it may appear as a single coccus. Several structures may be seen on a single erythrocyte at the height of infection, and at other times there may be only one organism on a cell. The rod-shaped forms, if present, are usually located around the periphery of the erythrocyte. In infection in the cat, organisms are seldom seen free in the intercellular spaces, whereas in severe infections in dogs they may be observed in the intercellular areas.

Haemobartonella felis, cat: Feline infectious anemia, produced by *H. felis*,[91] varies from mild to severe, depending upon the number of infective organisms present and the resistance or susceptibility of the host. In a typical infection, hemoglobin levels usually fall to less than 7 gm/dl, and packed cell volumes are usually less than 18 per cent. The erythrocytes are usually macrocytic and normochromic. The mean corpuscular volume is increased, and the mean corpuscular hemoglobin concentration remains within the normal range. The majority of these macrocytes are young forms of erythrocytes and in many instances may be reticulocytes. Howell-Jolly bodies, polychromatophilia, nucleated erythrocytes, and anisocytosis are almost always present. Although Howell-Jolly bodies are commonly observed in the red blood cells of normal cats, they have a tendency to increase in association with this infection. Care must be taken to differentiate these inclusion bodies from the parasite.

Since there is a marked fluctuation in the number of parasites appearing in peripheral blood during acute stages of the condition, repeated examinations are often necessary to demonstrate the organism.[38] Several periods of borderline anemia may occur before acute anemia appears. This probably represents a series of attacks by the parasite, during which the number of organisms increases. These increases are often followed by a decrease to a point at which no parasites can be demonstrated. If a practitioner suspects the existence of this parasitic disease, periodic examinations of the blood for the presence of H. felis should be made.

Haemobartonella canis, dog: Anemia may be produced in the dog by H. canis.[7,100] Clinical anemia produced by this organism probably does not occur frequently in intact animals, although such cases have been suspected and intact animals can be infected experimentally. If anemia occurs in association with this organism, it is usually mild and often will go unobserved. Many animals may be carriers of H. canis and following splenectomy may become ill with the acute infection. In splenectomized animals, the anemia develops quite rapidly in the acute form of the disease.

Benjamin and Lumb[1] described a chronic form of haemobartonellosis in which organisms were found periodically in the blood. A marked anemia developed with the total erythrocyte count dropping as low as 900,000, the PCV as low as 9 per cent, and the hemoglobin as low as 2 gm. Typical morphological alterations in the blood occurred and included the appearance of nucleated erythrocytes, anisocytosis, and polychromatophilia. As the animal began to recover from this anemia, macrocytosis was evident. During the period when parasites were demonstrated, the total leukocyte count varied from normal to a slight leukopenia. Leukopenia appears to be associated with depressed formation of all blood cells.

Haemoproteus. *Haemoproteus* sp., birds: A number of species of this genus attack turkeys, pigeons, ducks, and other fowl. Gametocytes are found in erythrocytes along with black pigment and are halter-shaped when mature (Fig. 20–3). The parasite completes the schizogonous phase of its life cycle in endothelial cells. Blood-sucking arthropods transmit the organisms among birds, and sexual reproduction is completed in the invertebrate host, mostly hippoboscids and biting midges.

Hepatozoon. *Hepatozoon canis*, dog: H. canis can be identified in peripheral blood smears, the gametocyte stage occurring in neutrophils and monocytes. This parasite was previously thought to occur only in the Old World but has been reported to occur in dogs in Texas. Parasitemias ranged from 1 per cent to 60 per cent of the circulating neutrophils. The schizogonous phase of the H. canis life cycle occurs in the liver, spleen, and bone marrow, but confirmatory diagnosis is usually based upon demonstration of gametocytes in circulating leukocytes (Plate 20–1). Dogs become infected by ingesting *Rhipicephalus sanguineus*, the brown dog tick, containing sporulated oocysts of H. canis; ticks acquire their infection by ingesting gametocytes in circulating neutrophils.

Histoplasma. *Histoplasma capsulatum*, dogs: Histoplasma organisms produce a systemic mycosis in dogs and therefore have no rightful place in a discussion of hematozoan parasites; but because such organisms in leukocytes of the peripheral blood may be confused with protozoans, they are included. Organisms may be seen in the cytoplasm, in the nucleus, or in both; the staining properties of this organism with Romanowsky stains is not predictable (Fig. 20–3).

Leucocytozoon. *Leucocytozoon* sp., birds: Leucocytozoonosis is usually caused by *Leucocytozoon smithi* in turkeys, L. simondi in ducks and geese, and L. andrewsi in chickens. There are other species in this genus, some of which are associated with domestic fowl, but they will not be discussed. Gametocytes are found in erythrocytes in the peripheral blood (Fig. 20–3). The host cell is so badly distorted that there has been confusion concerning whether the parasites infect leukocytes or erythrocytes. The host cell becomes spindle shaped, as its nucleus is crowded to one side and becomes greatly elongated. Parasites are often more than 20 μm long.

Plasmodium. *Plasmodium* sp., birds: Plasmodium relictum and other species in this genus have been reported in a wide variety of birds. Parasites are seen in circulating erythrocytes (Fig. 20–3) and may be in any one of the following stages of development: merozoite, trophozoite, schizont, and gametocyte. Black pigment is often observed in association with parasites, especially in the gametocytes and schizonts.

Plasmodium sp., primates: There are many species of the genus *Plasmodium* that attack primates that are used as experimental animals. *Plasmodium cynomolgi* and P. knowlesi are perhaps the

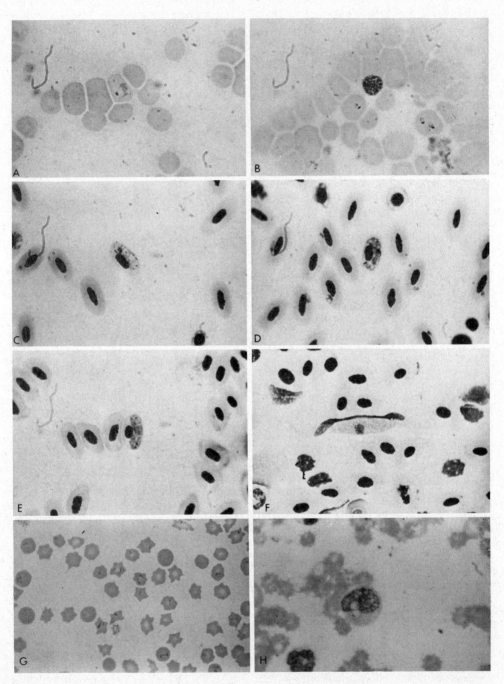

Figure 20–3. Avian and mammalian hematozoon parasites and *Histoplasma capsulatum*. A, *Plasmodium cynomolgi*, trophozoite from primates. B, *Plasmodium cynomolgi*, trophozoites and schizont from primates. C, *Plasmodium relictum*, gametocyte from bird. D, *Plasmodium relictum*, trophozoite and schizont from bird. E, *Haemoproteus* sp., gametocyte from bird. F, *Leucocytozoon* sp., gametocyte from duck. G, *Theileria* sp., trophozoite from deer. (Courtesy of Doctors R. G. Buckner and B. L. Glenn, College of Veterinary Medicine, Oklahoma State University, Stillwater.) H, *Histoplasma capsulatum*, from dog. Occasionally observed in peripheral leukocytes, this organism may be found in either the nucleus or cytoplasm of the host cell.

most commonly observed of these. These malarial parasites are morphologically quite similar to the plasmodia that parasitize human beings. Diagnosis can be made from properly stained peripheral blood films. Several stages occur in erythrocytes, and hemozoin is usually present (Fig. 20–3).

Toxoplasma. *Toxoplasma gondii*, many hosts: Trophozoites of this parasite are found in a wide variety of tissues in many hosts. They are crescent- or banana-shaped and may appear intercellularly in peripheral blood smears. (See also Figs. 20–79 and 20–80 for fecal oocysts.)

Theileria. *Theileria* sp., ruminants: Cattle, sheep, goats, and deer in the United States of America have been reported to harbor *Theileria mutans* (*Gonderia mutans*). The parasite does not produce disease problems of the same magnitude as those caused by *T. parva*, which infects African cattle and is the etiological agent of East Coast fever. In fact, many workers consider *T. mutans* to be nonpathogenic. *Theileria*-infected deer that have been splenectomized, however, may suffer disease. The organisms are small—0.5 to 2.0 µm—and are found in circulating erythrocytes (Fig. 20–3). The nucleus is usually deeply stained and is red; the cytoplasm is usually light blue on Romanowsky-stained preparations.

Cytauxzoon. *Cytauxzoon felis*, cats: A uniformly and rapidly fatal disease of domestic cats that was first recognized in Missouri in 1976 has since been reported from several parts of the United States; it is thought to be transmitted from bobcats (*Lynx rufus*) to domestic cats by ixodid ticks. Antemortem diagnosis can be confirmed by demonstration of piroplasms in erythrocytes of blood films stained with Romanowsky-type stains. Erythroparasitemia does not always occur, however, and when it does develop, the parasitemia commonly involves less than 5 per cent of the erythrocytes; there are reports of parasitemia reaching 25 to 28 per cent in terminally ill cats but such a high parasitemia would ordinarily occur only in splenectomized animals. The organisms are round to slightly oval, 1 to 5 µm in diameter, and contain a small, peripherally located, dark purple nucleus when stained with Wright's, Giemsa's, or similar preparations.

Unfortunately, diagnosis must often be made at necropsy. The characteristic histological lesion is occurrence of large (up to 75 µm) histiocytic macrophages containing intracytoplasmic schizonts in various organs. Typically the large macrophages are found in association with the endothelial lining of venous channels and sinusoids in lung, spleen, lymph nodes, and bone marrow. In terminally ill cats one may find these large parasitized cells in the peripheral blood. They are usually in the feather edge of a blood smear and their cytoplasm is packed with schizogenous stages.

Several other members of the genus *Cytauxzoon* are parasites of African ungulates.

Trypanosoma. *Trypanosoma theileri*, cattle: Fortunately, cattle in the United States are not afflicted with severely pathogenic trypanosomes. *Trypanosoma theileri* (*T. americanum* is probably a synonym) is only occasionally observed in peripheral blood of cattle but can be isolated rather commonly by culture methods. Some workers allege that the parasite is harmless under normal conditions but is capable of producing disease in cattle stressed in any of a variety of ways. The parasite is seen intercellularly and is quite large, 60 to 70 µm long.[56]

Trypanosoma melophagium, sheep: This is a nonpathogenic organism sometimes seen in peripheral blood. It is transmitted by the sheep ked, *Melophagus ovinus*.

Trypanosoma cruzi, dogs: Canine trypanosomiasis has been considered an exotic disease in dogs in the United States, though it was commonly observed in South American dogs. A report by Tippit[96] describes 15 indigenous cases observed in dogs from Texas, beginning in 1972. The parasite, which also causes severe cardiomyopathy in human beings, is transmitted by insects of the family Reduviidae. Diagnosis can be made by conventional blood smears. Culture techniques are also available, and serodiagnostic tests of several kinds, including complement fixation, have been used successfully.

EXAMINATION OF BLOOD FOR MICROFILARIAE

MODIFIED KNOTT'S TECHNIQUE

The reagents needed for this technique are:

1. Heparin (or other anticoagulant)
2. Formalin (2 per cent)
3. Methylene blue (1:1000 solution)

The equipment needed is a graduated ocular disc (calibrated ocular micrometer).

This method is the most useful, and perhaps the most reliable, technique available for recovering and identifying *Dirofilaria immitis* microfilariae and detecting microfilariae of other nematodes, such as *Dipetalonema* sp. and *Setaria* sp., in the peripheral blood.

Collect a sample of venous blood, do not allow it to clot, and use it promptly. Place 1 ml of whole blood in 10 ml of 2 per cent formalin, mix gently by inverting the closed tube twice, and centrifuge five to eight minutes at 1,500 rpm. Discard the supernatant fluid by careful inversion of the tube and stain sediment with an equal amount of 1:1,000 methylene blue. Pipette mixture onto two glass microscope slides, apply 22 × 40 mm coverslips, and examine at 100×. Blue-stained, elongated microfilariae are readily visible, and length and width must be determined for positive identification. Microfilariae found in canine blood may be those of *Dirofilaria immitis* or those of *Dipetalonema* species (most considered to be *D. reconditum*). The latter nematode apparently is harmless, which emphasizes the need for a definitive diagnosis. Measurements for identification are given in the table at the end of this chapter (see Table 20–9). Measurements made from samples that are not fresh are unreliable for diagnosis, since morphology may not remain constant when samples are allowed to stand.

OTHER TECHNIQUES

A number of other techniques have been utilized in attempts to differentiate microfilariae quickly. Differentiation usually has been based upon motility, the number of microfilariae present, and the shape of the tail and other morphological landmarks. These techniques have been used with varying degrees of success and are presented here without judgment as to their reliability. As stated previously, the author considers the modification of Knott's technique presented earlier to be the most reliable method available.

Filter Technique. Commercially available kits have made the filter technique more generally accessible and have helped to standardize this method. Manufacturers' products and instructions vary slightly. One must be certain to adhere carefully to the directions provided with whatever product is selected.

Microcapillary Tube Test (Capillary Hematocrit Tube Test). Differentiation of microfilariae utilizing this test alone is based upon comparison of motility of the microfilariae. Blood that has been collected with an anticoagulant is placed in capillary tubes and spun in a microhematocrit centrifuge. The microfilariae will be found in the serum portion of the separated sample, and differentiation is based upon the number of organisms present and their motility. Many workers apparently utilize the microcapillary tube test for screening purposes only. When microfilariae are found, the Knott's or other technique is employed to determine which species is present.

Cephalic Hook Detection. Blood is collected, preferably from a marginal ear vein, and thick smears are prepared. After air drying, slides are placed in tap water for two minutes (or less) to remove hemoglobin. Slides are transferred, while still wet, to a solution of 1:50 dilution of 1 per cent brilliant cresyl blue (the stock solution and the diluted stain are prepared in 0.8 per cent sodium chloride). After staining, the slides are rinsed twice in saline, and a coverslip edged with petrolatum is applied while the slide is still wet. The preparation is examined at $430 \times$ and under oil immersion. *Dipetalonema* microfilariae possess an anterior (cephalic) hook, whereas *Dirofilaria* microfilariae do not. *Dirofilaria* microfilar-

iae do, however, possess a fine spine at the anterior end that should not be confused with the cephalic hook.

Histochemical Differentiation. A method to detect acid phosphatase activity in microfilariae was described by Chalifoux and Hunt,[12] but it is considered too involved for use in most practice settings. (See Appendix for technique.) A naphthol AS-TR-phosphate method is used to detect acid phosphatase activity; enzyme activity is restricted to two distinct, well-circumscribed zones in *Dirofilaria immitis* but is rather uniformly distributed throughout the body of *Dipetalonema reconditum*.

Serological Diagnosis. A number of serological techniques designed to detect immunoglobulins produced in response to filarial antigens have been developed. Impetus for perfecting these immunological techniques comes in large part from a need to confirm diagnoses of so-called occult infections, i.e., those in which infected dogs are amicrofilaremic. Some of these serological tests are utilized routinely in diagnostic laboratories and certain of them have been adapted as kits that are available from commercial firms. If one chooses to use these techniques it is essential that manufacturers' instructions be followed explicitly. It remains to be determined how well standardized these tests are and to what extent interpretation of results can be relied upon.

Because the quantity of specific antibody does not discriminate between resolved and active infections, attempts have been made to develop tests to detect filarial antigen in peripheral blood. Such a test would be especially valuable for identification of infected but amicrofilaremic animals. Assays have been developed and one has been adapted as a commercially available kit. Like the kits designed to detect filarial antibody, there has not been adequate time to assess the reliability of the test in private clinical settings.

EXAMINATION OF SOLUTIONS FOR PARASITIC ARTHROPODS

Many arthropods function indirectly in disease, in that they transmit but do not produce disease conditions; some inflict injury by bites, stings, or other activities, and still other species are parasites. Some are both parasites and mechanical and/or biological vectors of disease. The following discussion concerns primarily those that are parasites.

MITES

Definitive diagnosis of mite-induced conditions may be made by finding parasites or their eggs. Several common mites are described in Table 20–1 and Figures 20–4 to 20–15.

TABLE 20–1. Mites

Scientific Name	Common Name and Host	Identification
Demodex spp. (D. bovis, D. canis, D. caprae, D. cati, D. equi, D. ovis, D. phylloides)	Red mange mite. Ox, dog, goat, cat, horse, sheep, and pig, respectively	Elongate, no body hairs, abdomen transversely striated; legs anterior to midbody and very short (Fig. 20–4).
Sarcoptes scabiei (varieties: bovis, canis, caprae, equi, ovis, suis, and vulpis)	Sarcoptic mange mite. Ox, dog, goat, horse, sheep, pig, and fox, respectively	Anus terminal. Legs short, not extending past body margin; legs 1 and 2 with sucker on long, unjointed stalk, female; and on legs 1, 2, and 4, male (Fig. 20–5).
Notoedres cati	Notoedric mange mite. Cat, fox, rabbit	Anus dorsal; leg morphology same as Sarcoptes (Figs. 20–6 and 20–7).
Psoroptes ovis	Scabies, or scab mite. Sheep, ox, horse	Anus terminal. Legs extend beyond body margin; legs 1, 2, and 4 with sucker on long, jointed stalk, female; and on legs 1, 2, and 3, male (Figs. 20–8 and 20–9).
P. cuniculi	Sheep, goat, horse, rabbit	
Chorioptes spp. (C. bovis, C. cuniculi, C. caprae, C. equi, C. ovis)	Foot, leg, and tail mange mite. Ox, rabbit, goat, horse, and sheep, respectively	Anus terminal. Legs extend beyond body margin: legs 1, 2, and 4 with sucker on short, unjointed stalk, female; and on legs 1, 2, 3, and 4, male, but leg 4 very small (Figs. 20–10 and 20–11).
Otodectes cyanotis	Ear mange mite. Dog, cat, fox	Anus terminal. Legs extend beyond body margin (except 4th of female): legs 1 and 2 with sucker on short unjointed stalk, female; and on legs 1, 2, 3, and 4, male (Figs. 20–12 and 20–13).
Raillietia auris	Ear mange mite. Ox	Adults 1.5 mm long.
Pneumonyssoides caninum	Nasal or sinus mite. Dog	Mite white, legs long with paired terminal claws; adults 2 mm (Fig. 20–14).
Psorergates ovis	Itch or Australian itch mite. Sheep	Legs spaced equidistantly; 0.189 mm by 0.162 mm.
Cheyletiella parasitivorax	Rabbit fur mite. Dog, cat, rabbit	Body oval, less than 1 mm; large, clawlike, serrated pedipalpi (Fig. 20–15).
Trombicula spp.	Chiggers or redbugs. Horse, ox, dog, humans, fowl, and others	Red to orange, 6 legs; only larval stage parasitic.

Because of the location of these organisms, intimately associated with or in the skin, scrapings of the infected area must be made. In general, it is best to scrape at the edge of the lesion rather than the center because organisms are more commonly found around the periphery. To make an adequate examination, the skin must be scraped deeply, even to draw blood. If tissue is dry or scaly, use a small amount of oil or glycerine on the scraping instrument.

Mix the scrapings with mineral oil on a microscope slide, apply coverslip, and examine. If material is too dense for ready examination, add one or two drops of a 10 per cent solution of potassium hydroxide, allow to stand a few minutes, then examine. This procedure will clear debris and mites; then parasites may be seen more easily. At times it may be necessary to digest epithelial debris and concentrate parasites by levitation. Please refer to the following paragraph for a description of the technique.

Digestion-Concentration Technique. The reagents needed for this technique are 5 per cent potassium hydroxide and saturated sucrose solution.

This technique is most useful in recovering mites and lice that cause epidermal hyperplasia and for concentrating parasites from animals with exfoliative lesions.

1. Mix scrapings with 5 per cent potassium hydroxide (digesting solution); use about 10 volumes of solution to 1 volume of detritus.
2. Heat gently in a beaker or flask covered by a funnel; the condensate should return to the digesting solution.
3. When hair has dissolved, remove mixture from heat and allow to cool.
4. Centrifuge and discard supernatant fluid.
5. Resuspend sediment in water and centrifuge again.
6. Discard supernatant fluid and examine sediment. If no parasites are found, concentrate (step 7).
7. Resuspend sediment in saturated sucrose solution (concentrating solution) and centrifuge.
8. Remove parasites from top of solution with a wire loop or other implement.

Text continued on page 392

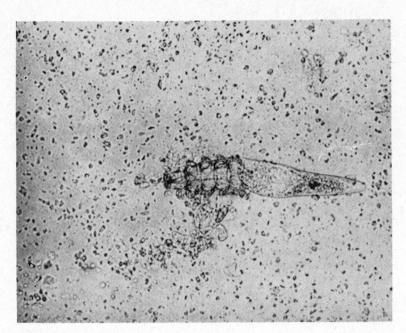

Figure 20-4. Demodex sp. Notice elongated body, absence of body hairs, and short legs. High power.

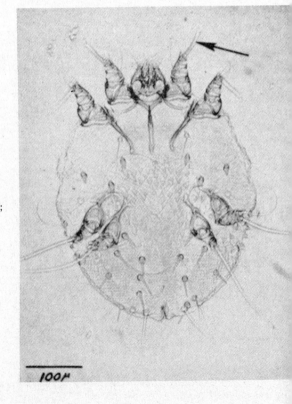

Figure 20-5. Female Sarcoptes sp. containing egg; the stalk (arrow) is long.

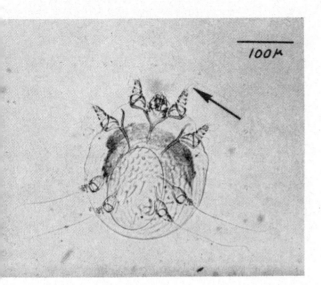

Figure 20–6. Female *Notoedres* sp. containing egg; the stalk (arrow) is medium long.

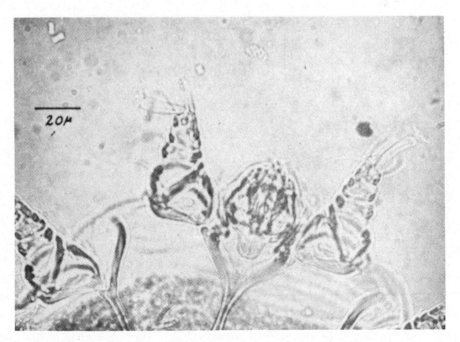

Figure 20–7. *Notoedres* sp. showing detail of suckers on unjointed stalk.

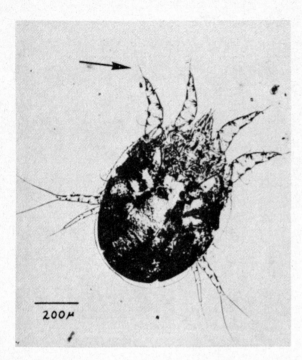

Figure 20–8. Female *Psoroptes* sp. showing suckers on long, jointed stalks (arrow).

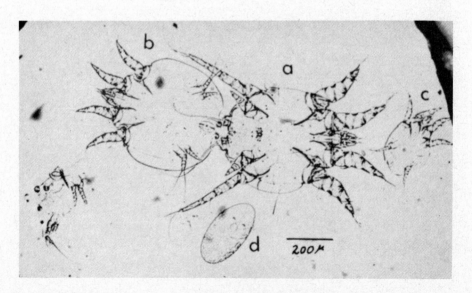

Figure 20–9. *Psoroptes* sp., male (a) with nymph (b) attached, larva (c), and egg (d).

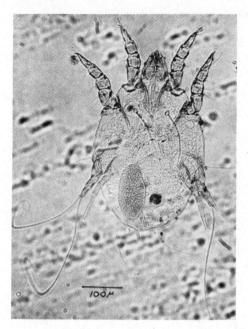

Figure 20–10. Female *Chorioptes* sp. containing egg.

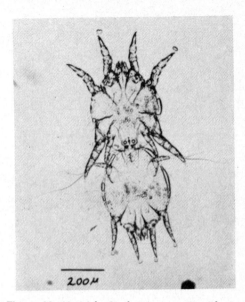

Figure 20–12. Male *Otodectes cyanotis* with nymph attached.

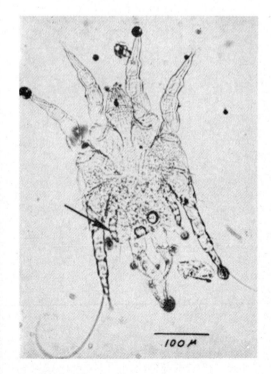

Figure 20–11. Male *Chorioptes* sp. Notice very small fourth legs (arrow).

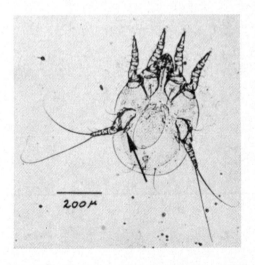

Figure 20–13. Female *Otodectes cyanotis* containing egg; notice very small fourth (arrow).

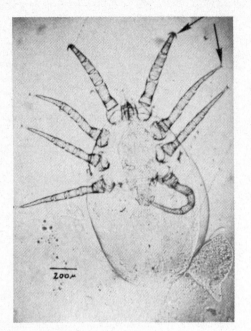

Figure 20–14. *Pneumonyssoides caninum;* notice paired, terminal claws (arrows).

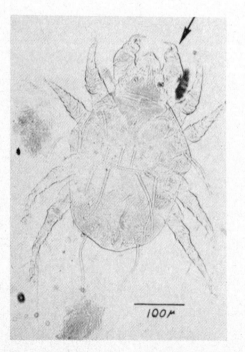

Figure 20–15. *Cheyletiella parasitivorax;* notice large pedipalpi (arrow) with claw-like tips.

Ticks

Ticks may be located and removed from hosts by hand. Adult stages of most hard ticks (Ixodidae) are located easily, nymphs are less obvious, and larvae are exceedingly difficult to see. Descriptions of several common hard ticks may be found in Table 20–2 and Figures 20–16 to 20–18. A larval tick is shown in Figure 20–19.

Certain ticks have preferential locations on hosts, and attention should be given to these areas. Ticks affecting dogs are found frequently between the toes, in the ears, and on the neck. Some soft ticks (Argasidae) are intermittent feeders and *Otobius* sp., which affect cattle and other animals, are found in the ears as immature forms that vary greatly in size and color; the adults are not parasitic (Table 20–3). It may be necessary to inspect the premises, and this is certainly a recommended procedure when dealing with *Rhipicephalus sanguineus, Otobius megnini,* and *Argas persicus.*

Fleas

Descriptions of several common fleas are found in Table 20–4 and Figures 20–20 to 20–23.

Adult fleas may be removed from animals in the same manner as described for lice. Dusting a host with rotenone or other insecticide may be helpful. The fleas are stupefied or killed. Fleas will fall off if the hair is raised by rubbing. In general, they are large enough to be seen with the unaided eye. It may be desirable, however, to look for flea larvae and pupae. The sweepings from floors of dwellings occupied by suspected hosts may be sieved, using medium mesh, and the sieved material examined at low power. The larvae, which hatch from eggs, are rather small, legless, caterpillar-like organisms (Fig. 20–24). They are whitish to slightly brown and have a few long hairs on all the segments of the body. They move by twisting motion and appear to dislike light. Occasionally, they may be found in the hair of extremely dirty dogs and cats, but usually they are in the sleeping quarters or in the grass surrounding areas where the animals are found. The brownish pupae are inclosed in semi-transparent cocoons and show some characteristic markings of adults. The larvae form cocoons by sticking together bits of sand or organic material with a loose network of silken threads. In the immediate vicinity of infested animals, one may find eggs, larvae, cocoons, or adults.

Hypersensitivity to the bites of fleas is a common problem in dogs and cats. A radioimmunoassay has been developed to detect allergen-specific antibodies (IgE and IgG) in serum, but it is not yet in general use. Dogs and cats parasitized by helminths often have high levels of IgE and that fact may complicate serological assessment of flea-induced hypersensitivity.

TABLE 20-2. Hard Ticks

Scientific Name	Common Name	Host and Distribution in U.S.A.	Identification
Amblyomma americanum	Lone star tick	East of central Texas to Atlantic coast, north to Iowa. Dogs, birds, and humans.	Female easily recognized by conspicuous silvery white spot at tip of scutum.
Amblyomma cajennense	Cayenne tick	Southern Texas, south to Argentina. Livestock, deer, dogs, and humans.	Scutum ornate with pale markings in extensive pattern; coxa I of female with internal spur about one-half length of external spur.
Amblyomma maculatum	Gulf Coast tick	South Carolina westward to Texas. Livestock, deer, birds, dogs, and humans.	Spurs on 2nd, 3rd, and 4th pairs of legs; pale markings more diffuse than on female of lone star tick.
Boophilus annulatus	Cattle tick fever	South of 37° North latitude. Largely eradicated in U.S. Livestock and deer. Recently reappeared in southwest.	One-host species; larva, nymph, and adult on cattle or deer. Recognized by short palpi, each with dorsal and lateral ridge on each segment, hexagonal basis capituli, and margin of abdomen without festoons.
Boophilus microplus	Southern cattle tick	Rarely Florida and Texas. Cattle and deer.	
Dermacentor albipictus	Winter tick	It is widely distributed throughout North America. Large domestic animals, wild animals, and humans.	One-host tick; oval spiracular plates with very large goblets.
Dermacentor occidentalis	Pacific Coast tick	Pacific Coast region, U.S. Wild mammals and livestock.	Basis capituli with conspicuous tooth-like projections (cornua) on posterior margin.
Dermacentor variabilis	American dog tick	East of line drawn from 105th meridian south to western Texas, and in California. Dogs, small mammals, large mammals, and humans.	Mouth parts and basis capituli subequal length. Scutum with pale white or yellowish markings; basis capituli parallel-sided.
Dermacentor andersoni	Rocky Mountain tick, wood tick	Western states, to northern Arizona and New Mexico. Livestock, wild mammals, and humans.	Similar to American dog tick but adults, in general, have paler coloring and larger goblets on the spiracular plates.
Haemaphysalis leporispalustris	Rabbit tick	Widely distributed in U.S.A. Rabbits, small mammals, and birds.	Small, inornate, no eyes, but with festoons. Second article of palpus produced laterally (Fig. 20-16).
Ixodes scapularis	Black-legged tick	Texas and Oklahoma eastward. Mammals, birds, and humans.	Anal groove extends from side to side of body and in front (diagnostic) of anus. Most species in genus have enlarged clublike palpi (Fig. 20-17).
Rhipicephalus sanguineus	Brown dog tick	Throughout most of U.S.A. Dogs, and occasionally other mammals.	Reddish brown, hexagonal basis capituli, with festoons. Male with both (diagnostic) adanal plates and accessory plates (Fig. 20-28).

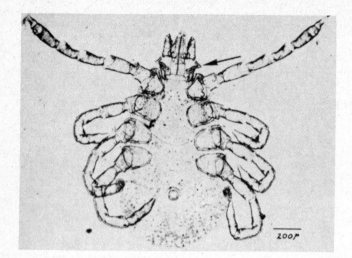

Figure 20–16. *Haemaphysalis* sp.: notice second article of palpus produced laterally (arrow).

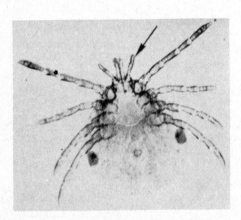

Figure 20–17. *Ixodes scapularis* nymph; notice long palpi (arrow). Approximately × 7.

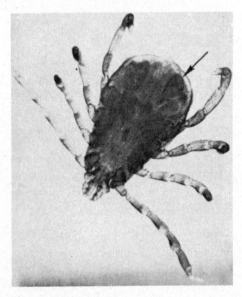

Figure 20–18. Male *Rhipicephalus sanguineus*; notice adanal plate (arrow).

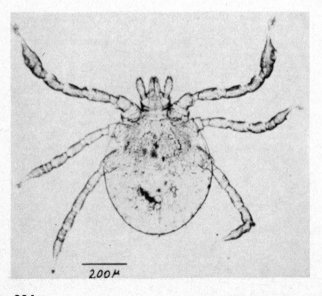

Figure 20–19. Larval tick with six legs (nymphs and adults have eight).

TABLE 20–3. Soft Ticks

Scientific Name	Common Name	Host and Distribution in U.S.A.	Identification
Argas persicus	Fowl tick ("Blue bug")	Found mainly in the southern tier of states. Fowl.	Body flattened, with sharp sutural line dividing decidedly dorsal and ventral surfaces of body.
Ornithodoros hermsi	Herm's relapsing fever tick	Idaho, Oregon, Washington, California, Nevada, and Colorado. Chipmunks and humans.	Ticks of genus *Ornithodoros* have a globular body without the specific sutural line of Argas. Body surface roughened by tiny protuberances called mammillae. Toothed hypostome.
Ornithodoros parkeri	Parker's relapsing fever tick	Found in western states. Humans and rodents.	
Ornithodoros turicata	Relapsing fever tick	Found in southern tier of states, also Kansas and Oklahoma. Man, rodents, and pigs.	
Otobius megnini	Spinose ear tick	Mostly southwestern and western U.S.A. Livestock, large wild mammals, and humans.	Larva and nymph spinose, parasitic in ears; adult freeliving, not spinose, hypostome without teeth.

TABLE 20–4. Fleas

Scientific Name	Common Name and Host	Identification
Ctenocephalides felis	Cat flea; principally cats, dogs, and other carnivores.	Species of *Ctenocephalides* have both genal and prontoal ctenidia. Head height about one-half length, forms an acute anterodorsal angle. Spines I and II in genal comb same length.
Ctenocephalides canis	Dog flea; principally dogs, cats, and other carnivores.	Head height and length subequal, front margin has less acute angle than that of cat flea. Spine I of genal comb much shorter than Spine II (Figs. 20–20 and 20–21).
Pulex irritans	Human flea; humans, pigs, and dogs (also on other—coyote, prairie dog, etc.)	Ctenidia or combs absent, ocular bristle insertion beneath eye, no vertical, rod-like thickenings of mesopleuron.
Pulex simulans	Similar to above.	Similar to above (Fig. 20–22).
Xenopsylla cheopis	Oriental rat flea; rats major host; other mammals may serve. Chief vector of bubonic plague and murine typhus.	No ctenidia or combs; ocular bristle insertion in front of eye; mesopleuron divided by vertical rod-like thickening. Females easily recognized by pigmented (unique for U.S.A. siphonapterans) spermatheca.
Echidnophaga gallinacea	Stick-tight flea; usually domestic fowl, cats, dogs, rabbits; also on rats, ground squirrels, horses, and humans.	No ctenidia or combs. Front margin of head angular, thorax contracted (Fig. 20–23).
Tunga penetrans	Chigoe; humans; dogs, and perhaps a few other animals.	The male small, female large and globose; remains attached in one location for long period.

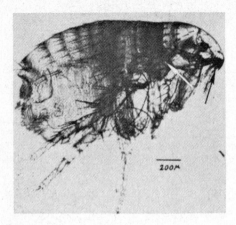

Figure 20–20. Female *Ctenocephalides* sp.; notice ctenidia (arrow).

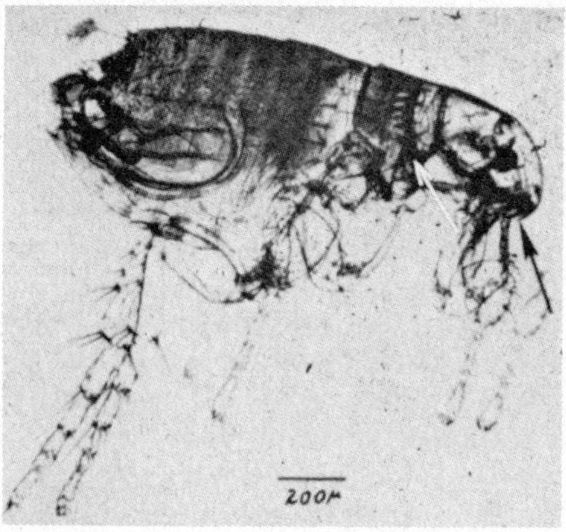

Figure 20–21. Male *Ctenocephalides*; notice ctenidia (arrow).

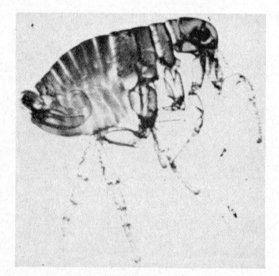

Figure 20–22. Male *Pulex simulans.*

LARVAL FLIES

The critical aspects of myiasis, as to lesions and symptoms, will vary with the body part affected, with the species of fly involved, and with the number of maggots present. Sometimes it is possible to make a specific diagnosis on the basis of the location of the parasites in some hosts. However, symptoms of intestinal myiasis are not specific, and even cutaneous myiasis may present problems insofar as specific diagnosis is concerned. Cutaneous myiasis usually causes a painful ulcer or sore of long standing. Nasal myiasis may cause obstruction of the nasal passages, severe irritation, and in some cases facial edema. Aural myiasis, particularly when the middle ear is involved, may lead to brain damage. Ophthalmomyiasis will lead not only to severe irritation and pain but sometimes to blindness.

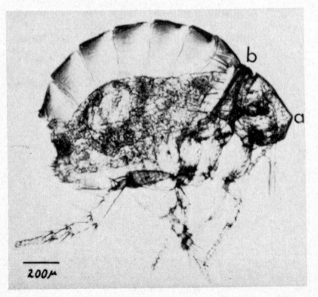

Figure 20–23. *Echidonophaga gallinacea;* notice angular head (a) and reduced (telescoped) thorax (b).

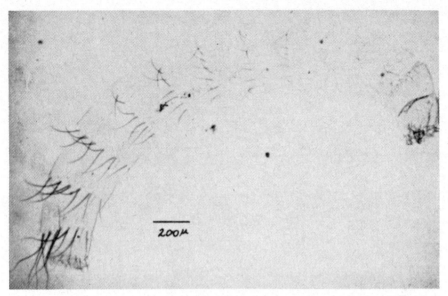

Figure 20–24. Larval flea.

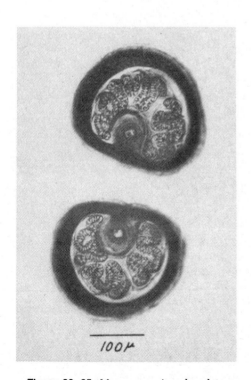

Figure 20–25. *Musca* sp. spiracular plates.

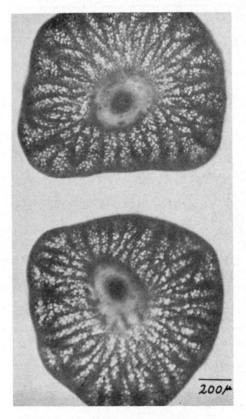

Figure 20–26. *Oestrus ovis* spiracular plates.

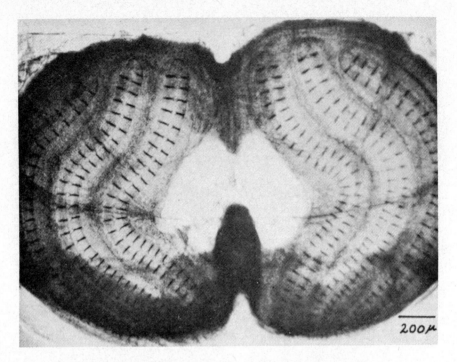

Figure 20–27. *Gastrophilus* sp. spiracular plates.

A definitive diagnosis of myiasis can be made only upon finding and identifying the larvae responsible. Maggots may be removed from the lesion to a container of moist sand in an attempt to secure adult flies. The maggots may burrow into the sand and pupate, and the adult flies that emerge may then be used for identification. Precise specific identification is much easier if one has the adult fly, though specialists can make a diagnosis on the basis of larvae alone.

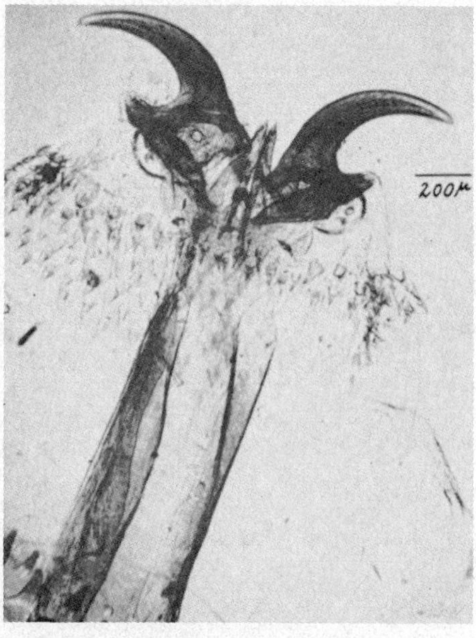

If the diagnosis cannot be made upon knowledge of host specificity and anatomical location, dark chitinous plates (stigmal plates) situated on the posterior end of larvae may be useful to most veterinary practitioners. These plates contain the respiratory apertures (spiracles) arranged in a pattern characteristic of different flies or groups of flies (Figs. 20–25 to 20–27). In addition, the number and arrangement of spines on the larvae may be useful.

Grasp the larva with forceps and make a smooth cut across the posterior end with a sharp scalpel, removing the posterior end with the stigmal plates. Mount the specimen with cut surface in contact with the slide, add water or a clearing medium if desired, apply coverslip and examine at 100×.

Figure 20–28 shows the mouth hooks of a *Gastrophilus* organism.

LICE

Most species of lice and their eggs are large enough to be seen without the aid of magnification, although a reading glass may be helpful. Animals that are heavily parasitized generally exhibit rather characteristic rough hair coats. If the hair is rubbed in the direction opposite that in which it normally rests, biting lice will be seen to

Figure 20–28. *Gastrophilus* sp. mouth hooks.

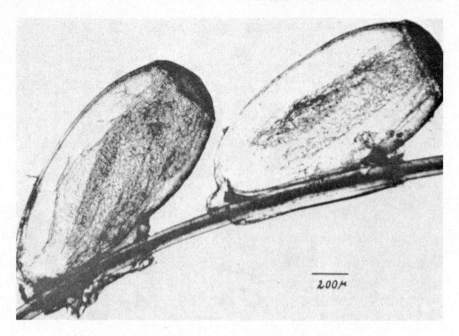

Figure 20–29. Louse eggs (nits) attached to hair.

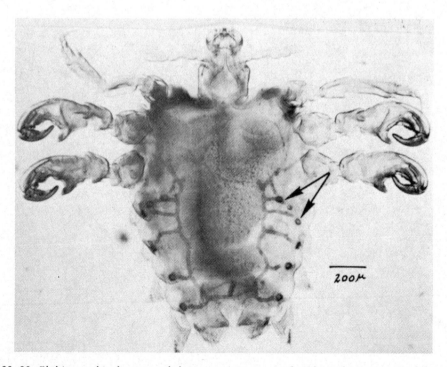

Figure 20–30. *Phthirus pubis*, human crab louse, sometimes mistaken for a domestic animal parasite. Notice arrangement of first three of six spiracles (arrows).

move about rapidly; sucking lice are more slug-gish. They may be recovered by catching individ-uals with forceps, by hand, or by combing. The eggs are attached to the hair and may be observed either grossly or microscopically (Fig. 20–29). Lice can be examined microscopically at several magnifications if mounted in water, oil, glycerine, or a clearing agent such as that indicated for mites. Hair may be clipped with a scissors and placed in a container, and the organisms may be re-moved. Alternatively, the clipped hair may be placed on white paper under an incandescent light. The heat of the light bulb will stimulate the organisms to crawl off. In addition to adult lice and eggs, one may find nymphs, which, in gen-eral, look like the adult except that they are smaller and paler. They do not possess mature sex organs. The human crab louse (Fig. 20–30) is sometimes mistaken for a domestic animal par-asite.

IDENTIFICATION OF LICE OF SPECIFIC SPECIES

LICE OF HORSES

There is contradictory information in the lit-erature concerning the lice *Trichodectes equi* (*Damalinia equi*) and *T. pilosus* (*D. pilosus*); *T. equi* is probably the more widely distributed. Both are less than 2 mm in length; *T. pilosus* is smaller. *Trichodectes pilosus* antennae are in-serted well forward on the head, about at level of

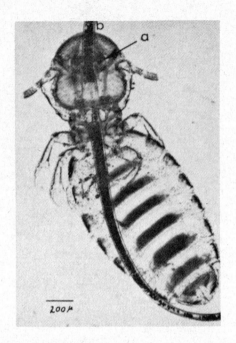

Figure 20–32. *Trichodectes equi;* notice mandibles (*a*) locked around horse hair (*b*).

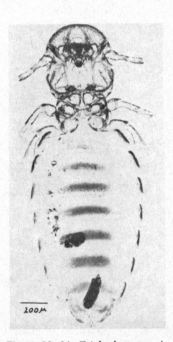

Figure 20–31. *Trichodectes equi.*

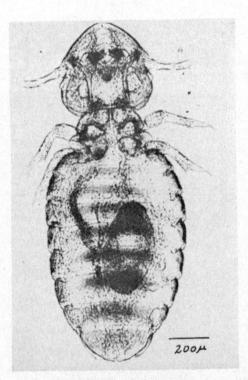

Figure 20–33. *Bovicola bovis.*

anterior border; antennae of *T. equi* are inserted about midway between anterior and posterior borders (Figs. 20–31 and 20–32).

LICE OF CATTLE

Chewing. *Bovicola bovis* (*Damalinia bovis*). *B. bovis* is the red louse of cattle. This organism has an anteriorly rounded head provided with mandible-like mouth parts (Fig. 20–33).

Sucking. *Haematopinus eurysternus*. *H. eurysternus*, the short-nosed ox louse, is longer than 2 mm. This louse has a broad thorax and abdomen, and a relatively short head with anterolateral blunt prolongations behind the antennae; eyes are absent (Fig. 20–34).

Haematopinus quadripertusus. *H. quadripertusus*, the tail louse or tail switch louse, is larger than, but similar to, *H. eurysternus*; it has five or six to eight or more setae at the margins of each abdominal segment.

Linognathus vituli. *L. vituli* is the long-nosed louse of cattle. Head and body are elongate, about 2 mm long; eyes are absent. The abdomen is membranous with numerous setae on the segments. The first pair of legs is smaller than other pairs (Fig. 20–35).

Solenopotes capillatus. *S. capillatus* is the tubercle-bearing louse of cattle (small blue louse or capillate louse). Females are about 1.5 mm long; males are smaller. The best differential characteristic is six pairs of abdominal spiracles, which open through short tubular openings; there is one row of bristles on each abdominal segment (Fig. 20–36).

LICE OF SHEEP AND GOATS

There is considerable confusion regarding species of lice on sheep and goats, and it would be impossible for the layman to differentiate them, except to distinguish chewing and sucking ones.

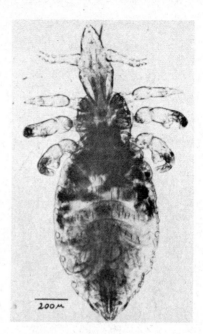

Figure 20–35. *Linognathus vituli.*

Chewing. *Bovicola ovis* (*Damalinia ovis*). *B. ovis* is the chewing or biting louse of sheep.

Bovicola caprae (*Damalinia caprae*). *B. caprae* is the chewing or biting louse of goats; it is also called the red louse (Fig. 20–37).

Sucking. *Linognathus africanus*. *L. africanus* is the African blue louse of sheep.

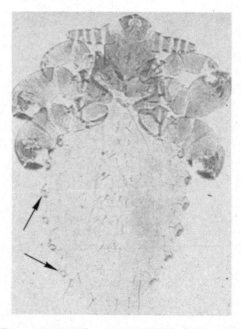

Figure 20–36. *Solenopotes capillatus;* notice large tubercles (arrows). About × 20.

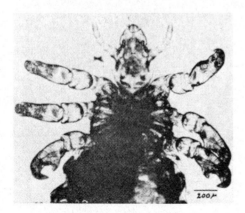

Figure 20–34. *Haematopinus eurysternus.*

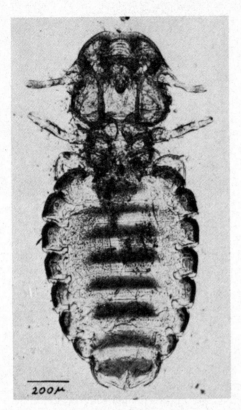

Figure 20–37. *Bovicola caprae.*

Linognathus pedalis. L. pedalis is the foot louse of sheep. Its head is as wide as it is long and not longer than the thorax; it is found on the legs and feet of sheep where there is no wool.

Linognathus stenopsis. L. stenopsis is the blue louse of goats.

Linognathus ovillus. L. ovillus is the body louse or blue louse of sheep. It occurs in New Zealand, Australia, and Scotland. Its head is much longer than it is wide and is also longer than the thorax.

LICE OF SWINE

Haematopinus suis. H. suis is the common hog louse. It is the only louse of swine. The head has small anterolateral prolongations behind the antennae; eyes are absent (Fig. 20–38).

LICE OF DOGS AND CATS

Chewing. *Trichodectes canis.* T. canis is the small biting louse of dogs. It is about 1.5 mm long and has a stubby, broad body. Its head is broad, with anterior and lateral margins well-rounded (Fig. 20–39).

Heterodoxus spiniger. H. spiniger, the biting louse of dogs, is more than 2 mm long. Its head, anterior to lateral antennal depressions, forms a roughly equilateral triangle, i.e., the head is pointed or "arrowhead shaped."

Felicola subrostrata. F. subrostrata is the biting louse of cats. Ranging from 0.98 to 1.29 mm long,

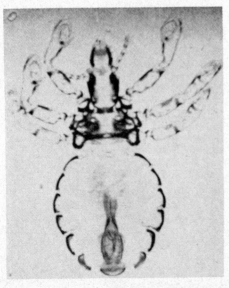

Figure 20–38. *Haematopinus suis.* About × 7.

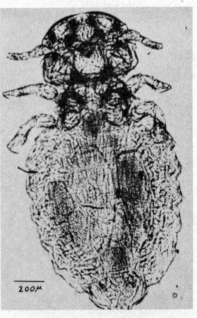

Figure 20–39. *Trichodectes canis.*

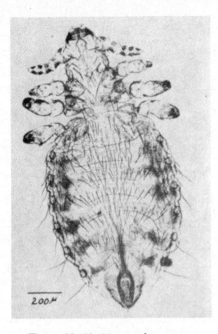

Figure 20-40. *Linognathus setosus.*

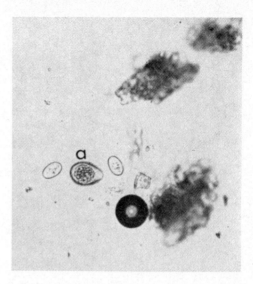

Figure 20-42. Two species of bovine coccidian oocysts; *Eimeria bukidnonensis* (a) is large and dark.

it has no pleural plates; antennae are alike in both sexes.

Sucking. *Linognathus setosus* (*Linognathus piliferus*). *L. setosus* is the suctorial louse of the dog. Eyes are absent, the abdomen is membranous with numerous setae on segments. The first pair of legs is the smallest (Fig. 20-40).

LICE OF RABBITS

Haemodipsus ventricosus. *H. ventricosus* is a sucking louse.

LICE OF GUINEA PIGS

Gyropus ovalis, Gliricola porcelli, and *Trimenopon hispidum.* These are all biting lice; they are exceedingly small and easily overlooked (Fig. 20-41).

SUMMARY OF HOST/PARASITE RELATIONSHIPS

Parasites commonly found in the various species of domestic animals are listed. See Table 20-5 (Figs. 20-42 to 20-53) for cattle; Table 20-6 (Figs. 20-54 to 20-68) for sheep and goats; Table 20-7 (Figs. 20-69 to 20-73) for horses; Table 20-8 (Figs. 20-74 to 20-77) for swine; and Table 20-9 (Figs. 20-78 to 20-95) for dogs and cats.

A tapeworm egg contaminating the feces of dogs and cats is shown in Figure 20-96, and a common contaminant found in the feces of many animals is demonstrated in Figure 20-97.

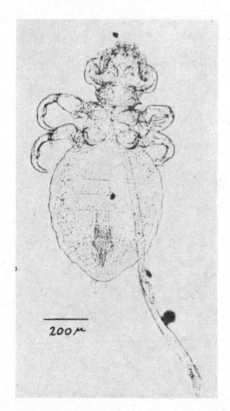

Figure 20-41. Guinea pig louse, Family Gyropidae.

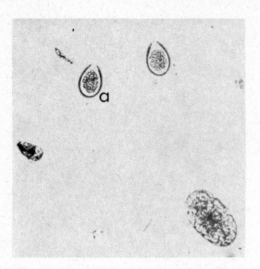

Figure 20–43. *Eimeria bukidnonensis* oocyst (a) compared with a trichostrongylid-type of nematode egg.

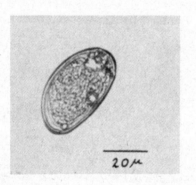

Figure 20–44. *Dicrocoelium dendriticum* egg.

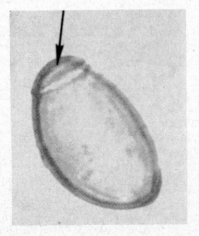

Figure 20–45. *Dicrocoelium dendriticum* egg shell; notice operculum (arrow). High power.

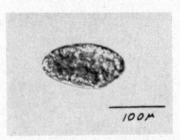

Figure 20–46. *Fasciola hepatica* egg, the contents of which are slightly distorted by fixation.

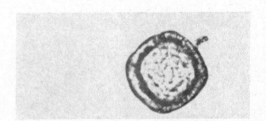

Figure 20–47. *Moniezia* sp. egg, three pairs of hooks obscured.

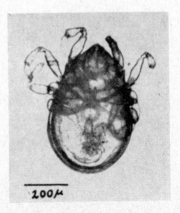

Figure 20–48. Oribatid mite, intermediate host for *Moniezia* sp., has chewing mouthparts.

TABLE 20–5. Cattle Parasites

Scientific Name	Common Name	Identification
Protozoans		
Eimeria spp. (*E. alabamensis, E. auburnensis, E. bovis, E. brasiliensis, E. bukidnonensis, E. canadensis, E. cylindrica, E. ellipsoidalis, E. subspherica, E. zurnii*)	Coccidia	Oocysts in feces. Mixed infections more common than "pure infection"; oocysts distinguishable, description given for two most pathogenic species: *E. zurnii*, colorless to pale grayish-lavender, spherical to bluntly ellipsoidal, no micropyle, 15–20 by 13–18 μm (mean 17.8 by 15.6 μm). *E. bovis* usually transparent, greenish-brown or yellowish-brown, shape not constant but strictly ovoid and blunted at narrow end; micropyle a lightened area at small end, 23–34 by 17–23 μm (mean 27.7 by 20.3 μm) (Figs. 20–42 and 20–43).
Cryptosporidium sp. (This parasite is known to occur in many species; young calves most often clinically affected; zoonotic potential significant especially for immunocompromised persons.)	Minute coccidia	Oocysts very small (4–6 μm), without sporocysts, with 8 naked sporozoites. (Thick-walled oocysts pass in feces; thin-walled ones rupture within intestine, leading to autogenous reinfection.)
Sarcocystis spp. (*S. cruzi*, acquired from dogs and other carnivores; *S. hirsuta*, acquired from cats; *S. hominis*, acquired from primates.)	Sarcocyst	Muscle
Toxoplasma gondii	Toxoplasma	Various tissues.
Buxtonella sulcata	Ciliate	Trophozoites in feces, 46–100 by 60–138 μm (mean, 72 by 100 μm); contain oval or bean-shaped macronucleus.
Trematodes		
Paramphistomum spp. Includes at least three species		Eggs have no color in shell and are somewhat attenuated at opercular end; underdeveloped when deposited; 132–160 by 68–99 μm.
P. microbothrioides (common)	Rumen fluke or cone fluke	
P. cervi (rare)		
P. liorchus (in certain Gulf Coast states)		
Dicrocoelium dendriticum	Lancet fluke	Eggs brown, 36–45 by 20–30 μm; contain a miracidium when deposited; have a conspicuous shoulder where operculum fits into shell (Figs. 20–44 and 20–45).
Fasciola gigantica	Giant liver fluke	
Fasciola hepatica	Common liver fluke	Eggs yellow to brown, operculate, undeveloped, usually in range of 130–150 by 63–90 μm. (First eggs from some flukes contain no color.) (Fig. 20–46).
Fascioloides magna	Large American fluke or large liver fluke	Eggs indistinguishable from those of *Fasciola hepatica.*
Cestodes		
Moniezia benedeni	Common tapeworm	Eggs usually square to cuboidal in shape, contain well-developed pyriform apparatus; measure 56–67 μm in diameter (Fig. 20–47).
Moniezia expansa	Common tapeworm	Eggs similar to those of *Moniezia benedeni*, but are usually triangular to subtriangular in shape (Fig. 20–47). Figure 20–48 shows an oribatid mite, which is an intermediate host for *Moniezia* spp.
Cysticercus tenuicollis (*Taenia hydatigena*)	Thin-necked bladder worm	Usually attached to liver, mesentery, omentum, body wall, and other abdominal organs.
Echinococcus granulosus	Hydatid cyst	Large cyst usually with multiple scoleces; in liver, lungs, and elsewhere.
Cysticercus bovis (*Taenia saginata*)	Beef measles	Heart and voluntary muscles; 7.5–10 by 4–6 mm. long.

Table continued on following page

TABLE 20–5. (*continued*)

Scientific Name	Common Name	Identification
	Nematodes	
Gonglyonema spp.	Gullet worms	Eggs thick-shelled, contain larva when deposited; measure 50–70 by 25–37 μm.
Haemonchus spp.	Large stomach worms or barber pole worms	Eggs are typical strongyle type, nearly transparent, thin-shelled, elliptical; usually deposited in 16- or 32-cell stage of development. Eggs average 78.5 by 45 μm, range 65–82 by 39–46 μm. It would be difficult to differentiate, even statistically, *Haemonchus* eggs from other stomach worm eggs with which they are often associated (Fig. 20–49).
Ostertagia spp. (*Ostertagia bisonis, O. lyrata, O. ostertagi, O. orloffi*)	Medium stomach worm, brown stomach worm, or brown hair worm	*O. ostertagi* eggs 70–84 by 40–50 μm. Statistically, there is little overlapping of size with *H. contortus*, but shapes are different as indicated by measurements; *H. contortus* 68–84 by 41–51 μm; *Ostertagia* spp. 83–103 by 46–52 μm.
Trichostrongylus axei	Stomach hair worm	Eggs 79–96 by 31–48 μm. Measurements not diagnostic, but eggs are large for size of worms; eggs similar to those of *Haemonchus, Ostertagia,* and *Cooperia* organisms.
Cooperia spp. (*Cooperia curticei, C. oncophora, C. pectinata, C. punctata, C. spatulata, C. bisonis*)	Cooperids	Eggs of *Cooperia* spp. characterized by having parallel sides. Size varies somewhat: *C. punctata* 69–83 by 29–34 μm. *C. pectinata* 67–80 by 31–38 μm; *C. curticei* 70–82 by 35–41 μm (Figs. 20–50 and 20–51).
Nematodirus helvetianus *Nematodirus spathiger*	Thread-necked strongyles	Eggs transparent, thick-shelled, oval, unusually large; leave host in 1–8 cell stage; cells refractory and dark. *Nematodirus spathiger* 181–230 by 91–107 μm. (see Fig. 20–59).
Bunostomum phlebotomum	Hookworm	Eggs strongyle-like but more truncate at ends. Cells of embryo dark and granular. 4–8 cell stage; 75–98 by 40–50 μm (Fig. 20–52).
Strongyloides papillosus	Threadworm	Eggs 52–65 by 31–36 μm; contain larva when passed in feces.
Trichostrongylus colubriformis *Trichostrongylus longispicularis*	Intestinal hair worm	Eggs typical strongyle type. *T. colubriformis* 73–101 by 34–47 μm.
Neoascaris vitulorum	Large roundworm	Eggs subglobular, 75–95 by 60–75 μm. Albuminous layer or covering thinner than that of *Ascaris lumbricoides* but rough or mamillated.
Oesophagostomum radiatum *Oesophagostomum venulosum*	Nodular worm	Eggs thin-shelled, strongyle-like, 8–16 cell stage. *O. radiatum* 70–76 by 36–40 μm (Fig. 20–53).
Trichuris discolor *Trichuris ovis*	Whipworm	Eggs brown, barrel-shaped, unsegmented; transparent plug at either pole; 70–80 by 30–42 μm including plugs.
Chabertia ovina	Large-mouthed bowel worm	Eggs strongyle-like; 80–105 by 47–59 μm.
Dictyocaulus viviparus	Cattle lungworm	Eggs hatch in air passages (sometimes digestive tract); larvae coughed up and usually swallowed, passed in feces. Diarrheic animals may pass eggs containing larva in the feces; usually larvae are passed.
Syngamus laryngeus	Throat worm	Eggs 78–110 by 43–46 μm; in 16-cell stage; unlike *S. trachea,* operculum absent.
Pelodera strongyloides	No common name	Saprophytic or facultative nematode in skin.
Stephanofilaria stilesi	No common name	In skin of abdomen. Adults and larvae may be recovered from coarsely chopped tissue using Baermann apparatus.
Setaria cervi	Abdominal worm	Microfilariae in bloodstream.
Linguatula serrata	Tongue worm larva or nymph	A sexually immature internal parasite found in lymph gland and other tissues. Bear heavy spines on segments. Nothing is shed from the host.

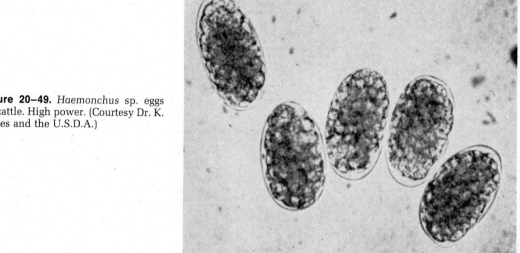

Figure 20–49. *Haemonchus* sp. eggs from cattle. High power. (Courtesy Dr. K. C. Kates and the U.S.D.A.)

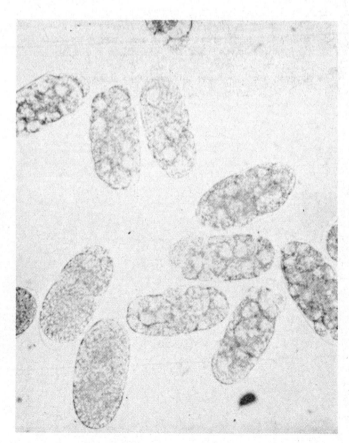

Figure 20–50. *Cooperia punctata* eggs. High power. (Courtesy Dr. K. C. Kates and the U.S.D.A.)

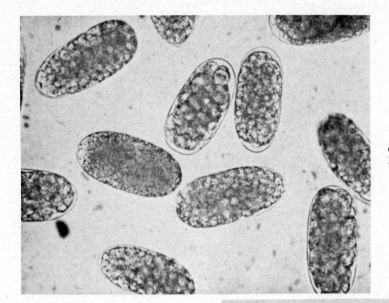

Figure 20–51. *Cooperia oncophora* eggs. High power. (Courtesy Dr. K. C. Kates and the U.S.D.A.)

Figure 20–52. *Bunostomum phlebotomum* eggs. High power. (Courtesy Dr. K. C. Kates and the U.S.D.A.)

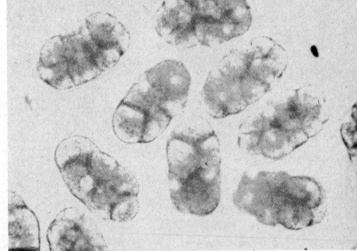

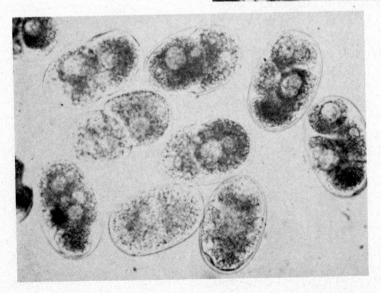

Figure 20–53. *Oesophagostomum radiatum* eggs. High power. (Courtesy Dr. K. C. Kates and the U.S.D.A.)

TABLE 20–6. Sheep and Goat Parasites

Scientific Name	Common Name	Identification
Protozoans		
Eimeria spp. (*E. ahsata, E. arloingi, E. christenseni, E. crandallis, E. faurei, E. granulosa, E. intricata, E. ninaekohlyakimovae, E. pallida, E. parva, E. punctata*)	Coccidia	Oocysts in feces. Mixed infections common, pathogenicity differs with combinations. *E. ahsata* quite pathogenic alone; oocysts pink, ellipsoidal, with micropyle and micropylar cap; 29–37 by 17–28 μm (mean 33.4 by 22.6 μm). *E. arloingi* very common; elongate, ellipsoidal, sometimes asymmetrical, with micropyle and micropylar cap; 17–42 by 13–37 μm (mean 27 by 18 μm). *E. parva* common; pale yellow to yellowish-green, subspherical, ellipsoidal or spherical, no micropyle; 12–22 by 10–18 μm (mean 16.5 by 14.1 μm).
Sarcocystis spp. (*S. ovicanis* acquired from dogs; *S. tenella* acquired from cats)	Sarcocyst	Muscle.
Toxoplasma gondii	Toxoplasma	Various tissues.
Trematodes		
Paragonimus spp.	Lung fluke	Usually a parasite of dogs, cats, and other carnivores.
Dicrocoelium dendriticum	Lancet fluke	Eggs described in Table 20–5.
Fasciola gigantica	Giant liver fluke	Eggs described in Table 20–5.
Fasciola hepatica	Common liver fluke	Eggs described in Table 20–5.
Fascioloides magna	Large American fluke	Eggs described in Table 20–5.
Cestodes		
Moniezia benedeni *Moniezia expansa*	Common tapeworm	Described in Table 20–5.
Thysanosoma actinioides	Fringed tapeworm	Terminal gravid segments on fecal pellets are 1.5–3 mm. wide; resemble miniature calcimine brushes. Eggs not in proglottids but piled up in capsules beside it. Each capsule contains 1–30 hexacanths, average 6. Capsule wall relatively thick, appears fibrous, and embryonic membranes are thin.
Cysticercus tenuicollis (*Taenia hydatigena*)	Thin-necked bladder worm	Liver, mesentery, and omentum; contains one scolex.
Echinococcus granulosus	Hydatid cyst	Usually liver and lungs but all organs liable; contains many scoleces and brood capsules, called hydatid sand. Some sterile.
Cysticercus ovis (*Taenia ovis*)	Sheep measles	Muscles.
Nematodes		
Gongylonema pulchrum *Gongylonema verrucosum*	Gullet worms	*G. pulchrum* in esophagus and *G. verrucosum* in rumen. Eggs 50–70 by 25–37 μm, thick-shelled, embryonated.
Haemonchus spp. (*H. contortus, H. placei, H. similis*)	Large stomach or barber-pole worm	Eggs strongyle-type, transparent, thin-shelled, elliptical, 16–32 cell stage. (Fig. 20–54). (See comments in Table 20–5).
Trichostrongylus axei	Stomach hair worm	See Table 20–5 (Fig. 20–55).
Marshallagia marshalli *Ostertagia circumcincta* *O. occidentalis, O. ostertagi* *O. trifurcata* *Pseudostergagia bullosa* *Teladorsagia davitani*	Medium stomach worms	*Marshallagia marshalli* eggs large, 178–217 by 75–100 μm, morula stage, i.e., usually more advanced than *Nematodirus*, which are similar. *Ostertagia circumcincta* 80–100 by 40–50 μm; *O. ostertagi* 70–84 by 40–50 μm (Figs. 20–56 and 20–57).
Nematodirus spp. (*N. abnormalis, N. filicollis, N. lanceolatus, N. rufaevastitatis, N. spathiger*)	Thread-necked strongyles	Eggs transparent, thick-shelled, oval, large in 1–8 cell stage, refractory and dark. *N. spathiger* 181–230 by 91–107 μm. *N. filicollis* 149–194 by 74–107 μm. Eggs not distinguishable by size alone. Ends in *N. spathiger* attenuated and thickened; in *N. filicollis* not attenuated and shell uniform thickness (Figs. 20–58 and 20–59).

Table continued on following page

TABLE 20–6. (*continued*)

Scientific Name	Common Name	Identification
Ascaris spp.	Large roundworm	Uncommon.
Bunostomum trigonocephalum	Hookworm	See Table 20–5 (Fig. 20–60).
Capillaria bovis	Capillarids	Bipolar opercula (Fig. 20–61).
Capillaria brevipes		
Cooperia spp. (*C. curticei, C. pectinata, C. punctata, C. oncophora, C. spatulata, C. bisonis*)	Cooperids	See Table 20–5 (Fig. 20–62).
Strongyloides papillosus	Threadworm	See Table 20–5 (Fig. 20–63).
Trichostrongylus spp. (*T. capricola, T. colubriformis, T. longispicularis, T. vitrinus*)	Intestinal hair worm	Eggs typical strongyle type. Those of *T. vitrinus* 93–118 by 41–52 μm. Measurements of others similar enough so that it is unreliable to attempt specific diagnosis (Fig. 20–64).
Oesophagostomum columbianum	Nodular worm	Refer to Table 20–5 for description (Figs. 20–65 and 20–66).
Oesophagostomum venulosum		
Skrjabinema caprae	Pinworm	Eggs with one side convex, the other almost straight; 58–63 by 30–34 μm.
Skrjabinema ovis		
Trichuris ovis	Whipworm	Brown egg with double operculum 70–80 by 30–42 μm (Fig. 20–67).
Chabertia ovina	Large-mouthed bowel worm	Eggs strongyle-like; 80–105 by 47–59 μm (Fig. 20–68).
Dictyocaulus filaria	Thread lungworm	Eggs 112–138 by 69–90 μm, usually hatch in lungs and larvae usually passed.
Muellerius capillaris	Hair lungworm	*M. capillaris* eggs 100 by 20 μm, hatch in alveoli; larvae passed are distinctive; 0.23–0.30 mm long, esophagus half length of worm, increasing progressively in size posteriorly, no conspicuous bulbs. Excretory duct immediately posterior to nerve ring. Posterior end undulatory, tapers to point, with dorsal spine near end. *Protostrongylus* has similar tail without spine. When together, distinguished on basis of size and difference in activity: both active in water, entire body of *Muellerius* and only ends of body of *Protostrongylus* involved in bending.
Protostrongylus rufescens	Red lungworm	
Syngamus laryngeus	Throat worm	See Table 20–5.
Elaeophora schneideri	Arterial worm	Adults in carotid and other arteries, but microfilariae under skin, usually head region where they cause ulcerative lesions.
Odocoileostrongylus tenuis (*Elaphostrongylus tenuis, Pneumostrongylus tenuis*)	Meningeal worm	Brain, meninges, and spinal cord.

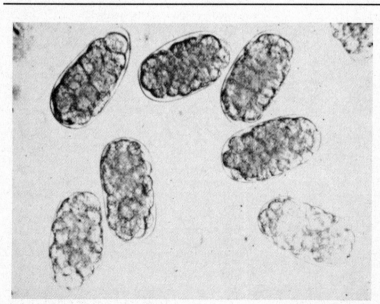

Figure 20–54. *Haemonchus contortus* eggs from sheep. High power. (Courtesy Dr. K. C. Kates, the U.S.D.A., and Am. J. Vet. Res. [Kates, K. C., and Shorb, D. A.: Am. J. Vet. Res., 4:54, 1943].)

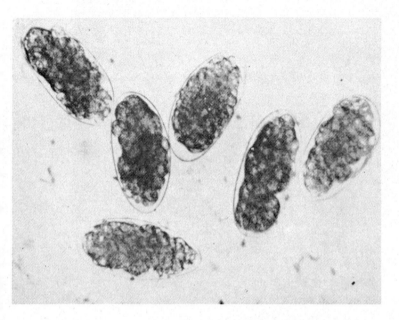

Figure 20–55. Trichostrongylus axei eggs. High power. (Courtesy Dr. K. C. Kates, the U.S.D.A., and Am. J. Vet. Res. [Kates, K. C., and Shorb, D. A.: Am. J. Vet. Res., 4:54, 1943].)

Figure 20–56. Marshallagia marshalli egg; the egg is near the morula stage. High power. (Courtesy Dr. K. C. Kates, the U.S.D.A., and Am. J. Vet Res. [Kates, K. C., and Shorb, D. A.: Am. J. Vet. Res., 4:54, 1943].)

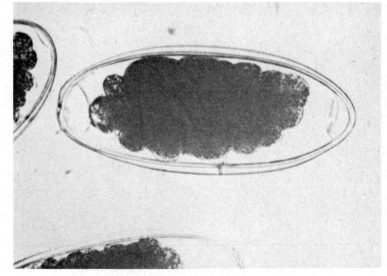

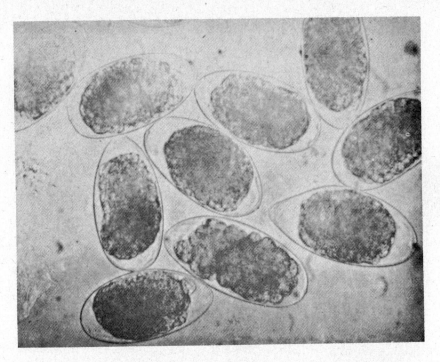

Figure 20–57. *Ostertagia circumcincta* eggs. High power. (Courtesy Dr. K. C. Kates, the U.S.D.A., and Am. J. Vet. Res. [Kates, K. C., and Shorb, D. A.: Am. J. Vet Res., 4:54, 1943].)

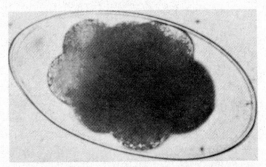

Figure 20–58. *Nematodirus filicollis* egg. High power. (Courtesy Dr. K. C. Kates, the U.S.D.A., and Am. J. Vet Res. [Kates, K. C., and Shorb, D. A.: Am. J. Vet. Res., 4:54, 1943].)

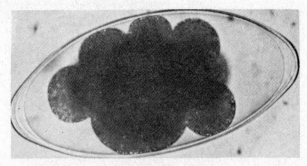

Figure 20–59. *Nematodirus spathiger* egg. High power. (Courtesy Dr. K. C. Kates, the U.S.D.A., and Am. J. Vet. Res. [Kates, K. C., and Shorb, D. A.: Am. J. Vet. Res., 4:54, 1943].)

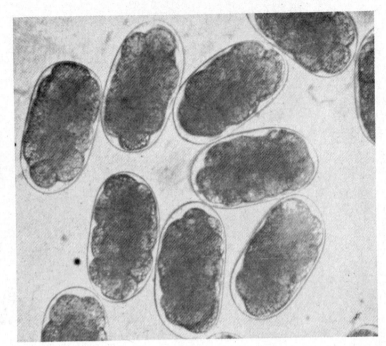

Figure 20–60. *Bunostomum tri-gonocephalum* eggs; notice truncate ends. High power. (Courtesy Dr. K. C. Kates, the U.S.D.A., and Am J. Vet Res. [Kates, K. C., and Shorb, D. A.: Am J. Vet. Res., 4:54, 1943].)

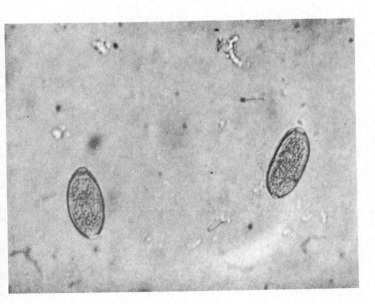

Figure 20–61. *Capillaria brevipes* eggs. High power. (Courtesy Dr. K. C. Kates, the U.S.D.A., and Am. J. Vet. Res. [Kates, K. C., and Shorb, D. A.: Am. J. Vet. Res., 4:54, 1943].)

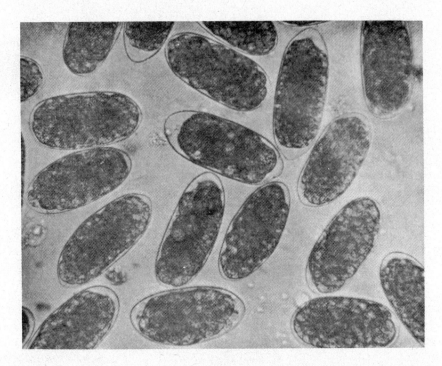

Figure 20–62. *Cooperia curticei* eggs. High power. (Courtesy Dr. K. C. Kates, the U.S.D.A., and Am. J. Vet. Res. [Kates, K. C., and Shorb, D. A.: Am. J. Vet. Res., 4:54, 1943].)

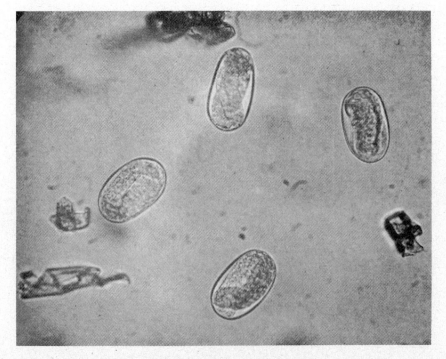

Figure 20–63. *Strongyloides papillosus* eggs. High power. (Courtesy Dr. K. C. Kates, the U.S.D.A., and Am. J. Vet. Res. [Kates, K. C., and Shorb, D. A.: Am. J. Vet. Res., 4:54, 1943].)

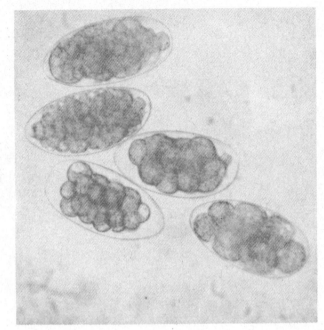

Figure 20–64. *Trichostrongylus colubriformis* eggs. High power. (Courtesy Dr. K. C. Kates, the U.S.D.A., and Am. J. Vet. Res. [Kates, K. C., and Shorb, D. A.: Am. J. Vet. Res., 4:54, 1943].)

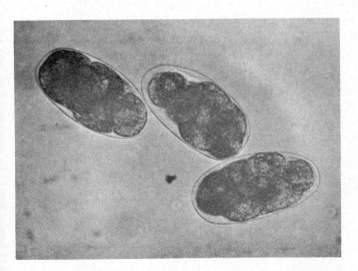

Figure 20–65. *Oesophagostomum columbianum* eggs. High power. (Courtesy Dr. K. C. Kates, the U.S.D.A., and Am. J. Vet. Res. [Kates, K. C., and Shorb, D. A.: Am. J. Vet. Res., 4:54, 1943].)

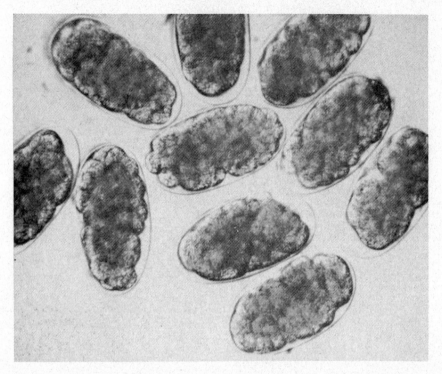

Figure 20–66. *Oesophagostomum venulosum* eggs. High power. (Courtesy Dr. K. C. Kates and the U.S.D.A.)

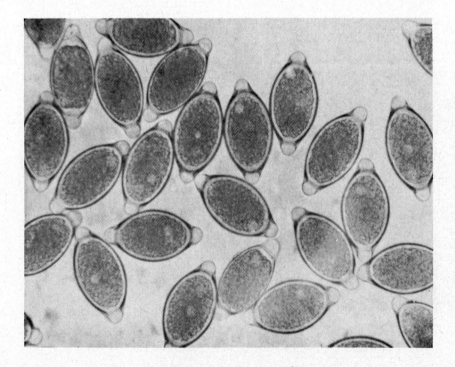

Figure 20–67. *Trichuris* sp. eggs from sheep. High power. (Courtesy Dr. K. C. Kates, the U.S.D.A., and Am. J. Vet. Res. [Kates, K. C., and Shorb, D. A.: Am. J. Vet. Res., 4:54, 1943].)

TABLE 20–7. Horse Parasites

Scientific Name	Common Name	Identification
Protozoans		
Tritrichomonas equi	Flagellate	Trophozoites in feces, 6 by 11 μm, 3 anterior flagella, undulating membrane.
Entamoeba gedoelsti	Amoeba	Trophozoites in feces, 7–13 μm; food vacuoles contain bacteria.
Klossiella equi	Coccidia	Kidney; described from histopathology studies.
Sarcocystis spp. (S. bertrami and S. fayeri, both acquired from dogs.)	Sarcocyst	Muscle.
Trematodes		
Fasciola gigantica (Hawaii and Puerto Rico only)	Giant liver fluke	See Table 20–5.
Cestodes		
Anoplocephala magna	Large horse tapeworm	Eggs rounded, contain pyriform apparatus 50–60 μm (Fig. 20–69).
Paranoplocephala mamillana	Dwarf horse tapeworm	Eggs contain pyriform apparatus; 80 by 50–60 μm (Fig. 20–69).
Anoplocephala perfoliata	Medium horse tapeworm	Eggs contain pyriform apparatus; 65–80 μm (Fig. 20–69).
Nematodes		
Draschia megastoma (Habronema megastoma)	Large stomach worm or large-mouthed stomach worm	Larvae.
Habronema microstoma	Small-mouthed stomach worm	Larvae.
Habronema muscae	Carter's stomach worm	Eggs weiner-shaped, transparent, thin-shelled, 40–50 μm by 10–20 μm, contain larvae. (Eggs and/or larvae destroyed by some flotation media.)
Trichostrongylus axei	Stomach hair worm	Eggs typical strongyle type; 79–96 by 31–48 μm.
Parascaris equorum	Large intestinal roundworm or horse ascarid	Eggs subglobular, 90–100 μm, shell layers thick, albuminous covering finely pitted, often not colored by gut contents like most ascarid eggs (Figs. 20–70 and 20–71).
Strongyloides westeri	Intestinal thread worm	Eggs relatively shorter and wider than most *Strongyloides* species; contain a larva. (Eggs of most *Strongyloides* sp. are from 45–55 by 26–35 μm.)
Strongylus equinus*	Large strongyle	Eggs 70–85 by 40–47 μm (Figs. 20–72 and 20–73).
Strongylus edentatus*	Toothless strongyle	
Strongylus vulgaris*	Single-toothed strongyle	Eggs 75–80 by 40–50 μm.
Oxyuris equi	Pinworm	Eggs 42 by 90 μm, operculate, one side somewhat flattened.
Probstmayria vivipara	Pinworm	Ovoviviparous, apparently multiplies in host.
Dictyocaulus arnfieldi	Lungworm	Eggs (48 by 98 μm) usually hatch in lungs; usually larvae 0.5 mm. long passed.
Setaria equina	Abdominal worm	Sheathed larvae circulate in bloodstream; periodicity may occur.
Onchocerca cervicalis (O. reticulata)	Neck thread worm	Ligamentum nuchae of horse; larvae probably circulate in bloodstream.

*All three of these species may be referred to as "large strongyles," "blood worms," "sclerostomes," or "palisade worms." There are approximately 40 species of worms referred to as the small strongyles or cylicostomes; most eggs of the species are indistinguishable from those of the large strongyles.

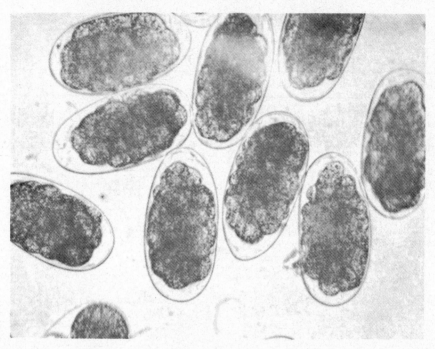

Figure 20–68. *Chabertia ovina* eggs. High power. (Courtesy Dr. K. C. Kates, the U.S.D.A., and Am J. Vet. Res. [Kates, K. C., and Shorb, D. A.: Am. J. Vet. Res., 4:54, 1943].)

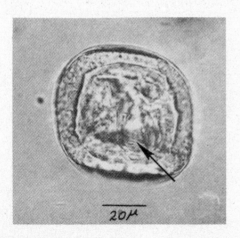

Figure 20–69. Anoplocephalan tapeworm egg from horse. Notice hooks (arrows).

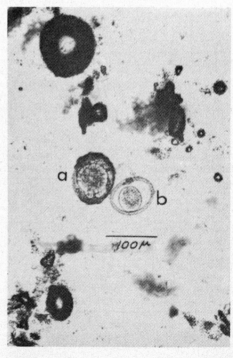

Figure 20–70. *Parascaris equorum* eggs with incomplete albuminous covering (*a*) and with no covering (*b*).

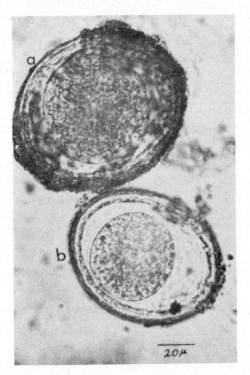

Figure 20–71. *Parascaris equorum* eggs with incomplete albuminous covering (*a*) and with no covering (*b*); variations are normal.

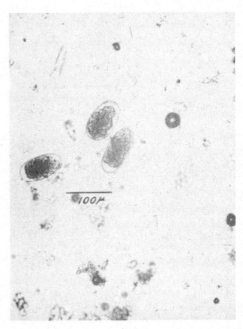

Figure 20–72. Strongyle eggs, horse.

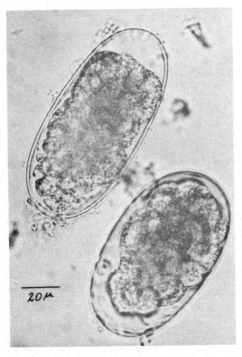

Figure 20–73. Strongyle eggs, horse.

TABLE 20–8. Swine Parasites

Scientific Name	Common Name	Identification
Protozoans		
Chilomastix mesnili	Flagellate	Trophozoites in feces, symmetrically pyriform, 6–24 by 3–10 μm; cysts lemon-shaped, 6.5–10 μm.
Giardia lamblia	No common name	Trophozoites in feces, usually 12–15 μm; cysts ovoid, 8–12 μm, contain 4 nuclei.
Tritrichomonas suis	Pig nasal trichomonad	Usually nasal passages or stomach, sometimes gut; trophozoites usually elongate, 9–16 by 2–6 μm.
Trichomonas buttreyi and T. rotunda	Cecal trichomonads	Cecum only; trophozoites in feces, average 9 by 5.8 μm (T. rotunda).
Endolimax nana	Amoeba	Trophozoites in feces, 6–15 μm (avg. 10 μm); cysts oval, thin-shelled, 5–14 μm (avg. 8–10 μm).
Entamoeba coli	Amoeba	Trophozoites in feces, 15–50 μ (usually 20–30 μm); cysts 10–33 μm, contain 8 nuclei.
Entamoeba suis	Amoeba	Trophozoites in feces, 5–25 μm.
Iodamoeba buetschlii	Amoeba	Commonest amoeba of swine; trophozoites in feces, 4–20 μm (usually 9–14); cysts 5–14 μm (usually 8–10 μm).
Eimeria spp. (E. debliecki, E. perminuta, E. polita, E. scabra, E. scrofae, E. spinosa)	Coccidia	Oocysts distinguishable; description given for commonest species; E. debliecki colorless to brownish, ovoid to ellipsoidal or subspherical, no micropyle; 13–29 by 13–19 μm.
Isospora suis	Coccidia	Oocysts in feces, brownish-yellow, subspherical to ellipsoidal (more ellipsoidal when sporulated), no micropyle; 20–24 by 18–21 μm (mean 22.5 by 19.4 μm).
Sarcocystis spp. (S. miescheriana acquired from dogs; S. porcifelis acquired from cats; S. suihominis acquired from human beings.)	Sarcocyst	Muscle.
Toxoplasma gondii	Toxoplasma	Various tissues.
Balantidium coli	Ciliate	Trophozoites in feces, ovoid, ciliated; subterminal cytostome at smaller end; 30–150 by 25–120 μm. Cysts spherical to ovoid, 40–60 μm.
Trematodes		
Paragonimus rudis (P. kellicotti, P. westermani)	Lung fluke	Eggs operculate, yellowish-brown, 75–118 by 42–67 μm, shell thickened at pole opposite operculum.
Fasciola gigantica	Giant liver fluke	See Table 20–5. (Hawaii, otherwise erratic.)
Fasciola hepatica	Common liver fluke	See Table 20–5. (Hawaii, otherwise erratic.)
Agamodistomum sp. (Alaria sp.)		Metacercariae, muscle of swine. (Florida and New York.)
Cestodes (immature only)		
Cysticercus tenuicollis (Taenia hydatigena)	Thin-necked bladder worm	In liver, mesentery, and omentum.
Echinococcus granulosus	Hydatid	Mainly in liver and lungs.
Cysticercus cellulosae (Taenia solium)	Pork bladder worm	Muscles.
Sparganum sp.	Larval pseudophyllidean tapeworm	Muscle and fascia.
Acanthocephalans		
Macracanthorhynchus hirudinaceus	Thornyheaded worm	Eggs have thick, layered shell, ellipsoidal, brownish, 50 by 100 μm; contains spiny larva when deposited (Fig. 20–74).
Nematodes		
Gongylonema pulchrum	Gullet worm	Eggs thick-shelled, 50–70 by 25–37μm; embryo.
Ascarops strongylina	Thick stomach worm	Eggs ellipsoidal, thick-shelled, 40 by 22 μm; larva.
Physocephalus sexalatus	Thick stomach worm	Eggs subcylindrical, thick-shelled, one end slightly depressed, larvated; 16 by 36 μm.

TABLE 20–8. (*continued*)

Scientific Name	Common Name	Identification
Hyostrongylus rubidus	Red stomach worm	Eggs 60–76 by 31–38 μm; usually "tadpole stage" larva. One pole more convex than other. (Measurement in literature, 36 by 45 μm, is erroneous.)
Ascaris lumbricoides	Large intestinal roundworm or giant intestinal round-worm	Eggs 45–75 by 35–50 μm, ovoid, shell thick, transparent, surrounded by coarsely mamillated albuminous covering (Figs. 20–75 and 20–76). (Unfertilized eggs show bizarre shapes and sizes; mistaken for debris by untrained observer.)
Globocephalus urosubulatus	Swine hookworm	Eggs strongyle type, 36 by 52 μm.
Strongyloides ransomi	Intestinal thread worm	Eggs thin-shelled, 53–57 by 30–34 μm; larvated.
Trichinella spiralis	Garbage worm	Adults in small intestine, larvae in muscles; stages in feces usually not observed.
Oesophagostomum dentatum (O. geogianum, O. brevicaudum, O. longicaudum)	Nodular worm	Eggs strongyle type, thin-shelled, 8–16 cells. *O. dentatum* eggs 30–45 by 60–80 μm; *O. brevicaudum* 30–45 by 52–67 μm.
Trichuris suis	Whipworm	Eggs brown, lemon-shaped, 50–56 by 21–25 μm; plug at poles; unsegmented.
Metastrongylus apri (M. pudendotectus, M. salmi)	Swine lungworm	Eggs thick-shelled, rough, 45–57 by 38–41 μm; larvated (Fig. 20–77).
Stephanurus dentatus	Kidney worm	Eggs in urine when shed. Eggs strongyle-like, thin-shelled, dark, 60 by 100 μm, passed in 32–64 cell stage.

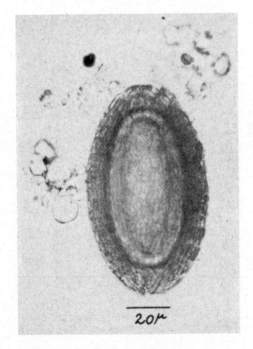

Figure 20–74. *Macracanthorhynchus hirudinaceus* egg; hooks indistinct at end.

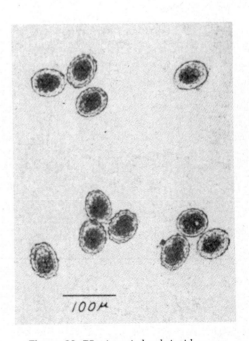

Figure 20–75. *Ascaris lumbricoides* eggs.

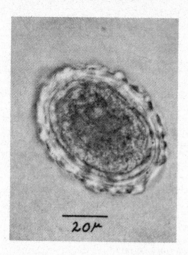

Figure 20–76. *Ascaris lumbricoides* egg.

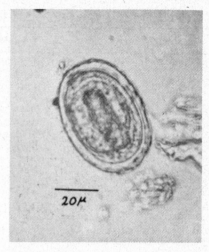

Figure 20–77. *Metastrongylus* sp. egg.

TABLE 20–9. Dog and Cat Parasites

Scientific Name	Common Name	Identification
	Protozoans	
Trichomonas sp.	Trichomonad	In feces; significance undetermined (Fig. 20–78).
Trichomonas canistomae	Trichomonad	Mouth; trophozoites pyriform, 7–12 by 3–4 μm; four anterior flagella, about length of body.
T. felistomae	Trichomonad	Mouth of cat; similar to or same as *T. canistomae*.
Giardia canis	No common name	Trophozoites 12–17 by 7–10 μm; cysts 9–13 by 7–9 μm.
Giardia cati	No common name	Trophozoites 10–18 by 5–9 μm (mean 13 by 7μm); cysts 7 by 10.5 μm; similar to or same as *G. canis*.
Isospora spp. (Dogs) Some 4 or 5 species assigned to the genus are found in dogs, including . . .	Coccidia*	
I. canis	Coccidia*	Oocyst 35–42 by 27–33 μm (mean 38 by 30 μm)
I. ohioensis	Coccidia*	Oocyst 20–27 by 15–24 μm (mean 23 by 19 μm)
I. wallacei (Previously called "small form" of *I. bigemina*)	Coccidia*	Oocyst 10–14 by 7–9 μm (Dubey,[21] considered sporulated small forms to be *I. cati*; Figs. 20–79 and 20–80.)
Sarcocystis spp. (Dogs) Some 7 or 8 species assigned to the genus are found in dogs, including . . .	Coccidia*	Sporocysts rather than oocysts passed in feces.
S. cruzi (Previously "large form" of *Isospora bigemina*?)	Coccidia*	Sporocyst 13–22 by 9–15 μm (mean 15–17 by 8–11 μm)
S. fayeri	Coccidia*	Sporocyst 11–13 by 7–9 μm (mean 12 by 8 μm)
Besnoitia, Hammondia, Isospora, Sarcocystis, and *Toxoplasma*	Coccidia* (Cat)	Five genera containing 12–15 species of coccidians that parasitize cats; common ones listed.
Isospora felis	Coccidia*	Oocyst 38–51 by 27–39 μm (mean 42 by 30.5 μm); Figs. 20–79, 20–80, and 20–81; see also Fig. 20–92.
I. rivolta	Coccidia*	Oocyst 21–28 by 18–23 μm (mean 25 by 21 μm); Figs. 20–79 and 20–80.
Toxoplasma gondii	Coccidia*	Oocyst 12–15 by 10–13 μm (mean 13 by 12 μm); Figs. 20–79 and 20–80.
Balantidium sp.	Ciliate	See Table 20–8. (When found, often associated with *Trichuris vulpis*.)
	Trematodes	
Alaria americana	No common name	Eggs 106–134 μm by 64–80 μm, unsegmented.
Alaria arisaemoides	No common name	Eggs 140 by 90 μm.
Alaria michiganensis	No common name	Eggs 80–104 by 76–80 μm.
Alaria canis	No common name	Eggs 107–133 by 77–99 μm (Fig. 20–82).

TABLE 20–9. (*continued*)

Scientific Name	Common Name	Identification
Nanophyetus salmincola	Salmon poisoning fluke	Eggs 78 by 45 μm, ovate to oval, light brown, indistinct operculum one end, blunt projection at other.
Paragonimus rudis (P. kellicotti, P. westermani)	Lung fluke	See Table 20–8.
Amphimerus pseudofelineus	No common name	Eggs 25–35 by 12–15 μm.
Metorchis conjunctus	No common name	Eggs operculate, 22–32 by 11–18 μm, embryonated.
Platynosomum fastosum	No common name	Eggs 42 by 27 μm.
Eurytrema procyonis	Pancreatic fluke	Eggs oval, lemon-yellow, operculate, 45–53 by 29–36 μm.
	Cestodes	
Dipylidium caninum	Double-pored tapeworm	Proglottids active in feces, singly or in groups; if ruptured, eggs confined to clusters or capsules (Fig. 20–83).
Echinococcus granulosus	Hydatid tapeworm	Eggs *Taenia*-like, may be slightly ovoid, 32–36 by 25–30 μm.
Taenia pisiformis	No common name	Eggs taenioid, diameter 45 μm. Segments in feces usually flaccid (Fig. 20–84).
Taenia ovis	No common name	Eggs taenioid. Segments have prominent raised genital pore (Fig. 20–84).
Taenia hydatigena	No common name	Eggs taenioid. Gravid segments 10–14 by 4–7 mm. (Fig. 20–84).
Hydatigera taeniaeformis (Taenia taeniaeformis)	No common name	Eggs taenioid (Fig. 20–84).
Multiceps multiceps	No common name	Eggs taenioid (Fig. 20–84).
Multiceps serialis	No common name	Eggs taenioid. Gravid segments 8–12 by 3–4 mm. (Fig. 20–78).
Dibothriocephalus latus (Diphyllobothrium latum)	Broad fish tapeworm	Eggs unsegmented, operculate, ends rounded, 70 by 45 μm.
Mesocestoides spp.	No common name	Eggs of *M. variabilis* 20–25 μm, *M. lineatus* 40–60 by 35–43 μm. Unlike all other cyclophyllideans, genital atrium on ventral, median surface.
	Acanthocephalans	
Oncicola canis	No common name	Eggs 59–71 by 40–50 μm. Larva in egg has hooks at one end.
	Nematodes	
Spirocerca lupi	Esophageal worm	Eggs 30–37 by 11–15 μm, thick-shelled, sides parallel, ends bluntly rounded, larvated.
Physaloptera spp. (P. praeputialis, P. felidis, P. rara)	Stomach worm	Eggs similar, smooth, thick-shelled, broadly oval, colorless, larvated, 42–53 by 29–35 μm (Fig. 20–85).
Ancylostoma caninum	Hookworm	Eggs 55–74 by 37–43 μm, elliptical, thin-shelled, transparent, 8-cell stage (Fig. 20–86).
Ancylostoma tubaeforme	Hookworm	Like *A. caninum*, but infects cats.
Ancylostoma braziliense	Hookworm	Eggs 75–95 by 41–45 μm.
Uncinaria stenocephala	Hookworm	Eggs 71–93 by 37–55 μm.
Toxascaris leonina	Large intestinal roundworm	Eggs 75–85 by 60–75 μm, slightly oval, smooth shell (Figs. 20–87 and 20–88).
Toxocara canis	Large intestinal roundworm	Eggs 75–85 μm, sub-globose to oval; shell thick and pitted (Figs. 20–87 and 20–88).
Toxocara cati (T. mystax)	Cat ascarid	Eggs 65–75 μm, sub-globose; thin shell delicately pitted (Figs. 20–89 and 20–90).
Strongyloides stercoralis, var. canis (S. canis)†	No common name	First stage (rhabditiform) larva in feces. Larva with esophagus broad anteriorly, then constricted in the nerve ring area and terminated by a bulb having the same diameter as the anterior part. No other larvae with these characteristics in fresh feces, unless there are contaminants. If sample is several hours old, hookworm larvae, similar grossly, may be present. Using high dry magnification, they can be differentiated by buccal or mouth cavity characteristics; small, rounded, thin-walled and cup-like in *Strongyloides* and long, parallel-sided and thick-walled in hookworm (Fig. 20–91).

Table continued on following page

TABLE 20–9. (*continued*)

Scientific Name	Common Name	Identification
Strongyloides tumefaciens	Cat strongyloides	Probably only larvae are found in feces.
Trichuris vulpis	Whipworm	Eggs yellowish, lemon-shaped, 72–89 by 37–40 μm, plug at pole (Figs. 20–92 and 20–93).
Pelodera strongyloides	No common name	A facultative parasite. All stages with rhabditiform esophagus associated with skin lesions.
Dipetalonema reconditum	No common name	Microfilariae in bloodstream, 269–283 by 4.3–4.8 μm.
Dirofilaria immitis	Heartworm	Microfilariae in bloodstream, 307–322 by 6.7–7.1 μm (Fig. 20–94).
Dracunculus insignis	Guinea worm	Larvae shed from pustular skin lesions.
Thelazia californiensis	Eye worm	Larvae and adults in tear ducts and under eyelids; larvae shed in tears.
Aelurostrongylus abstrusus	Cat lungworm	Eggs 71–105 by 62–101 μm, unsegmented when laid, but hatch, and larvae passed in feces. Measure 349–401 by 17 μm; excretory pore 96 μm from anterior end; esophagus approximately one-half length of larva, constricted midway between its two ends; constriction surrounded by prominent nerve ring; tail S-shaped with one or two small subterminal projections.
Capillaria aerophila	Fox lungworm	Eggs similar to whipworm, oval, yellowish-brown, surface roughened by fine granules or pits, plug or cap at poles, 58–79 by 29–40 μm. (Fig. 20–95).
Filaroides osleri	Dog and fox lungworm or tracheal worm	Eggs 80 by 50 μm, thin-shelled, colorless, larvated. (May hatch in the worm's uterus.)
Capillaria plica	Bladder worm	Eggs in urine, nearly colorless, slightly roughened, plug at poles, characteristic of capillarids, 65 by 25 μm.
Capillaria feliscati	Bladder worm	May not be a valid species.
Dioctophyma renale	Giant kidney worm	Eggs in urine, ellipsoidal, brownish, thick-shelled, sculptured depressions or pits on all parts except poles, 70–84 by 40–52 μm.
Capillaria hepatica	No common name	Eggs similar to other capillarids but shell perforated by minute pores, giving striated appearance; 51–66 by 30–35 μm. Eggs retained in liver, do not escape but are freed when host is eaten by another animal and eggs deposited in feces. There is no means of antemortem diagnosis.
Ollulanus tricuspis	No common name	Worms ovoviviparous, larvae develop to third stage in uterus. When discharged, they may complete development in same host, or be discharged in vomitus, producing infection in cat that ingests it. One of the smallest nematodes affecting animals.
Linguatula serrata	Tongue worm	Eggs 90 by 70 μm, oval, relatively thick-shelled, yellowish, contain larva with four ventral hooklike structures that are probably vestigial legs. Eggs may escape by nostrils when sneezing, by mouth when coughing, or may be swallowed and passed in feces.

*The classification of coccidians is in flux.

†Larvae may be collected with Baermann apparatus or by adding a small mass of feces, size of a bean, carefully (without dissociation), to watch glass type of containers nearly full of water. Several should be set up and kept under warm conditions under a light bulb for 15 to 30 minutes, then examined; larvae will usually escape from fecal mass and be active in the water. Identifications also may be secured by culturing feces. Mix fecal material, half and half, with sand, charcoal, or sphagnum moss and add enough water to make the mass moist but not sloppy. Transfer and keep sample in a suitable glass container after the bottom has been covered by a couple of moist filter papers. Cover with a glass plate or suitable lid and incubate at room temperature for 36 hours. If sample is an active culture, larvae accumulate on various parts of mass or in the moist filter paper. If larvae are present in limited numbers and not readily observed, they may be recovered by use of the Baermann apparatus. Such a culture usually contains three types of individuals: immature and mature free-living males and females and filariform third-stage infective larvae. Females are larger than males, resemble the first-stage rhabditiform larvae but are larger, and eggs containing larvae fill the uteri; males otherwise like females but without eggs and with prominent spicules and gubernaculum. The third-stage filariform larva, which is infective, is very small and thin and exceedingly simple anatomically but with diagnostic structures. The esophagus is approximately half the length of the body, and the tail is blunt but if examined under high power, appears bipartite or tripartite, a condition not found in any free-living stages.

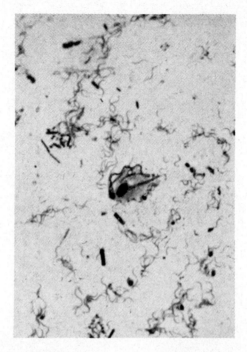

Figure 20–78. *Trichomonas* sp. trophozoite from dog feces; Wright's stain.

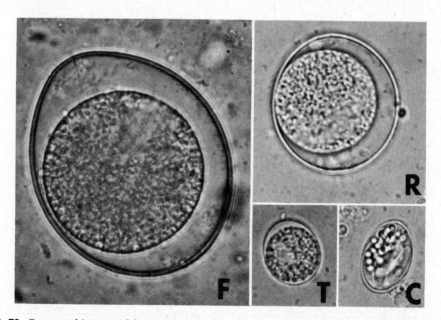

Figure 20–79. Oocysts of *Isospora felis* (F), *I. rivolta* (R), *Toxoplasma gondii* (T), and *Isospora cati* (C); the first three coccidia are excreted unsporulated, whereas *Isospora cati* is excreted sporulated, usually as a free sporocyst. (Courtesy Dr. J. P. Dubey and J.A.V.M.A. [Dubey, J. P.: J.A.V.M.A., *162*:873, 1973].)

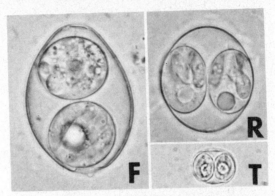

Figure 20–80. Sporulated oocysts of *Isospora felis* (F), *I. rivolta* (R), and *Toxoplasma gondii* (T). There are two sporocysts in each oocyst, and each sporocyst contains four sporozoites. The sporozoites lie at different levels and are clearly visible in *Isospora felis* and *I. rivolta* oocysts, but are barely visible in *Toxoplasma gondii* oocysts. (Courtesy Dr. J. P. Dubey and J.A.V.M.A. [Dubey, J. P., J.A.V.M.A., 162:873, 1973].)

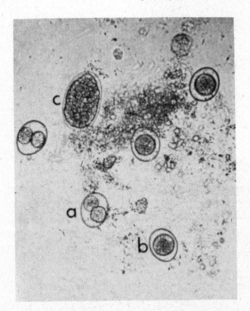

Figure 20–81. *Isospora felis* oocysts, sporulated (*a*) and unsporulated (*b*); and hookworm egg (*c*).

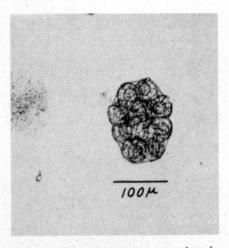

Figure 20–83. *Dipylidium caninum*, packet of eggs.

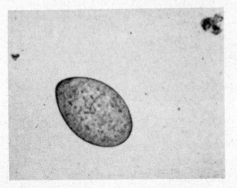

Figure 20–82. *Alaria* sp. egg. (Courtesy Department of Laboratory Medicine, Kansas State University.)

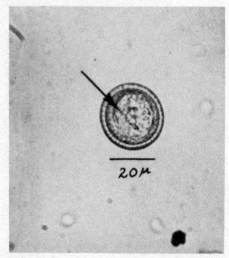

Figure 20–84. *Taenia* sp. egg; two of six hooks visible (arrow).

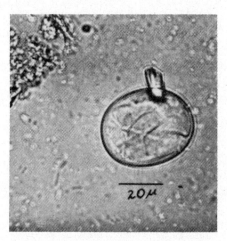

Figure 20–85. *Physaloptera* sp. egg. (Debris overlapping shell.)

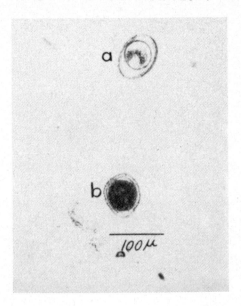

Figure 20–87. Ascarid eggs; *Toxascaris leonina* (a) and *Toxocara canis* (b).

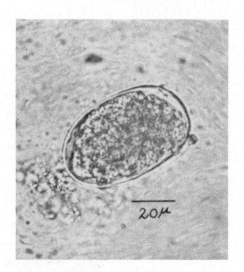

Figure 20–86. *Ancylostoma* sp. egg.

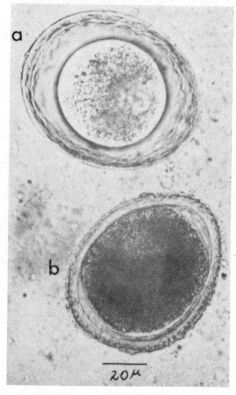

Figure 20–88. Ascarid eggs; *Toxascaris leonina* (a) and *Toxocara canis* (b).

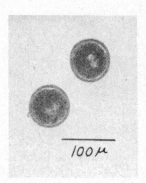

Figure 20–89. *Toxocara cati* eggs.

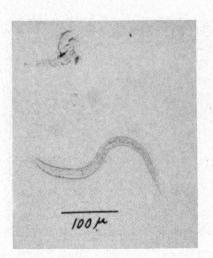

Figure 20–91. *Strongyloides* sp. rhabditiform larva.

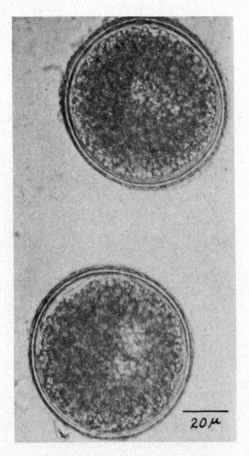

Figure 20–90. *Toxocara cati* eggs.

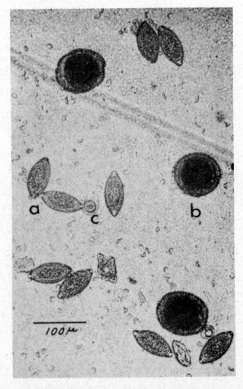

Figure 20–92. *Trichuris vulpis* eggs (a), *Toxocara canis* egg (b), and *Isospora felis* oocyst (c).

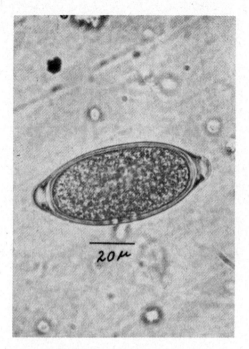

Figure 20–93. *Trichuris vulpis* egg.

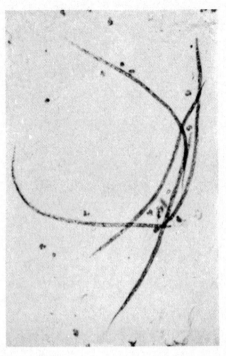

Figure 20–94. *Dirofilaria immitis* microfilariae, fixed and stained.

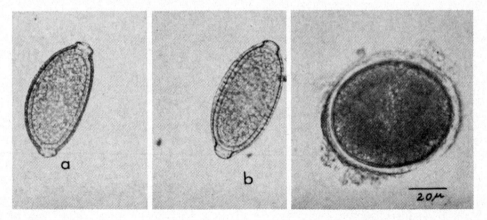

Figure 20–95. Capillarid and ascarid eggs. Notice variation in shape of capillarid eggs (*a*) and (*b*); the variations are normal.

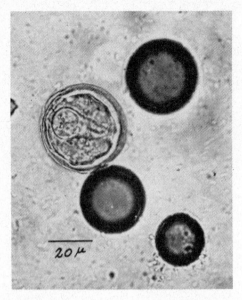

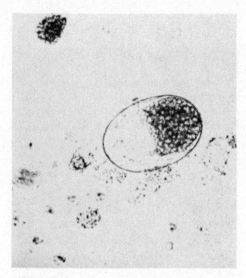

Figure 20–97. Grain mite egg; a common contaminant in domestic animal feces and often confused with hookworm eggs, especially in the dog.

Figure 20–96. *Cittotaenia* sp. egg from cat feces; this fecal contaminant is fairly common since the lagomorph, which is the host of the parasite, is eaten by dogs and cats.

SELECTED REFERENCES

1. Alcaino, H. A., and Baker, N. F.: Comparison of two flotation methods for detection of parasite eggs in feces. J.A.V.M.A., *164*:620, 1974.
2. Barker, R. W., Hoch, A. L., Buckner, R. G., and Hair, J. A.: Hematological changes in white-tailed deer fawns, *Odocoileus virginianus*, infested with *Theileria*-infected lone star ticks. J. Parasitol., *59*:1091, 1973.
3. Beaver, P. C.: The standardization of fecal smears for estimating egg production and worm burden. J. Parasitol., *36*:451, 1950.
4. Becklund, W. W.: Revised check list of internal and external parasites of domestic animals in the United States and possessions and in Canada. Am. J. Vet. Res., *25*:1380, 1964.
5. Bell, D. S., Pounden, W. D., Edington, B. H., and Bentley, O. G.: *Psorergates ovis*—a cause of itchiness in sheep. J.A.V.M.A., *120*:117, 1952.
6. Benbrook, E. A., and Sloss, M. W.: *Veterinary Clinical Parasitology*, Iowa State University Press, Ames, 1961.
7. Benjamin, M. N., and Lumb, W. V.: *Haemobartonella canis* infection in a dog. J.A.V.M.A., *135*:388, 1959.
8. Besch, E. D.: Notes on the morphology of *Pneumonyssoides caninum* (Chandler and Ruhe, 1940) Fain, 1955 (Acarina: Halarachnidae). J. Parasitol., *46*:351, 1960.
9. Blouin, E. F., Kocan, A. A., Glenn, B. L., and Kocan, K. M.: Transmission of *Cytauxzoon felis* Kier, 1979 from bobcats, *Felis rufus* (Schreber), to domestic cats by *Dermacentor variabilis* (Say). J. Wildlife Dis., *20*:241, 1984.
10. Carter, G. B., Seamer, J., and Snape, T.: Diagnosis of tropical canine pancytopaenia (*Ehrlichia canis* infection) by immunofluorescence. Research in Vet. Sci., *12*:318, 1971.
11. Caveness, F. E., and Jensen, H. J.: Modification of the centrifugal flotation technique for the isolation and concentration of nematodes and their eggs from soil and plant tissue. Proc. Helm. Soc. Washington, *22*:87, 1955.
12. Chalifoux, L., and Hunt, D. D.: Histochemical differentiation of *Dirofilaria immitis* and *Dipetalonema reconditum*. J.A.V.M.A., *158*:601, 1971.
13. Chandler, A. C., and Read, C. P.: *Introduction to Parasitology*, 10th ed., John Wiley and Sons, Inc., New York, 1961.
14. Christensen, J. F.: Species differentiation in the coccidia from the domestic sheep. J. Parasitol., *24*:453, 1938.
15. Coffin, D. L.: *Manual of Veterinary Clinical Pathology*, 3rd ed., Comstock Publishing Associates, Ithaca, 1953.
16. Cooley, R. A., and Kohls, G. M.: The genus *Amblyomma* (Ixodidae) in the United States. J. Parasitol., *30*:77, 1944.
17. Cooper, K. W.: The occurrence of the mite *Cheyletiella parasitivorax* (Mégnin) in North America, with notes on its synonymy and "parasitic" habit. J. Parasitol. *32*:480, 1946.
18. Craig, T. M., Smallwood, J. E., Knauer, K. W., and McGrath, J. P.: *Hepatozoon canis* infection in dogs: Clinical, radiographic, and hematologic findings. J.A.V.M.A., *173*:967, 1978.
19. Crosby, R. G.: Differential diagnosis of nematode

ova in cattle. *In* Threlkeld, W. L.: *Some Nematode Parasites of Domestic Animals.* Published by author. Blacksburg, Va., 1958.

20. Denton, J. F.: Studies on the life history of *Eurytrema procyonis* Denton, 1942. J. Parasitol., 30:277, 1944.

21. Dubey, J. P.: Feline toxoplasmosis and coccidiosis: A survey of domiciled and stray cats. J.A.V.M.A., 162:873, 1973.

22. Dubey, J. P.: A review of *Sarcocystis* of domestic animals and of other coccidia of cats and dogs. J.A.V.M.A., 169:1061, 1976.

23. Dubey, J. P.: *Toxoplasma, Hammondia, Besnoitia, Sarcocystis,* and other tissue cyst-forming coccidia of man and animals. *In* Kreier, J. P.: *Parasitic Protozoa* (Volume III), Academic Press, New York, pp. 101–237, 1977.

24. Dubey, J. P., Weisbrode, S. E., and Rogers, W. A.: Canine coccidiosis attributed to an *Isospora ohioensis*-like organism: A case report. J.A.V.M.A., 173:185, 1978.

25. Ehrenford, F. A.: Differentiation of the ova of *Ancylostoma caninum* and *Uncinaria stenocephala* in dogs. Am. J. Vet. Res., 14:578, 1953.

26. Elsdon-Dew, R.: Zinc sulphate flotation of faeces. Trans. Roy. Soc. Trop. Med. Hyg., 41:213, 1947.

27. Ewing, S. A.: Observations on leukocytic inclusion bodies from dogs infected with *Babesia canis.* J.A.V.M.A., 143:503, 1963.

28. Ewing, S. A.: Correspondence. J.A.V.M.A., 144:4, 1964.

29. Ewing, S. A.: Differentiation of hematozoan parasites of dogs. Proc. U.S. Livestock Sanitary Assoc., Sixty-ninth Annual Meeting: p. 524, 1965.

30. Ewing, S. A., and Buckner, R. G.: Observations on the incubation period and persistence of *Ehrlichia* sp. in experimentally infected dogs. Vet. Med./Sm. Animal Clin., 60:152, 1965a.

31. Ewing, S. A., and Buckner, R. G.: Manifestations of babesiosis, ehrlichiosis and combined infections in the dog. Am. J. Vet. Res., 26:815, 1965b.

32. Ewing, S. A., Roberson, W. R., Buckner, R. G., and Hayat, C. S.: A new strain of *Ehrlichia canis.* J.A.V.M.A., 159:1771, 1971.

33. Farwell, G. E., LeGrand, E. K., and Cobb, C. C.: Clinical observations on *Babesia gibsoni* and *Babesia canis* infections in dogs. J.A.V.M.A., 180:507, 1982.

34. Faust, E. C., Sawitz, W., Tobie, J. E., Odom, V., Peres, C., and Lincicome, D. R.: Comparative efficiency of various technics for the diagnosis of protozoa and helminths in feces. J. Parasitol., 25:241, 1939.

35. Ferris, G. F., and Stojanovich, C. J.: *The Sucking Lice,* Memoirs Pacific Coast Entomol. Soc., Vol. I, 1951.

36. Fitzgerald, P. R., Hammond, D. M., and Shupe, J. L.: The role of cultures in immediate and delayed examination of preputial samples for *Trichomonas foetus.* Vet. Med., 49:409, 1954.

37. Fitzgerald, P. R., Hammond, D. M., Miner, M. L., and Binns, W.: Relative efficacy of various methods of obtaining preputial samples for diagnosis of trichomoniasis in bulls. Am. J. Vet. Res., 13:452, 1952.

38. Flint, J. C., Roepke, M. H., and Jensen, R.: Feline infectious anemia. I. Clinical aspects. Am. J. Vet. Res., 19:164, 1958; II. Experimental cases. *Ibid.,* 20:33, 1959.

39. Georgi, J. R.: *Parasitology for Veterinarians,* 4th ed. W. B. Saunders, Philadelphia, 1985.

40. Glenn, B. L., Kocan, A. A., and Blouin, E. F.: Cytauxzoonosis in bobcats. J.A.V.M.A., 183:1155, 1983.

41. Glenn, B. L., and Stair, E. L.: Cytauxzoonosis in domestic cats: Report of two cases in Oklahoma, with a review and discussion of the disease. J.A.V.M.A., 184:822, 1984.

42. Gordon, H. M., and Whitlock, H. V.: A new technic for counting nematode eggs in sheep faeces. Austr. Counc. Sci. Indust. Res. J., 12:50, 1939.

43. Greene, C. E., Burgdorfer, W., Cavagnolo, R., Philip, R. N., and Peacock, M. G.: Rocky Mountain spotted fever in dogs and its differentiation from canine ehrlichiosis. J.A.V.M.A., 186:465, 1985.

44. Halliwell, R. E. W., and Longino, S. J.: IgE and IgG antibodies to flea antigen in differing dog populations. Vet. Immunol. Immunopathol., 8:215, 1985.

45. Hamilton, R. G., and Scott, A. L.: Immunoradiometric assay for quantitation of *Dirofilaria immitis* antigen in dogs with heartworm infections. Am. J. Vet. Res., 45:2055, 1984.

46. Hammond, D. M., and Bartlett, D. E.: Patterns of fluctuations in numbers of *Trichomonas foetus* occurring in the bovine vagina during initial infections. I. Correlation with time of exposure and with subsequent estrus cycles. Am. J. Vet. Res., 26:84, 1945.

47. Hammond, D. M., and Bartlett, D. E.: The relative value of sedimentation and of saline-egg culture in the examination of bovine vaginal and preputial samples for *Trichomonas foetus.* J.A.V.M.A., 104:10, 1964.

48. Holland, C. J., Ristic, M., Cole, A. I., Johnson, P., Baker, G., and Goetz, T.: Isolation, experimental transmission, and characterization of causative agent of Potomac horse fever. Science 227:522, 1985.

49. James, M. T.: *The Flies that Cause Myiasis in Man,* U.S. Department of Agriculture, Miscellaneous Publication No. 631, 1947.

50. Kates, K. C., and Shorb, D. A.: Identification of eggs of nematodes parasitic in domestic sheep. Am. J. Vet. Res., 4:54, 1943.

51. Keller, A. E.: A comparison of the efficiency of the Stoll egg-counting technique with the simple smear method in diagnosis of hookworm. Am. J. Hyg., 20:307, 1934.

52. Kirkpatrick, C. E., and Farrell, J. P.: Cryptosporidiosis. The Compendium on Continuing Education for the Practicing Veterinarian, 6:S155, 1984.

53. Knott, J. I.: Method for making microfilarial surveys on day blood. Trans. Roy. Soc. Trop. Med. Hyg., 33:191, 1939.

54. Koutz, F. R.: *Demodex folliculorum* studies. II. Comparison of various diagnostic methods. Speculum, 6:8, 1953.

55. Krull, W. H.: The identification of *Thysanosoma actinioides* infections in sheep by examination of fecal pellets. Trans. Am. Microsc. Soc., 65:351, 1946.

56. Kudo, R. R.: *Protozoology,* Charles C Thomas, Springfield, 1954.

57. Lapage, G.: *Veterinary Parasitology,* Charles C Thomas, Springfield, 1956.

58. Lapage, G.: *Monnig's Veterinary Helminthology and Entomology*, 4th ed. The Williams & Wilkins Co., Baltimore, 1959.

59. Lesser, E.: Modification of the formalin-ether fecal concentration technique for use with swine feces. J. Parasitol., 44:318, 1958.

60. Levine, N. D.: *Protozoan Parasites of Domestic Animals and of Man*, Burgess Publishing Co., Minneapolis, 1961.

61. Levine, N. D.: *Protozoan Parasites of Domestic Animals and of Man*. 2nd ed., Burgess Publishing Co., Minneapolis, 1973.

62. Levine, N. D., and Clark, D. T.: Correction factors for fecal consistency in making nematode egg counts of sheep feces. J. Parasitol., 42:658, 1956.

63. Levine, N. D., Mehra, K. N., Clark, D. T., and Aves, I. J.: Comparison of nematode egg counting techniques for cattle and sheep feces. Am. J. Vet. Res., 21:511, 1960.

64. Lindsey, J. R.: Identification of canine microfilariae. J.A.V.M.A., 146:1106, 1965.

65. Morgan, B. B., and Hawkins, P. A.: *Veterinary Helminthology*, Burgess Publishing Co., Minneapolis, 1953.

66. Morgan, D. O.: The helminth parasites of the goat in Britain, including an account of *Skrjabinema ovis* (Skrjabin, 1915), Werestchagin, 1926. J. Helminthol., 8:69, 1930.

67. Newton, W. L., and Wright, W. H.: The occurrence of a dog filariid other than *Dirofilaria immitis* in the United States. J. Parasitol., 42:246, 1956.

68. Newton, W. L., and Wright, W. H.: A reevaluation of the canine filariasis problem in the United States, Vet. Med., 52:75, 1957.

69. Olsen, S. J., and Roth, H.: On the mite *Cheyletiella parasitivorax* occurring on cats, as a facultative parasite of man. J. Parasitol., 33:444, 1947.

70. Otto, G. F., Hewitt, R., and Strahan, D. E.: A simplified zinc sulfate levitation method of fecal examination for protozoan cysts and hookworm eggs. Am. J. Hyg., 33:32, 1941.

71. Pratt, H. D.: *Mites of Public Health Importance and Their Control*, Public Health Service Publication No. 772, Insect Control Series, Part IX, 1963.

72. Pratt, H. D., and Littig, K. S.: *Ticks of Public Health Importance and Their Control*, Public Health Service Publication No. 772, Insect Control Series, Part X, 1962.

73. Pratt, H. D., and Wiseman, J. S.: *Fleas of Public Health Importance and Their Control*, Public Health Service Publication No. 772, Insect Control Series, Part VII, 1962.

74. Prestwood, A. K.: Cryptosporidium and cryptosporidiosis: Life cycle and diagnosis. Georgia Vet. 36(6):8, 1984.

75. Richardson, U. F., and Kendall, S. B.: *Veterinary Protozoology*, Oliver and Boyd, London, 1963.

76. Ristic, M., Huxsoll, D. L., Weisiger, R. M., Hildebrandt, P. K., and Nyindo, M. B. A.: Serological diagnosis of tropical canine pancytopenia by indirect immunofluorescence. Infection and Immunity, 6:226, 1972.

77. Ritchie, L. S., Pan, C., and Hunter III, G. W.: A comparison of the zinc sulfate and MGL (formalin-ether) technics, J. Parasitol., 38(Sec. 2):16, 1952.

78. Sanford, S. E.: Porcine neonatal coccidiosis: Clinical, pathologic, epidemiologic, and diagnostic features. Calif. Vet., 37:26, 1983.

79. Sawyer, T. K., Rubin, E. F., and Jackson, R. F.: The cephalic hook of microfilariae of *Dipetalonema reconditum* in the differentiation of canine microfilariae. Proc. Helm. Soc., Washington, 32:15, 1965.

80. Sawyer, T. K., Weinstein, P. P., and Bloch, J.: Canine filariasis—the influence of the method of treatment on measurements of microfilariae in blood samples. Am. J. Vet. Res., 24:395, 1963.

81. Schalm, O. W., and Jain, N. C.: Detection of microfilariae using the capillary hematocrit tube. Calif. Vet., 20:14, 1966.

82. Sheather, A. L.: The detection of intestinal protozoa and mange parasites by a flotation technic. J. Comp. Path. Therap., 36:266, 1923.

83. Sheather, A. L.: The detection of worm eggs and protozoa in the faeces of animals. Vet. Rec., 4:553, 1924.

84. Shorb, D. A.: A method of separating infective larvae of *Haemonchus contortus* (Trichostrongylidae) from free-living nematodes. Proc. Helm. Soc., Washington, 4:52, 1937.

85. Shorb, D. A.: Differentiation of eggs of various genera of nematodes parasitic in domestic ruminants in the United States. U.S. Department of Agriculture Tech. Bull No. 694, 1939.

86. Shorb, D. A.: A comparative study of eggs of various species of nematodes parasitic in domestic ruminants. J. Parasitol., 26:223, 1940.

87. Sloss, M. W., and Kemp, R. L.: *Veterinary Clinical Parasitology*, 5th ed., Iowa State Univ. Press, Ames, 1978.

88. Splitter, E. J.: *Eperythrozoon suis*, the etiologic agent of ictero-anemia or an anaplasmosis-like disease in swine. Am. J. Vet. Res., 11:324, 1950a.

89. Splitter, E. J.: *Eperythrozoon suis* n. sp. and *Eperythrozoon parvum* n. sp.—two new blood parasites of swine. Science, 111:513, 1950b.

90. Splitter, E. J., and Williamson, R. L.: Eperythrozoonosis in swine. A preliminary report. J.A.V.M.A., 116:360, 1950.

91. Splitter, E. J., Castro, E. R., and Kanawyer, W. L.: Feline infectious anemia. Vet. Med., 51:17, 1956.

92. Stein, F. J., and Lawton, G. W.: Comparison of methods for diagnosis and differentiation of canine filariasis. J.A.V.M.A., 163:140, 1973.

93. Stoll, N. R.: Investigations on the control of hookworm disease. XV. An effective method of counting hookworm eggs in feces. Am. J. Hyg., 3:59, 1923.

94. Summers, W. A.: A modification of zinc sulfate centrifugal flotation method for recovery of helminth ova in formalinized feces. J. Parasitol., 28:345, 1942.

95. Tilley, L. P., and Wilkins, R. J.: The Difil Test Kit for detection of canine heartworm microfilariae. Vet. Med./Sm. Animal Clin., 69:288, 1974.

96. Tippit, T. S.: Canine trypanosomiasis (Chagas' Disease). Southwest Vet., 31:97, 1978.

97. Wagner, J. E.: A fatal cytauxzoonosis-like disease in cats. J.A.V.M.A., 168:585, 1976.

98. Watkins, R. G.: A concentration and staining technique for diagnosing equine piroplasmosis. J.A.V.M.A., 141:1330, 1962.

99. Weil, G. J., Malane, M. S., Powers, K. G., and Blair, L. S.: Monoclonal antibodies to parasite antigens found in the serum of *Dirofilaria immitis*–infected dogs. J. Immunol., 134:1185, 1985.

100. Weinman, D.: Infectious anemias due to *Bartonella* and related red cell parasites. Trans. Am. Philos. Soc., *33*:308, 1944.

101. Whitlock, H. V.: Some modifications of the McMaster helminth egg–counting technic and apparatus. Aust. Counc. Sci. Industr. Res. J., *21*:177, 1948.

102. Whitlock, J. H.: A practical dilution-egg-count procedure. J.A.V.M.A., *98*:466, 1941.

103. Whitlock, J. H.: *Diagnosis of Veterinary Parasitisms*, Lea & Febiger, Philadelphia, 1960.

104. Wightman, S. R., Kier, A. B., and Wagner, J. E.: Feline cytauxzoonosis: Clinical features of a newly described blood parasite disease. Feline Practice, *7*:23, 1977.

105. Wyckoff, J. H., and Bradley, R. E.: Diagnosis of *Fasciola hepatica* infection in beef calves by plasma enzyme analysis. Am. J. Vet. Res., *46*:1015, 1985.

106. Wykoff, D. E., and Ritchie, L. S.: Efficiency of the formalin-ether concentration technic. J. Parasitol., *38*(4, Sec. 2):15, 1952.

107. Wylie, J. P.: Detection of microfilariae by a filter technique. J.A.V.M.A., *156*:1403, 1970.

APPENDIX

EXAMINATION OF BLOOD AND BONE MARROW

WRIGHT'S STAIN FOR BLOOD AND BONE MARROW FILMS

Preparation of Wright's Stain

1. Place 0.1 gm of powdered Wright's stain in a mortar.
2. Add 60 ml of acetic acid–free absolute methyl alcohol, a few milliliters at a time, and grind the stain with a pestle while adding the alcohol.
3. Grind the stain for several minutes after all alcohol is added.
4. Transfer the stain to a tightly stoppered brown bottle and store in the dark for two to four weeks.
5. Filter through filter paper prior to use.

Commercial Wright's stain can be purchased in a liquid form and is recommended for use in most laboratories.

Staining Blood or Bone Marrow Films by Wright's Method

Phosphate buffer is prepared as follows:

$$3.80 \text{ gm } Na_2HPO_4$$
$$5.47 \text{ gm } KH_2PO_4$$

Dissolve in 500 ml distilled water and bring total volume to 1,000 ml. Use a volumetric flask for measuring.

If distilled water is used, it must be neutralized, using a few drops of hematoxylin as follows:

1. Rinse a clean test tube in the water to be used.

2. To 5.0 ml of distilled water add a few crystals of hematoxylin and read results as follows:

Neutral—becomes pale lavender in 10 seconds.

Acid—becomes yellow and remains yellow for more than five minutes.

Alkaline—becomes reddish-purple immediately or within one minute.

3. If the water is acid, add 1 per cent $KHCO_3$ drop by drop until the test indicates neutrality.
4. If the water is alkaline, add 1 per cent HCl and test until it indicates neutrality.
5. Neutral water should be prepared daily and stored in a tightly stoppered Pyrex bottle.

STAINING SLIDES

1. Place slide on staining rack and add sufficient Wright's stain to cover slide. To conserve stain, the area to be stained may be marked on the surface of the slide, using a wax marking pencil.
2. Allow undiluted stain to act for one to three minutes. The optimal time for this step should be established for each batch of stain. This is the fixation time.
3. Add an equal amount of neutral distilled water or buffer and mix thoroughly by blowing on the slide until a metallic sheen appears on the surface of the buffer-stain mixture.
4. Allow the diluted stain to react for two to five minutes. The exact time must be determined for each batch of stain, whether commercial or "homemade." In testing a new stain, it is suggested that a three-minute period be used and modified according to personal preference. The time must be extended to properly stain bone marrow films.
5. Float off the scum and stain with tap water or neutral distilled water, using a wash bottle or beaker. This is one of the most important steps in

the procedure and should be carried out as quickly as possible. Excessive washing will de-stain the slide.

WRIGHT-GIEMSA STAIN

Wright's stain may be modified by the addition of Giemsa stain as follows:

1. Grind 300 mg powdered Wright's stain and 30 mg powdered Giemsa stain in a mortar with 100 ml of absolute methyl alcohol.
2. Let the stain age for 24 to 48 hours; filter and use as indicated for Wright's standard method.

WRIGHT-LEISHMAN STAIN

The stain is prepared as follows:

1. Solution I. Place 0.6 gm of powdered Wright's stain, 5.0 ml of glycerin, and 300 ml of absolute methyl alcohol (acetone free) into a 500-ml Pyrex flask. Heat this mixture gently, using constant agitation until the solution reaches a temperature just below the boiling point. Caution must be observed to avoid ignition of the alcohol. Allow the solution to cool and repeat the heating process three or four times. Cool to room temperature and filter. Store in a tightly stoppered brown bottle.
2. Solution II. Prepare a solution of Leishman's stain in a similar manner, substituting 0.6 gm of Leishman's powdered stain.
3. Final staining solution is prepared by mixing three parts of Solution I with one part of Solution II.
4. Store in the same manner as Wright's stain.
5. Slides are stained in the same manner as for the standard Wright's technique, except that the staining time should be extended to six to eight minutes, depending on the batch of stain being used.

GIEMSA STAIN

1. Because of the difficulty sometimes encountered in the preparation of liquid Giemsa stain it is recommended that this stain be purchased in a liquid form.
2. Fix the blood film in absolute methyl alcohol for three to five minutes and allow it to air dry.
3. Fill a Coplin jar with Giemsa staining solution prepared by adding one drop of Giemsa liquid stain for every milliliter of neutral distilled water. Sufficient diluted stain should be used to completely cover the slides.
4. Place the dry, fixed blood film in the diluted stain and leave it for 30 minutes.

5. Wash the slide in neutral distilled water and air dry.

STAINING BLOOD OR BONE MARROW FILMS ON COVERSLIPS

Coplin Jar Method
1. Place the coverslip in the special small Coplin jar containing the staining solution (Wright's). The time of exposure must be determined for each batch of stain and will also vary depending upon the thickness of the film. The average time required is two minutes.
2. Using forceps, transfer the coverslip to a Coplin jar containing phosphate buffer and allow it to remain for two to three minutes. The buffer can be used for 10 to 15 coverslips before being replaced.
3. Wash the coverslip carefully. DO NOT OVERWASH. Air dry the coverslip and mount on a slide with a mounting medium.

RETICULOCYTE STAINING AND COUNTING

New methylene blue or brilliant cresyl blue vital stains are used to demonstrate the presence of reticulocytes.

New Methylene Blue
This stain is prepared as follows:

New methylene blue powder	0.5 gm
Potassium oxalate	1.6 gm
Distilled water	100.0 ml
Formalin	1.0 ml

Filter prior to use.

STAINING PROCEDURE

1. Mix equal parts of whole blood and stain in a small test tube and allow reaction to continue for 15 to 20 minutes.
2. Prepare a film of the stained blood in the usual manner on either a microslide or a coverslip.
3. The film may be examined immediately or counterstained, using any of the preceding methods.

Brilliant Cresyl Blue Stain
The stain is prepared as follows:

Brilliant cresyl blue powder	1.0 gm
Sodium citrate	0.4 gm
0.85 per cent saline	100.0 ml

Filter prior to use.

STAINING TECHNIQUE

1. Add equal quantities of blood and stain to a small test tube and allow mixture to react for five minutes.

2. Prepare a film of the mixture on a microslide or coverslip and allow it to air dry.

3. Counterstain with a Romanowsky type stain.

Examination of Stained Blood Film

Reticulocytes will have a blue-stained reticulum that may vary according to the age of the cell. Young reticulocytes have a more filamentous-appearing reticulum that is present in abundance. In older reticulocytes, the reticulum is condensed and less filamentous in appearance. In feline blood, the type of reticulocyte (I, II, or III) should be noted.

The reticulocyte count is expressed as a percentage determined by the examination of 500 to 1,000 erythrocytes. In order to facilitate counting, an etched disc may be used in the ocular to divide the microscopic field into small squares. The percentage of reticulocytes is calculated, using the formula:

Reticulocyte count in % =

$$\frac{\text{Number reticulocytes counted}}{\text{Number erythrocytes counted}} \times 100$$

HAYEM'S SOLUTION FOR TOTAL ERYTHROCYTE COUNT

Mercuric chloride	0.5 gm
Sodium sulfate crystals	5.0 gm
Sodium chloride	1.0 gm
Distilled water	100.0 ml

Filter prior to use. Store in a tightly stoppered bottle. This solution may cause agglutination of erythrocytes in some bloods, particularly ruminant blood. This solution is stable for two to three weeks only.

TECHNIQUE FOR TOTAL EOSINOPHIL COUNT

REAGENTS

Pilot's (phloxine) diluting fluid:

Propylene glycol	50.0 ml
Distilled water	40.0 ml
Phloxine (1 per cent stock)	10.0 ml
Sodium carbonate (10 per cent stock)	1.0 ml
Heparin sodium	100.0 units

Mix solutions, filter, keep in well-stoppered bottle. Discard after four weeks.

PROCEDURE

1. Draw blood into a white cell pipette to the 0.5 mark.
2. Wipe tip dry and adjust volume exactly.
3. Draw in Pilot's solution to the 11 mark.
4. Wipe tip dry and let stand for 15 minutes.
5. Shake pipette for three minutes.
6. Fill the hemocytometer, avoiding flooding. Fill both chambers.
7. Let stand under Petri dish on a damp paper towel for three minutes.
8. Count total eosinophils in all squares of both chambers.
9. Calculate the total eosinophils based on 1:20 dilution of the blood as follows: Average the count per square millimeter by dividing the total by 2. The average number of cells $\times$ 11.1 = total number of eosinophils per microliter.

Canine eosinophils are difficult to stain. The following solution is useful for counting dog eosinophils:

Eosin Y	250 mg
Phloxine	250 mg
Water	50 ml

Dissolve the solutions just listed and add:

Propylene glycol	50.0 ml
Formalin	0.5 ml
Phenol	0.5 ml

No filtering is required before use as just outlined.

TECHNIQUE FOR ERYTHROCYTE FRAGILITY TEST

REAGENTS

Sodium chloride (absolutely dry)
Distilled water

PROCEDURE

Prepare a 1.0 per cent solution of sodium chloride by adding 1 gm of sodium chloride to a 100-ml volumetric flask containing approximately 40 to 50 ml of distilled water. Dissolve and bring to 100 ml total volume, using distilled water.

1. Place 15 to 18 small test tubes in a rack.
2. For the dog, add 0.6 ml of saline and 0.4 ml of distilled water to the first tube. To the second tube add 0.58 ml saline and 0.42 ml of distilled water. Add decreasing amounts of saline (0.02 ml) to each tube until the last tube contains 0.30 per cent saline.
3. Draw the blood to be tested, using a dry syringe, and add one drop of blood to each tube. If blood with an anticoagulant is used, centrifuge the specimen, replace the plasma with 0.85 per

cent saline, and add one drop of the saline suspension of blood cells to the prepared saline tubes.

4. Allow the tubes to stand at room temperature for two hours.

5. Record the saline concentration for beginning hemolysis and complete hemolysis. A sample of normal blood should be tested simultaneously as a control method.

DIRECT COOMBS' TEST

REAGENTS

Erythrocytes from patient
Erythrocytes from a normal animal
Antiglobulin for animal species being tested
Isotonic saline

COLLECTION AND PREPARATION OF SPECIMEN

1. Collect approximately 4 ml of blood in EDTA or in a serum tube. Clotted specimens should be used if the sample is being sent to an outside laboratory for testing. A similar sample should be collected from a normal animal and treated in the same manner as outlined below.

2. EDTA blood: Centrifuge to remove RBC's and remove plasma.

3. Clotted blood: Remove serum from the clot. Add isotonic saline (2 to 3 ml) and gently break clot to release RBC's. Pour off saline containing RBC's, centrifuge, and decant the saline.

4. Pipette 0.1 ml of packed cells into a test tube (12 × 75 mm) and resuspend packed cells in 4.9 ml of isotonic saline.

5. Centrifuge, decant plasma, and resuspend in 4.9 ml isotonic saline. Resuspension should be accomplished with little damage to the RBC's.

6. Repeat step 5 until cells have been washed four times. The last tube should contain 5 ml of a 2 per cent RBC suspension.

7. Test specimens immediately after washing and as soon after collection as possible.

PROCEDURE (MACROTUBE)

1. Preparation of the dilutions of the antiglobulin:

a. Use three 12 × 75 mm tubes and identify with dilution to be used 1:2, 1:4, 1:8, and so on.

b. Pipette 0.1 ml of antiglobulin for each sample and control that will be tested into the tube labeled 1:2. (For example, if you have two specimens and a control, pipette 0.3 ml of antiglobulin in tube 1:2.)

c. Pipette 0.1 ml of isotonic saline for each sample to be run into each of the tubes 1:2, 1:4, 1:8, and so on. (If as above you have three tests, pipette 0.3 ml.)

d. Mix contents of tube 1:2 and transfer 0.1 ml from tube 1:2 into tube 1:4 and mix well. Transfer 0.1 ml from tube 1:4 into tube 1:8 and mix well. (As above if you have more than one specimen being tested, transfer 0.1 ml per specimen.)

2. Testing:

a. Label four 12 × 75 mm test tubes for each specimen or control to be tested. Label each set as C (for control) or a number for the specimen being tested. Label tubes with S, 1:2, 1:4, 1:8, and so forth.

b. Pipette 0.1 ml of washed negative control cells into the tubes labeled CS, C1:2, C1:4, and C1:8. Note: additional dilutions may be used and should be labeled accordingly.

c. For each patient to be tested add 0.1 ml of washed cells into tubes labeled with the specimen number; for example: P1–S, P1–1:2, P1–1:4, P1–1:8.

d. Place 0.1 ml of isotonic saline in each tube labeled –S.

e. Place 0.1 ml of antiglobulin reagent dilutions 1:2, 1:4, and 1:8 into each of the tubes labeled with this dilution.

f. Mix all tubes gently and incubate at 37° C for exactly 30 minutes.

g. Following incubation observe each tube for agglutination. There should be no agglutination in the S (saline control) tubes. Agglutination of the RBC's will occur in any tubes that are positive. If the agglutination is not obvious it should be checked microscopically. Results are reported as the highest dilution in which agglutination occurred.

PROCEDURE FOR MICROTITER PLATES

1. Cells and dilutions of the antiglobulin are prepared in the manner described above.

2. Because of the small volume used, commercially available microdilution loops and droppers simplify the test and are recommended.

3. Each specimen to be tested requires four or more wells, depending on the antiglobulin dilutions being used.

4. Drop 0.05 ml of isotonic saline into four or more consecutive wells for each patient to be tested plus one row for the saline control.

5. Drop 0.05 ml of the antiglobulin reagent stock solution into the second well of each row.

6. Using a microdilution loop, mix the reagent and saline in the second well of each row. Transfer 0.05 ml with the loop into the third well and mix. Subsequent dilutions are prepared in the same manner, transferring 0.05 ml each time into the next well. The procedure is repeated for each row of wells being used.

7. Add 0.05 ml of negative control cells into each well in row 1.

8. Add 0.05 ml of patient cells into each well in row 2. Repeat for each patient being tested.

9. Mix the cells and antiglobulin dilutions by shaking the microtiter tray.

10. Incubate at 37° C for 30 minutes.

11. Observe the wells for agglutination by stirring samples with a toothpick. View the wells for the presence of agglutination. Negative samples, including the saline controls, will remain in suspension while positive samples will have distinct clumping of the RBC's. DO NOT READ THE SETTLING PATTERNS TO DETERMINE PRESENCE OR ABSENCE OF AGGLUTINATION. If in doubt, place material on a glass slide and examine microscopically.

If the clinician suspects that the antibody is of class IgM the test should be conducted at 4° C.

INDIRECT COOMBS' TEST

REAGENTS

Serum from patient
Erythrocytes from a normal animal
Isotonic saline
Antiglobulin for animal species being tested

PROCEDURE

1. Wash erythrocytes from normal animal and prepare a 5 per cent suspension of washed cells in saline.

2. Prepare three tubes and label them "test," "control 1," and "control 2."

3. Add two drops of the red cell suspension to each tube.

4. Add four to eight drops of fresh patient serum to the tube labeled "test."

5. Add four to eight drops of isotonic saline to tube "control 1."

6. Add four to eight drops of fresh serum from normal animal to tube "control 2."

7. Incubate all tubes for 30 minutes at 37° C.

8. Wash cells from each tube at least three times with isotonic saline to remove any trace of serum.

9. After last wash, subject cells to the direct test as previously outlined.

10. There should be no agglutination, macroscopic or microscopic, in either control tube, but if antibodies were present in patient serum, agglutination will occur.

Note: False positive results are not uncommon with either the direct or indirect Coombs' test. Commercial antiglobulins may contain antibodies to erythrocytes, and agglutination will develop in control tubes containing uncoated normal erythrocytes. False positives will also occur if the tubes are over-centrifuged; therefore, speeds over 1,000 revolutions per minute (rpm) should be avoided. If possible, all tests should be accompanied by positive and negative controls.

LUPUS ERYTHEMATOSUS CELL TEST— CLOTTED BLOOD METHOD

1. Obtain blood by venipuncture and permit it to clot while remaining at room temperature for two to three hours.

2. Rim the clot and transfer clot and serum to a special sieve (Scientific Products, Div. American Hospital Supply Corp., Evanston, Illinois).

3. Mash the clot plus serum through the sieve and collect the material into a Petri dish.

4. Fill two Wintrobe hematocrit tubes with the sieved material.

5. Incubate the Wintrobe tubes for 2 to $2\frac{1}{2}$ hours at 37° C.

6. Centrifuge for five to 10 minutes at 1,000 rpm.

7. Remove serum and make smears (four or five) from the buffy coat.

8. Stain the buffy coat smear with a Romanowsky-Type stain.

9. Examine smears carefully for the presence of LE cells. Slides containing two or more classical lupus erythematosus (LE) cells should be considered positive.

Note: A typical LE cell is a neutrophilic leukocyte that has ingested a mass of nuclear material. This nuclear material appears as an intracytoplasmic homogeneous red-purple body. The phagocytosed mass is almost completely homogeneous and stains redder than does unaltered chromatin. The nucleus is pushed to one side of the cell and is distorted. These phagocytic cells are usually larger than normal cells.

Slides containing LE cells may also have other abnormalities. Free masses of homogeneous material may be observed as varying-sized globules. Rosettes are frequently present, as neutrophils surround these globules. These rosettes probably represent an intermediate stage in the development of the true LE cell.

REAGENTS USED IN STUDY OF BLOOD COAGULATION

REES-ECKER DILUTING FLUID FOR THROMBOCYTE COUNT

REAGENTS

Sodium citrate	3.8	gm
Formalin (40 per cent solution)	0.2	ml
Brilliant cresyl blue	0.05	gm
Water	100.0	ml

Store in closed bottle in refrigerator and filter before use.

ONE-STAGE PROTHROMBIN TIME

REAGENTS

Thromboplastin: This reagent is commercially prepared and is usually in the form of a suspension of acetone-dried extract of brain tissue. As most preparations are made from rabbit brain, this will not work with avian plasma. Thromboplastin from chicken brain is needed for tests on avian plasma.

Calcium chloride, 0.02 M: Many preparations are available in which the thromboplastin and calcium are mixed and ready for use.

Plasma control

PROCEDURE

1. Place test tubes in a water bath.
2. Add 0.2 ml of thromboplastin-calcium mixture to each tube, or add 0.1 ml thromboplastin and 0.1 ml calcium chloride.
3. Allow tubes to warm for about 30 seconds.
4. Taking one tube at a time, add 0.1 ml of sample plasma by blowing it quickly into the thromboplastin mixture. Start stop watch at the same time.
5. Keep tube in water bath for 10 seconds but continuously and gently agitate it.
6. Remove tube, hold it in front of a bright light, and tilt it slightly every second until a clot appears. Stop the watch at this point.
7. Each sample should be run in duplicate and the results averaged.
8. A normal control must be included in each batch of tests. The results are reported in seconds, and the results of the control time should also be recorded.

PROTHROMBIN CONSUMPTION

REAGENTS

Thromboplastin: commercially prepared
Calcium chloride, 0.02 M (often incorporated with thromboplastin)
Plasma control
Patient's serum

PROCEDURE

1. Place test tubes in a water bath.
2. Add 0.2 ml of thromboplastin-calcium mixture to each tube, or add 0.1 ml of thromboplastin and 0.1 ml of calcium chloride.
3. Allow tubes to warm in the water bath.
4. Taking one tube at a time, add 0.1 ml of sample serum by blowing it quickly into the thromboplastin mixture, starting the stop watch at the same time.
5. Keep tube in water bath for 10 seconds but continuously and gently agitate it.

6. Remove tube, hold it in front of a bright light, and tilt it slightly every second until a clot appears. At the first appearance of a clot, stop the stop watch.
7. Each sample should be run in duplicate and the results averaged.
8. A normal control must be included with each batch of tests.

LIVER FUNCTION TESTS

TESTS DEPENDENT ON HEPATIC SECRETION AND EXCRETION

VAN DEN BERGH'S REACTION

Reagents

1. Sulfanilic acid (solution A): Dissolve 100 mg sulfanilic acid in 1.5 ml HCl in a 100-ml volumetric flask and dilute to volume with distilled water.
2. Sodium nitrite, 5 per cent: Dissolve 5 gm sodium nitrite in distilled water and dilute to 100 ml with distilled water.
3. Sodium nitrite, 0.5 per cent (solution B): Dilute 1 ml 5 per cent sodium nitrite to 10 ml with distilled water. Make fresh just prior to use.
4. Diazo reagent: Mix 0.3 ml solution B with 10 ml Solution A. Make fresh prior to use.
5. Dilute hydrochloric acid: Dilute 1.5 ml HCl by adding distilled water to a total volume of 100 ml.
6. Methyl alcohol
7. Standard solution
8. Control solution
9. Diazo blank. Dilute 60 ml of concentrated hydrochloric acid to a volume of 1 liter with water.

Procedure

TOTAL BILIRUBIN

1. Label two tubes, one blank and one sample, for each unknown, standard, and control.
2. Add 5 ml methyl alcohol and 1 ml diazo blank solution to blank tube.
3. Add 5 ml methyl alcohol and 1 ml diazo reagent to the sample tube.
4. Dilute 1 ml of serum or plasma by adding to 9 ml distilled water.
5. Add 4 ml diluted serum or plasma to each tube.
6. Insert a stopper and shake well.
7. Let stand for exactly 30 minutes.
8. Set photometer on zero optical density or 100 per cent transmittance and read at 540 nm against blank.

DIRECT BILIRUBIN

1. Label two test tubes for each unknown standard and control, one blank and one sample.
2. Add 5 ml of distilled water and 1 ml diazo blank solution to the test tube.
3. Add 5 ml distilled water and 1 ml diazo reagent to the sample tube.
4. Add 4 ml diluted serum or plasma to each tube.
5. Insert a stopper and shake contents well.
6. Let stand for exactly five minutes.
7. Read in a cuvette at a wavelength of 540 nm with a reading of 100 per cent transmittance or zero optical density with the blank tube.

Calculations

As with others, use the standard formula.

The indirect bilirubin value is calculated by subtracting the direct bilirubin value from the total bilirubin value.

EHRLICH'S TEST FOR URINE UROBILINOGEN

REAGENTS

Ehrlich's reagent:

Paradimethylaminobenzaldehyde	10.0 gm
Concentrated HCl	75.0 ml
Distilled water	75.0 ml

Urine

PROCEDURE

1. Place 10 ml of urine in a test tube. If the urine has been stored in the refrigerator, it should be warmed to room temperature.
2. Add 1 ml of Ehrlich's reagent, and mix.
3. Allow to stand from three to five minutes, at the end of which time a cherry red color appears if urobilin is present in abnormal quantity. If the tube is held at a slight angle over a white paper and the liquid examined through the mouth of the tube, the color is easier to observe.
4. If no color appears, the tube should be allowed to stand longer, then if no color appears it should be heated and re-examined.
5. A semiquantitative test can be performed by diluting the urine and making readings.

MODIFICATION OF EHRLICH'S TEST

REAGENTS

Ehrlich's reagent as above
Saturated sodium acetate solution (requires 2 or 3 pounds of analytical grade anhydrous or triple-hydrated sodium acetate for each liter of distilled water)

Ascorbic acid power
Standard phenolsulfonphthalein (PSP) dye solution prepared by dissolving 20 mg of phenol red in 100 ml of 0.05 per cent NaOH
Working standard: Dilute stock PSP dye solution 1:100 with 0.05 per cent NaOH. This is equivalent to a solution of urobilinogen aldehyde containing 0.346 mg of urobilinogen/100 ml of final colored solution in the method.

PROCEDURE

1. Measure the volume of a two-hour urine sample.
2. Test urine for bilirubin. If there is more than a trace, mix 2.0 ml of 10 per cent $BaCl_2$ solution with 8.0 ml of urine and filter. If this step is required, the final result must be multiplied by 1.25.
3. Add 100 mg of ascorbic acid to 10 ml of urine. If the solution is cloudy, it must be centrifuged.
4. Label one tube "B" for blank and one "U" for unknown and add 1.5 ml of urine to each.
5. Prepare a fresh mixture of one volume of Ehrlich's reagent and two volumes of saturated sodium acetate.
6. Add 4.5 ml of the reagent in step 5 to tube B and mix.
7. To the U tube add 1.5 ml of Ehrlich's reagent, mix, add 3.0 ml of saturated sodium acetate, and mix well.
8. Within five minutes of step 7, measure the absorbance of U and B at 525 nm. against water set at zero.
9. Measure absorbance of the working standard of PSP against water at the same wavelength.
10. Make calculations as follows:

Ehrlich units/100 ml urine =

$$\frac{^AU - ^AB}{A_S} \times 0.346 \times \frac{6.0}{1.5} = \frac{^AU - ^AB}{A_S} \times 1.38$$

and

Ehrlich units/2 hr =

$$\frac{^AU - ^AB}{A_S} \times 0.0138 \times \text{Urine volume in ml}$$

Note: Multiply answer by 1.25 if bilirubin was removed by $BaCl_2$.

TEST FOR BILIRUBIN IN URINE

REAGENTS

Ictotest Tablets (Ames Co., Elkhart, Indiana)

PROCEDURE

1. Place five drops of urine in one square of the special test mat.
2. Place reagent tablet in the center of the moistened area.

3. Flow two drops of water onto the tablet.
4. Interpretation:

Negative: Mat shows no blue or purple color within 30 seconds. A slight red or pink color that may sometimes appear should be reported as negative.

Positive: Mat around tablet turns blue or purple. The amount of bilirubin present is proportionate to the speed and intensity of the color reaction.

BROMSULPHALEIN (SULFOBROMOPHTHALEIN)

REAGENTS

0.05 N sodium hydroxide (NaOH)

PROCEDURE

1. Pipette 0.5 ml of the serum of plasma drawn prior to the injection of the dye into a cuvette.
2. Into a second cuvette, pipette 0.5 ml of the serum sample drawn at the selected time interval. (If more than one postinjection sample is obtained, it should be added to a third cuvette in the same amount.)
3. To each of the cuvettes add 5.0 ml of the 0.05 N NaOH and mix by inverting.
4. Read in a spectrophotometer at 575 nm with the reference blank (serum prior to injection plus the NaOH) set at 100 per cent transmittance.
5. Compare reading obtained to a chart prepared, using known quantities of the dye in NaOH.

PLASMA PROTEINS

TOTAL PROTEIN

Biuret Method
REAGENT

Biuret reagent

Rochelle salt	45 gm
(sodium potassium tartrate)	
Copper sulfate ($CuSO_4 \cdot 5H_2O$)	15 gm
Potassium iodide	5 gm
0.2 N NaOH (q.s.)	1000 ml

Dissolve Rochelle salt in about 400 ml of 0.2 N NaOH. Add copper sulfate and dissolve completely. Add potassium iodide, dissolve, and add 0.2 N NaOH to the 1-liter mark in the volumetric flask.

Reagent tablets containing measured amounts of the dry reagents are available commercially (Scientific Products Co., Evanston, Illinois). The tablets are dissolved in 70 ml of distilled water and 30 ml of 10 per cent NaOH. Stable biuret solutions are available.

Normal saline

NaCl	8.5 gm
Distilled water	1000.0 ml

TECHNIQUE OF TEST

1. Place 4.9 ml of 0.85 per cent NaCl into three chemically clean tubes marked "test," "standard," and "control."
2. Add 5 ml of 0.85 per cent NaCl to a tube labeled "blank."
3. Add 0.1 ml of unknown serum to tube marked "test."
4. Add 0.1 ml of standard to tube marked "standard."
5. Add 0.1 ml of control to tube marked "control."
6. Add 5 ml of biuret reagent to all tubes and mix well.
7. Incubate in a water bath at 37° C for 30 minutes.
8. Transfer solutions to matched cuvettes and read in a spectrophotometer at 545 nm against the reagent blank. If matched cuvettes are not available, a single cuvette may be used if it is carefully rinsed between solutions, using 2 to 3 ml of the solution to be tested. Calculation of the total serum protein is determined by use of the formula:

$$\frac{\text{Optical density unknown}}{\text{Optical density standard}} \times$$

Concentration of standard (gm/dl)
$$= \text{Total protein (gm/dl)}$$

ALBUMIN:GLOBULIN RATIO

Biuret Method
REAGENTS

Biuret reagent
Ether (ACS)
Sodium chloride solution, 0.85 per cent
Sodium sulfate solution, 22.6 per cent
Aerosol-OT solution, 10 per cent

Biuret reagent is prepared as previously described.

Sodium sulfate (22.6 per cent) is prepared by placing 226 gm of anhydrous sodium sulfate in a 1-liter volumetric flask. Warm 1 liter of distilled water to 37° C. Add warmed distilled water to the sodium sulfate and shake to dissolve. When sodium sulfate is dissolved, adjust volume to 1 liter. Store at 37° C to avoid crystallization.

TECHNIQUE OF TEST

1. Pipette 0.5 ml of serum or plasma into a 12-ml heavy-walled centrifuge tube.
2. Pipette 0.5 ml of control serum into a second tube and 0.5 ml of a standard into a third tube.

3. Add 9.5 ml of 22.6 per cent sodium sulfate to each tube. Mix by inverting.

4. Immediately after mixing unknown, pipette 2 ml into a test tube or cuvette marked "TP" (total protein).

5. Immediately after mixing standard, pipette 2 ml into a second tube or cuvette and mark "S-TP" (standard-total protein). Complete the same procedure for the control, marking the tube "C-TP" (control-total protein).

6. To the remaining 8 ml of the unknown, standard, and control solutions, add 0.1 ml aerosol and 2 to 3 ml of ether.

7. Stopper and shake vigorously about 20 times.

8. Allow to stand for several minutes or until globulin rises to interface.

9. Centrifuge 10 minutes at about 2,000 rpm so that a firm mat is formed at the ether-serum sulfate interface.

10. Title the tube marked "TP" and insert pipette without disturbing the globulin mat. Withdraw 2 ml of clear liquid and place it in a tube marked "ALB."

11. Repeat same procedure for standard, marking it "ST-ALB," and for control, marking it "C-ALB."

12. BLANK: To another tube or cuvette add 2 ml of sodium sulfate.

13. To each of the other three tubes add 8 ml of biuret reagent and mix.

14. Let stand 30 minutes at room temperature or 10 minutes at 30° C and read at 540 nm. Adjust reading of blank for 100 per cent transmittance or zero optical density.

Calculations are made as follows:

$$\frac{\text{Density of unknown}}{\text{Density of control}} \times \frac{\text{Value (total protein}}{\text{of control)}}$$

$$= \text{Total protein value of unknown}$$

To determine the albumin (A) content, substitute the albumin value for the total protein value of the control. Globulin (G) value is determined by subtracting the albumin value from the total protein value. The A:G ratio is determined by dividing the total albumin value by the value for total globulin.

ZINC SULFATE TURBIDITY TEST FOR GLOBULINS

REAGENTS

Zinc sulfate (ZnSO$_4$·7H$_2$O)	205 mg
Boiled distilled water	1,000 ml

Store in aspirator bottle with soda lime tube inserted into the stopper.

PROCEDURE

1. Add 6.0 ml ZnSO$_4$ solution to a test tube.

2. Add 0.1 ml of hemolysis-free serum to each tube.

3. Shake tubes gently.

4. Allow tubes to stand at room temperature for one hour.

5. Remix and read in a spectrophotometer at 485 nm. (Spectrophotometer is blanked with distilled water.)

INTERPRETATION IN THE HORSE

1. With spectrophotometer:
Optical density (O.D.) > 0.45 = foal ingested enough colostral antibody to give serum value of at least 400 mg/dl.
O.D. < 0.45 = probably inadequate immunoglobulin G (IgG) colostral transfer.

2. Without use of spectrophotometer:
Turbidity becomes visible at an OD of 0.4 to 0.5, which would be equal to 400 to 500 mg of IgG/dl.
Colostral-deficient foals have an IgG concentration of less than 400 mg/dl.

3. By comparison with dam:
Conduct ZnSO$_4$ turbidity test on serum from both dam and foal.
If foal has adequate colostral IgG, the turbidity of both will be approximately equal, with the foal's concentration only slightly less than that of the dam.

RENAL FUNCTION TESTS

NONPROTEIN NITROGENOUS SUBSTANCES

Mercury Combining Power
REAGENTS

10 per cent trichloroacetic acid: Add 10 gm of trichloracetic acid to 50 ml of distilled water. Dissolve and dilute to 100 ml.

5 per cent mercuric chloride: Dissolve 5 gm of mercuric chloride in 50 ml of distilled water and dilute to 100 ml.

Saturated solution of sodium carbonate.

PROCEDURE

1. Add equal quantities of whole blood and trichloracetic acid (5 ml each). Add the blood drop by drop to the acid, mixing thoroughly.

2. Centrifuge for five minutes, or filter.

3. Pour off the clear supernatant or filtrate into a clean tube.

4. Place 5 ml of the supernatant or filtrate into a small (50-ml) beaker.

5. Add 1.5 ml of 5 per cent mercuric chloride to the filtrate and mix completely.

6. Add additional mercuric chloride a few drops at a time. Test a small quantity of the mix-

ture by placing a drop of the mixture on a spot plate and adding one drop of the saturated sodium carbonate. This should be continued until a drop of the mixture and a drop of the sodium carbonate result in a dark brown precipitate.

7. Calculate the *blood urea** level by recording the total quantity of mercuric chloride required to result in a brown precipitate. Each 0.1 ml of mercuric chloride is equal to a blood urea value of 4 mg/dl.

Urograph†
REAGENTS

Urograph (BUN-O-Graph) strips
Serum or plasma

PROCEDURE

1. With a long-tipped pipette, place 0.2 ml serum or plasma in a 10 × 75 mm test tube. *Avoid wetting sides of the tubes.*
2. Into tube containing sample, place one strip with the taped end down. Do not touch the indicator band with the fingers. Be sure strip is centered in the bottom of the tube. Be sure strip is not bent and touches the tube only at the top and bottom. Let stand for 30 minutes at room temperature, away from drafts.
3. At 30 minutes, remove strip from tube and measure with a millimeter rule the height of the color change on the indicator band. This distance is quantitatively proportional to the urea nitrogen concentration. No color change indicates less than 10 mg/dl. A hair-breadth of color indicates 10 mg/dl. For levels greater than 10 mg. each 0.5 mm of color represents an additional 2.5 mg/dl urea nitrogen.

CREATININE

Folin-Wu Method
REAGENTS

10 per cent sodium tungstate: 100 gm sodium tungstate ($Na_2WO_4 \cdot H_2O$). Place about 600 ml of water in a 1-liter volumetric flask. Add sodium tungstate. Dilute to volume with distilled water.

2/3 N sulfuric acid: 18.3 ml concentrated sulfuric acid. Add concentrated sulfuric acid to approximately 800 ml of distilled water in a volumetric flask. Dilute to volume with distilled water.

10 per cent sodium hydroxide: 100 gm sodium hydroxide. Dissolve sodium hydroxide in distilled water. Dilute to 1 liter.

---

*Blood urea value is approximately twice the value for urea nitrogen.

†Warner Chilcott Labs., Morris Plains, New Jersey

Buffered picric acid solution: 11.7 gm picric acid, 2 N sodium hydroxide. Place picric acid in 900 ml distilled water in a 1-liter flask. Adjust pH to 2.0 by adding 2 N sodium hydroxide. Let stand overnight and adjust pH again. Dilute to 1-liter mark with distilled water.

Alkaline picrate: Place 36 ml of buffered picric acid solution (previously described) in flask; add 4 ml of 10 per cent NaOH. Make fresh daily.
  Standard solution
  Control solution

PROCEDURE

1. Pipette 16 ml 2/3 N sulfuric acid into three 50-ml flasks.
2. Add 2 ml unknown serum, control, and standard solutions into respective flasks.
3. Mix well.
4. Add 2 ml 10 per cent sodium tungstate to each flask. Stopper and shake vigorously.*
5. Filter or centrifuge.
6. Transfer 5 ml of the clear protein-free filtrate to a small, properly labeled flask.
7. Add 5.0 ml of distilled water to a fourth flask and label "blank."
8. Add 2.5 ml of alkaline picrate to each flask.
9. Transfer to cuvettes after 15 minutes at room temperature to allow complete color development.
10. Set spectrophotometer to zero optical density with the blank at a wavelength of 520 nm.
11. Read within five minutes.
12. Make calculation using the following formula:

$$\frac{\text{Optical density of unknown}}{\text{Optical density of standard}}$$

$$\times \text{ Mg creatinine in standard}$$
$$= \text{ Mg creatinine/dl serum.}$$

Serum Creatinine Using Lloyd's Reagent
REAGENTS

Picric acid: 9.16 gm of anhydrous or 10.17 gm reagent grade picric acid (containing 10 to 12 per cent added water) is dissolved and made up to 1,000 ml in a volumetric flask.

Sodium hydroxide: Dissolve 30 gm of NaOH up to 1 liter with distilled water.

Oxalic acid: Saturated aqueous solution.

Lloyd's reagent (an aluminum silicate): Use approximately 100-mg aliquots of powder for each adsorption, or, alternatively, use 1 ml of a 10 per cent aqueous suspension.

Stock creatinine standard: 1.5 mg/ml in 0.1 N HCl. Stable indefinitely in refrigerator.

---

*A stable tungstic acid solution is available commercially and may be used.

Working creatinine standard: Dilute stock standard 1:100 with distilled water to create a 15 µg/ml solution. Must be prepared fresh daily.

PROCEDURE

1. Place 2.0 ml of serum in a test tube and add 3.0 ml of water, 1 ml of 10 per cent sodium tungstate, and 2.0 ml of 2/3 N sulfuric acid. Mix and refrigerate.
2. Set up three tubes as follows:
   B (blank)—5.0 ml distilled water
   S (standard)—4.0 ml distilled water and 1.0 ml of working creatinine standard
   U (unknown)—4.0 ml distilled water and 1.0 ml of protein-free filtrate
3. Add 0.5 ml of saturated aqueous oxalic acid to each tube.
4. Add Lloyd's reagent to each tube (100 mg of powder or 1.0 ml of a 10 per cent aqueous suspension).
5. Close tubes and shake intermittently for 10 minutes.
6. Centrifuge, decant, and drain tubes.
7. To each tube add 3.0 ml of distilled water, 1.0 ml picric acid, and 1.0 ml 0.75 N NaOH.
8. Close each tube and shake intermittently for 10 minutes.
9. Centrifuge all tubes.
10. Decant supernate, and at least 20 minutes after completion of step 8, read at 520 nm against reagent blank.
11. Make calculation as follows:

$$\frac{^AU}{^AS} \times 2 = mg\ creatinine/dl\ serum$$

Sodium Sulfanilate Determination
REAGENTS

Trichloroacetic acid, 50 per cent solution
The following solutions can be made as stock solutions and diluted to proper concentrations each day:
0.1 per cent sodium nitrite
0.5 per cent ammonium sulfamate
0.1 per cent N (1-naphthyl) ethylenediamine dihydrochloride

PROCEDURE

1. Place 1 ml of whole blood in a test tube and add 8 ml of distilled water.
2. Add 1 ml of 50 per cent trichloroacetic acid and mix well.
3. Filter or centrifuge and collect filtrate or centrifugate.
4. Place 5 ml of filtrate or centrifugate in a test tube and add 1 ml of 0.1 per cent sodium nitrite and mix.
5. After three minutes, add 1.0 ml of the 0.5 per cent ammonium sulfamate and mix.

6. After two minutes, add 1 ml of the 0.1 per cent N (1-naphthyl) ethylenediamine dihydrochloride and mix.
7. Wait one minute and read against a distilled water blank at 540 nm.
8. Calculations are made against a standard curve prepared from dilutions of a 1 per cent sodium sulfanilate stock solution in a range from 0 to 3.5 mg/100 ml and plotted against percentage transmission.

DETERMINATION OF PHENOLSULFONPHTHALEIN IN URINE

REAGENTS

2.5 N sodium hydroxide: Prepare a 10 per cent solution of sodium hydroxide.

PROCEDURE

1. Wash urine specimens into a properly labeled 1,000-ml volumetric flask.
2. Dilute to approximately 500 ml with distilled water.
3. Add 10 per cent (2.5 N) NaOH until the maximum purplish-red color is obtained. It will usually require approximately 1.0 ml.
4. Dilute to the 1,000-ml mark with distilled water and mix by inversion.
5. If the specimens are clear, pour into cuvettes. If the specimens are the least bit cloudy, they should be filtered, then poured into the cuvettes.
6. Read all tubes in a spectrophotometer at 550 nm with a water reference blank set at 100 per cent transmittance or zero optical density.
7. Compare readings obtained with the standard curve or chart prepared by plotting the per cent transmittance or optical density of known concentrations of the dye in distilled water with enough NaOH added to produce maximum color.

PANCREATIC FUNCTION TESTS

SERUM LIPASE

Sigma Titrimetric Method*
REAGENTS

Lipase substrate: This is a stabilized olive oil emulsion that should be stored in the refrigerator but not frozen. Probably stable for at least six months.
TRIS buffer: This is a buffer at pH 8.0 and should be stored in the refrigerator.
Ethyl alcohol, 95 per cent
Thymolphthalein indicator solution
Sodium hydroxide, 0.050 N

---

*Sigma Chemical Co., St. Louis, Mo.

PROCEDURE

1. Into each of two test tubes pipette the following:

    2.5 ml water

    3.0 ml lipase substrate (shake vigorously before pipetting)

    1.0 ml TRIS buffer

2. Add 1.0 ml of serum to one test tube and mark "test." Mark the other tube "blank." Stopper both tubes with clean rubber stoppers. Shake vigorously for five seconds.

3. Note the time, and place both tubes in a constant temperature water bath at 37° C. Incubate for six hours.

4. Pour contents of "blank" tube into a flask labeled "blank" and contents of "test" tube into a second clean flask labeled "test."

5. Into each of the two tubes pipette 3.0 ml of 95 per cent ethyl alcohol. Shake and pour into their respective flasks.

6. To each flask add four drops of thymolphthalein indicator solution.

7. Set up a 5- or 10-ml buret graduated to 0.05 ml. A pipette similarly marked will suffice.

8. Titrate each flask to a slight but definite blue color (not dark blue). The "blank" and the "test" must be titrated to the same color intensity. Read buret after each titration; record value. Subtract "initial" reading from "final" reading for each titration.

9. Subtract the "blank" NaOH value from the "test" NaOH value. The Sigma-Tietz units of lipase are exactly equal to the number of milliliters of 0.05 N NaOH required to neutralize the free fatty acid liberated during the six-hour incubation of the test.

ROE AND BYLER METHOD

REAGENTS

Substrate-buffer: Dissolve 1.21 gm TRIS (hydroxymethyl)aminomethane (Fisher Scientific Co., St. Louis, Missouri) and 1.0 gm of sodium benzoate in 500 ml distilled water. Place this solution in a blender and add 10.0 gm acacia and 50 ml USP olive oil. Homogenize for 10 minutes. Allow it to stand at room temperature for 5 hours and using a pH meter adjust pH to 8.5 by adding dropwise 1 N HCl or 1 N NaOH. Store in refrigerator at 4° C. Test pH at least monthly.

Indicator: Dissolve 1 gm phenolphthalein in 25 ml of 95 per cent ethyl alcohol.

Sodium hydroxide: 0.01 N solution prepared from commercial 1 N stock solution.

95 per cent ethyl alcohol

PROCEDURE

1. Place 1 ml of test serum in a 150-ml beaker and refrigerate (to be used later as a control).

2. Add 10 ml of substrate-buffer to two 40-ml test tubes labeled "U" (unknown) and "C" (control).

3. Place tubes in a water bath at 37° C for five minutes.

4. Add 1 ml of test serum to tube labeled "U" and mix.

5. Incubate both tubes in water bath at 37° C for one hour.

6. Empty contents of tube labeled "U" into a 150-ml beaker containing 30 ml of 95 per cent ethyl alcohol.

7. Remove beaker containing 1 ml of serum from refrigerator and add 30 ml of 95 per cent ethyl alcohol and contents of tube labeled "C."

Note: To facilitate complete removal of incubated substrate-buffer, pour contents between tube and beaker several times in steps 6 and 7.

8. Add 3 drops of phenolphthalein indicator to each beaker.

9. Titrate the control mixture with 0.01 N NaOH. Add NaOH a drop at a time while gently swirling the beaker. Titrate to a faint but definite pink that persists. Record milliliters of NaOH required to reach the endpoint.

10. Titrate the unknown mixture in the same manner.

11. Calculate as follows:

Ml NaOH for unknown − ml NaOH for control × 10 = Roe-Byler units of activity.

SERUM AMYLASE TEST

REAGENTS

Buffered starch substrate (pH 7.0):

Anhydrous disodium phosphate	13.3 gm
Benzoic acid	4.3 gm

Dissolve in approximately 250 ml distilled water and bring to a boil. Mix separately 200 mg soluble starch (Merck or Baker) in 5 ml of cold water and add to the boiling mixture, rinsing beaker with additional cold water. Continue boiling for one minute. Cool to room temperature and dilute to 500 ml with distilled water.

Stock solution of iodine (0.1 N): Dissolve 3.567 gm of potassium iodate and 45.0 gm of potassium iodide in approximately 800 ml of water. Slowly add 9 ml of concentrated hydrochloric acid, mixing constantly. Dilute to 1000 ml with water.

Working solution of iodine: Dissolve 25 gm of potassium fluoride in approximately 350 ml of water in a volumetric flask. Add 50 ml of the stock solution of iodine and dilute to the 500 mark with water.

Saline solution, 0.9 per cent.

PROCEDURE

1. Dilute the serum 1:25 with 0.9 per cent saline solution.

2. Place 5 ml starch substrate into two 100-ml volumetric flasks marked "test" and "control."

3. Place flask marked "test" in a water bath at 37° C for five minutes.

4. Add 1 ml diluted serum to substrate in warmed flask and return to water bath for exactly 8.5 minutes of incubation.

5. At end of incubation period, add 5 ml of working iodine solution to both flasks, with thorough mixing.

6. Dilute to 100 ml volume, using distilled water and mix well by inversion.

7. Measure optical density of test and control solutions in a 19 × 105 mm cuvette at 660 nm on a spectrophotometer, using a water reference blank.

8. Units of amylase are determined by the formula:

$$\frac{\text{OD of control} - \text{OD of test}}{\text{OD of control}} \times 2{,}000$$

$$= \text{Amylase units}$$

Amylochrome* Technique for Amylase Activity in Serum or Urine

REAGENTS

Diluent: Dissolve contents of one packet of crystalline diluent in deionized or distilled water and dilute to 250 ml in a volumetric flask. Store in a refrigerator and discard after two months.

Reagent blank: Incubate one substrate tablet with 2.0 ml distilled water for 15 minutes, add 8.0 ml diluent solution and centrifuge. This solution is used to zero the photometer and is stable for two weeks at room temperature.

PROCEDURE

1. Add one blue substrate tablet to 1.9 ml distilled water in a 15 × 125 mm test tube. Mix well by vortexing and warm to 37° C.

2. Add 0.1 ml serum or urine and again mix by vortexing. Incubate exactly 15 minutes at 37° C.

Note: Canine serum should be diluted 1:3 or 1:5. Heparinized plasma will give the same results, but oxalate, citrate, and ethylenediaminetetraacetic acid (EDTA) plasma may give low results.

3. Add 8.0 ml diluent to the tube to stop the reaction.

4. Mix well and centrifuge to obtain a clear supernatant that is transferred to a cuvette.

5. Read absorbance (optical density) at 625 nm against the reagent blank.

6. Determine amylase activity using the calibration reference curve prepared according to instructions accompanying the kit. Multiply results by the dilution factor.

---

*Roche Diagnostics, Nutley, N.J.

BT-PABA:XYLOSE TEST FOR INTESTINAL ABSORPTIVE FUNCTION

The techniques, doses, and timing of samples for this test are presented in Chapter 8. The chemical analyses on plasma samples are as follows:

Plasma PABA

MATERIALS

"Bentiromide" (BT-PABA powder)*
Sodium nitrite ($NaNO_2$) (Sigma No. 2252)
Ammonium sulfamate (Sigma No. A4630)
N-(1-naphthyl) ethylene diamine dihydrochloride (NED) (Sigma No. N9125)
PABA (free acid) (Sigma No. A9878)
Trichloroacetic acid (Sigma No. 4885)
Note: These chemicals are available from other sources. Sigma Chemical Company's address is PO Box 14508, St. Louis Mo 63178.
Appropriate size cuvette
Spectrophotometer

REAGENTS

1. Ammonium sulfamate—Dissolve 2.5 gm in 500 ml of distilled water. This reagent is stable for several weeks.

2. Sodium nitrite—Dissolve 100 mg $NaNO_2$ in 100 ml distilled water. Must be prepared fresh daily.

3. NED—Dissolve 100 mg N-(1-naphthyl) ethylene diamine dihydrochloride in 100 ml distilled water. Store in brown bottle in refrigerator. Stable for one week.

4. PABA (free-acid)—Prepare a series of standards 25, 50, 100, 200, 400, 800 µg/dl and prepare a standard curve using the method outlined below.

5. Trichloroacetic acid (TCA)—Dissolve 50 gm in 100 ml of distilled water. Stable for several weeks. (Saturated solutions of TCA are commercially available and can be diluted to 50 per cent.)

TEST PROCEDURE

1. Add one part of 50 per cent TCA to nine parts of plasma. (Heparinized plasma is preferred but EDTA plasma is satisfactory. DO NOT USE SERUM.)

2. Mix (vortex) this mixture thoroughly and let it stand for 10 minutes and centrifuge to obtain a clear protein-free filtrate (PFF).

3. In appropriate-size cuvettes place the following:

> BLANK—4 ml 10 per cent TCA
> TESTS—4 ml PFF
> STANDARD—4 ml of appropriate standard (100 or 200 µg/dl)

---

*Available from Adria Laboratories, PO Box 16529, Columbus, Ohio 43216.

4. Add 0.8 ml of $NaNO_2$ solution, mix, and let stand 3 minutes.

5. Add 0.8 ml NED solution, mix, and let stand 10 minutes.

6. Read at 540 nm with the blank set at 100 per cent (0 OD).

7. Record optical density (absorbance) or per cent T and compare to standard curve or calculate using the formula:

$$PABA/\mu g/dl = \frac{\text{Absorbance test}}{\text{Absorbance standard}}$$

$$\times \text{ Conc of standard}$$

Analysis for D-Xylose

MATERIALS

Thiourea (Sigma No. T7875)
Glacial acetic acid
p-Bromoaniline (Sigma No. B0755)
D-Xylose (Sigma No. X1599)
Benzoic acid (Sigma No. B3250)
Trichloroacetic acid

REAGENTS

1. p-Bromoaniline: Prepare a saturated solution of thiourea by placing about 4 gm of thiourea in 100 ml of glacial acetic acid and shaking thoroughly. Decant the supernatant. Dissolve 2 gm p-bromoaniline in 100 ml of the decanted thiourea solution. Place in a dark bottle. Stable for a week.

2. Benzoic acid: Dissolve 3 gm benzoic acid crystals in 1000 ml distilled water.

3. Stock standard (200 mg xylose/dl): Place 200 mg of D-xylose in a 100-ml volumetric flask and dissolve in and fill up to volume with 0.3 per cent benzoic acid.

4. Working standard (0.1 mg/dl): Dilute stock standard 1:20 with saturated benzoic acid.

5. Trichloroacetic acid (TCA): Prepare 50 per cent solution by adding 50 gm to 100 ml distilled water.

TEST PROCEDURE

1. Prepare a protein-free filtrate by adding 1 part of 50 per cent TCA to 9 parts of plasma. Mix (vortex) thoroughly: centrifuge and decant the protein-free filtrate (PFF).

2. Place 0.5 ml of standard into two tubes. Label one tube "blank" and the other "test." Do the same for PFF from the patient using two tubes for each filtrate. Label in the same fashion.

3. Add 2.5 ml of p-bromoaniline solution to each tube and mix.

4. Place all tubes marked "test" in a water bath at 70° C for 10 minutes. Place all tubes marked "blank" in the dark at room temperature.

5. Remove tubes from water bath and cool to room temperature in running water.

6. Place all tubes ("test" and "blank") in the dark for 70 minutes.

7. After 79 minutes read the "test" against its appropriate "blank" at a wavelength of 520 nm.

8. Record the absorbance and calculate as follows:

mg xylose/dl

$$= \frac{\text{absorbance test}}{\text{absorbance (standard, 0.1 mg/ml)}} \times 100$$

Note: If the tests and the blanks are all read against water at 100 per cent T (0.0 OD), the absorbance of the blank must be subtracted from that of the test before making the calculation.

MINERAL BALANCE AND PARATHYROID FUNCTION

CALCIUM

Ferro-Ham Method

REAGENTS

Chloranilic acid: Dissolve 4 gm sodium hydroxide in 600 to 700 ml distilled water. Add 11 gm chloranilic acid and sufficient distilled water to make 1 liter.

Agitate for one minute or until acid is dissolved. pH should be between 3.5 and 7.0; if it is higher than 7.0, add additional 1-gm quantities of chloranilic acid to reduce pH below 7.0. Filter through a fine pad.

Isopropyl alcohol: Dilute 50 ml isopropyl alcohol to 100 ml with distilled water.

Tetrasodium ethylenediaminetetraacetate (EDTA): Prepare a 5 per cent solution by dissolving 5 gm in distilled water and adjusting volume to 100 ml.

Standard solution
Control solution
All of these items can be purchased commercially.

PROCEDURE

1. Pipette 2 ml of serum, standard, and control into appropriately marked heavy-walled 12-ml centrifuge tubes.

2. To each tube add 1 ml chloranilic acid solution, agitating constantly.

3. Allow tubes to stand for at least 30 minutes.

4. Centrifuge at approximately 1,800 rpm for 10 minutes.

5. Decant the supernatant and allow the tubes to drain for two to three minutes on some absorbent paper such as filter paper or a paper towel.

6. Wipe the lip of the tube dry with cotton gauze.

7. Wash precipitate with 6 to 7 ml of isopropyl alcohol. A fine stream from a plastic wash bottle

should be used. Break up the sediment and re-suspend it.

8. Centrifuge and drain as before.

9. Add two drops (0.1 ml) distilled water to each precipitate.

10. Break up precipitate by striking bottom of tube sharply against palm of hand until mat breaks loose and precipitate is suspended in water. If this is not successful, a clean dry applicator stick may be used to loosen the precipitate.

11. Add 6 ml of the EDTA solution to each tube.

12. Stopper tubes and invert several times until precipitate is completely dissolved. Do not shake too vigorously.

13. Transfer the solution to a cuvette and read at 520 nm after adjusting to 100 per cent transmittance or zero optical density. This color is stable for as long as five days.

14. Make calculations as follows:

$$\frac{\text{Density of unknown}}{\text{Density of standard}}$$

$$\times \text{Concentration of standard} = \text{Mg calcium/dl}$$

Fiske-SubbaRow Method (Gomori Modification)

REAGENTS (REAGENTS ARE AVAILABLE COMMERCIALLY)

10 per cent trichloroacetic acid: Dissolve 10 gm trichloroacetic acid in distilled water and dilute to 100 ml with distilled water.

10 N sulfuric acid: Add slowly with stirring 105 ml concentrated sulfuric acid to 270 ml distilled water. Cool before using.

5 per cent sodium molybdate: Dissolve 25 gm sodium molybdate in 500 ml distilled water. Filter if not clear.

Molybdate-sulfuric acid: Add 250 ml 10 N sulfuric acid to the sodium molybdate. Mix thoroughly and dilute to 1 liter with distilled water.

Elon reducing solution: Dissolve 1 gm Elon (p-methyl amino phenol) in 100 ml 3 per cent sodium bisulfite. This solution is stable for several months in the refrigerator.

Standard phosphate solution

Control solution

PROCEDURE

1. Pipette 1 ml unknown serum, control solution, and standard solution into small flasks and label accordingly.

2. Add 9 ml trichloroacetic acid to each tube and mix thoroughly.

3. Let stand five to 10 minutes and centrifuge for 10 minutes or filter through Whatman No. 1 paper.

4. Pipette 4 ml of each filtrate into tubes and label "unknown," "standard," and "control."

5. Pipette 4 ml trichloroacetic acid into another tube and label "blank."

6. Add 1 ml of molybdate-sulfuric acid reagent to each tube.

7. Add 0.5 ml Elon reducing solution to each tube and mix by inverting.

8. Let stand 30 to 45 minutes and read at 700 nm after adjusting the reading of the blank for 100 per cent transmittance or zero optical density.

9. Calculate as follows:

$$\frac{\text{Density of unknown}}{\text{Density of standard}} \times \text{Mg P in standard}$$

$$= \text{Mg/dl of P in serum}$$

STAINS FOR DIAGNOSTIC CYTOLOGY

New Methylene Blue Stain

New methylene blue	0.5 gm
Saline, 0.85 per cent	99 ml
Formalin, 40 per cent	1 ml

Filter and store in a brown bottle.

Papanicolaou Stain

REAGENTS

Harris hematoxylin—stock solution

Hematoxylin	2.5 gm
Ammonium sulfate	50 gm
Ethyl alcohol	25 ml
Distilled water	500 ml
Mercuric oxide	0.25 gm

TECHNIQUE

1. Dissolve hematoxylin in alcohol.

2. To 500 ml water in a Pyrex beaker add 50 gm of ammonium sulfate and heat to boiling point.

3. Add hematoxylin solution to ammonium sulfate solution and bring it back to a full boil.

4. Immediately add 0.25 gm of mercuric oxide.

5. Swirl quickly until a black-purple color appears in a few seconds.

6. Quickly place beaker in cold water to cool as rapidly as possible.

7. When cold, filter into a brown bottle.

8. The stock solution of Harris hematoxylin must age at least two weeks before use.

Harris Hematoxylin—Working Solution

To 1000 ml of stock Harris hematoxylin add 4 ml of glacial acetic acid.

Orange G

Stock solution: Dissolve 10 gm of orange G in water and bring to 100 ml total volume.

Working solution:

Orange G stock solution	25	ml
Ethyl alcohol, 95 per cent	25	ml
Phosphotungstic acid	0.075	gm

EA-65 Stock Solution

Prepare 10 per cent aqueous solution to:

1. Light green S.F. yellowish
2. Bismark brown
3. Eosin Y

EA-65 Alcohol Solutions from Stock Aqueous Solutions

Prepare the following:

1. Light green S.F. yellowish—0.05 per cent solution in 95 per cent ethyl alcohol.
2. Bismark brown—0.05 per cent solution in 95 per cent ethyl alcohol.
3. Eosin Y—0.5 per cent solution in 95 per cent ethyl alcohol.

EA-65 Staining Solution

Light green S.F. yellowish alcohol solution	90 ml
Bismark brown alcohol solution	20 ml
Eosin Y alcohol solution	90 ml
Phosphotungstic acid	1.2 gm

Filter and store in a brown bottle.

STAINING PROCEDURE

1. After fixation of slide, transfer directly into 80 per cent alcohol and through 70 per cent and 50 per cent alcohol solution to distilled water.
2. Stain in working solution of Harris hematoxylin for 45 seconds.
3. Using three separate containers, gently but thoroughly rinse in successive containers of water.
4. Rinse slide in 50 per cent alcohol.
5. Rinse in 70 per cent, 80 per cent, and 95 per cent alcohol solutions.
6. Stain in working solution of orange G for one minute, 15 seconds.
7. Using 95 per cent alcohol in three separate containers, rinse slide three times.
8. Stain in EA-65 staining solution for three minutes.
9. Rinse three times in 95 per cent alcohol using three separate containers.
10. Dehydrate using absolute alcohol.
11. Clear with a mixture of equal parts of absolute alcohol and xylene.
12. Rinse in two changes of xylene.
13. Mount in a suitable mounting medium.

STAINING FOR VIRUS INCLUSION BODIES

Infectious Canine Hepatitis

REAGENTS

Wright's stain
Buffer
Water

TECHNIQUE

1. Cut blocks of liver tissue approximately 1 cm square and blot the surface on a piece of filter paper or paper towel.
2. Carefully clean a microslide by dipping it in alcohol and wiping it dry with a piece of lintless cloth, such as cheesecloth.
3. Gently press the slide on the cut surface of the block tissue from which the excess blood has been blotted. Lift the slide without any lateral movement.
4. Make four or five impressions on a slide.
5. Several slides should be prepared, using a fresh block of tissue for each slide.
6. Air dry the imprints and stain by Wright's method as for blood smears but allow the stain to react longer (approximately five minutes for undiluted stain and 15 minutes for buffer and stain).
7. Rinse in water and stand on the end to dry.
8. Examine under the microscope, using low power to locate an area in which hepatic cells may be clearly observed. Switch to the oil immersion lens and look for inclusion bodies that will appear as dark basophilic bodies within the nuclei. The inclusion bodies are considerably larger than nucleoli that may be present in some hepatic cells.

Shorr Stain

Inclusion bodies in the cells from an animal with canine distemper are difficult to demonstrate, but the Shorr stain has been reported to be effective.

REAGENTS

Shorr staining solution: can be purchased in prepared form
Harris hematoxylin: can also be purchased in a prepared form
Ammonia water

Tap water	1000 ml
Strong ammonia water	2.0 to 3.0 ml

1 per cent acid alcohol

Concentrated hydrochloric acid	1.0 ml
Ethyl alcohol, 70 per cent	99.0 ml

TECHNIQUE

1. Prepare a blood film or tissue scraping from the urinary bladder, trachea, or conjunctiva.
2. Dry five to 10 minutes, fix in alcohol for one minute, and rinse in water.
3. Stain in Harris's hematoxylin for three to five minutes.
4. Rinse in water.
5. Differentiate in 1 per cent acid alcohol until there is no hematoxylin in the cytoplasm of the cells when examined under the microscope.
6. Place the sections in ammonia water until they turn blue and check with the microscope.
7. Wash for 10 minutes in running tap water.

8. Place slides in Shorr staining solution for one minute.

9. Wash in 95 per cent alcohol and check with the microscope. Connective tissue stains clear light green when the differentiation is complete.

10. Rinse several times in absolute alcohol, clear in two to four changes of xylene, and mount the coverslip.

11. The inclusion bodies will stain a brilliant red, whereas the nuclei stain blue and the erythrocytes orange-red.

IMMUNOLOGY TECHNIQUES

Some of the immunology techniques (Coombs' tests) have been described in the section on Examination of Blood and Bone Marrow.

ANTINUCLEAR ANTIBODY (ANA) TEST

MATERIAL REQUIRED

Serum from the patient
Negative control serum
Positive control serum
Fluorescein-labeled antiglobulin (available from a variety of sources including VMRD Inc., Pullman, Washington; Miles Laboratories, Elkhart, Indiana; Cappell Laboratories, West Chester, Pennsylvania; and other laboratories).

Tissue culture cells grown on a glass microscope slide. (These are commercially available from many scientific supply companies that serve the medical professions.)

Microscope equipped with an ultraviolet light source

Most commercially prepared tissue or cell-culture slides come complete with directions. Those should be followed. The general procedure is outlined below.

1. Prepare appropriate dilutions of the patient serum: usually 1:5, 1:10, 1:20, and 1:40. Serum dilutions being used will depend on the laboratory. We use a 1:10 dilution for screening all samples.

2. Add an appropriate amount of diluted serum from the patient, a negative control, and a positive control, to three separate areas on the cell-culture slide.

3. Incubate for 30 minutes at room temperature.

4. Wash for 10 minutes in phosphate-buffered saline. This is done by placing slide in three changes of phosphate-buffered saline.

5. Remove as much of the buffer as possible by giving the slide a quick flip.

6. Add the species-specific fluorescein-specific antiglobulin to the slide and incubate for 30 minutes.

7. Wash for 10 minutes in phosphate-buffer saline as described above.

8. A counterstain such as Evans Blue can be used if desired.

9. Place a small quantity of phosphate-buffered glycerol on slide, apply a coverslip, and view slide using microscope equipped with an ultraviolet light source.

10. A positive test is the appearance of an apple-green fluorescence in the nucleus of the cells. The pattern of fluorescence may vary. Four patterns have been described: rim, speckled, nucleolar, and diffuse. The control area and the negative serum should be negative. Negative tests are reported when there is no fluorescence of the nucleus. Occasional specimens with pale perinuclear fluorescence are observed but should be considered negative.

MICROBIOLOGIC TECHNIQUES

STAINS AND INDICATORS

GRAM'S STAINING METHOD

REAGENTS

Gentian violet

Crystal violet (85 per cent dye content)	4.0 gm
Ethyl alcohol (95 per cent)	20.0 ml
Dissolve the crystal violet in the alcohol	
Ammonium oxalate	0.8 gm
Distilled water	80.0 ml

Dissolve the ammonium oxalate in the water and dilute the concentrated crystal violet solution 1:10 with distilled water; mix one part of the diluted crystal violet solution with four parts of the ammonium oxalate solution.

Gram's iodine

Iodine	1.0 gm
Potassium iodide	2.0 gm
Distilled water	300.0 ml

This solution should be prepared fresh every two to three weeks.

Safranin

Prepare a 2.5 per cent solution of safranin in 95 per cent alcohol.

Safranin (2.5 per cent solution)	10.0 ml
Distilled water	100.0 ml

Ethyl alcohol (95 per cent) or equal parts of 95 per cent alcohol and acetone.

TECHNIQUE

1. Prepare a slide and allow it to dry. The slide is then fixed by *gently* heating the slide over a low flame of a Bunsen burner.
2. Cool slide and stain for 1½ to 2 minutes with gentian violet.
3. Wash with water.
4. Treat with Gram's iodine for at least one minute.
5. Wash with water.
6. Decolorize for a few seconds with 95 per cent alcohol or a mixture of equal parts of 95 per cent ethyl alcohol and acetone.
7. Wash with water.
8. Counterstain with the safranin solution for ½ to 1 minute.
9. Wash, blot dry, and examine under the oil immersion lens.

HISS CAPSULE STAIN

REAGENTS

Serum
Hiss stain: Prepare a saturated solution of gentian violet in alcohol (95 per cent). Dilute 5 ml of saturated gentian violet in 95 ml of distilled water.
Copper sulfate, 20 per cent solution in water.

TECHNIQUE

1. Mix material to be stained with equal amount of serum and make a thin smear.
2. Air dry the smear.
3. Fix either in the flame or in 1:10 diluted commercial formalin.
4. Cover with Hiss stain and heat to steaming for a few seconds.
5. Wash off the stain with the copper sulfate solution.
6. Dry in the air and examine under the oil immersion lens.
7. Bacterial bodies, cells, and background stain purple. Capsules are colorless or pale lavender.

SPORE STAIN (DORNER)

REAGENTS

Ziehl-Neelsen carbolfuchsin: Alcoholic basic fuchsin (saturated solution) is prepared by dissolving 3 gm of basic fuchsin in 100 ml of 95 per cent ethyl alcohol. Five per cent phenol is prepared by dissolving 5 gm of phenol in 100 ml distilled water. Mix 10 ml of alcoholic basic fuchsin and 90 ml of 5 per cent phenol, let stand for 24 hours, and filter.
Dorner solution:

Nigrosin	10.0 gm
Distilled water	100.0 ml

Boil 30 minutes in an Erlenmeyer flask and add 0.5 ml of formalin as a preservative. Filter twice through double filter paper and store in serological test tubes in 5-ml quantities. Stopper the tubes with aluminum foiled corks.

TECHNIQUE

1. Make a heavy suspension of the organisms in three or four drops of water.
2. Add three to four drops of Ziehl-Neelsen carbolfuchsin.
3. Boil the mixture for 10 to 15 minutes in a water bath.
4. Mix a loopful of preparation on a slide with a loopful of Dorner solution.
5. Prepare a thin smear and allow it to dry.
6. Examine under the microscope. Spores are red, the background is gray, and the vegetative cell is unstained.

ACID-FAST STAIN

REAGENTS

Ziehl-Neelsen carbolfuchsin (prepared as detailed previously)
Acid-alcohol:

Concentrated hydrochloric acid	2.0 ml
Ethyl alcohol (95 per cent)	98.0 ml

Methylene blue: Prepare a saturated solution of methylene blue by adding 1.5 gm of methylene blue powder to 100 ml of 95 per cent ethyl alcohol. To dissolve, rub the powder with a small quantity of alcohol, slowly adding the alcohol as the powder dissolves.

Distilled water	100.0 ml
Potassium hydroxide (10 per cent solution)	0.1 ml
Saturated alcoholic solution of methylene blue	30.0 ml

Filter through filter paper and dilute 1:20 with distilled water prior to use.

TECHNIQUE

1. Prepare a smear of the suspected material and after drying, heat fix.
2. Cover the smear with Ziehl-Neelsen carbolfuchsin and steam gently for five minutes.
3. Wash with tap water.
4. Decolorize with acid-alcohol until the film is colorless.
5. Wash with water.
6. Counterstain with methylene blue for 5 to 20 seconds, depending upon the thickness of the smear.
7. Wash with water and dry.

INDICATORS FOR CARBOHYDRATES

Bromthymol Blue

REAGENTS

Bromthymol blue powder
N/20 sodium hydroxide
Distilled water

TECHNIQUE

1. Dissolve 0.4 gm bromthymol blue in 12.8 ml N/20 NaOH by grinding in a mortar.
2. Dilute to 100 ml with distilled water.
3. Use 2 to 5 ml for each liter of culture medium.
4. The pH range is 6.1—yellow, 7.7—blue.

Andrade's Indicator

REAGENTS

Acid fuchsin
Distilled water
1 N sodium hydroxide

TECHNIQUE

1. Dissolve 0.5 gm of acid fuchsin in 100 ml of distilled water.
2. Add 16 ml of 1 N NaOH and the mixture will decolorize.
3. It may be necessary to add one or two drops of NaOH after several hours if the fuchsin is not decolorized.
4. Use 10 ml of indicator for each 1,000 ml of medium.
5. The indicator is colorless and will not produce any change in the color of the carbohydrate medium. Acid production is indicated by the appearance of a red to pink color.

"STRING OF PEARLS" TEST FOR BACILLUS ANTHRACIS

REAGENTS

Tryptose agar
Penicillin G

TECHNIQUE

1. Prepare a 24-hour broth culture of the suspected organism.
2. Prepare an agar plate or slant containing tryptose agar with 0.05 to 0.5 unit of penicillin G/ml.
3. Streak the 24-hour culture of the suspected organism on the tryptose-penicillin agar.
4. Incubate for three to six hours at 37° C.
5. Carefully place a coverslip over the developing growth.

6. Using the oil immersion objective, examine the bacterial growth.
Bacillus anthracis will form chains of spheres resembling a string of beads. Other bacilli form strands of rods.

MODIFIED STRING OF PEARLS TEST*

1. Streak suspected material (blood, tissue, or bacterial colony) on the surface of a plate containing Mueller-Hinton agar.
2. Place a penicillin-impregnated disc on the surface of the streaked agar.
3. Place a glass coverslip over the streaked area adjacent to the penicillin disc.
4. Incubate $2\frac{1}{2}$ to 3 hours at 37° C.
5. Examine the area under the coverslip with a microscope.
6. If *Bacillus anthracis* is present, typical chains of swollen, rounded cells will be observed.

COAGULASE TEST FOR STAPHYLOCOCCI

REAGENTS

Brain-heart infusion broth or other good nutrient broth.
Rabbit plasma.

TECHNIQUE

1. Grow the suspected staphylococcus in a tube of brain-heart infusion or other good nutrient broth for 24 hours.
2. Prepare a 1:5 dilution of rabbit plasma or reconstitute dried plasma.
3. Add 0.5 ml of the plasma to a sterile test tube.
4. Add two to four drops of the 24-hour broth culture of the organism to the plasma and incubate at 37° C.
5. Most coagulase-positive staphylococci will clot the plasma within two hours. However, a second reading should be made in four hours. If no coagulation takes place, the test should be considered negative.

SLIDE TECHNIQUE

1. Prepare a homogeneous suspension of the suspected organism in a drop of water on a slide with minimum spreading.
2. Mix a large loopful of the plasma with the suspension.

---

*Bailie, W. E., and Stowe, E. C. Simplified test for identification of *Bacillus anthracis*. Proceedings Abstracts, Annual Meeting Am Soc. Microbiol., American Society for Microbiology, Washington, D.C., 1977.

3. Coagulase-positive staphylococci will produce macroscopic clumping within five to 15 seconds. Delayed clumping is not indicative of a positive test.

REAGENTS USED IN DIAGNOSIS OF MASTITIS

BROMTHYMOL BLUE SOLUTION

REAGENTS

Bromthymol blue	1.0 gm
N/100 sodium hydroxide	160.0 ml
Distilled water	590.0 ml

BROMCRESOL PURPLE SOLUTION

REAGENTS

Bromcresol purple powder	0.9 gm
Distilled water	100.0 ml

CHLORIDE TEST SOLUTIONS

Solution A

Silver nitrate	1.3415 gm
Distilled water	1000.0 ml

Solution B

Potassium chromate	10.0 gm
Distilled water	100.0 ml

NEWMAN-LAMPERT STAIN

REAGENTS

Certified powdered methylene blue	1.12 gm
Ethyl alcohol (95 per cent)	54.0 ml
Tetrachloroethane (Eastman Kodak Co.)	40.0 ml
Glacial acetic acid	6.0 ml

EDWARD'S MEDIUM

REAGENTS

Meat extract agar at pH 7.4	1,000.0 ml
Crystal violet, 0.1 per cent aqueous solution	2.0 ml
Esculin	1.0 gm
Sterile bovine blood	50.0 ml

Put esculin into solution by boiling it in a small quantity of water, then add it to the melted cooled agar at the same time the blood is added.

SODIUM AZIDE–CRYSTAL VIOLET BLOOD AGAR

Blood agar base at pH 6.8	1,000.0 ml
Crystal violet, 0.1 per cent aqueous solution	2.0 ml
Sodium azide	0.5 gm
Sterile citrated or defibrinated bovine blood	50.0 ml

Similar results can be obtained using a prepared kit. (Leukocyte Acid phosphatase Kit, Sigma Chemical Co., St. Louis, MO, Kit No. 386A). The microfilarae are isolated and a glass slide prepared and stained following directions furnished with the kit. The results are interpreted as explained above.

HISTOCHEMICAL STAIN FOR DIFFERENTIATING DIROFILARIA FROM DIPETALONEMA[1]

REAGENTS

1. Michaelis veronal acetate buffer, pH 10.0

Sodium acetate ($NaC_2H_3O_2 \cdot 3H_2O$)	9.714 gm
Sodium barbital	14.714 gm
Distilled water	500 ml

Store at 4° C.
2. Naphthol AS-TR-phosphate

Naphthol AS-TR-phosphate, sodium salt[2]	0.05 gm
N,N-Dimethyl-formamide[3]	5.0 ml

Prepare fresh.
3. Pararosanilin

Pararosanilin hydrochloride[4]	1.0 gm
Distilled water	20.0 ml
Concentrated HCl	5.0 ml

Add Pararosanilin to water, heat to dissolve. Add HCl and cool. Store at 4° C. (This solution is stable for six months.)
4. Sodium Nitrite, 4 per cent

Sodium Nitrite ($NaNO_2$)	4.0 gm
Distilled water	100.0 ml

Keeps well at room temperature or at 4° C. (This solution is stable for six months.)
5. 1 per cent methyl green in phosphate buffer
   A. 0.2 M sodium phosphate

Na_2HPO_4	23.396 gm
Distilled water	1.000 ml

   B. 0.1 M citric acid

C_3H_4 (OH) $(COOH)_3 \cdot H_2O$	21.011 gm
Distilled water	1.000 ml

   Working solution

Solution A	77.1 ml
Solution B	122.9 ml
Methyl green[5]	2.0 gm

Keeps well at room temperature.

Substrate

Add 20 ml of solution 1 and 50 ml of distilled water to a Coplin jar. Add 4 ml of solution 2. (This mixture can be prepared and stored at 4° C for 4 weeks.) Using a separate test tube, mix 3.2 ml of each of solutions 3 and 4 and add to the mixture in the Coplin jar. Adjust the pH to 5.0 using 0.1 N NaOH. This substrate solution must be prepared fresh before each use.

Procedure

1. Use clotted blood. Loosen the clot from the sides of the test tube. Wash the clot in an equal quantity of distilled water.
2. Collect the water and serum in a clean test tube.
3. Centrifuge the water serum mixture for five minutes at approximately 1000 g.
4. Discard the supernatant, leaving a drop in the bottom of the tube.
5. Shake the remaining drop to resuspend the sediment and examine sediment under a microscope to detect microfilariae.
6. If microfilariae are present, use this material to prepare a smear on a glass slide and proceed with the next steps.
7. Incubate smears in the substrate for one hour at 37° C or for two hours at room temperature (25° C).

8. Rinse slides in distilled water.
9. Counterstain in solution 5 for two or three minutes. (This step can be eliminated if the parasites are numerous.)
10. Rinse slides in distilled water.
11. Dehydrate in 95 per cent and then absolute ethyl alcohol.
12. Rinse in xylene and mount in Permount. (The slides can also be examined wet.)

Interpretation

Dirofilaria immitis—Presence of two distinct red bands or spots in the areas of the excretory and anal pores.

Dipetalonema reconditum—Red over all or almost all of the body.

References

1. Chalifoux, L., and Hunt, R. D.: Histochemical differentiation of *Dirofilaria immitis* and *Dipetalonema reconditum*. J.A.V.M.A., *158*:601, 1971.
2. Catalog No. N6125, Sigma Chemical Co., St. Louis, MO.
3. Catalog No. D4254, Sigma Chemical Co., St. Louis, MO.
4. Catalog No. P3750, Sigma Chemical Co., St. Louis, MO.
5. Catalog No. M5015, Sigma Chemical Co., St. Louis, MO.

CONVERSION OF CONVENTIONAL UNITS TO SI UNITS — BLOOD AND SERUM

Component	Conventional Units	×	Factor	=	Recommended SI Units
Albumin	g/dl		10		g/L
Ammonia	μg/dl		0.554		μmol/L
Amylase	Somogyi units		1.85		U/L
Base excess	mEq/L		1		mmol/L
Bicarbonate	mmol or mEq/l		1		mmol/L
Bilirubin	mg/dl		17.1		μmol/L
BSP (dog and cat)	Percent retention		0.01		Fraction retention
Calcium	mg/dl		0.25		mmol/L
Carbon dioxide	mM		1		mmol/L
Chloride	mEq/L		1		mmol/L
Cholesterol	mg/dl		0.026		mmol/L
Cholinesterase	IU/L		1		U/L
Cortisol	μg/dl		27.6		mmol/L
Creatine kinase	U/L		1		U/L
Creatinine	mg/dl		88.4		μmol/l
Cr. clearance	ml/min		0.0167		ml/sec
Electrophoresis protein	gm/dl		10		g/L
Fibrinogen	mg/dl		0.01		g/L
Gamma GT	IU/L		1		U/L
Globulins	g/dl		10		g/L
Glucose	mg/dl		0.055		mmol/L
Haptoglobin	mg/dl		0.01		g/L
Hemoglobin	g/dl		10		g/L
Iron binding	μg/dl		0.179		μmol/L
Iron, total	μg/dl		0.179		μmol/L
Lipase	mIU/ml		1		U/L
Lipase	Cherry-Crandall units		278		U/L
Magnesium	mEq/L		0.5		mmol/L
Magnesium	mg/dl		0.41		mmol/L
Osmolality	Osm/Kg		1		mmol/L
Phosphatase, alkaline	IU/L		1		U/L
Phosphorus (inorganic)	mg/dl		0.01		g/L
Potassium	mEq/L		1		mmol/L
Protein, total	g/dl		10		g/L
Sodium	mEq/L		1		mmol/L
T$_4$ (RIA)	μg/dl		13		mmol/L
Transferases	IU/L		1		U/L
Urea nitrogen	mg/dl		0.357		mmol/L
Uric acid	mg/dl		0.059		mmol/L
Xylose absorption	mg/dl		0.067		mmol/L

INDEX

Italic numbers refer to illustrations; (t) indicates tables.